Feline Oncology

A Comprehensive Guide to Compassionate Care

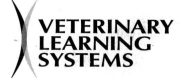

VETERINARY
LEARNING
SYSTEMS

Feline Oncology

A Comprehensive Guide to Compassionate Care

Gregory K. Ogilvie, DVM
Diplomate ACVIM
(Specialties of Internal Medicine and Oncology)
Professor and Head of Medical Oncology
Animal Cancer Center
Department of Clinical Sciences
College of Veterinary Medicine and Biomedical Sciences
Colorado State University
Fort Collins, Colorado

Antony S. Moore, MVSc
Diplomate ACVIM
(Specialty of Oncology)
Professor and Head of the Harrington Oncology Program
Tufts University School of Veterinary Medicine
North Grafton, Massachusetts

Designed and Published by Veterinary Learning Systems

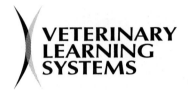

275 Phillips Boulevard
Trenton, NJ 08618
A division of MediMedia USA

Editor: Yvonne Stecher
Managing Editor: Cheryl Hobbs
Designed and Produced by: Veterinary Learning Systems
Bioillustrator: Felecia Paras, Biomedical Visuals, Columbus, Ohio

The authors would like to thank the following individuals for sharing their photos, slides, illustrations and/or personal experience.

J. Berg, Tufts University; M. Brown, Veterinary Referral Centre, Little Falls, NJ; S.M. Cotter, Tufts University; K. Cronin, New England Veterinary Oncology Group, Massachusetts; W. Dernell, Colorado State University; A. Evans, Tufts University; L. Freeman, Tufts University; A.E. Frimberger, Tufts University; D. Greco, Colorado State University; M. Kent, University of Georgia; L. Kleine, Tufts University; K. Kraus, Tufts University; B.R. Madewell, University of California, Davis; R. Malik, University of Sydney; Beth Mellor, Tufts University; R. Meuller, Colorado State University; G. Nesbitt, Tufts University; D. Penninck, Tufts University; K.M. Rassnick, Cornell University; D. Ruslander, North Carolina State University; W. Shapiro, University of California, Davis; G.H. Theilen, University of California, Davis; A. Théon, University of California, Davis; A. Tidwell, Tufts University; D. Twedt, Colorado State University; S.J. Withrow, Colorado State University

NOTICE: Every effort has been made to ensure that the drug dosage schedules and current therapy contained herein are accurate and in accord with the standards accepted at the time of publication. However, as new research and experience broadens our knowledge, changes in treatment and drug therapy occur. Therefore the reader is advised to check the product information sheet included in the package of each drug he/she plans to administer to be certain that changes have not been made in the recommended dose or in the contraindication. This is of particular importance in regard to new or infrequently used drugs.

Printed in the U.S.A.
Library of Congress Control Number: 2001099170

ISBN 1-884254-53-5

9   8   7   6   5   4   3   2   1

DEDICATION

To my beautiful daughter Torrie—
Lover of the piano and piccolo, harp and horses.
You bring wonder and delight to every day of my life!

Gregory K. Ogilvie

—

To all the cats that have enriched my life:
Pyewacket, Samai, Tao, Dara, Woota,
Bluebottle, Jack, Trevor, Nigel, Spiny Norman,
Athena, Eubie, Hotchkiss, Jerome,
and most of all Mungo.

Antony S. Moore

ACKNOWLEDGMENTS

This book would not have met its goal of being a practical, up-to-date resource for the progressive practicing veterinarian without the magic of very special friend and coauthor of this book, Dr. Tony Moore. Professionally, Tony is known world-wide as an accomplished clinician-scientist, a veterinary oncologist, and a true renaissance man. These pages reflect Tony's critical eye, humor, and intelligence that spring from his "outside" life as an athlete, gardener, apiarist, connoisseur of fine foods and wine, lover and collector of old books, kind and sensitive human being, and above all, a special friend to many, as well as husband and father extraordinaire. A special thought of appreciation and recognition goes to Tony's gifted wife Angela, who gave a great deal of her time as a veterinary oncologist and scientist to see this text become reality, and their young son Alexander, who has the most remarkable parents a child could ever imagine.

A second person who must not go unnoticed is critical reviewer, content editor, and critical analyst, Dr. Kathy L. Mitchener. Kathy carefully reviewed each page of this book with her heart and mind, while always challenging us both to reach our goal of providing up-to-date, practical information that touches the very reason we practice veterinary medicine: the human-animal bond. Kathy has placed meaning and energy into the words "compassionate care" and is the very reason why those words mean so much to many, including me. In short, Dr. Mitchener was the angel behind this book's every page and the guardian of our intent to ensure that this book provides an opportunity for practitioners to care from their hearts as well as from the science. More than that, Kathy has been an unrestrained source of boundless enthusiasm and a special friend to us both.

Another remarkable person who must be recognized is Catherine Hageman, who breathed life into every section of the book with her insight, heart, and editorial skill. She allowed us to fulfill our dream of providing clarity and accuracy to every page. Catherine has not only become a trusted and valued colleague and friend, but a person who has an extraordinary future in veterinary medicine.

Each page of this book has been critically reviewed by a small army of people too numerous to mention but including individuals from private practice, Colorado State University, Blackwell Sciences, and Veterinary Learning Systems. My thanks to all of them, with special thoughts of appreciation for the extraordinary efforts of Dr. Robin Downing, Mr. Keith Farquhar, and Heather Appleton. A special thanks must go to all the wonderful people at Veterinary Learning Systems who believed in our dream and made sure that the dream stayed alive, including but not limited to Cheryl Hobbs, Yvonne Stecher, Michelle Taylor, and Dr. Beth Thompson.

The pages of this book directly or indirectly reflect the knowledge, experience, and wisdom of a number of people who have impacted my life tremendously: Dr. Susan Cotter, my residency mentor and heroine, gently guided me to understand the magic and mysteries of feline medicine. Another heroine, Dr. Jean Holzworth, ignited my love for cats during our time together at Angell Memorial Animal Hospital. Drs. S. J. Withrow, Edward L. Gillette, Rod Straw, Dennis Macy, Sue LaRue, Barbara Powers, and Sue Lana all have contributed significantly to this book with their support, knowledge, and friendship. The pages of this book also reflect the enthusiasm and knowledge of medical residents and veterinary students who kept me running to keep up with them while I attempted to provide them with some mentorship. Special recognition goes to former and current medical oncology residents and friends: Drs. Donna Vicini, M. K. Klein, David Vail, Robyn Elmslie, Steve Atwater, Joyce Obradovich, Phyllis Ciekot, Phillip Bergman, Elizabeth McNiel, Karina Valerius, Christine Anderson, Victoria Bregazzi, Nicole Liebman, Mary Kay Blake, Kim Selting, Kathy Kazmierski, and Monika Jankowski. Finally, thank you to the greatest professors I have ever had: Mouse and, above all, Fieldler.

Last, but not least, a special acknowledgment must go to my parents, Bev and Stan, who gave me the gift of independence to achieve my heart's desires, and to my wife Karla and daughter Torrie, who have graced my life and granted me the time and opportunity to complete this book.

Gregory K. Ogilvie

ACKNOWLEDGMENTS

This book is certainly a culmination of my veterinary interests over the past 20 years. Since a brief, and probably misguided, period during which I had thought to become an equine practitioner, my professional life has always been happiest when involved with cats. The foundation for this enjoyment is the role cats have played in my personal life since I was born. It is to these cats that this book is dedicated. In addition, cats have interesting diseases. And, as every veterinarian knows, they are different than dogs—in the way you handle them, the way they handle you, and the consequences of a mistake in either of those activities.

I owe a debt of gratitude to the veterinarians who first introduced me to the joys of cat practice, David Watson and Deborah Middleton, who showed me how to handle cats professionally and kindly; David Watson also acted as my patient mentor while I worked on my Master's Thesis in feline hematology. The lessons from those people are as fresh today as when I learned them. It was my respect for the outstanding work of Susan Cotter that led me to Tufts Veterinary School more than 12 years ago and, despite all my efforts, I find I still know only a fraction of what she has learned about cats. My admiration for her professional strength continues unabated.

I also want to recognize the inspiration for many of my chapters in this book. Dr. Jean Holzworth, whom I have never had the privilege of meeting, believes that there is knowledge in every piece of literature that has been written. I have tried to be true to this belief and was assisted by two excellent librarians in this regard. Jean Maguire made obtaining articles from Algerian veterinary journals from the 1940s seem effortless, and her support, as well as more recently that of Nancy Boucher, have made this book as complete as it could be. The other inspiration and a source for much of the information cited in this book is the chapter by Jim Carpenter in Holzworth's *Diseases of the Cat*. This chapter stands alone as an original work and contains probably the largest amount of primary information about cat cancer in publication. I am indebted to his effort.

Angela Frimberger has been a constant source of support, both personally and as a translator of all the German and Dutch articles (of which there are many) cited in this book. Without her, this book might never have happened. She shares a love of cats, which we hope to pass on to our son, Alexander.

Other people who have supported this book are Dominique Penninck, who helped translate French articles and provided illustrations, Mauricio Solano, who helped with Portuguese and Spanish, and Ken Rassnick and David Ruslander, who provided critical input and illustrations. I am grateful to many others whose slides were made available for this book. Those people are acknowledged individually with their illustrations.

Finally, my coauthor, Greg Ogilvie, provided the original idea for this book, seeing the need for it in the veterinary world. As always, he has been supportive and a tireless worker. I hope to continue our collaboration and friendship in the future.

The literature regarding feline oncology is not as scant as it might first appear. There are gems within case reports and "What's your diagnosis?" presentations. More recently, there have been large, well-designed studies that provide a wealth of information for the veterinary practitioner, but there is room for still more information. I would encourage all those who read this book to consider contributing their knowledge and observations to the literature—if you find it interesting, then it is certain that someone else will also.

Antony S. Moore

ABOUT THE AUTHORS

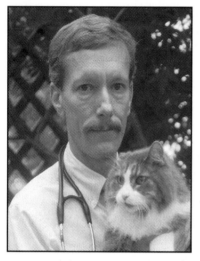

Gregory K. Ogilvie is a full Professor, Internist, Head of Medical Oncology, and Director of the Medical Oncology Research Laboratory at the Animal Cancer Center at Colorado State University (CSU). He practices oncology and teaches his students not only about medicine but also about the importance of special care for cancer patients. Dr. Ogilvie received his DVM from CSU and was awarded a National Institutes of Health Fellowship at the University of Wisconsin. He was in private practice in Connecticut before completing a residency at Tufts University/Angell Memorial Animal Hospital. Dr. Ogilvie is board certified in the specialties of both Internal Medicine and Oncology by the American College of Veterinary Internal Medicine. Along with Dr. Antony S. Moore, he is coauthor of *Managing the Veterinary Cancer Patient: A Practice Manual* (Veterinary Learning Systems, 1995; in English, French, and Japanese); he has also written over 150 peer-reviewed articles and chapters, as well as more than 120 scientific abstracts. He has been awarded two international patents and is the recipient of many awards, including the Arnold O. Beckman Research Award, the Beecham Research Award, the Purina Small Animal Research Award, the Scheidy Memorial Research Award, and the AVMA/American Kennel Club Award. Dr. Ogilvie's teaching skills have also been frequently recognized. He is the recipient of the Outstanding Teachers Award (University of Illinois, 1984–1988), the Norden Distinguished Teacher Award (CSU, 1987 and 1988), the MSD Agvet Award for Creativity in Teaching, and the SCAVMA Award for "Dedication to Students and the Profession" (1993 and 1994); he was also named Outstanding Companion Animal Speaker for 1999 at the North American Veterinary Conference. He has been recognized with the Cycle Award, the American Veterinary Medical Association's "Veterinarian of the Year-1995," the American Animal Hospital Association's "Veterinarian of the Year-1996," the Colorado Veterinary Medical Association Outstanding Faculty Award (1996), the 1999 SHARE Human Animal Bond Companion Animal Award, and the George Glover Gallery of Contemporary Faculty at CSU (2001). Dr. Ogilvie speaks worldwide about oncology and the importance of animals to people. He is a certified ski instructor and enjoys camping, SCUBA diving, and long distance cycling. Since 1987, he has volunteered as a counselor at the Sky High Hope Camp for children with cancer. His greatest joy is his daughter, Torrie.

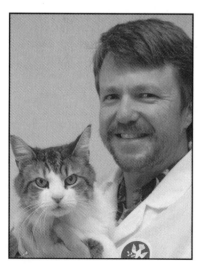

Dr. Antony S. Moore is a full Professor and Head of the Harrington Oncology Program at Tufts University School of Veterinary Medicine (TUSVM). He is board certified in the specialty of Oncology by the American College of Veterinary Internal Medicine. Dr. Moore received his veterinary degree in 1981 and a Master's degree in feline hematology, both from the University of Sydney, Australia. In 1988, he received the Robert S. Brodey Clinical Research Award for veterinary clinical oncology. Dr. Moore has spoken at national meetings within the United States and at international meetings in Europe, Australia, and Japan. He has received the MSD AgVet Award for creativity in teaching and established the Pet Loss Support Hotline at TUSVM as a training program for students as well as a resource for pet owners throughout the country. Dr. Moore actively pursues clinical research in the field of veterinary chemotherapy and is particularly interested in the epidemiology of common cancers in cats and dogs. His outside interests include entomology, SCUBA diving, hiking, contemporary fiction, book collecting, and running.

FOREWORD

This handbook is designed to provide veterinary practitioners with clinically relevant details about the diagnosis and management of the feline cancer patient in an easy-to-read format. The book is a response to readers of the companion book, *Managing the Veterinary Cancer Patient: A Practice Manual*, who demanded more detailed information about the species they love: the cat. There is no question that our knowledge base and the subsequent volume of literature are somewhat limited compared to what is available in canine medicine. However, for the first time in veterinary medicine, this book compiles a staggering amount of detail about feline oncology in one reference. The contents are divided into eight major sections. Each chapter is organized and subdivided by major headings, which facilitates easy access to practical information and the most common problems encountered in clinical feline oncology. A clinical briefing is included at the beginning of each chapter or section to give the reader information about the most commonly asked clinical questions. Key points are also included throughout the text to reinforce facts that, in many cases, are critical to the successful management of the feline cancer patient.

The first section, entitled **Compassionate Care for the Feline Cancer Patient**, reviews the approach to the cat with cancer. The goal is to direct the reader to meet the medical needs of their patients while meeting the nonmedical needs of the client or caregiver.

The second section, **Biopsy,** is devoted to important diagnostic procedures that can be performed in private practice. This step-by-step, highly illustrated section provides the busy practitioner with an easy reference guide for executing diagnostic methods essential for the management of the feline cancer patient. Also included in the chapter on Clinical Cytology and Neoplasia is a section of color plates and accompanying illustrations that will assist the practitioner in general cytologic interpretation.

The third section, **Common Therapeutic and Supportive Procedures,** details practical and important information needed to treat and support a cat with cancer. Topics include such therapeutic modalities as safe handling and administration of chemotherapeutic agents as well as the use of biologic response modifiers, radiation therapy, and hyperthermia. A chapter on complementary and alternative medicine can assist practitioners who wish to provide integrative care. Management of complications of cancer in cats, such as pain, vomiting, and side effects of treatment, is discussed and is a key part of providing compassionate care. Information about the nutritional needs of cats with cancer is provided. Also helpful is a list of toxicities associated with some commercially available anticancer drugs and hormones.

The fourth section, **Oncologic Emergencies,** is essential for veterinarians who deal with cancer. This "bottom line" section focuses on the diagnosis and treatment of life-threatening problems that can arise during the course of cancer and its treatment. Tables provide easy access to information on drugs and dosages that may be needed in an emergency situation.

The fifth section focuses on the diagnosis and management of **Paraneoplastic Syndromes**. These problems may complicate the management of cats with cancer. In many cases, the successful diagnosis and management of paraneoplastic conditions can impact the patient's quality of life and survival as much as the management of the malignant condition itself.

The sixth section is directed at the **Management of Specific Diseases.** Extraordinary efforts have been made to provide only the most important, up-to-date, and clinically relevant data to assist the practitioner in understanding how to determine the extent of cancer and how best to treat affected cats.

The seventh section contains an **Abridged Formulary** to assist busy practitioners in meeting the needs of the feline patient.

Finally, the eighth section, **Client Information Series,** provides material that can be photocopied and distributed to clients and caregivers to empower them with information and knowledge about cancer.

This manual is a comprehensive reference guide to the management of the most common natural cause of death in cats: cancer. Our hope is that it will prove to be an easy-to-use, practical resource for the progressive practitioner who seeks the very best for his or her patients. We are confident that this book will be so useful that there will be a demand for a second edition to capture the avalanche of new, as yet unpublished, information about cats and their cancers.

The authors, editors, and publisher of this manual have made every effort to ensure that all therapeutic modalities are recommended in accordance with accepted standards at the time of publication and that all drug dosages and regimens are correct. Nevertheless, anyone not familiar with cancer treatment should consult a veterinary oncologist before administering or prescribing any form of cancer treatment.

G. K. Ogilvie
A. S. Moore

CONTENTS

SECTION I: COMPASSIONATE CARE FOR THE FELINE CANCER PATIENT

OVERVIEW

Gregory K. Ogilvie and Antony S. Moore

1

CLINICAL BRIEFING

Three Steps of Cancer Care	Step 1: Dispel the myths: The caregiver's, the team's, and yours.
	Step 2: Establish the team, including the caregiver.
	Step 3: Deliver compassionate care.
TLC Approach (Staging)	**T**: Obtain a **T**issue diagnosis.
	L: Determine the **L**ocation of the cancer.
	C: Determine the cat's **C**ondition and general health.
Commandments of Cancer Care	Do not let your patient hurt, vomit, or starve.

BACKGROUND

Cancer is both the number one natural cause of death in geriatric cats and, according to a recent Morris Animal Foundation study, the number one health concern of pet owners. Therefore care of the cancer patient must be considered a major part of any progressive veterinary practice.

In addition, in recent years there has been a heightened awareness of the value and necessity of the relationship between people and their cats. The human-animal bond, or simply "the bond," is a major driving force behind advances in veterinary medicine. As medical and surgical advances have become available, recognition of the bond, both by clients and veterinarians, has driven the need for, as well as supply of, advanced care for beloved cats. This is especially true of cancer treatment. To support the bond, the veterinarian and the veterinary health care team must provide specialized care that is at the same time compassionate as well. Today, owners—and in particular, caregivers of cats with cancer—are willing to seek out advanced care for their pets and do so to ensure not only quantity but also quality of life.

The caregiver, the veterinarian, and the veterinary health care team often have preconceived notions about cancer and its treatment. In approaching feline patients with cancer, one must first dispel these negative notions regarding the disease and the efficacy and toxicity of cancer therapy. Within the past 10 years, tremendous advances have resulted in improved response rates, disease-free intervals, and survival times. Despite these strides in feline cancer care, many caregivers and veterinarians are not aware that a large percentage of cats with cancer can be cured or at least rendered free of their diseases for significant periods. In most situations, cats undergoing cancer treatment experience limited to no decrease in the quality of their life. Advances in palliative therapy and support for feline cancer patients have resulted in good quality of life for these patients while undergoing treatment. The objectives of this chapter are to examine how clients and the veterinary health care team perceive cancer, dispel the myths associated with cancer treatment, and replace these myths with accurate concepts about how cats with cancer and their caregivers should be approached, supported, and treated.

THREE STEPS OF CANCER CARE

There are three simple steps to treating the cancer patient and incorporating compassionate cancer care into a practice. We can only truly understand the wonder of the care of the cancer patient and the client/caregiver when we recognize and master these three steps.

Step One: Dispel the Myths

The first step is to face cancer head-on and dispel the myths of the disease. Too often the client, staff, and even the veterinarian perceive cancer and its therapy as something dark and hopeless. However, cancer itself is not as big or as dark as it seems. The truth is that fears and misconceptions envelop the disease in a cloud that obscures true understanding and vision and blocks out all hope. Surgical procedures such as amputations and "ectomies" are perceived as traumatic to both clients and health care givers. We imagine chemotherapy protocols fraught with horrible side effects. We fear the price of too many treatments, and we worry that treatment options would be financially and physically debilitating and result only in rather limited life expectancies. Is it all "worth it," we wonder?

Clients appear on our doorsteps frightened and out of control, holding in their arms a precious family member stricken with what they consider the worst of all possible diseases. In their minds, cancer is a one word death sentence. Their heads spin with anxieties and uncertainties.

KEY POINT

Cancer steals hope from the veterinary health care team and the caregiver. Empowering each member of the veterinary health care team, including the caregiver, with information is the first step toward providing compassionate care.

They are afraid of losing a loved one and they cling to every possible hope for treatment. They may recall a previous, personal experience with cancer too difficult to even express. They are deeply troubled that they may "put their friend through" a long and difficult treatment to gain additional time, and they feel selfish and guilty. They are worried about both financial and quality of life issues. They fear they will make a wrong decision and are frightened of how painful diagnostic procedures and treatment may be. They are also afraid the disease may be even worse than they can imagine. Yet they come to our doorsteps with the hope of returning to their pet the unconditional love and dignity that have graced their lifetime together.

The first big step to providing compassionate cancer care is dispelling the myths for our clients. We also must realize that these same fears exist in the veterinary staff, including ourselves. In the examination room, there are two parties—veterinary health care professionals (veterinarians and their staff) and the client or caregiver, each of whom drags his or her own misperceptions, prejudgments, and preconceived notions that can stifle the hope in cancer care. In the middle is a precious pet, which in many instances is beyond any describable value. The dialogue that begins in that room will impact its life and the bond shared with its caregiver. Thus we must first identify the misperceptions and myths existing within all team members and then work to dispel them. In all cancer care facilities, the single most important goal of therapy must be quality of life. True, small sacrifices in quality sometimes might have to be made, but those must be temporary and made only to gain significant additional length of life. We must assure our staff members, the caregiver, and ourselves that quality time during cancer therapy is a reality, and through each step of that care we must always work to maintain that quality. It is then that hope begins to supplant the myths and misperceptions.

Step Two: Establish the Team

The second step of compassionate cancer care is as vital as the first. A dedicated, trained, cohesive, caring veterinary health care team is essential to adequately care for the feline cancer patient and the caregiver. All members of the staff—veterinarians, technicians, nurses, and front office personnel—must understand that they play a vital role in the care of the cancer patient and the loving people who bring us these patients (Figure 1-1). Everyone must be united in philosophy and in the ultimate goal of cancer care—quality of life. Each veterinarian within a facility must be prepared to accept his or her role as part of the team, and then the team must reach out beyond the walls of the practice whenever appropriate to specialists and consultants such as pathologists, pharmacists, and veterinary oncologists. Finally, the most vital links to the team are the caregivers themselves. They must be incorporated into this team through education, encouragement, and empowerment to provide day-to-day care for the patient. Without their input, attention, and ongoing assessment, care of the cancer patient will not be optimal.

Once the caring team is forged to include at least the vet-

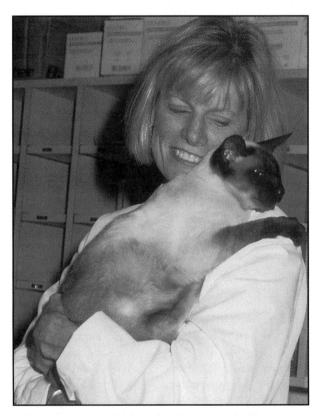

Figure 1-1: The role of each member of the veterinary health care team is to meet the medical needs of the patient and the nonmedical needs of the caregiver. Working to make sure that the feline patient is free of pain and nausea and that there is adequate nutritional support not only medically supports the cancer patient but also meets the needs and concerns of the caregiver.

erinarian, veterinary health care staff, and caregiver and we shed ourselves of the misperceptions of cancer, we begin to conquer the emotional component of this disease. Once stripped of its emotional cloak, cancer is attackable, diagnosable, treatable or manageable, and in many cases curable. Now we are prepared for the third step.

Step Three: Delivering the Care

Compassionate care is the single most important term in cancer medicine. It is the outward manifestation of caring with science and the heart. Compassionate care is a direct response to one's recognition and understanding of the bond. The first phase of compassionate care is to understand the disease and the health status of the patient through the "TLC approach." The second phase is providing caring support of the feline cancer patient by responding to the cat's needs and the client's concerns through the "Commandments of Cancer Care." The last phase is providing direct therapy for the underlying disease using the appropriate tools at hand, such as surgery, chemotherapy, or radiation therapy. Each phase is interdependent on the others.

TLC APPROACH TO CANCER: STAGING THE PATIENT

Each cancer patient and caregiver must be approached with tender loving care or "TLC." In the field of cancer care, the acronym takes on a second meaning that is just as important as the first: It describes the process of diagnosing and assessing the individual patient's cancer and its consequences to the body. TLC introduces us to the enemy (cancer) and is an essential prelude to effectively designing a treatment strategy. The three components are:

- **Tissue diagnosis**—Each tumor is different and unique, and each must be identified with a biopsy.
- **Location of the tumor**—Once the tumor type is named and, where appropriate, given a grade by an experienced, highly trained histopathologist, it must be located. Location is essentially the stage of disease or the extent of the malignancy locally and at distant sites through the metastatic process. Although this assessment will vary among tumor types, in general, the process of staging begins with a thorough physical examination to identify any enlarged lymph nodes or other obvious areas of cancer spread, a complete blood count, chemistry profile, urinalysis, thoracic radiographs (right and left laterals and a ventral-dorsal view), and abdominal radiographs. In addition, ancillary diagnostics such as ultrasonography, computerized tomography, magnetic resonance imaging, or other more specialized tests may be required.
- **Condition of the patient**—Finally, the patient's condition must be assessed. Any neoplastic process may re-

sult in a number of paraneoplastic conditions that affect the well-being of the cancer patient. In addition, these cats are generally geriatric patients, which have the potential for a number of underlying conditions and problems that may adversely affect their health or the potential success or course of therapy. It is all too easy to claim that "the patient has cancer; that's why it's sick." In many instances, correcting underlying problems such as renal failure, urinary tract infections, heart disease, and metabolic disturbances may significantly improve the overall health of the patient and thus improve the potential for successful cancer care.

Once the patient has been "TLC'd," appropriate options for therapy and prognosis are determined. The owner is given the power of information and education regarding the name of the disease, its extent, the many options for care, and the prognosis. The veterinary health care team is given the information they need to formulate an appropriate plan of care and then to prevent and/or treat potential problems.

KEY POINT

Staging the patient by determining the histologic diagnosis of the tumor, the extent of the primary tumor and metastases, and the condition of the patient is essential to treating the cat with cancer.

COMMANDMENTS OF CANCER CARE

As a plan of treatment (either for cure or control/management) is being developed, three commandments of cancer care must be followed. These commandments are a direct response to the caregiver's three greatest concerns about what cancer care may "look" like:

- **Do Not Let Them Hurt!**—Providing active, preemptive, and ongoing pain management for the cat with cancer is absolutely imperative. This reassures the caregiver that quality of life is optimal. Management can include oral medications (morphine, codeine, feldene, carprofen, or others) or transdermal delivery systems for fentanyl. The most important principle is that our caregivers know in advance that the veterinary health care team will not tolerate any pain. We work together to recognize, prevent, and manage it.
- **Do Not Let Them Vomit!**—This commandment strikes at the preconceived and unfounded fear that cats on chemotherapy often experience extreme amounts of nausea. This simply is not true. With recent advances in cancer care, nausea and vomiting no longer are commonly associated with chemotherapy. Moreover, we

have the tools to control these problems should they occur. Dispensing oral medication such as metoclopramide to the caregiver each and every time a potentially nauseating drug is administered empowers the caregiver to prevent this symptom at home. In addition, we must be prepared to stop vomiting should it occur, ensuring that medications and supportive care are immediately available. Stocking drugs such as ondansetron hydrochloride and dolasetron mesylate, although costly, will provide this level of assurance for all members of the team.

- **Do Not Let Them Starve!**—This final directive is just as vital as the first two. In the minds of many caregivers, patients undergoing cancer care often appear cachectic and weak. Today, we have the benefit of years of research into the metabolic alterations of cancer and have gained the ability to counteract them nutritionally. In addition, using the team approach and providing care that assures our patients will eat are vitally important. This includes basic nursing care (e.g., warming food, providing aromatic foods and comfortable environments), medicinal appetite stimulants, and, when needed, assisted feeding techniques such as esophagostomy, gastrostomy, or jejunostomy tube placement. All these components of nutritional care must be available early in the course of disease, and weight loss must not be tolerated, particularly in cats, which have few reserves due to their small size. To our caregivers, appetite is a vital, objective assessment of quality of life that must not be overlooked or left to chance.

EUTHANASIA, PET LOSS, AND BEREAVEMENT

While cancer is the most curable of all chronic diseases in the cat, death due to the tumor or to euthanasia is still an ever-present facet of clinical practice. More clients leave a practice as a result of an unpleasant experience over the loss of a pet than for any other reason. Managing this difficult aspect of compassionate care involves adequate preparation as well as ongoing dialogue between the entire veterinary health care team and the caregivers prior to, as well as at the time of, death and euthanasia.

Many clients believe they can more comfortably and rationally discuss euthanasia before a decision must be made. Therefore it is advisable to have open and frank discussions well in advance of the actual event about the euthanasia process, options for care of the cat's remains, and the inevitable grief.

Most clients ask how they will know when it is time to euthanize their pet. Each owner bases his or her decision on unique criteria. However, despite the variety of individual criteria, the decision usually is made at approximately the same time. While it is tempting to respond to the question,

"What would you do if it were your cat, doc?," most experts believe that the veterinarian and the health care team should take the role of educator and leave the ultimate decision to the client. When contemplating euthanasia, the cat caregiver should consider quality of life issues. Caregivers can be encouraged to define objective parameters for quality of life, such as appetite, kinds of activity, and energy level, that they can assess at home. It is very helpful for them to keep some sort of written or conscious record of their cat's home "lifestyle." These definitions and measured observations provide caregivers a means by which to assess their pet's quality of life and a system to determine if the quality is changing.

Questions you might want to ask a client include:

- "Do the good days and times outnumber the bad?"
- "Is your pet able to do the things that have made it happy in the past?"
- "Describe a day in the life of your pet."

In addition, consideration should be given to financial issues, probability and duration of response to treatment, side effects and toxicity of treatment, and the amount of time required for treatment. Once the client has decided to euthanize his or her cat, the veterinary health care team should actively support this decision. This support can happen in a number of ways, such as validating the client's decision or assisting the client in understanding the euthanasia and bereavement processes.

The manner in which caregivers work through the euthanasia process is extremely important to the total life experience with their pet. It is also important in their relationship with the veterinarian and the health care team. Studies have shown that this process can profoundly affect the memories and actions of a caregiver for months to years after the actual time of euthanasia. During this experience, the veterinary health care team must support the caregivers and their families and friends. This support includes allowing caregivers to make as many decisions as possible, ideally long in advance of the actual event. By supporting the caregivers and allowing them to be active decision-makers, the veterinary health care team provides a sense of empowerment during a time that would otherwise be marked by feelings of helplessness and defeat.

Caregivers need to first understand how a patient is euthanized. Providing information regarding the physical process and what to expect as their beloved cat dies will help to dispel fears and preconceived ideas about death. With your guidance, caregivers may wish to choose the site, time, and lighting of the euthanasia process, as well as guide its tempo. They may wish to organize the presence of family and friends, the reading of poetry or books, or the reciting of favorite stories about their beloved pet. Whenever possible, a secluded comfortable location should be selected with a private entrance and exit to preclude any embarrassing situations, such as having the tearful client walk through a waiting room full of healthy cats and their caregivers. Time should be set aside for not only the caregiver and family but for the health care team as well to say goodbye prior to and after euthanasia. Also, make sure the caregiver has thought in advance of how he or she will get home safely.

It is important that children not be "sheltered" from the decision-making process. Many studies demonstrate that excluding children or making up stories (e.g., "Fluffy ran away") is destructive in the long run. An open and honest discussion with children is imperative. They should be allowed the chance to say goodbye to their pet, too.

Understanding of death and euthanasia is dependent on age and maturity. A good rule of thumb is to answer the children's questions in the manner in which they are asked. Many good references are available to help parents explain death and euthanasia to their children. In addition, many veterinary schools offer Pet Loss Support Hotlines that can be a source of advice and comfort during the grieving process (see Section VIII, Client Information Series, for additional information).

In addition, the caregiver and family may wish to create transition or remembrance objects to help them work through their grief. Transition objects are physical items that help the clients adjust to the loss of their cat. Examples are photographs, paw imprints made with ink on paper or baked into clay, hair clippings, or the cat's collar.

Finally, it is necessary to discuss openly and frankly—yet compassionately—what will be done with the cat's remains. Burial, cremation, or disposal by your facility are viable options. If burial or cremation is considered, a choice of urns or coffins may be important to some clients. Ideally, all of these decisions can be made early in the course of treatment, but for many clients, the final details will have to wait until they are prepared to consider the choices.

Today, most clients wish to be present during the euthanasia process. Hospital staff should be trained and prepared to be present during this emotional time. The patient should be prepared before the actual euthanasia process. Preplacement of an indwelling catheter within the distal extremity reduces the need to acquire vascular access in a cat at the time when the client's expectations and tensions are highest. Placement in the medial saphenous vein allows good access to a vein often not used for previous therapy. When the euthanasia solution is delivered, the veterinarian should provide some distance for personal space so the owner can comfortably hold the pet without having to watch the needle and syringe.

The veterinarian and the health care team should review with the caregiver what to expect before, during, and after euthanasia. While euthanasia can be performed with a vari-

ety of drugs, many veterinarians are convinced that thiopental (18 mg/kg IV over 10–30 seconds) followed immediately by pentobarbital (88 mg/kg IV over 10 seconds) results in a smooth, effortless transition to a state of death. It may be necessary to premedicate certain patients with a tranquilizer prior to catheter placement or the euthanasia procedure. Clients and other caregivers should be encouraged to be present in whatever manner they feel comfortable during the euthanasia process. If an owner decides not to be present, that decision should be supported as well. A detailed review of what may happen is important. Inform the owner that his or her cat may lose bladder and bowel control and may not close its eyes due to a total state of relaxation. Most clients accept and readily understand. A towel or other absorbent object may be placed under the cat to capture any bodily excretions.

After the process is reviewed with the client, the catheter is placed, the location, setting, and rituals are designed, and the time for euthanasia arrives. While every veterinarian has his or her own style and procedures, many feel it is important for other team members to be present or at least to say their goodbyes. The process may be reviewed briefly one more time before the catheter is checked for patency and the drugs are injected and the heart is stopped. It is very important for the attending veterinarian to listen to the heart for an appropriate period and then indicate when the heart has stopped and the beloved cat has died. A gentle touch and an offer of facial tissues are appropriate, affirmative, and supportive gestures. They tell a client that a display of emotion is accepted by everyone, including the attending clinician. At this point, client and friends and family may wish to spend time alone with their cat. Many veterinarians do not have clients deal with paying bills at this time but prefer instead to mail them the charges.

Follow-up communication can be very important for the client and the veterinary health care team. Cards, letters, or flowers can be sent by everyone involved and can be important not only for the client but for closure for the entire team as well. Adding a picture of the patient to a scrapbook or a bulletin board of beloved pets may also be of value in memorializing important patients.

There is no single way for clients or the team to work through their grief. Ideally, clients should be made aware of pet loss support groups, pet loss hotlines, or local specialists who are knowledgeable about loss and receptive to helping people who have lost a beloved pet. These support services, even if not used, provide a sense of validation for the caregiver's loss and grief and can be of lasting benefit to everyone involved.

* * *

Cancer, a disease shrouded with misconceptions, a disease poorly understood and feared, can become a cornerstone for a progressive veterinary practice—one that embraces a compassionate care approach, develops a working health care team, and fosters the bond between caregivers and their pets.

SUMMARY

Once the philosophy and mindset of cancer care are embraced and a team is built, compassionate care of the cancer patient becomes a vivid reality. The cat with cancer is cared for, and the needs and concerns of the caregiver are attended to. This nurturing environment not only offers the best care for the patient, it provides an atmosphere of healing and hope for both the patient and the caregiver as well. The medical needs are met, the patient and the tumor are adequately assessed and evaluated, options for care are examined and weighed, a treatment plan is selected, and the care then begins. The goal of this approach is ensuring quality of life for a precious family member—there is no doubt that quantity of life will also be the reality.

It is at this place that the veterinary health care team is most effective and most successful. The goal is achieving moments of time for a caregiver to share with that most precious cat that they have entrusted within our care. The victorious outcome is prolonging and enhancing the bond.

BIBLIOGRAPHY

Downing R. *Pets Living with Cancer: A Pet Owner's Resource.* Denver, American Animal Hospital Association, 2000.

Mitchener KL, Ogilvie GK: Rekindling the bond. *Vet Econ* 40:30–36, 1999.

Mitchener KL, Ogilvie GK: Giving cancer patients hope. *Vet Econ* 40:84–88, 1999.

Slater MR, Barton CL, Rogers KS, et al: Factors affecting treatment decisions and satisfaction of owners of cats with cancer. *JAVMA* 208:1248–1252, 1996.

THEORY AND PRACTICE OF TUMOR BIOPSY

Gregory K. Ogilvie and Antony S. Moore

2

CLINICAL BRIEFING

Indications	A biopsy should be performed prior to definitive therapy if the results will: ● Alter the type of therapy to be employed, or ● Influence an owner's willingness to treat his or her cat.
Guidelines	● Biopsy should be performed only after consultation with the surgeon who will perform the definitive surgery. ● Obtain as large a sample as possible. ● DO NOT use electrocautery or surgical instruments that can potentially crush or otherwise damage tissues. ● Place each biopsy sample in a separate, properly labeled container. ● Submit the entire lesion that has been resected and properly prepared for fixation whenever possible. ● Consider submitting portions of the lesion for culture and sensitivity testing or other analysis. ● Submit the biopsy to a highly qualified veterinary pathologist. Biopsies are best analyzed by an anatomic pathologist and cytology samples by a clinical pathologist.

The three golden rules in feline oncology are biopsy, biopsy, biopsy! To determine prognosis, treatment options, and palliative care, one must know the histopathologic name and, in many instances, the grade of the cancer.[1-4] These rules are the key to successful management of almost any cat with cancer. A biopsy prior to the definitive procedure is critical in feline oncology because "salvage" procedures are much less likely to be successful in cats than in other species; therefore the definitive treatment must be handled correctly the *first time*. In addition, the cat is smaller, and in some cases, because of the advanced stage of many malignancies, its physical condition is likely to be more fragile; thus the definitive procedures must be planned with care.

A minor limitation in feline oncology biopsy procedures is the size of the cat versus the large size of the instruments designed for biopsies in human medicine. This challenge rarely precludes obtaining tissues for biopsy but does require some creative planning.

SUMMARY GUIDELINES FOR OBTAINING A SUCCESSFUL BIOPSY SAMPLE

● Biopsy should be performed only after consultation with the surgeon who will perform the definitive surgery to formulate a correct plan for the biopsy such that follow-up surgical procedures will not be made more difficult or less potentially successful (Figure 2-1).

● Obtain as large of a sample as possible.
● DO NOT over use electrocautery energy or any surgical instruments that can potentially crush or otherwise damage tissues.
● Ensure that the tissue is adequately fixed in a 10% buffered neutral formalin solution.
● Place each biopsy sample in a separate container and properly label each container.
● Submit the entire lesion, whenever possible, after it has been resected and properly prepared for fixation.
● Consider submitting portions of the lesion for culture and sensitivity testing or other analysis.
● Submit the biopsy to a highly qualified veterinary pathologist. Remember that an anatomic pathologist can best evaluate biopsies and a clinical pathologist can best analyze cytology.

The biopsy is one of the most important procedures performed when evaluating a cat with cancer. Biopsy results must be interpreted carefully in conjunction with results of other diagnostic procedures such as blood work, radiography, and other imaging modalities. A biopsy specimen is of value only if it is properly collected and prepared and then interpreted by a highly trained pathologist who is willing to use all available clinical information to arrive at an accurate diagnosis.

Each biopsy should be performed with the assumption

that the lesion is malignant. Therefore the procedure should be performed so that the entire surgical field, including all tissues or tissue planes that may have been dis-

KEY POINT

The biopsy provides the entire health care team with the first vital piece of information in developing a plan of action. This is the first phase of restoring the sense of power, which is often lost when cancer is mentioned.

turbed and any postbiopsy hemorrhage/hematoma, can be removed during subsequent surgery. Second surgeries performed to remove the tumor and surrounding tissues frequently involve at least one fascial layer below the tumor and all tissues disturbed by previous surgery (Figure 2-2).

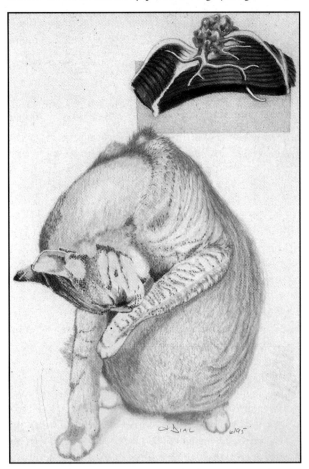

Figure 2-1: *A biopsy procedure has the potential to disturb fascial planes and tumor architecture, which could complicate definitive surgical procedures. When performing a biopsy, attention must be given to the three-dimensional nature of the tumor and surrounding tissue. The inset demonstrates how the multiple "fingers" of a vaccine-associated sarcoma can complicate an excisional biopsy.*

Several types of biopsies exist, including needle core biopsies, incisional (wedge) biopsies, and excisional biopsies. A small core of tissue is obtained with a needle core biopsy, whereas a portion of the tumor is removed for an incisional biopsy. Incisional biopsies are generally taken at the junction of normal and abnormal tissue and are preferred in cases where a punch or needle biopsy cannot provide an adequate tissue sample for analysis. Regardless of the type, the biopsy procedure must be performed correctly to avoid compromising subsequent curative resection. An excisional biopsy, which removes the entire tumor, is preferred in cases in which knowledge of the tissue type will not influence the definitive procedure or treatment plan (e.g., a solitary lung mass or a splenic mass).

KEY POINT

The biopsy is one of the most important procedures performed when evaluating a cat with cancer.

As mentioned, the biopsy should be performed prior to definitive therapy if the results will:

- Alter the type of therapy to be employed or
- Influence an owner's willingness to treat his or her cat.[1]

For example, if biopsy results indicate a benign basal cell tumor, the clinician can confidently proceed with a small resection; if, however, the biopsy results reveal that the mass is a high-grade vaccine-associated sarcoma, which is a more aggressive tumor, then wide surgical resection with 2 to 3 cm margins around the periphery of the tumor is required and adjunctive therapy may be recommended. For financial and/or emotional reasons, some owners may be more willing to treat a cat with a benign basal cell tumor than one with a more malignant vaccine-associated sarcoma.

GUIDELINES[1,2]

1. *Biopsies DO NOT negatively influence the survival of the patient when taken appropriately.* The myth that the biopsy procedure causes cancer cells to spread throughout the cat's body, resulting in early demise of the patient, is not supported in the scientific literature.
2. *A biopsy should be performed after consultation with the surgeon who will perform the definitive surgery (Figure 2-1).* This gives the surgeon the information needed to ensure that the lesion and the entire biopsy tract are removed to allow for adequate resection of the mass and biopsy site without "spilling" or "seeding" tumor cells into the surgical field. In addition, the biopsy incision should be oriented to cause the least amount of tension on the skin, thereby simplifying any subsequent definitive surgical

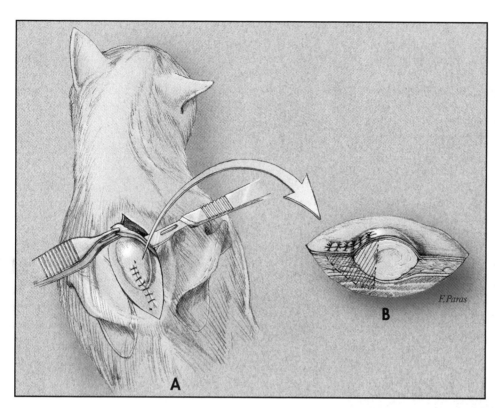

Figure 2-2: *Vaccine-associated sarcoma being removed (**A**). An incisional biopsy had previously been taken from the junction of normal and abnormal tissue. Note that in the definitive tumor removal, an elliptic "birds-eye" incision is made to include a "cuff" of normal tissue on all sides of the tumor. Tissue removed (**B**) includes the entire previous biopsy tract, the tumor with a "cuff" of normal tissue, and one fascial layer below the tumor margin.*

procedure(s). In general, the direction of the incision should be made like the stripes on a tiger to minimize skin tension and maximize the amount of tissue that can be removed around the tumor (Figure 2-3); there are, however, some exceptions, such as the presence of odd-shaped tumors in areas where the skin is tight.

3. *Obtain as large a sample as possible to assist the pathologist in making a correct diagnosis.* With an incisional biopsy, the juncture of normal and abnormal tissue is an ideal site for collecting samples of the tumor. Osteosarcoma (or any tumor involving bone) is an exception to this rule. When this tumor type is suspected, biopsy specimens should be taken from the center of the tumor because the periphery of the lesion is primarily composed of reactive bone. Ulcerated, necrotic tissue should not be collected unless absolutely necessary because secondary pathologic lesions may obscure the primary diagnosis. In addition, if needle core biopsies are obtained, multiple samples (at least three to five) should be taken throughout the tumor.

4. *Original architecture of the tissue sample should be maintained, and thus electrocautery, lasers, or surgical instruments that crush or otherwise damage tissues should not be used.*

5. *Ensure that the tissue is adequately fixed in 10% buffered neutral formalin (1 part tissue to 10 parts fixative).* Fresh tissue should be placed in fixative for 24 to 48 hours. Although most pathologists prefer 10% buffered formalin, such fixatives as Zenker's or Bouin's can be used for special purposes (e.g., optic tissue). For best results, tissue

samples should not be thicker than 1 cm to ensure proper exposure to the fixative. If an excisional biopsy is performed and the entire sample is larger than 1 cm, it can be cut like a loaf of bread to allow proper exposure of the tissue to the fixative (Figure 2-4). The exception to this rule is brain tissue, which can be fixed intact without the "bread-loafing" technique. Very thin samples should be avoided because the fixation process can distort the tissue architecture. The tissue should not be exposed to heat, cold, or water at any time.

6. *Each biopsy specimen should be placed into a separate, properly labeled container.* The container should be labeled on its side rather than the lid to prevent mix-ups if the tops are switched. If multiple samples are collected, all containers should be labeled *before* the procedure to reduce the chance of confusing samples.

7. *When possible, all resected tissue should be properly prepared and submitted for appropriate analysis.* This enables the pathologist to examine the tissue for completeness of removal ("clean" or "dirty" margins) and architectural detail. Trimming the biopsy specimen or submitting only a small section means that this valuable information may be lost. However, if mailing costs must be reduced, smaller, adequately fixed representative tissue samples can be sent in just enough formalin to keep them moist. Tissues that are adequately fixed in formalin can be placed in sealable sandwich bags with a formalin-saturated paper towel or sponge. If only a portion of the

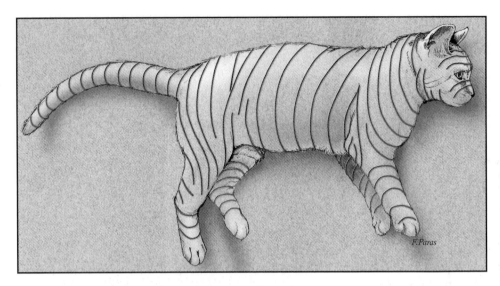

Figure 2-3: *When a biopsy or definitive procedure is performed, incisions should be made to minimize tension on the skin. Generally, an incision made like the stripes on a tiger will minimize skin tension and maximize the amount of tissue surrounding the tumor that can be removed.*

sample is submitted, the original tissue should be kept by the attending clinician in the event that additional samples are needed. Overfixation may decrease the chances of successful immunohistochemistry. All margins should be marked with ink or suture and submitted to determine adequacy of surgical excision (Figure 2-5). Again, if decreasing the size of sample submission is necessary, margins can be submitted separately.

8. *After a biopsy sample has been obtained, consideration should be given to submitting portions for culture and sensitivity testing or alternate analysis (e.g., electron microscopy).* For best results, it is essential to plan which types of samples are to be submitted and analyzed before preparing the biopsy sample. Once the tissue is in the formalin, other tests or analyses may not be possible.

9. *Biopsy specimens should be submitted to a highly qualified veterinary pathologist who is willing to work with the clinician.* In addition:
   —The pathologist should be given a detailed history and a complete account of all relevant clinical material (Figure 2-4C).
   —Margins should be identified with ink or suture. The pathologist will then have all the information necessary to make an accurate diagnosis.
   —It is important for the clinician and pathologist to work together to help coordinate the clinical picture with the diagnosis. If the two do not match, then the clinician and pathologist should work together to reevaluate all case information, including histopathology. This cooperative interaction is essential for the cat's benefit and allows for a more successful plan of action.
   —Board-certified, anatomic pathologists are best qualified to analyze histopathologic specimens, whereas board-certified clinical pathologists are most appropriate to evaluate cytology, hematology, and biochemical problems.

CONTRAINDICATIONS

In each case, the risks and benefits of the biopsy procedure should be evaluated and clearly described to the owner. In most cases, risks are minimal. Uncontrollable hemorrhage is the most common complication with all biopsy procedures with the possible exception of bone marrow aspiration. Therefore hemostatic abnormalities should be identified and corrected before each biopsy. Aseptic technique is critical to avoid the uncommon but serious complications of infection at the biopsy site and/or sepsis in the patient. Lastly, a biopsy should not be performed if it could potentially put the success of a definitive procedure at risk. For example, an incisional biopsy of a primary lung tumor or mass on the spleen may contaminate the entire chest or abdominal cavity with tumor cells, which is why primary lung tumors or splenic masses are usually removed during one definitive surgical procedure (i.e., an excisional biopsy). Note that diffusely enlarged spleens are most often caused by lymphoma or mast cell tumor and are often diagnosed by transabdominal fine-needle aspiration cytology.

BIOPSY AS A PRELUDE TO DEFINITIVE THERAPY

Frequently quoted is the saying, "Our eyes are not microscopes." A palpable, persistent mass is the most common indication for biopsy as a prelude to definitive therapy.[1-3] As accuracy and sensitivity of diagnostic tests (e.g., ultrasonography, computed tomography, magnetic resonance imaging) improves, biopsies are being performed with increasing frequency to clarify the diagnosis of visualized yet nonpalpable masses.

When developing a diagnostic strategy for a cat with cancer, the clinician must consider subsequent disease management.[3] Cats are often diagnosed with advanced, frequently malignant disease, and the formulation of appropriate diagnostic and therapeutic strategies early in the course of the

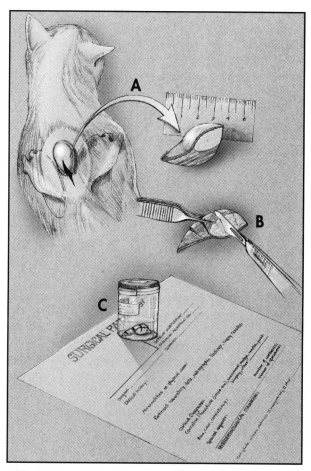

Figure 2-4: *Vaccine-associated sarcomas often require an incisional biopsy at the junction of normal and abnormal tissue (**A**). Tissues larger than 1 cm in diameter should be incompletely incised like a loaf of bread, leaving one side uncut to retain the tumor's spatial relationship (**B**). The slices should be made 1 cm apart to allow for adequate penetration of the fixative. For the most accurate diagnosis, submit the entire properly fixed and prepared specimen with a detailed history and description (**C**).*

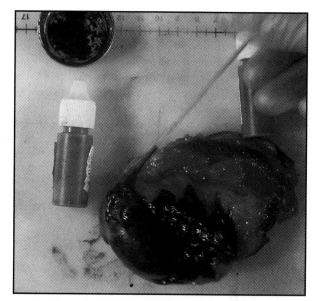

Figure 2-5: *Marking the margins of the sample to be submitted with various colored inks allows the pathologist to determine if all abnormal tissue has been removed.*

BIOPSY

disease is essential. The first step toward diagnosing most palpable lesions is fine-needle aspiration cytology. If the cytologic diagnosis strongly suggests a malignant condition or is highly suggestive of a particular condition (e.g., soft tissue sarcoma), a definitive procedure such as surgical removal can be planned. In addition, this tentative diagnosis can help guide the staging procedure ahead. Fine-needle aspiration cytology can also confirm the presence of a benign process, eliminating the need for further diagnostic steps.

If fine-needle aspiration cytology is not definitive, then an incisional biopsy should be performed, guided or executed by the surgeon who will perform the definitive surgery. Before collecting a biopsy sample, standard diagnostic tests can be performed to identify any concurrent disease or clinically evident metastatic disease.

Staging is accomplished through certain diagnostic tests that determine the extent of the neoplastic disorder. The staging scheme differs for each neoplastic disease but should include a complete blood count, biochemical profile, urinalysis, serology for feline leukemia virus and feline immunodeficiency virus, serum T_4 determination, thoracic radiographs, and cytologic evaluation of regional lymph nodes. Discussions regarding additional diagnostic steps in specific staging schemes are included in the review of each individual disease.

Each biopsy should be performed with the assumption that the lesion is malignant. Therefore the biopsy should be done so that the entire surgical field, including all tissues or tissue planes that may have been disturbed as well as any postbiopsy hemorrhage/hematoma, can be removed by subsequent surgery. Second surgeries performed to remove the tumor and surrounding tissues frequently involve going at least one fascial layer below the tumor and all tissues disturbed by the previous surgery (Figure 2-1).

REFERENCES

1. Ogilvie GK, Moore AS: *Managing the Veterinary Cancer Patient: A Practice Manual.* Trenton, NJ, Veterinary Learning Systems, 1995, pp 1-47.
2. Withrow SJ, MacEwen EG: The biopsy, in *Small Animal Clinical Oncology.* Philadelphia, WB Saunders, 1996, pp 52-57.
3. Morrison WB, Hamilton TA, Hahn KA, et al: Diagnosis of neoplasia, in Slatter D (ed): *Textbook of Small Animal Surgery,* ed 2. Philadelphia, WB Saunders, 1993, pp 2036–2048.
4. Wolmark N: Biopsy as a prelude to a definitive operative therapy for breast cancer, in Wittes RE (ed): *Manual of Oncologic Therapeutics 1991/1992.* Philadelphia, JB Lippincott, 1991, pp 5–8.

SKIN BIOPSY

Gregory K. Ogilvie and Antony S. Moore

3

CLINICAL BRIEFING

Methods	Benefits
Punch biopsy	Outpatient diagnostic procedure; quick and simple.
Incisional biopsy	Diagnostic and allows surgeon to plan definitive procedure.
Excisional biopsy	Potentially therapeutic and diagnostic.
Needle core biopsy	Diagnostic and allows surgeon to plan definitive procedure, done on outpatient basis; quick, and simple, minimal recovery.

A skin biopsy is essential to diagnose and evaluate potentially malignant skin conditions. *Punch, incisional, excisional,* and *needle core biopsies* are employed.[1-3]

PUNCH BIOPSY[1-3]

Biopsy punches are available as expensive reusable instruments or inexpensive disposable units; the latter may be reused after appropriate sterilization until they become dull. They are available in diameters ranging from 2 to 6 mm (Figure 3-1). Generally, taking a larger biopsy specimen is preferred so that the pathologist has an adequate sample from which to make a histologic diagnosis. When possible, multiple samples at the juncture between normal and abnormal tissue should be biopsied. Punch biopsies are usually inadequate for obtaining tissue below the dermis because subcutaneous tissue is rarely obtained in the average punch biopsy of the skin.

Indication: Identification of any dermal or epidermal lesion of unknown etiology.

Contraindications/Complications: Coagulopathies; lidocaine toxicities (unlikely).

Benefits: General anesthesia is not required; simple outpatient procedure.

Limitation: Small tissue samples obtained may not be diagnostic.

Equipment: Sedation and analgesia should be considered (Table 3-1); 2% lidocaine and 8.4% bicarbonate (50:50); Baker's biopsy instrument; standard surgical instruments; suture material.

Technique (Figure 3-2).

1. Clip the hair and prepare the site with proper aseptic surgical technique.

2. Dilute 2% lidocaine 50:50 with 8.4% bicarbonate to reduce stinging on injection. Using a 25-ga needle, approximately 0.25 to 1 ml of this local anesthetic agent is injected around the lesion. It is important to make sure that injection of lidocaine does not distort or disturb the normal architecture of the tissue to be biopsied.

3. The biopsy area is surgically scrubbed a final time after the lidocaine is injected.

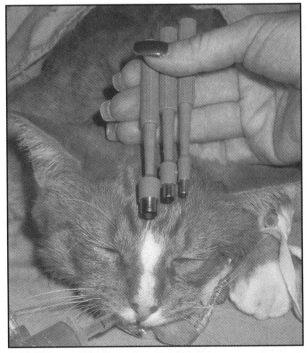

Figure 3-1: *Several sizes of punch biopsy instruments are available. Consideration should be given to obtaining as large a sample as possible from the margin of normal and abnormal tissue.*

TABLE 3-1
Sedation and Analgesia for a Punch Biopsy

Sedative or Preemptive Medication Options	Anesthesia	Perioperative Analgesia Options	Postoperative Analgesia Options
• Medetomidine (5–20 μg/kg IM) or xylazine (0.5–1 mg/kg IM) + butorphanol (0.2 mg/kg IM)	• Usually not necessary	• Topical or local blocks with lidocaine (<11 mg/kg) or bupivacaine (<4 mg/kg)	• NSAIDs • If NSAIDs not adequate, consider adding opioid agonist-antagonist drugs
• Acepromazine (0.025–0.05 mg/kg IV) + butorphanol (0.2–0.4 mg/kg IV)			
• Diazepam (0.2 mg/kg IV) + butorphanol (0.2 mg/kg IV)			
• Propofol (2–6 mg/kg IV)			
• Ketamine (5 mg/kg IV) + diazepam (0.2 mg/kg IV)			

Adapted from Tranquilli W, Grimm K, Flaggella A, et al: *A Roundtable Discussion: Rethinking Your Approach to Sedation, Anesthesia, and Analgesia* [monograph]. Lenexa, KS, Veterinary Medicine Publishing, 1997.

4. Stretch the skin of the site to be biopsied between the thumb and index finger.
5. Place the biopsy punch instrument at a right angle to the skin surface (Figure 3-3).
6. Rotate the punch instrument in one direction and, at the same time, apply firm downward pressure until the subcutis is reached.
7. Angle the punch almost parallel with the skin while still applying pressure along the long axis of the instrument.
8. Rotate the punch to sever at least part of the base of the biopsied tissue.
9. Remove the punch instrument and gently elevate the core of tissue with the point of a needle; sever the base that is still attached with a scalpel blade or a pair of iris scissors.
10. Place one or two sutures as needed to close the defect, depending on the size of the punch taken.

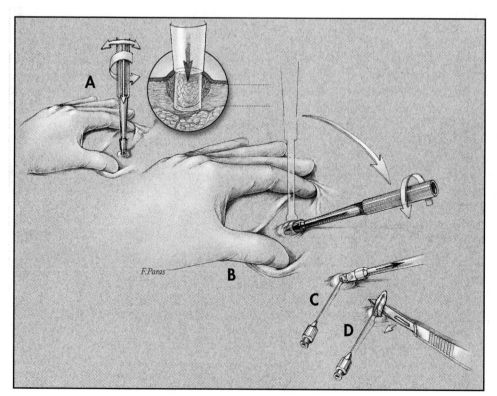

Figure 3-2: *A punch biopsy procedure begins by injecting lidocaine around the area to be biopsied, being careful not to alter tissue architecture of interest. The skin is then stretched between the thumb and index finger. The biopsy punch (e.g., Baker's biopsy punch) is placed at a right angle to the skin surface (**A**). The punch is rotated in one direction; at the same time, firm downward pressure is applied until the subcutis is reached. The punch is then angled almost parallel with the skin while still applying pressure along the long axis of the biopsy punch (**B**). The punch is rotated to sever at least part of the base of the biopsied material. The punch is removed (**C**), and the core of tissue is gently elevated with the point of a needle and severed at the base with a scalpel (**D**).*

F. Paras

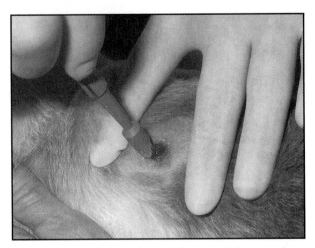

Figure 3-3: After injecting lidocaine and preparing the biopsy site, the punch biopsy instrument is placed at a 90 degree angle to the stretched skin. Note that the punch is located at the junction of normal and abnormal skin.

Supportive Care: Oral analgesics; periodic cleansing of the surgery site; consider the use of an Elizabethan collar to prevent self-trauma.

INCISIONAL BIOPSY[1–3]

In some cases, an incisional biopsy is preferred to a punch biopsy because larger sections of tissue can be obtained for histologic diagnosis. In addition, if the lesion is biopsied at the junction of the normal and abnormal tissue, a "wedge" of tissue is obtained that retains a larger section of the tissue's architecture. This makes it easier for the histopathologist to see characteristics of malignancy, such as invasion into the normal tissue.

Indication: Identification of dermal, epidermal, or subcutaneous lesion of unknown etiology.

Contraindications: Coagulopathies; cats that are at high risk for general anesthesia.

Benefit: Larger tissue sample often results in a more accurate diagnosis.

Limitations: General anesthesia is often needed; not a definitive procedure.

Equipment: Sedation and general anesthesia (Table 3-2); standard surgical instruments; suture material.

Technique (Figure 3-4A):
1. Perform routine screening tests to identify problems such as coagulopathies and metabolic disease.
2. Place the cat under general anesthesia.
3. Surgically prepare the area with clipping and strict aseptic technique, and then properly drape the site. An elliptical or wedge incision is made at the margin of normal and abnormal tissue. Care is taken to obtain adequate tissue and to ensure that a subsequent definitive surgery can remove the tumor and the incisional biopsy area successfully.
4. Vessels going to and from the tissue to be biopsied are carefully identified and ligated.
5. The specimen is lifted and severed at the base with either scissors or a scalpel blade.
6. The incision is sutured for closure.

Supportive Care: Oral or parenteral analgesics for several days to weeks; periodic cleansing of the surgery site.

EXCISIONAL BIOPSY[1–3]

An excisional biopsy should be performed for histologic diagnosis of a lesion that is small and located in an anatom-

TABLE 3-2
Sedation, Anesthesia, and Analgesia for Incisional and Excisional Biopsies

Sedative or Preemptive Medication Options	Anesthesia Options	Perioperative Analgesia Options	Postoperative Analgesia Options
• Medetomidine (10–15 µg/kg IM) + butorphanol (0.2 mg/kg IM)	• Thiopental (2–10 mg/kg IV to effect)	• Topical or local blocks with lidocaine (<11 mg/kg) or bupivacaine (<4 mg/kg)	• NSAIDs
• Acepromazine (0.025–0.05 mg/kg IM or SQ) + butorphanol (0.2–0.4 mg/kg IM or SQ)	• Propofol (1–3 mg/kg IV to effect)		• If NSAIDs not adequate, consider adding opioid agonist-antagonist drugs
• Butorphanol (0.2–0.4 mg/kg IV) + ketamine (5 mg/kg IV) + diazepam (0.2 mg/kg IV)	• Ketamine (1–4 mg/kg IV to effect)		• Acupuncture
• Butorphanol (0.2–0.4 mg/kg IM) + Telazol® (2–4 mg/kg IM)	• Telazol® (1–2 mg/kg IV to effect)		
• Butorphanol (0.2–0.4 mg/kg IV) + propofol (3–6 mg/kg IV to effect)	• Mask or chamber induction		

Adapted from Tranquilli W, Grimm K, Flaggella A, et al: *A Roundtable Discussion: Rethinking Your Approach to Sedation, Anesthesia, and Analgesia* [monograph]. Lenexa, KS, Veterinary Medicine Publishing, 1997.

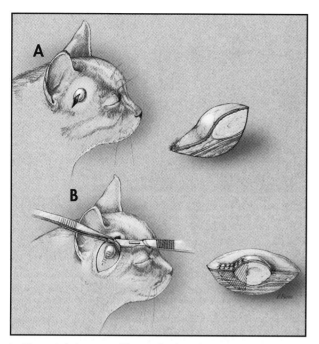

Figure 3-4: An incisional biopsy taken from the margin of normal and abnormal tissue (**A**). When performing an incisional biopsy, keep in mind that the entire tumor and the biopsy tract will need to be removed in a subsequent definitive procedure. In a definitive tumor removal after incisional biopsy (performed in the same manner as an excisional biopsy), the entire tumor is removed (**B**). Wide margins are obtained through the use of an elliptical "bird's-eye" incision and the tissue removed includes one fascial plane below the tumor.

lateral abdominal wall). In nearly all cats, an excisional biopsy is preceded by fine-needle aspiration cytology and/or incisional biopsy to give the surgeon as much information as possible about the characteristics of the tumor prior to removal. For example, a vaccine-associated sarcoma requires wide surgical margins (2 to 3 cm), whereas a benign basal cell tumor can be excised with smaller margins.

Indication: Identification of dermal, epidermal, or subcutaneous lesion of unknown etiology.

Contraindications: Coagulopathies; cats that are at high risk for general anesthesia.

Benefit: Larger tissue sample often results in a more accurate diagnosis.

Limitation: Requires general anesthesia; may make definitive second procedure more difficult to achieve.

Equipment: Sedation and general anesthesia (Table 3-2); standard surgical instruments; suture material.

Technique (Figure 3-4B): This biopsy is performed in the same manner as an incisional biopsy except the lesion, along with adequate margins, is excised completely.

Supportive Care: Oral or parenteral analgesics for days to weeks; periodic cleansing of the surgery site.

> ### KEY POINT
>
> *An excisional biopsy should be performed on a lesion that is small and in an anatomic location that will permit wide surgical removal.*

ic location where wide surgical removal is possible but will not compromise the normal tissue around it (e.g., cutaneous basal cell tumor <0.5 cm in diameter located on the

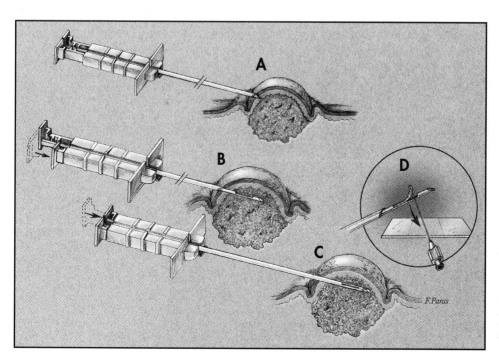

Figure 3-5: A needle core biopsy is accomplished by making a stab incision through the skin with a No. 11 surgical blade after the skin and underlying structures are anesthetized locally with 0.25 to 0.5 ml of lidocaine. A needle biopsy instrument is then advanced through the skin to the periphery of the lesion (**A**). The stylet is advanced into the tissue to be biopsied (**B**), and the outer cannula is advanced over the stylet to "cut" off the tissue left in the notch of the stylet (**C**). The entire instrument is removed from the incision, and the tissue is teased out of the stylet using a 22 ga needle (**D**).

BIOPSY

NEEDLE CORE BIOPSY

Needle core biopsy is generally safe and quick and can be performed on an awake, cooperative cat on an outpatient basis when appropriate analgesia and sedation are used.[1] Unless medically contraindicated, analgesics are used prior to and after the biopsy procedure. Generally, histopathology results are more accurate than those of fine-needle aspiration cytology but are not as accurate as the results of an excisional or incisional biopsy due to the size of tissue sample obtained. Needle core biopsy instruments, especially the spring-loaded models that can be adjusted to obtain tissue from different depths, are preferred.

KEY POINT

Needle core biopsy is generally safe and quick and can be performed on an awake, cooperative cat as an outpatient using appropriate analgesia and, when indicated, sedation.

Indication: Identification of a skin or subcutaneous lesion of unexplained etiology.

Contraindications/Complications: Coagulopathies; lidocaine toxicity (unlikely).

Benefit: General anesthesia is not required, so the procedure can be performed on an outpatient basis.

Limitation: The small tissue samples obtained may not be diagnostic.

Equipment: Sedation and analgesia should be considered (Table 2-1); No. 11 surgical blade; 2% lidocaine; needle core biopsy instrument.

Technique (Figures 3-5 and 3-6):
1. The cutaneous or subcutaneous lesion is grasped by an assistant and immobilized, and the biopsy site is prepared with surgical scrub for an aseptic procedure.
2. Approximately 0.25 to 1 ml of 2% lidocaine is injected around the lesion to be biopsied while trying not to disturb the architecture of the tissue to be evaluated with the lidocaine. (The lidocaine will sting less upon injection if diluted 50:50 with 8.4% bicarbonate.)

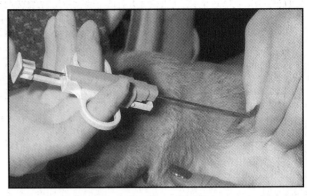

Figure 3-6: *A spring-loaded needle core biopsy instrument is placed against the skin over the abnormal tissue to be sampled. When the notch in the stylet has been advanced into the abnormal tissue, pushing the plunger will automatically close the outer cannula over the sample.*

3. Using a No. 11 surgical blade, make a stab incision in the skin to allow easy entry of the needle core biopsy instrument.
4. Advance the needle core biopsy instrument through the incision to the outer portion of the lesion to be biopsied. In the case of the skin, the instrument is advanced just into the tissue to be biopsied.
5. Obtain three to five biopsy specimens from the suspect tissue through the same stab incision. This will allow the histopathologist to evaluate a sample of tissue from various portions of the mass, enhancing the probability of making an accurate diagnosis. These individual biopsies are best obtained by redirecting the needle within the mass.
6. The needle biopsy specimens are fixed in 10% buffered formalin, as described previously. A separate container should be used and labeled accordingly for each lesion.
7. The stab incision is sutured only if indicated by the size and depth.

Supportive Care: Oral analgesics for several days; periodic cleansing of the surgery site.

REFERENCES

1. Ogilvie GK, Moore AS: *Managing the Veterinary Cancer Patient: A Practice Manual.* Trenton, NJ, Veterinary Learning Systems, 1995, pp 1–47.
2. Morrison WB, Hamilton TA, Hahn KA, et al: Diagnosis of neoplasia, in Slatter D (ed): *Textbook of Small Animal Surgery,* ed 2. Philadelphia, WB Saunders, 1993, pp 2036–2048.
3. Sober AJ: Skin biopsy in the diagnosis and management of malignancy, in Wittes RE (ed): *Manual of Oncologic Therapeutics 1991/1992.* Philadelphia, JB Lippincott, 1991, pp 1–5.

4

LYMPH NODE BIOPSY

Gregory K. Ogilvie and Antony S. Moore

C L I N I C A L B R I E F I N G	
Methods	**Benefits**
Lymph node excision	Pathologist can evaluate complete nodal architecture.
Needle core biopsy	Outpatient diagnostic procedure; quick and simple.

Lymph node biopsy is often important in the diagnosis, staging, and proper therapeutic management of the cat with cancer.[1-3] Excisional or needle core biopsy is frequently performed after fine-needle aspiration cytology suggests the presence of disease. Despite the accuracy of fine-needle aspiration cytology in determining the presence of diseases such as lymphoma or metastatic solid tumors, a histopathologic diagnosis is always recommended prior to initiation of therapy. A completely excised lymph node will allow the histopathologist to assess subtle architectural changes not always present in tissue obtained by needle core biopsy. In each case, adequate tissue must be obtained for histopathologic diagnosis and for special stains, if indicated. If other lymph nodes are enlarged, the submandibular lymph nodes should be avoided; they often are reactive in the normal cat because they drain the oral cavity, where the bacterial count is usually quite high. These reactive cells are sometimes misdiagnosed as neoplastic cells. Whenever a malignancy is suspected, the biopsy should be planned so that the entire biopsy "tract" can be removed by the definitive surgery. This is because the biopsy procedure can "seed" the operative field with tumor cells if the principle of en bloc dissection is violated. As with all biopsies, the surgeon who will perform the definitive surgery should be consulted prior to the biopsy to ensure that incisions are properly placed for a subsequent definitive procedure.

KEY POINT

When possible, the submandibular lymph nodes should not be biopsied; they are often reactive because they drain the oral cavity, where the bacterial count is usually high.

LYMPH NODE EXCISION

The type of biopsy done on the lymph node will depend on each case; however, an excisional biopsy should be performed when possible[1-3] because this allows the pathologist

to determine the architecture of the entire lymph node and whether capsular invasion exists. This is especially valuable in cats, in which lymphoma must be differentiated from lymph node hyperplasia.

Lymph node excisions are commonly performed in cats that have lymphadenopathy, especially when lymphoma or other malignant conditions are suspected. A lymph node that is not easily seen or palpated by the casual observer should not be considered for removal. Hair should be clipped prior to surgery; however, the amount of hair clipped should not be excessive, because cats receiving chemotherapy often have slow hair regrowth. In addition, antineoplastic agents can cause alopecia, which makes the surgical site cosmetically noticeable for weeks to months after the procedure.

Indication: Lymphadenopathy of unexplained etiology.

Contraindications: Coagulopathies; cats that are at high risk for complications due to anesthesia.

Benefit: An accurate histopathologic diagnosis can be obtained because the entire lymph node architecture is present.

Limitation: Requires general anesthesia.

Equipment: Sedation and general anesthesia (Table 4-1); standard surgical instruments; suture material.

Technique:

1. Place the cat under general anesthesia after routine screening tests are performed to identify problems such as coagulopathies and metabolic disease.
2. Clip the hair; prepare the surgical site using proper aseptic technique.
3. After the region is draped, make an incision over the enlarged lymph node.
4. Carefully identify and ligate the vessels going to and from the lymph node to be excised.
5. After the lymph node is removed, subcutaneous tissue is closed with absorbable suture and the skin is closed with either absorbable or nonabsorbable suture.

TABLE 4-1
Sedation, Anesthesia, and Analgesia for a Lymph Node Biopsy

Sedative or Preemptive Medication	Anesthesia	Perioperative Analgesia Options	Postoperative Analgesia Options
• Medetomidine (10–15 μg/kg IM) + butorphanol (0.2 mg/kg IM)	• Thiopental (2–10 mg/kg IV to effect)	• Topical or local blocks with lidocaine (<11 mg/kg) or bupivacaine (<4 mg/kg)	• NSAIDs
• Acepromazine (0.025–0.05 mg/kg IM or SQ) + butorphanol (0.2–0.4 mg/kg IM or SQ)	• Propofol (1–3 mg/kg IV to effect)	• Postoperative analgesia prn	• If NSAIDs not adequate, consider adding opioid agonist-antagonist drugs
• Butorphanol (0.2–0.4 mg/kg IV) + ketamine (5 mg/kg IV) + diazepam (0.2 mg/kg IV)	• Ketamine (1–4 mg/kg IV to effect)	• Acupuncture	• Acupuncture
• Butorphanol (0.2–0.4 mg/kg IM) + Telazol® (2–4 mg/kg IM)	• Telazol® (1–2 mg/kg IV to effect)		
• Butorphanol (0.2–0.4 mg/kg IV) + propofol (3–6 mg/kg IV to effect)	• Mask or chamber induction		

Adapted from Tranquilli W, Grimm K, Flaggella A, et al: *A Roundtable Discussion: Rethinking Your Approach to Sedation, Anesthesia, and Analgesia* [monograph]. Lenexa, KS, Veterinary Medicine Publishing, 1997.

Supportive Care: Oral or parenteral analgesics for days to weeks; periodic cleansing of the surgery site.

NEEDLE CORE BIOPSY
See discussion of procedure in Chapter 3.

REFERENCES

1. Ogilvie GK, Moore AS: *Managing the Veterinary Cancer Patient: A Practice Manual.* Trenton, NJ, Veterinary Learning Systems, 1995, pp 1–47.

2. Morrison WB, Hamilton TA, Hahn KA, et al: Diagnosis of neoplasia, in Slatter D (ed): *Textbook of Small Animal Surgery,* ed 2. Philadelphia, WB Saunders, 1993, pp 2036–2048.

3. Avis F: Lymph node biopsy, in Wittes RE (ed): *Manual of Oncologic Therapeutics 1991/1992.* Philadelphia, JB Lippincott, 1991, pp 8–9.

RESPIRATORY TRACT BIOPSY

Gregory K. Ogilvie and Antony S. Moore

5

THORACIC CAVITY

CLINICAL BRIEFING

Methods	Benefits
Bronchoscopy	Visualization of lesions and a directed biopsy allow more accurate diagnosis.
Transthoracic aspirate	Quick, simple, and inexpensive method of diagnosing pleural and pulmonary lesions.
Transtracheal/ Transendotracheal wash	Relatively quick and simple method of diagnosing some lesions confined to the airways.

DIAGNOSTICS

Bronchoscopy is used commonly to diagnose primary lung tumors in humans; however, in feline medicine, lung tumors are not often diagnosed successfully with this approach,[1-5] possibly because cats rarely have primary lung tumors arising from the major airways. Metastatic tumors often arise in the pulmonary parenchyma. Therefore transendotracheal tube washes are often not successful in obtaining a sample of primary or metastatic tumors of the pulmonary parenchyma. Primary lung tumors of cats are frequently limited to the pulmonary parenchyma and must be accessed via techniques that can sample pulmonary tissue from outside of the airways. Bronchoscopy is helpful in the diagnosis of metastatic neoplastic conditions that shed tumor cells into the major airways. This technique is usual-

KEY POINT

Extreme care should be used to prevent overinflation of the lungs or overdosing the cat on inhalant anesthetic gases during bronchoscopy.

ly of more value in nonneoplastic conditions of the lungs and major airways.[1-4] Transthoracic needle aspiration, with or without imaging guidance, may be helpful in successfully obtaining cells or tissue samples from the peripheral pulmonary parenchyma when bronchoscopy is unproductive. Cats often have pleural effusion associated with primary or metastatic pulmonary neoplasia; therefore thoracocentesis and fluid cytology can be of diagnostic help. If these methods fail, an open biopsy via thoracotomy may be successful.

Bronchoscopy[1,2,4]

The flexible fiberoptic bronchoscope has proven to be superior to the rigid bronchoscope because it does not limit lung visualization but rather permits visualization of the respiratory tract in a wide view and is more effective in obtaining significant amounts of diagnostic tissue. In addition, a large variety of brushes, biopsy instruments, and grasping forceps can be introduced through the bronchoscope to obtain tissue or cytologic samples. It is estimated that more than 90% of all tumors located in the airways and 50% of peripheral lung tumors can be diagnosed with this modality when the procedure is performed by an experienced operator.[1-5] The benefits of imaging and biopsies guided by the bronchoscope include the ability to explore a large portion of the lungs and upper respiratory tract and to obtain tissue or cells from localized areas.[6] Disadvantages include the need for general anesthesia, inability to obtain tissue samples larger than those that can be obtained through a 1 to 2 mm channel, and the complication of secretions from the respiratory tract obscuring visualization. When possible, multiple biopsy specimens should be obtained to increase the probability of an accurate diagnosis. If large pieces of tissue are obtained, the tissue should not be extracted through the biopsy channel of the endoscope. Instead, with the biopsy instrument still extended through the biopsy port, the endoscope is removed from the trachea and endotracheal tube.

Indications: Exploration of any disease that appears to involve the airways or alveoli, including primary or metastatic lung tumors.

Contraindications: Coagulopathies; cats that are at high risk for general anesthesia, including patients with limited pulmonary function.

TABLE 5-1
Sedation, Anesthesia, and Analgesia for Bronchoscopy and Transthoracic Aspiration

Sedative or Preemptive Medication Options	Anesthesia Options	Postoperative Analgesia Options
• Medetomidine (10–15 µg/kg IM) + butorphanol (0.2 mg/kg IM)	• Thiopental (2–10 mg/kg IV to effect)	• NSAIDs
• Acepromazine (0.025–0.05 mg/kg IM or SQ) + butorphanol (0.2–0.4 mg/kg IM or SQ)	• Propofol (1–3 mg/kg IV to effect)	• If NSAIDs not adequate, consider adding opioid agonist-antagonist drugs
• Butorphanol (0.2–0.4 mg/kg IV) + ketamine (5 mg/kg IV) + diazepam (0.2 mg/kg IV)	• Ketamine (1–4 mg/kg IV to effect)	• Acupuncture
• Butorphanol (0.2–0.4 mg/kg IM) + Telazol® (2–4 mg/kg IM)	• Telazol® (1–2 mg/kg IV to effect)	
• Butorphanol (0.2–0.4 mg/kg IV) + propofol (3–6 mg/kg IV to effect)	• Mask or chamber induction	

Adapted from Tranquilli W, Grimm K, Flaggella A, et al: *A Roundtable Discussion: Rethinking Your Approach to Sedation, Anesthesia, and Analgesia* [monograph]. Lenexa, KS, Veterinary Medicine Publishing, 1997.

Benefits: Relatively minimal risk; noninvasive procedure.

Limitations: Requires general anesthesia (Table 5-1); the small tissue samples obtained may not be diagnostic

Equipment (Figure 5-1): There are many fiberoptic endoscopes available for performance of bronchoscopy (see Box on next page); adapters can be used to pass the bronchoscope down into the respiratory tract when oxygen and inhalant anesthetic gases are being used.

Complications: Rare; can include bleeding, which usually stops spontaneously. If brisk bleeding persists, introduce a Fogarty balloon catheter to occlude the opening. In humans, the risk of pneumothorax is reported to be less than 1% and, when it occurs, usually follows a transbronchial biopsy of peripheral lymph nodes.

Technique:

1. After tests have been carried out to ensure the absence of life-threatening diseases, general anesthesia with endotracheal intubation is performed.
2. After the cat is well oxygenated, one end of a Y-piece adapter specifically designed for bronchoscopy is attached to the endotracheal tube and the other end is fixed to the anesthesia machine.
3. The bronchoscope is inserted through the open end of the Y-piece and down the trachea. If the bronchoscope compromises adequate endotracheal space for normal respiration, then oxygen, with or without anesthetic gases, can be advanced down the bronchoscope. A systematic exploration of the respiratory tree is performed (Figure 5-2).

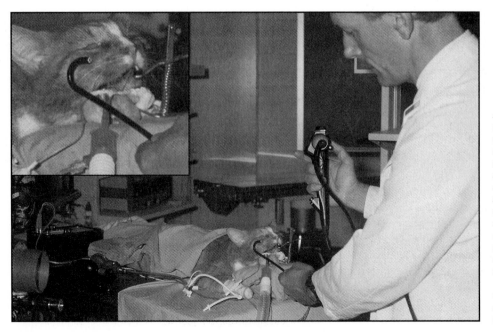

Figure 5-1: In the absence of a bronchoscope, a larger endoscope can be used to examine the upper respiratory and digestive tracts. The tip of this endoscope is placed alongside the cat's head to demonstrate the relative size of the scope. An examination of the area behind the soft palate and above the hard palate can be accomplished by placing the bronchoscope in the cat's mouth and then retroflexing the instrument above the soft palate. This bronchoscope is retroflexed near the patient to demonstrate appropriate configuration of the tip of the scope.

Selection of an Endoscope

The endoscope should:

- Have an instrument port and channel
- At least be bidirectional
- Bend more than 100 degrees in at least one direction
- Have an external light source

Instruments that should be available for the endoscopic procedure and that can pass through the instrument port are cytology brushes, biopsy forceps, and graspers. Adult or pediatric endoscopes (5 mm in diameter) can be inserted into the trachea of cats.

4. Suspect lesions are first sampled with the cytology brush for evaluation and then biopsied for histopathology. If a diffuse lesion is suspected, bronchoalveolar lavage is performed. A catheter is introduced down the bronchoscope into the area to be sampled, then sterile saline (5 to 10 ml 0.9% NaCl) is injected into the area and immediately withdrawn for culture and cytologic evaluation. This procedure can be repeated several times.

Supportive Care: Monitor respiration; oral analgesics are occasionally indicated.

Transthoracic Aspiration[2–4]

Transthoracic aspiration cytology and thoracocentesis are procedures to remove or sample pleural fluid or tissue within the lung for diagnostic or therapeutic reasons. Fluoroscopy and occasionally ultrasonography are generally used to guide the biopsy of pulmonary, parenchymal, pleural, and mediastinal lesions. Ultrasonography is effective when the tissue to be examined is surrounded by either fluid or other tissue, but not if it is surrounded by air. In cases that cannot be defined clearly by fluoroscopy or ultrasonography, computerized tomography imaging (CT) or magnetic resonance imaging (MRI) can be used to guide tissue sampling. In one study of human patients that included over 400 percutaneously biopsied pulmonary lesions, the accuracy of the procedure was determined to be 96.5%.[4] Ultrasound-guided fine-needle aspiration or blind aspiration was successful in obtaining diagnostic samples from 20 of 25 cats in one series. Fluoroscopic- or CT-guided aspiration may be the most accurate for small or less peripheral lesions.

Indications: Investigation of any masses, lesions, or fluid accumulations within or around the pulmonary parenchyma that are not near or associated with the heart or blood vessels.

Contraindications/Complications: Coagulopathies, poor pulmonary reserve, and pulmonary arterial hypertension; complications are rare (<10%) but include hemothorax and pneumothorax; placement of a chest tube may be required to resolve these problems.

Benefit: Cells or fluid can be acquired with limited risk and without a thoracotomy.

Limitations: Requires general anesthesia or tranquilization (Table 5-1); may cause pneumothorax or hemothorax.

Equipment: 2% lidocaine; 3 to 12 ml syringe; 22 ga 1.5 inch needle.

KEY POINT

Transthoracic needle aspiration, with or without imaging guidance, may be helpful in successfully obtaining cells or tissue samples from the peripheral pulmonary parenchyma when bronchoscopy is unproductive.

Technique (Figure 5-3):

1. After routine screening tests have been performed to identify problems such as coagulopathies, metabolic disease, or organ failure, the cat is placed under general anesthesia or tranquilized.
2. The lesions are identified with fluoroscopy, ultrasonography, or CT imaging. The hair is clipped, and the site is prepared with a surgical scrub and aseptic technique. A surgical drape is placed to enhance sterility.

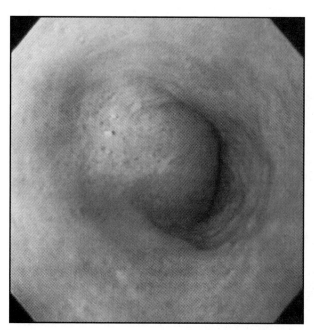

Figure 5-2: *Methodic examination of the respiratory tree can locate tumors such as this bronchial adenocarcinoma compressing the terminal bronchioles. (Courtesy of D. Twedt)*

Cats considered at high risk for general anesthesia, including patients with limited pulmonary function, should not undergo transthoracic aspiration or bronchoscopy.

3. If tranquilization is used instead of general anesthesia, the skin and underlying tissue, up to the pleura, are anesthetized with 2% lidocaine (0.5–1 ml) that has been diluted with 8.4% bicarbonate at a ratio of 50:50.
4. A 22 ga needle attached to a 3 to 12 ml syringe is advanced through the skin and intercostal muscles. This can be done blind but is best done using additional imaging techniques such as a fluoroscope, ultrasonography, or CT. Care is taken to avoid the heart and great vessels. Pneumothorax is always a potential complication but is not commonly a major concern if appropriate care is taken during the procedure. If fluid is to be sampled, a three-way stopcock is attached between the syringe and needle to facilitate removal of large amounts of fluid.
5. Tissue is aspirated while the needle is advanced through the lesion. To prevent injury of normal lung tissue, the needle is inserted and the mass aspirated over a relatively short period. The pressure is eliminated prior to removing the needle from the mass and chest cavity to prevent aspirating the acquired cells into the syringe where they may be unrecoverable. The syringe is then removed from the needle and filled with air. After the needle is reattached to the syringe, the material in the needle is forcefully expelled onto a clean microscope slide. If indicated, the material is gently spread over the slide to obtain a single layer of cells for subsequent analysis. If fluid or sufficient tissue is removed, slides are made, and fluid is saved for culture and sensitivity. The remaining fluid is saved in two tubes, an EDTA tube and a red top tube without anticoagulant, for subsequent submission to a clinical pathologist for analysis.
6. The cat is observed carefully for respiratory difficulty for several hours. Ideally, a thoracic radiograph is taken to ensure that hemothorax or pneumothorax has not developed after the procedure. In addition, the cat should be rested for 24 to 48 hours.

Supportive Care: Monitor respiration for hours to days; oral analgesics as indicated.

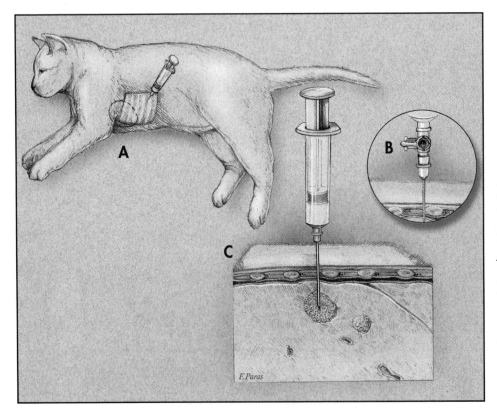

Figure 5-3: A transthoracic lung aspiration is accomplished with a 22 ga needle attached to a 3 to 12 ml syringe, which is advanced through the skin and intercostal muscles (A), ideally using fluoroscopic, ultrasonographic, or CT guidance. If fluid is to be sampled, a three-way stopcock is attached between the syringe and needle to facilitate removal of large amounts of fluid (B). In addition, it is advisable to use a 35 or 60 ml syringe. Tissue is quickly aspirated while the needle is advanced through the lesion (C). The pressure is eliminated prior to removing the needle from the mass and chest cavity.

NASAL CAVITY

C L I N I C A L B R I E F I N G	
Methods	*Benefits*
Rhinoscopy	Visualization of lesion and a biopsy especially valuable to differentiate tumor from infectious or inflammatory causes.
Curette biopsy	Biopsy method especially valuable for cats.

NASAL BIOPSY[1,4]

A nasal biopsy should be considered for every cat with a facial deformity, unilateral or bilateral epistaxis, or epiphora of unknown etiology. A nasal tumor or rhinitis of either fungal, viral, or bacterial origin must be suspected in many of these cases. A biopsy is required in each case before appropriate therapy can be recommended. Suspect tumors in cats can be biopsied using equipment that is relatively inexpensive and quite effective. Although fiberoptic examinations (Figure 5-4) and nasal flushes are valuable in some cases, they are not as rewarding as biopsy cup or curette techniques. Regardless of the procedure, general anesthesia is required for all cats. Each cat should be biopsied through the external nares to reduce surgical exposure through the skin, which could contaminate these structures with tumor cells from the nasal cavity. Biopsy of nasal tumors frequently involves the use of a bone curette or a relatively small "cup" biopsy instrument. Although biopsy through a bronchoscope or a cystoscope is relatively easy to accomplish, the size of the tissue sample obtained through these instruments often is inadequate for an accurate diagnosis. In part, this is because the tissue removed by these methods is superficial and the underlying true pathology frequently is obscured by septic inflammation. Note, however, that a bronchoscope is ideal for identifying lesions in the trachea (Figure 5-5). In addition, the bronchoscope can be retroflexed over the soft palate to clearly visualize the caudal nasal airways (Figure 5-1).

KEY POINT

The biopsy instrument should never be passed farther caudal than the medial canthus of either eye to prevent entering the cribriform plate and the brain.

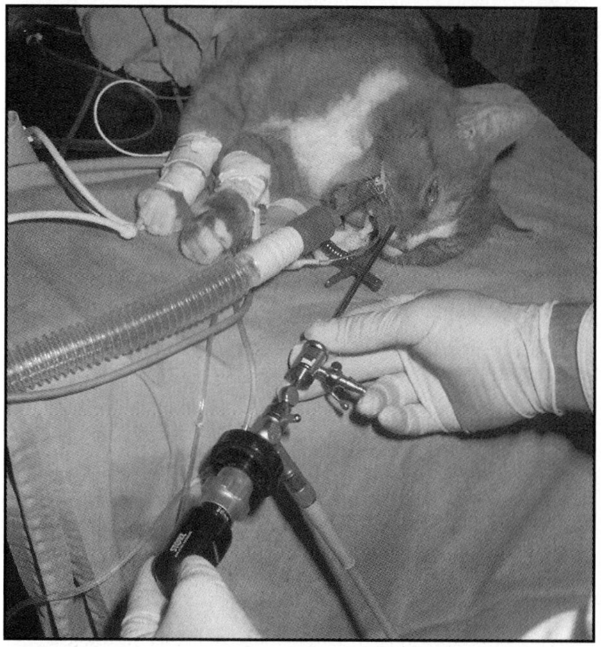

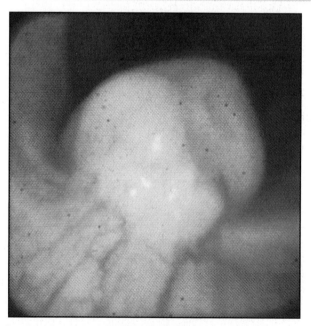

Figure 5-4: *A cytoscopic fiberoptic examination of the rostral nasal airways can provide information as to the size, location, and nature of a tumor. While this information is valuable, a biopsy specimen should be obtained for histopathologic analysis.*

Figure 5-5: *Bronchoscopy is an excellent method of localizing lesions in the respiratory tract, such as this tracheal oncocytoma. The tumor can be characterized as to size and location while a biopsy sample is readily obtained. (Courtesy of D. Twedt)*

TABLE 5-2
Sedation, Anesthesia, and Analgesia for Nasal Biopsy

Sedative or Preemptive Medication Options	Anesthesia Options	Perioperative Analgesia Options	Postoperative Analgesia Options
• Medetomidine (10–15 μg/kg IM) + butorphanol (0.2 mg/kg IM) • Acepromazine (0.025–0.05 mg/kg IM) + butorphanol (0.2–0.4 mg/kg IM) • Telazol® (2–4 mg/kg IM or IV) • Telazol®/ketamine/xylazine mixture (0.1 ml/5 kg IM)[a] • Ketamine (5–10 mg/kg IM) + medetomidine (30–50 μg/kg IM) • Ketamine (5–10 mg/kg IM) + xylazine (1 mg/kg IM)	• Thiopental (2–10 mg/kg IV to effect) • Propofol (1–3 mg/kg IV to effect) • Ketamine (1–4 mg/kg IV to effect) • Telazol® (1–2 mg/kg IV to effect) • Mask or chamber induction	• Topical or local blocks with lidocaine (<11 mg/kg) or bupivacaine (<4 mg/kg) administered in the nasal cavity • Postoperative analgesia prn	• NSAIDs • Opioid agonist oral preparations • Butorphanol syrup (1 ml of 1% butorphanol in 1 oz of Pet-Tinic™ syrup or fish-flavored base at a dose of 1 ml/4.5 kg) • Opioid-NSAID combinations • Acupuncture

Adapted from Tranquilli W, Grimm K, Flaggella A, et al: *A Roundtable Discussion: Rethinking Your Approach to Sedation, Anesthesia, and Analgesia* [monograph]. Lenexa, KS, Veterinary Medicine Publishing, 1997.
[a]Mixture of 1 ml 10% xylazine and 4 ml of ketamine as a diluent in a vial of Telazol®.

Indication: Examination of any undiagnosed nasal problem, especially when the cat has epiphora and epistaxis and/or facial deformity.

Contraindications: Coagulopathies; cats that are at high risk for general anesthesia.

Benefit: The large tissue sample that can be obtained leads to more accurate diagnosis.

Limitation: Requires general anesthesia.

Equipment: Sedation and general anesthesia (Table 5-2); small to medium-sized bone curette (Figure 5-6A) or "cup" biopsy instrument (Figure 5-6B).

Technique (Figure 5-7):

1. The cat is placed under general anesthesia after routine screening tests have been performed to identify clinical

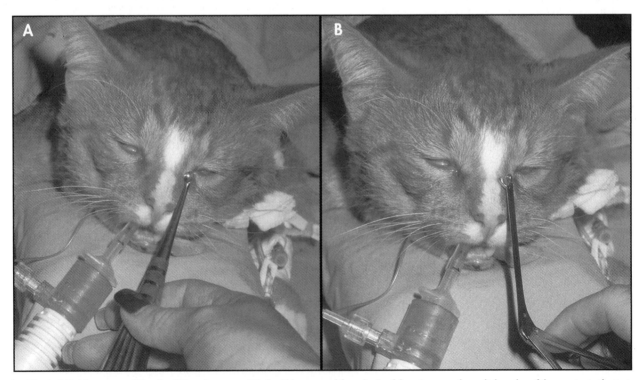

Figure 5-6: *A bone curette (A) or "cup" biopsy instrument (B) should be measured from the tip of the cat's nose to the medial canthus of the eye prior to the start of the nasal biopsy procedure. A piece of tape or some other marker should then be placed on the curette to indicate the maximum point of insertion.*

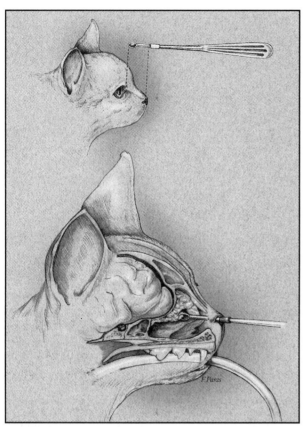

Figure 5-7: Biopsies in cats can be performed by passing a small to medium-sized bone curette into the nasal cavity no farther caudal than the medial canthus of the eye. This cannula is used to "scoop out" the tumor.

problems, such as coagulopathies, metabolic disease, or organ failure.

2. The nasal lesion is identified with skull radiographs or (preferably) CT imaging. The most valuable skull radiograph is an intraoral exposure, which is best made with nonscreen film placed inside the mouth to allow imaging of the caudal aspect of the nasal cavity. General anesthesia is required for this procedure.

3. Dilute 0.5 to 1 ml of 2% lidocaine 50:50 with 8.4% bicarbonate. The solution is then flushed up into the biopsy site by placing a tomcat or soft catheter, without the needle, through the nasal passage to the level of the lesion. This may reduce local discomfort and allow a lighter plane of anesthesia.

4. Before each biopsy, it is essential to "premeasure" from the nares to the medial canthus of the eye. The largest bone currette that can be passed up the opening of the nasal cavity should be measured and marked with tape or a marking pen. The curette is used to scoop or scrape the tumor into the instrument before it is removed from the nasal cavity. Small biopsy "cup" instruments can be used to pinch off portions of the tumor. The tumor should be placed into formalin for subsequent analysis.

5. Mild to moderate hemorrhage is expected and will subside within a relatively short period. If hemorrhage is excessive, ipsilateral carotid artery ligation should assist in reducing the bleeding. Hematocrit levels should be monitored hourly until all bleeding has stopped.

Supportive Care: Clean nose free of any crusting, dried material or moist exudates; provide oral or parenteral analgesics for days to weeks as needed.

REFERENCES

1. Ogilvie GK, Moore AS: *Managing the Veterinary Cancer Patient: A Practice Manual.* Trenton, NJ, Veterinary Learning Systems, 1995, pp 1–47.

2. Morrison WB, Hamilton TA, Hahn KA, et al: Diagnosis of neoplasia, in Slatter D (ed): *Textbook of Small Animal Surgery,* ed 2. Philadelphia, WB Saunders, 1993, pp 2036–2048.

3. Martini N: Diagnostic procedures relating to the thorax, in Wittes RE (ed): *Manual of Oncologic Therapeutics 1991/1992.* Philadelphia, JB Lippincott, 1991, pp 9–10.

4. Westcott JL: Direct percutaneous needle aspiration of localized pulmonary lesions: Results in 422 patients. *Radiology* 137:31–35, 1985.

5. Withrow SJ: Diseases of the respiratory system, in Withrow SJ, MacEwen EG (eds): *Clinical Veterinary Oncology.* Philadelphia, JB Lippincott, 1989, pp 215–233.

6. Hahn KA, McEntee MF: Primary lung tumors in cats: 86 cases (1979–1994). *JAVMA* 211:1257–1260, 1997.

BONE MARROW ASPIRATION AND BIOPSY

6

Gregory K. Ogilvie and Antony S. Moore

<table>
<tr><td colspan="2" align="center">**C L I N I C A L   B R I E F I N G**</td></tr>
<tr><td>*Methods*</td><td>*Benefits*</td></tr>
<tr><td>**Illinois or Rosenthal needle aspirate**</td><td>Relatively quick and simple outpatient procedure for obtaining marrow for cytology.</td></tr>
<tr><td>**Jamshidi needle biopsy**</td><td>Simple method of obtaining marrow core aspirates and biopsies in anesthetized cats.</td></tr>
</table>

Bone marrow aspiration and biopsy are essential procedures for determining cytologic and histologic abnormalities of the bone marrow caused by a wide variety of neoplastic, infectious, and myelodysplastic conditions.[1-3] Bone marrow aspiration and biopsy are indicated when an abnormality in the production of blood cells is suspected or when attempting to stage a cat with a hematopoietic malignancy.

Bone marrow aspiration is performed to acquire a monolayer of cells for individual evaluation.[1-3] Aspiration is therefore good for evaluating the cytology of the bone marrow versus the undisturbed architecture, which can be examined when a bone marrow biopsy is performed. To identify a wide variety of malignant and nonmalignant disorders, Romanovsky (including Wright's and Giemsa) stains are preferred. When the cytologic diagnosis of a cell type is not certain, additional special stains (including myeloperoxidase, Sudan black, and periodic acid-Schiff) can be used. Bone marrow biopsies are beneficial for determining bone marrow cellularity, the presence and extent of fibrosis or granulomatous conditions, and the presence of nonhematopoietic malignancies.

KEY POINT

Bone marrow aspiration and biopsy are essential procedures for determining cytologic and histologic abnormalities of the bone marrow caused by a wide variety of neoplastic, infectious, and myelodysplastic conditions.

TABLE 6-1
Sedation, Anesthesia, and Analgesia for Bone Marrow Aspiration or Biopsy

Sedative or Preemptive Medication Options	Anesthesia Options	Perioperative Anesthesia Options	Postoperative Anesthesia Options
• Medetomidine (10–15 µg/kg IM) + butorphanol (0.2 mg/kg IM)	• Thiopental (2–10 mg/kg IV to effect)	• Topical or local blocks with lidocaine (<11 mg/kg) or bupivacaine (<4 mg/kg)	• NSAIDs
• Acepromazine (0.025–0.05 mg/kg IM or SQ) + butorphanol (0.2–0.4 mg/kg IM or SQ)	• Propofol (1–3 mg/kg IV to effect)		• If NSAIDs not adequate, consider adding opioid agonist-antagonist drugs
• Butorphanol (0.2–0.4 mg/kg IV) + ketamine (5 mg/kg IV) + diazepam (0.2 mg/kg IV)	• Ketamine (1–4 mg/kg IV to effect)		• Acupuncture
• Butorphanol (0.2–0.4 mg/kg IM) + Telazol® (2–4 mg/kg IM)	• Telazol® (1–2 mg/kg IV to effect)		
• Butorphanol (0.2–0.4 mg/kg IV) + propofol (3–6 mg/kg IV to effect)	• Mask or chamber induction		

Adapted from Tranquilli W, Grimm K, Flaggella A, et al: *A Roundtable Discussion: Rethinking Your Approach to Sedation, Anesthesia, and Analgesia* [monograph]. Lenexa, KS, Veterinary Medicine Publishing, 1997.

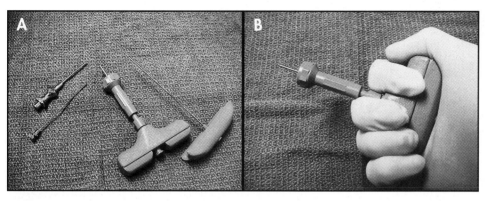

*Figure 6-1: Examples of bone marrow needles with the stylets removed (**A**). The plastic handle on the bone marrow needle allows for better control and ease of placement of the needle (**B**).*

Indications: Blood cell production abnormality; staging procedure for a hematopoietic or nonhematopoietic malignancy.

Contraindications: Coagulopathies.

Benefits: Aspiration can provide a sample for individual cell analysis, whereas a biopsy can provide tissue to analyze cellularity, architecture, and content; often, this can be done using local anesthesia with systemic analgesia and/or tranquilization (Table 6-1).

Limitation: A single sample may not be representative of the entire bone marrow.

Equipment: No. 11 surgical blade; 2% lidocaine; 6 to 12 ml syringe; 18 ga Illinois or Rosenthal bone marrow needle (Figure 6-1); microscope slides; EDTA container; sedation or anesthesia is preferred with local anesthesia.

Technique[1-3] (Figure 6-2):

1. The hair is clipped, the microscope slides are cleaned and made ready for the sample to be processed, as it will clot quickly, and the bone marrow aspiration site is prepared with a surgical scrub. Preferred sites and positioning in the cat include:
   —Dorsocranial or lateral aspects of iliac crest (cat is in sternal or lateral recumbency).
   —Greater trochanter of the femur (cat is in lateral recumbency).
   —Greater tubercle of the proximal aspect of the head of the humerus (cat is in lateral recumbency).

2. Using a 25 ga needle, approximately 0.5 to 1 ml of the local anesthetic agent, lidocaine (2%), is injected in and around the site where the bone marrow needle is to be introduced. Care is taken to inject lidocaine (2%) in and around all of the tissues that extend from the skin to the periosteum. The lidocaine will sting less upon injection if it is diluted 50:50 with 8.4% bicarbonate.

3. The biopsy area is scrubbed one more time after the li-

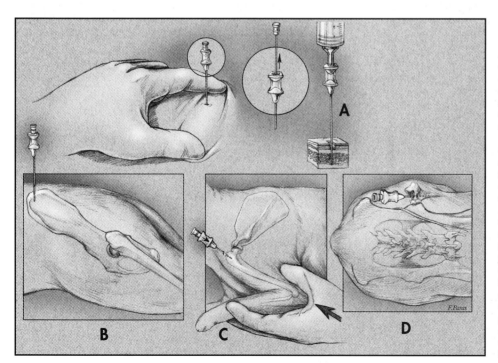

*Figure 6-2: A bone marrow sample is acquired by advancing a bone marrow needle, with the stylet in place, through one stab incision in the skin. A 1 inch, 18 ga bone marrow needle is advanced into the bone using a corkscrew motion. When the needle is fixed within the bone, the stylet is removed and the syringe is affixed (**A**). The bone marrow sample is then aspirated briskly into the 6 to 12 ml syringe and placed on slides and/or in a 1.5 ml EDTA tube. The bone marrow needle is placed through the cortex of bone into the bone marrow, where the stylet is removed prior to aspiration of a small amount of marrow contents. Three ideal locations for bone marrow aspiration are the dorsocranial aspect of the iliac crest (**B**), the greater tubercle of the proximal aspect of the head of the humerus (**C**), and the greater trochanter of the femur (**D**).*

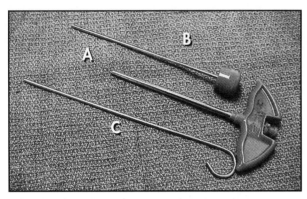

Figure 6-3: A Jamshidi or bone marrow biopsy needle (**A**) with the stylet (**B**) removed from the instrument. The smaller wire (**C**) is used to push the biopsy specimen from the needle after the needle has been removed from the bone.

docaine injection. A surgical drape should be applied for sterility.

4. The bone marrow site is identified, the skin is stretched between the thumb and index finger, and a small stab incision is made with a No. 11 surgical blade in the area blocked with lidocaine.

5. The bone marrow needle, with the stylet in place, is advanced into the stab incision and through the skin, subcutaneous tissue, and muscle all the way to the bone. It is crucial to keep the stylet in place because it has a tendency to back out during the procedure. An 18 ga Illinois or Rosenthal needle is preferred for most cats. After a sample is obtained for cytologic evaluation, a 14 ga Jamshidi (bone marrow biopsy instrument) needle is

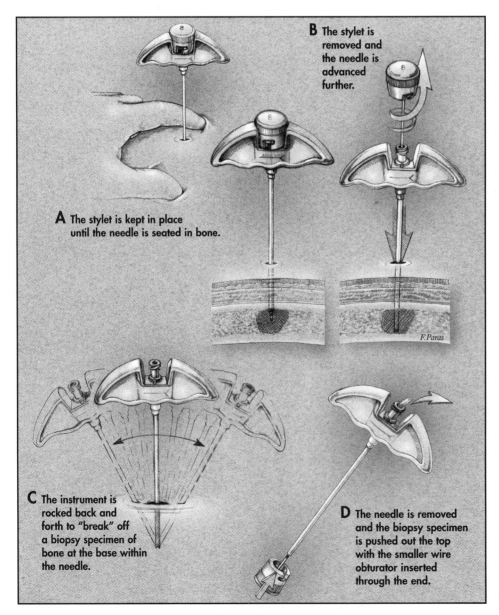

A The stylet is kept in place until the needle is seated in bone.

B The stylet is removed and the needle is advanced further.

F.Paras

C The instrument is rocked back and forth to "break" off a biopsy specimen of bone at the base within the needle.

D The needle is removed and the biopsy specimen is pushed out the top with the smaller wire obturator inserted through the end.

Figure 6-4: Outline of the procedure for obtaining a bone marrow core biopsy.

used to collect a biopsy specimen, if required.

6. With the stylet in place, the bone marrow needle is advanced into the bone, using a corkscrew motion. The instrument should not be allowed to wobble and should be fixed firmly into the bone like a nail that has been securely hammered into wood. When the needle is firmly fixed within the bone, the stylet is removed and the syringe is affixed. Many clinical pathologists suggest rinsing the syringe and bone marrow needle with EDTA before the procedure to reduce clotting of the bone marrow sample. Heparin should never be used.

7. The bone marrow sample is aspirated briskly into the 6 to 12 ml syringe; usually, 0.5 to 1 ml of marrow is adequate. The aspiration may be accompanied by a few seconds of pain, but this can be prevented by the use of oral or parenteral analgesics such as fentanyl, butorphanol, morphine, carprofen, or other analgesics.

8. If a sample is not obtained, the stylet is replaced in the bone marrow needle, and the instrument is then advanced further into the bone for a second attempt at aspirating marrow. Once marrow has been obtained, smears are prepared. This can be done in a number of ways:

—The marrow and blood are expelled into a small Petri dish that contains a few drops of EDTA. The marrow-rich spicules are placed on a slide or coverslip and then spread between slides or coverslips to make a monolayer of cells. Make sure the slides have been cleaned and are ready for the sample to be processed, as it will clot quickly.

—A portion of the marrow sample is placed on the proximal portion of the slide; the slide is tipped downward to allow the blood to run down and off the slide. The spicules and heavier nucleated cells do not run off and are used for subsequent slide preparation.

—Marrow can be spread into a monolayer like a routine blood smear.

—The first two methods may enhance the ability to evaluate the nucleated cell population of the bone marrow specimen.

A biopsy of a bone lesion or the bone marrow can be obtained with the Jamshidi (bone marrow biopsy instrument) needle (Figure 6-3) or the bone marrow needle after aspiration is performed (Figure 6-4). For biopsy, the stylet is removed. After the aspiration, the instrument is advanced as described earlier. The needle is then rocked back and forth at a 90 degree angle. In humans, premedication usually is not necessary if local anesthesia is adequate because pain is usually minimal. The purpose of the rocking movement is to sever the bone in the needle from its base. The biopsy instrument is then removed, and a smaller wire obturator is used to retrograde the biopsy piece out of the top end of the biopsy instrument. Cytology and histopathology can then be performed on this tissue. Direct pressure should be applied to the site for several minutes to prevent hematoma formation. The small incision may be sutured or glued closed.

Supportive Care: Oral or parenteral analgesics for hours to days may be indicated.

REFERENCES

1. Ogilvie GK, Moore AS: *Managing the Veterinary Cancer Patient: A Practice Manual.* Trenton, NJ, Veterinary Learning Systems, 1995, pp 1–47.

2. Morrison WB, Hamilton TA, Hahn KA, et al: Diagnosis of neoplasia, in Slatter D (ed): *Textbook of Small Animal Surgery*, ed 2. Philadelphia, WB Saunders, 1993, pp 2036–2048.

3. Lee EJ, Schiffer CA: Bone marrow aspiration and biopsy, in Wittes RE (ed): *Manual of Oncologic Therapeutics 1991/1992.* Philadelphia, JB Lippincott, 1991, pp 24–26.

LOWER UROGENITAL TRACT BIOPSY

Gregory K. Ogilvie and Antony S. Moore

7

CLINICAL BRIEFING	
Methods	*Benefits*
Cystotomy bladder biopsy	Surgical procedure allows for visual staging of tumor.
Open-ended catheter bladder biopsy	Relatively inexpensive procedure for obtaining biopsy.
Flexible or rigid fiberoptic cystoscopy	Visualization of lesion and direction of biopsy enhances diagnosis.

Biopsies of the lower urogenital tract are common procedures for the practitioner. Bladder tumors can be biopsied by laparotomy or with a less invasive procedure, such as using cystoscopy.[1,2] Pediatric bronchoscopes, rigid cystoscopes, or arthroscopes of the smallest size are the only instruments suitable for cystoscopy in cats (see below). The prostate, while rarely sampled, is usually biopsied via laparotomy, although it can be biopsied percutaneously, especially when guided with concurrent imaging.[1,2] Testicular biopsies can be performed by castration or, rarely, through fine-needle aspiration cytology.[1]

Cats with microhematuria or gross hematuria, with or without stranguria and dysuria, that cannot be resolved with antibiotic therapy must be evaluated for a bladder tumor.[1,2] Transitional cell carcinoma, although relatively uncommon, is the most common bladder tumor in cats. Other differentials causing the above clinical signs, including uroliths, must be ruled out. In each case, a biopsy is required to make an appropriate diagnosis. Prior to the biopsy, a double-contrast cystogram and/or bladder ultrasonography is essential to localize and characterize the lesion. The most common method for nonsurgical biopsy of the bladder is cystoscopy with a rigid or flexible fiberoptic endoscope. A more practical and less expensive method is to use an open-ended urinary catheter that is advanced against the tumor; the tumor is vigorously aspirated into the catheter and the entire instrument is then retracted, hopefully with a piece of tumor held within the catheter lumen.

CATHETER BIOPSY OF THE BLADDER

Indication: Any undiagnosed persistent bladder problem, especially in a cat with cystitis or hematuria, that is unresponsive to standard therapy.

Contraindications/Complications: Coagulopathies; cats that are at high risk for general anesthesia; this technique

is more challenging in female cats.

Benefit: Tissue samples can be obtained without surgery and often result in an accurate diagnosis; no risk of tracking tumor cells through the abdomen.

Limitations: Requires general anesthesia.

Equipment: 12 ml syringe and open-ended tomcat urinary catheter; general anesthesia (Table 7-1) is preferred.

KEY POINT

Care should be taken to prevent overinflation and potential rupture of the bladder. In addition, biopsies should be taken with the understanding that the bladder wall is likely to be friable due to the presence of the underlying disease.

Technique (Figure 7-1):
1. After routine screening tests have been performed to identify problems such as coagulopathies, metabolic disease, or organ failure, the cat is placed under general anesthesia.
2. The bladder or urethral lesion is identified with ultrasonography or a double-contrast cystogram.
3. The catheter should be "premeasured" so the length to be advanced does not exceed the measurement from the area of the distal urethra to the level of the tumor, which generally is not further forward than the caudal two mammary glands. This precaution reduces the risk of bladder perforation.
4. The open-ended tomcat catheter is advanced through the urethra and then forcefully into the tumor. This is best accomplished with ultrasonographic or fluoroscopic guidance or by palpating the mass per abdomen.

TABLE 7-1
Sedation, Anesthesia, and Analgesia for a Bladder Biopsy Using a Catheter

Sedative or Preemptive Medication Options	Anesthesia	Postoperative Analgesia Options
• Medetomidine (10–15 µg/kg IM) + butorphanol (0.2 mg/kg IM)	• Thiopental (2–10 mg/kg IV to effect)	• NSAIDs
• Acepromazine (0.025–0.05 mg/kg IM or SQ) + butorphanol (0.2–0.4 mg/kg IM or SQ)	• Propofol (1–3 mg/kg IV to effect)	• If NSAIDs not adequate, consider adding opioid agonist-antagonist drugs
• Butorphanol (0.2–0.4 mg/kg IV) + ketamine (5 mg/kg IV) + diazepam (0.2 mg/kg IV)	• Ketamine (1–4 mg/kg IV to effect)	• Acupuncture
• Butorphanol (0.2–0.4 mg/kg IM) + Telazol® (2–4 mg/kg IM)	• Telazol® (1–2 mg/kg IV to effect)	
• Butorphanol (0.2–0.4 mg/kg IV) + propofol (3–6 mg/kg IV to effect)	• Mask or chamber induction	

Adapted from Tranquilli W, Grimm K, Flaggella A, et al: *A Roundtable Discussion: Rethinking Your Approach to Sedation, Anesthesia, and Analgesia* [monograph]. Lenexa, KS, Veterinary Medicine Publishing, 1997.

5. Once the tumor has been entered, suction is applied while the instrument is withdrawn. Tissue that has been suctioned into the catheter and torn off during removal of the catheter is expelled and placed in 10% formalin for subsequent fixation and analysis. If impression smears are desired for cytology, those should be taken before the tissue is formalinized. Note that formalin fumes will alter cytologic characteristics.

Supportive Care: Oral analgesics may be needed.

FIBEROPTIC OR RIGID CYSTOSCOPIC BIOPSY[1,2]

Indications: Any disease that appears to involve the urethra or bladder.

Contraindications: Coagulopathies; cats that are at high risk for general anesthesia, including cats with limited pulmonary or cardiovascular function (due to insufflation of the bladder, venous return to the heart can be reduced and compress the diaphragm, compromising the ability to inspire easily); procedure is restricted to medi-

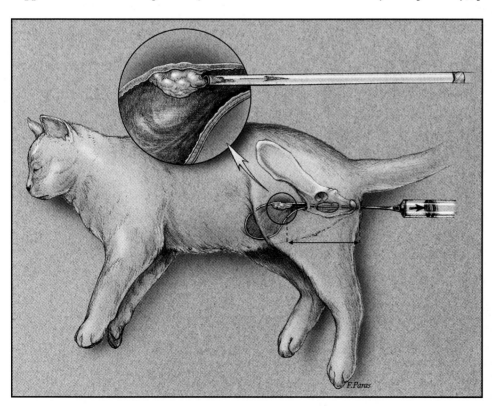

Figure 7-1: *Biopsy of a bladder tumor can be accomplished by advancing a catheter with an open end into the tumor. Suction is applied to aspirate a plug of tumor into the catheter (inset). The catheter is removed while suction is maintained to ensure that the tissue stays in the catheter.*

TABLE 7-2
Sedation, Anesthesia, and Analgesia for Cystoscopy

Sedative or Preemptive Medication Options	Anesthesia Options	Postoperative Analgesia Options
• Medetomidine (10–15 µg/kg IM) + butorphanol (0.2 mg/kg IM) • Acepromazine (0.025–0.05 mg/kg IM) + butorphanol (0.2–0.4 mg/kg IM) • Telazol® (2–4 mg/kg IV or IM) • Telazol®/ketamine/xylazine mixture (0.1 ml/5 kg IM)*a* • Ketamine (5–10 mg/kg IM) + medetomidine (30–50 µg/kg IM) • Ketamine + xylazine (1 mg/kg IM)	• Thiopental (2–10 mg/kg IV to effect) • Propofol (1–3 mg/kg IV to effect) • Ketamine (1–4 mg/kg IV to effect) • Telazol® (1–2 mg/kg IV to effect) • Mask or chamber induction	• NSAIDs • Opioid agonist oral preparations • Butorphanol syrup (1 ml of 1% butorphanol in 1 oz of Pet-Tinic™ syrup or fish-flavored base at a dose of 1 ml/4.5 kg) • Opioid-NSAID combinations • Acupuncture

Adapted from Tranquilli W, Grimm K, Flaggella A, et al: *A Roundtable Discussion: Rethinking Your Approach to Sedation, Anesthesia, and Analgesia* [monograph]. Lenexa, KS, Veterinary Medicine Publishing, 1997.
*a*Mixture of 1 ml 10% xylazine and 4 ml of ketamine as a diluent in a vial of Telazol®.

um to large female cats or large males that have had a perineal urethrostomy.

Complications: Very rare but can include bleeding (which usually stops spontaneously) and bladder rupture.

Benefits: Relatively minimal risk.

Limitations: Requires general anesthesia (Table 7-2) at the time of laparotomy.

Equipment: Few fiberoptic endoscopes are small enough for cystoscopy of the cat; pediatric bronchoscopes, rigid cystoscopes, or arthroscopes of the smallest size are often good choices; pediatric bronchoscopes (<5 mm in diameter) can be inserted into the urethra of most large male

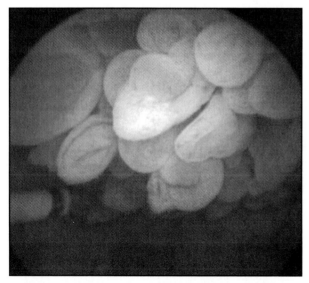

Figure 7-2: *Endoscopic view of a bladder biopsy being taken. Several "pinch" samples should be taken from different locations within the lesion. This lesion was diagnosed histologically as transitional cell carcinoma. (Courtesy of D. Twedt)*

cats that have had a perineal urethrostomy; the endoscope should have an instrument port and channel, be at least bidirectional, bend more than 100 degrees in at least one direction, and have an external light source; cytology brushes and biopsy forceps should be of a size and type that will pass through the instrument port with the scope in a flexed position.

Technique (Figure 7-2):

1. After tests are done to ensure the absence of life-threatening diseases, general anesthesia or other chemical restraint is administered.

2. A routine laparotomy is performed; the bladder is identified and packed off, and a small incision is made into the bladder to introduce the fiberoptic instrument.

3. Using aseptic technique, the rigid or flexible fiberoptic endoscope is inserted through the bladder rent (or through the urethra of a male cat with a perineal urethrostomy). Urine is suctioned off, and a judicious amount of carbon dioxide, air, or sterile water is insufflated into the bladder to enhance visualization of any pathology.

4. Suspect lesions are first sampled with the cytology brush for cytologic evaluation and then biopsied for histopathology. If a diffuse lesion is suspected, random samples are acquired. After biopsies are performed, the air is suctioned off, and the instrument is removed; in the case of a laparotomy, the bladder rent and the abdomen are closed routinely.

Supportive Care: Oral analgesics may be needed in some cases.

REFERENCES

1. Ogilvie GK, Moore AS: *Managing the Veterinary Cancer Patient: A Practice Manual.* Trenton, NJ, Veterinary Learning Systems. 1995, pp 1–47.

2. Morrison WB, Hamilton TA, Hahn KA, et al: Diagnosis of neoplasia, in Slatter D (ed): *Textbook of Small Animal Surgery,* ed 2. Philadelphia, WB Saunders, 1993, pp 2036–2048.

DIGESTIVE SYSTEM BIOPSY

Gregory K. Ogilvie and Antony S. Moore

8

Surgical exploration and biopsy remain the most complete method of exploring the digestive system in the cat. The oral cavity is readily accessible; however, planning of correct placement of the surgical biopsy tract is critical for long-term care of the cat with cancer. The biopsy is crucial not only to obtain a definitive diagnosis but also to ensure that definitive surgery can be performed subsequently with minimal cosmetic and functional alterations to the cat.[1] Surgical exploration of the abdomen and chest is more invasive than fiberoptic endoscopy and may be associated with greater risks. Although exploratory surgery has many benefits, endoscopic examination of the gastrointestinal (GI) tract is a common, effective, low risk means of diagnosing malignant conditions of this organ system.[1-5] In addition, with endoscopy, benign conditions that mimic malignancy can be identified for subsequent treatment.[1,5] Flexible fiberoptic endoscopes can be used to examine all areas of the esophagus, stomach, proximal duodenum, rectum, and colon. Rigid endoscopes or proctoscopes can be used to examine portions of the esophagus, rectum, and most of the descending colon. Laparoscopy has the advantage of evaluating many organs of the abdomen with very little trauma to the cat. The techniques of oral biopsy, upper and lower GI endoscopy, and abdominal laparoscopy are discussed separately.

BIOPSY OF THE ORAL CAVITY

CLINICAL BRIEFING

Methods	Benefits
Excisional biopsy	Diagnostic and therapeutic; requires knowledge of extent of disease prior to surgery.
Incisional biopsy	Diagnosis allows logical planning of definitive therapeutic procedure.

Biopsy of an oral cavity lesion is essential because almost all of the tumors in this area have different prognoses and treatments, despite similar gross appearances. Before an oral lesion is biopsied, radiographs should be taken to determine the presence of bone invasion. This is essential information for the pathologist and the surgeon. For example, a pathologist would consider a diagnosis of a low grade fibrosarcoma rather than a fibroma if radiographs suggested the presence of bone involvement, despite the fact that the biopsy finding was consistent with a diagnosis of fibroma. Similarly, a mandibulectomy or a maxillectomy would be the surgical approach if bone were involved. Whenever a tooth is removed in a cat, a biopsy should be considered to rule out the presence of cancer as an underlying cause. Before a biopsy is planned, the surgeon who will perform the definitive procedure should be consulted to ensure that the biopsy does not compromise the success of the procedure or the health of the cat. If the biopsy involves tissues essential for closure or if the tumor is seeded into an area too large to resect, a successful outcome of the definitive procedure may not be possible. Although an excisional biopsy is an option, an incisional biopsy is more frequently performed to guide the decision for a definitive procedure.

Indication: Identification of an oral mass of unexplained etiology.

Contraindications: Coagulopathies; cats that are at high risk for general anesthesia.

Benefit: An accurate histopathologic evaluation can be obtained because part or all of the oral mass can be sampled.

Equipment: General anesthesia (Table 8-1); standard surgical instruments.

Technique:

1. After routine screening tests have been performed to identify problems such as coagulopathies and metabolic disease, the cat is placed under general anesthesia. An endotracheal tube with a properly fitting cuff is placed and secured to prevent aspiration of blood or other oral contents.

2. The oral mass is radiographed. When possible, intraoral radiographs should be acquired in addition to other views. More specific details regarding this technique are outlined in Chapter 41.

3. After a nerve block is placed and/or parenteral analgesics are started, an incision is made over the oral mass, and a section of the lesion is taken at the junction of normal

TABLE 8-1
Sedation, Anesthesia, and Analgesia for Oral Biopsy

Sedative or Preemptive Medication Options	Anesthesia Options	Perioperative Analgesia Options	Postoperative Analgesia Options
• Medetomidine (10–15 µg/kg IM) + butorphanol (0.2 mg/kg IM)	• Thiopental (2–10 mg/kg IV to effect)	• Topical or local blocks with lidocaine (<11 mg/kg) or bupivacaine (<4 mg/kg for procedures such as mandibular nerve block for dentals and mandibulectomies	• NSAIDs
• Acepromazine (0.025–0.05 mg/kg IM or SQ) + butorphanol (0.2–0.4 mg/kg IM or SQ)	• Propofol (1–3 mg/kg IV to effect)		• If NSAIDs not adequate, consider adding opioid agonist-antagonist drugs
• Butorphanol (0.2–0.4 mg/kg IV) + ketamine (5 mg/kg IV) + diazepam (0.2 mg/kg IV)	• Ketamine (1–4 mg/kg IV to effect)		• Acupuncture
• Butorphanol (0.2–0.4 mg/kg IM) + Telazol® (2–4 mg/kg IM)	• Telazol® (1–2 mg/kg IV to effect)	• Postoperative analgesia prn	
• Butorphanol (0.2–0.4 mg/kg IV) + propofol (3–6 mg/kg IV to effect)	• Mask or chamber induction	• Acupuncture	

Adapted from: Tranquilli W, Grimm K, Flaggella A, et al: *A Roundtable Discussion: Rethinking Your Approach to Sedation, Anesthesia, and Analgesia* [monograph]. Lenexa, KS, Veterinary Medicine Publishing, 1997.

and abnormal tissue. Care is taken not to biopsy through normal lip or skin, as this tissue may be needed for reconstructive surgical techniques. Options include excisional or incisional biopsy procedures.

4. Any bleeding that occurs is stopped with ligation, cautery, or in the case of an open bone biopsy, bone wax. Bleeding usually subsides within 5 to 10 minutes.

5. After the oral mass is removed, surrounding tissue is sutured if possible. Keep in mind that the oral cavity is a contaminated area.

6. The oral tumor should then be adequately fixed in 10% formalin.

Supportive Care: Oral or parenteral analgesics may be indicated and soft food should be offered for a period of days.

UPPER AND LOWER GASTROINTESTINAL BIOPSY

CLINICAL BRIEFING

Methods	Benefits
Surgical exploration and biopsy	Allows visual determination of extent of disease and directed biopsy.
Fiberoptic endoscopic biopsy	Allows noninvasive visualization of the GI tract; useful for specifically directing biopsy.
Ultrasound-guided biopsy	Allows visualization of the entire gastrointestinal tract and other intraabdominal organs.

UPPER GASTROINTESTINAL ENDOSCOPY[5]

Indications for upper GI endoscopy include, but are not limited to, regurgitation, dysphagia, retching, nausea, vomiting, hematemesis, diarrhea, melena, and any mass-like lesions identified in the esophagus, stomach, or upper duodenum. The diagnostic accuracy of flexible endoscopic biopsies is approximately 95% in humans, but it may be lower in cats. Accuracy is highest with intraluminal diseases regardless of whether they are focal or diffuse, benign or malignant. Less

diagnostic accuracy is seen with infiltrating cancers such as lymphoma, in which a full thickness biopsy often is ideal to make a diagnosis. Since cats can have inflammatory bowel disease that may progress to lymphoma, multiple biopsies are indicated to maximize the chance of diagnosing the disease. In addition, endoscopy is ideal for rechecks of an intraluminal lesion. A veterinary pathologist who is interested and experienced in examining endoscopic biopsies is essential to the success of this type of diagnostic procedure.

Indications: Any disease that appears to involve the esophagus, stomach, or upper duodenum.

Contraindications: Coagulopathies; cats that are at high risk for general anesthesia.

KEY POINT

Care must be taken to avoid overdistention when performing upper GI endoscopy, as this can result in compromised blood return to the heart and rupture of the stomach or intestines.

Complications: Very rare but can include bleeding, which usually stops spontaneously; if brisk bleeding persists, introducing a Fogarty balloon catheter to occlude the bleeding vessel is recommended; if perforation occurs, emergency surgery to repair the rent or to resect the section of bowel should be performed (in humans, the risk of perforation of the bowel is reported to be <0.1%).

Benefits: Minimal risk; noninvasive.

Limitations: Requires general anesthesia (Table 8-2); biopsy samples are superficial and, therefore, may miss deeper pathology.

Equipment: There are many fiberoptic endoscopes on the market for performance of upper GI endoscopy (Figure 8-1); the flexible fiberoptic endoscope should have an instrument port and channel, be at least bidirectional, bend more than 100 degrees in at least one direction, and have an external light source, suction, and water insufflation capability; cytology brushes, biopsy forceps,

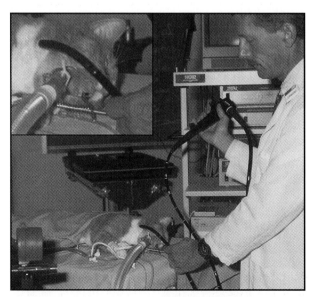

Figure 8-1: *Endoscopy can be a valuable tool for locating and characterizing lesions in the upper gastrointestinal tract, particularly intraluminal lesions. The inset shows the size of the instrument relative to the patient.*

and graspers that can pass through the instrument port with the endoscope in a flexed position should be available; adult or pediatric fiberoptic endoscopes 5 to 8 mm in diameter and at least as long as 150 cm can be inserted into the duodenum of most cats.

Technique (Figure 8-2):

1. Cats should be fasted for 6 to 8 hours before upper GI endoscopy. After tests are performed to ensure the absence of life-threatening diseases, general anesthesia with endotracheal intubation is performed. A mouth gag is used to prevent the cat from biting the endoscope.

2. The endoscope is inserted through the mouth and down into the esophagus. Carbon dioxide or air is insufflated into the structure to be examined. If excessive fluid is encountered, it is aspirated. Systematic examination of the esophagus, lower esophageal sphincter, stomach (Figure 8-3), and proximal duodenum (Figure 8-4) are performed.

3. Suspect lesions are first sampled with the cytology brush for cytologic evaluation and then biopsied for histopathology. It is necessary to collect a minimum of five biopsy samples for histopathologic analysis.

Supportive Care: Antiemetics or intestinal protectants may be helpful; in some cases, analgesics may be indicated.

LOWER GASTROINTESTINAL ENDOSCOPY[1,4]

In selected cats, indications for endoscopic evaluation of the rectum, colon, and ileum include diarrhea, dyschezia, constipation, and/or a mass in the lower intestinal tract. Because it allows greater visualization of the colon (Figure 8-5) and rectum, lower GI flexible fiberoptic endoscopy is surpassing rigid sigmoidoscopy in popularity. The rigid scope is more effective in evaluating the large bowel. Both instruments provide a means of examining the mucosal surface of the entire large bowel in great detail. Pinch biopsies can be taken for subsequent evaluation by a veterinary histopathologist. Although the procedure is best accomplished with the cat under general anesthesia, chemical tranquilization with analgesia may be adequate for selected cats.

Indications: Any disease that appears to involve the colon or rectum, especially those of the mucosal surface.

Contraindications: Coagulopathies; cats that are at high risk for general anesthesia or tranquilization; cats with fulminant, severe colitis may be at increased risk for perforation.

Complications: Very rare but can include bleeding, which usually stops spontaneously; if brisk bleeding persists, the introduction of a Fogarty balloon catheter to occlude the bleeding vessels is recommended; if bowel perforation occurs, emergency surgery to repair the rent or to resect the section of bowel should be performed (in

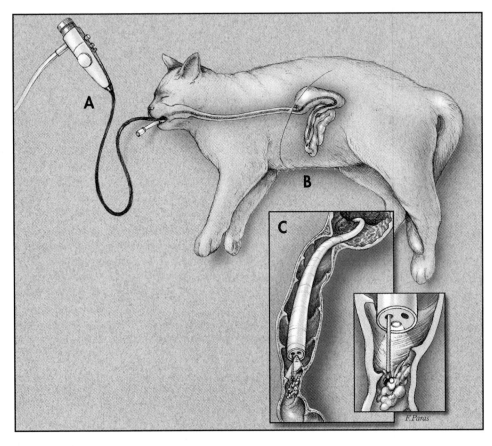

Figure 8-2: *A flexible endoscope (**A**) can be used to localize, characterize, and biopsy esophageal, gastric, or upper duodenal (**B**) tumors or lesions. The cat is given general anesthesia and is placed on its right side. In each case, multiple biopsy specimens (**C**) should be acquired to ensure that an accurate diagnosis is made.*

humans, the risk of perforating the bowel is reported to be <0.5%, which is higher than for the upper GI tract).

Benefits: Minimal risk; noninvasive.

Limitations: Requires general anesthesia or tranquilization with analgesia; procedure is generally effective only for diagnosing diseases that affect the lumen of the colon or rectum.

Equipment: There are many fiberoptic endoscopes on the market for performing lower GI endoscopy; the flexible fiberoptic endoscope should have an instrument port and channel, be at least bidirectional, bend more than 100 degrees in one direction, and have an external light source, suction, and water insufflator; adult or pediatric fiberoptic endoscopes 5 to 8 mm in diameter and longer than 1 m can be inserted into the colon and advanced to the level of the cecum of most cats; a skilled operator can occasionally pass the scope into the ileum; the rigid scope should be 25 cm in length and have a light source;

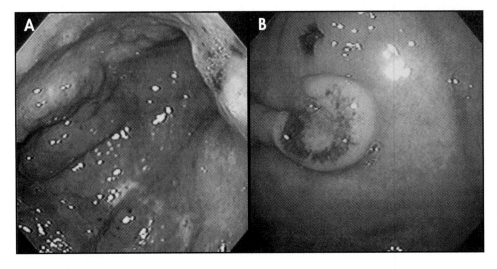

Figure 8-3: *Systematic endoscopic evaluation of the gastric mucosa can allow visualization of lesions, such as this gastric lymphoma (**A**) and pyloric lymphoma (**B**). (Courtesy of D. Twedt)*

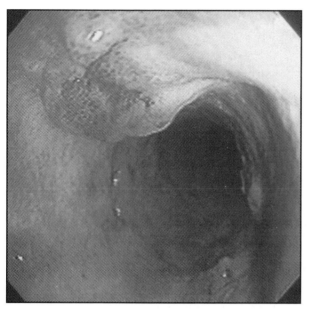

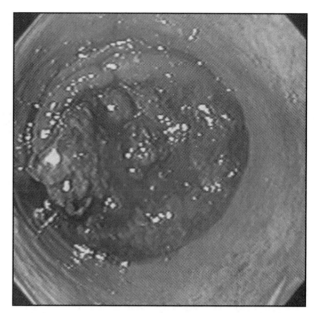

Figure 8-4: *Systematic endoscopic evaluation of the upper GI tract can allow visualization of lesions, such as this duodenal lymphoma. (Courtesy of D. Twedt)*

Figure 8-5: *Flexible fiberoptic endoscopic view of colonic adenocarcinoma. (Courtesy of D. Twedt)*

cytology brushes, biopsy forceps, and graspers that can pass through the instrument port with the flexible fiberoptic endoscope in a flexed position should be available; these same biopsy instruments can be used with a rigid scope; mare uterine biopsy instruments should be used with extreme care because of the high risk of perforating the colon or rectum.

Technique (Figure 8-6):

1. Preparation requires that the cat fast for 24 to 36 hours and be administered warm water enemas. In some cases,

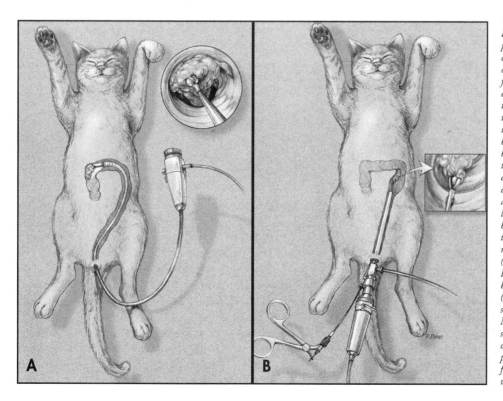

Figure 8-6: *Colonoscopy can be performed with either a flexible endoscope (A) or a rigid proctoscope or cystoscope (B). The flexible fiberoptic endoscope is more effective for exploring the area of the ileocecocolic junction and the transverse colon. The biopsy instrument is extended through the biopsy port to take small pinch biopsies (inset, Figure 8-6A) in the transverse colon. The rigid endoscope may be more effective for draining the colon of feces, blood, and fluid and for introducing larger biopsy instruments. Larger biopsy specimens can be taken from the descending colon by extending rigid biopsy instruments (instrument shown on lower left, Figure 8-6B) to the lesion to be biopsied. The tissue is grasped (inset, Figure 8-6B), and several samples are taken from the mass. Note that the flexible endoscope shown has an eyepiece for the operator to use, while the rigid proctoscope shown has only fiberoptic video output for visualization.*

a GI lavage solution containing polyethylene glycol as the main nonabsorbable solute (e.g., Golytely®, Colyte®) may be used. This is given at a dosage of 25 ml/kg via orogastric tube, twice, 1 hour apart, 12 to 18 hours prior to the endoscopy procedure (giving metoclopramide 30 minutes before the solution is administered may decrease distention and nausea). Care should be taken not to administer phosphate-containing enemas (e.g., Fleet® enemas) to cats due to the potential for inducing serious, adverse effects, including acute collapse and death. The cat is given the opportunity to eliminate all fecal material before the procedure is performed. After diagnostics are performed to ensure the absence of life-threatening diseases, general anesthesia or tranquilization is performed.

2. The endoscope is inserted through the anus and into the colon. Insufflation of carbon dioxide or air allows adequate visualization of the colon and proximal rectum. If liquid material is present, it is suctioned out. The lower GI tract is systematically examined.

3. Suspect lesions are first sampled with the cytology brush for cytologic evaluation and then biopsied for histopathology. A minimum of five biopsy samples are acquired for histopathologic analysis.

Supportive Care: Low-residue food may be helpful for some; analgesics may be indicated in select cases.

INTESTINAL ULTRASONOGRAPHY

Ultrasonography is often superior to contrast radiography in identifying a mass involving the intestinal wall, although it may be difficult to locate the lesion to a specific area of the bowel.[6-9] Ultrasonography may identify intraabdominal metastases, such as in the liver, that are not suspected on radiography. Ultrasonography may also identify enlarged regional lymph nodes and guide a needle biopsy for definitive diagnosis. An ultrasound-guided automated 18 ga "tru-cut" needle is available in 23 and 11 mm lengths, enabling biopsy of thickened intestinal wall with little risk of perforation. Limitations of ultrasonography include a poor ability to visualize peritoneal tumor seeding even in the presence of ascites. It is important to remember that barium will interfere with the diagnostic accuracy of ultrasonography. Ultrasonography is therefore best performed prior to administration of barium. Despite these limitations, ultrasonography is probably the imaging modality of choice for intestinal tumors.

LIVER BIOPSY[1-3]

C L I N I C A L B R I E F I N G	
Methods	*Benefits*
Surgical exploration	Allows visual determination of extent of disease and directed biopsy.
Ultrasound-guided biopsy	Allows visualization of disease and directs biopsy.
Transabdominal percutaneous biopsy	Relatively easy and safe method for obtaining liver tissue.
Keyhole liver biopsy	Allows liver to be isolated and stabilized for blind biopsy.
Laparoscopy	Allows direct visualization of abdominal contents and visually directed biopsy.

A liver biopsy is a common procedure to determine the histologic characteristics of a tumor or a nonmalignant condition after laboratory work and routine imaging methods have determined that the liver is abnormal.[1-4] Liver biopsies are accurately performed with ultrasonographic or fluoroscopic guidance.[2,4] More accurate biopsies are being performed as CT imaging becomes more commonly used in feline practice. Other methods of obtaining a liver biopsy include direct visualization by laparoscopy or by open surgical biopsy. An unguided (blind) percutaneous biopsy is generally not recommended, as ultrasonography is widely available and makes the procedure much safer. In all types of liver biopsies, the most common complication is bleeding from the biopsy site. Therefore before a liver biopsy is performed, hematocrit, platelet count, and an activated clotting time (ACT) or a one-step partial thromboplastin time (OSPTT) and an activated partial thromboplastin time (APTT) should be determined to identify cats that may be at high risk for bleeding after the procedure. In addition, cats should be kept quiet after the procedure and a hematocrit measured to compare with that obtained before the procedure.

TRANSABDOMINAL PERCUTANEOUS LIVER BIOPSY[1-3]

Indication: Evaluation and diagnosis of malignant and nonmalignant liver disease.

Contraindications: Coagulopathies; cats that are at high risk for general anesthesia or tranquilization.

Benefits: Aspiration can only provide a sample for individ-

KEY POINT

To prevent lacerating the liver and underlying structures, ultrasonography, if available, should be used to direct the biopsy equipment.

---

ual cell analysis, whereas a biopsy can provide tissue to analyze the cellularity, architecture, and content of the liver section; the procedure can often be done with local anesthesia, systemic analgesia, and tranquilization (Table 8-2); if there are any concerns about the cat's ability to lie quietly on its back, general anesthesia should be performed.

Limitation: Single samples taken may not be representative of the entire liver.

Equipment: Standard surgical instruments; needle biopsy instrument.

Technique:

1. The cat should be positioned in dorsal recumbency, and its right side tilted slightly down toward the table surface. Ideally, the caudal aspect of the cat should be lowered to allow the liver to "fall" caudally for easier access by the biopsy procedure. An area of hair 4 to 6 cm in diameter, encompassing the xyphoid process and the ventral left costal arch, is clipped, and the liver biopsy site is

TABLE 8-2
Sedation, Anesthesia, and Analgesia for Liver Biopsy or Laparoscopy

Procedure, Level of Pain	Sedative or Preemptive Medication Options	Anesthesia Options	Perioperative Anesthesia Options	Postoperative Anesthesia Options
Minor Surgery, Minor Pain	• Medetomidine (10–15 µg/kg IM) + butorphanol (0.2 mg/kg IM) • Acepromazine (0.025–0.05 mg/kg IM or SQ) + butorphanol (0.2–0.4 mg/kg IM or SQ) • Butorphanol (0.2–0.4 mg/kg IV) + ketamine (5 mg/kg IV) + diazepam (0.2 mg/kg IV) • Butorphanol (0.2–0.4 mg/kg IM) + Telazol® (1–4 mg/kg IM) • Butorphanol (0.2–0.4 mg/kg IV) + propofol (3–6 mg/kg IV to effect)	• Thiopental (2–10 mg/kg IV to effect) • Propofol (1–3 mg/kg IV to effect) • Ketamine (1–4 mg/kg IV to effect) • Telazol® (1–2 mg/kg IV to effect) • Mask or chamber induction	• Topical or local blocks with lidocaine (< 11 mg/kg) or bupivacaine (< 4 mg/kg) • Postoperative analgesia prn • Acupuncture	• NSAIDs • If NSAIDs not adequate, consider adding opioid agonist-antagonist drugs • Acupuncture
Moderate Surgery, Moderate Pain	• Medetomidine (10–15 µg/kg IM) + butorphanol (0.2 mg/kg IM) • Acepromazine (0.025–0.05 mg/kg IM) + butorphanol (0.2–0.4 mg/kg IM) • Telazol® (2-4 mg/kg IV or IM) • Telazol®/ketamine/xylazine mixture[a] (0.1 ml/5 kg IM) • Ketamine (5–10 mg/kg IM) + medetomidine (30-50 µg/kg IM) • Ketamine (5–10 mg/kg IM) + xylazine (1 mg/kg IM)	See above	See above	• NSAIDs • Opioid agonist oral preparations • Butorphanol syrup (1 ml of 1% butorphanol in 1 oz of Pet-Tinic™ syrup or fish-flavored base given at a dose of 1 ml/4.5 kg) • Opioid-NSAID combinations • Acupuncture

Adapted from Tranquilli W, Grimm K, Flaggella A, et al: *A Roundtable Discussion: Rethinking Your Approach to Sedation, Anesthesia, and Analgesia* [monograph]. Lenexa, KS, Veterinary Medicine Publishing, 1997.

[a]Mixture of 1 ml of 10% xylazine and 4 ml of ketamine as a diluent in a vial of Telazol®.

prepared with a surgical scrub.

2. Using a 25 ga needle, approximately 0.5 to 2 ml of the local anesthetic agent lidocaine is injected in and around the site where the biopsy needle is to be introduced. The lidocaine (2%) will sting less upon injection if it is diluted 50:50 with 8.4% bicarbonate.

3. The area to be biopsied is scrubbed a final time after the lidocaine is injected. A surgical drape can be applied for sterility.

4. Using aseptic surgical technique, the operator then makes a small stab incision with a No. 11 surgical blade at a point to (hopefully) be directed by ultrasonography.

5. Preferably using ultrasound guidance, the needle core biopsy instrument is advanced into the subcutaneous tissue and then just through the abdominal wall.

6. At least five biopsy specimens are obtained; one piece of tissue is submitted for bacterial culture and sensitivity and the others are submitted for histopathology and special analyses such as for copper levels.

7. The cat is placed in sternal recumbency and is observed for 24 to 48 hours for signs of bleeding or other complications. This technique has a very high likelihood of obtaining diagnostic quality tissue and has a mortality rate of approximately 1% in humans.

Supportive Care: Oral or parenteral analgesics are indicated.

KEYHOLE LIVER BIOPSY[1-4]

In the keyhole method, after the cat is prepared using the same methods as noted previously, a sterile gloved index finger is inserted through the abdominal musculature at the same site that is used for the percutaneous biopsy technique and the abdominal wall is bluntly dissected. After the finger is introduced into the abdomen through this blunt dissection, the liver is palpated and stabilized against the abdominal wall for subsequent biopsy, as noted previously. Compassionate care is optimal when preoperative and postoperative analgesics are employed to the point that healing and discomfort are not issues.

LAPAROSCOPIC LIVER BIOPSY[1-3]

In the hands of an experienced endoscopist, laparoscopic liver biopsy takes approximately 5 to 10 minutes from the time the abdomen is insufflated to the time of closure. With this method, the liver can be directly visualized for specific localization of lesions. The method is well described[1-3] and varies slightly depending on the equipment used. This procedure may be accomplished using either general anesthesia or local anesthesia with tranquilizers and analgesics. The site for insertion of the laparoscope can be on the midline or, more commonly, the right lateral abdominal wall just caudal to the ribs and ventral to the lateral spinous processes. Choosing the appropriate site of insertion depends on the area of the abdomen that is to be explored and biopsied.

KEY POINT

When undertaking any biopsy procedure, compassionate care is optimal when preoperative and postoperative analgesics are employed such that discomfort is minimized.

Indications: Evaluation and diagnosis of malignant and nonmalignant liver disease; determining the extent of the neoplastic processes.

Contraindications: Coagulopathies; cats with significantly compromised cardiovascular or respiratory systems (due to insufflation of the abdomen, venous return to the heart can be reduced and compress the diaphragm, compromising the ability to inspire easily).

Benefits: Biopsy can be selectively performed to acquire tissue to analyze cellularity, architecture, and content; in selected cases, the procedure can be done with local anesthesia, systemic analgesia, and tranquilization (Table 8-2); if there are any concerns about the cat's ability to lie quietly, however, general anesthesia should be performed.

Limitations: Small biopsy samples may not be representative of the entire liver; because this procedure allows visualization of lesions on the surface of all visible organs, lesions below the surface of each organ may be overlooked.

Equipment: Standard surgical instruments; laparoscope and laparoscopic biopsy instruments; Verres needle; trocar and cannula assembly.

Technique (Figure 8-7):

1. General anesthesia or tranquilizers with analgesic properties (e.g., butorphanol, fentanyl, morphine, or oxymorphone; Table 8-2) are administered. Compassionate care is optimal when preoperative and postoperative analgesics are employed such that discomfort is minimized.

2. If a lateral approach is used, the cat is placed with the left side down. If the patient is tranquilized, gentle but firm restraint of the limbs is applied so that the cat cannot change position during the procedure, ideally with an assistant nearby to calm the cat. The hair is clipped and the site prepared with a surgical scrub from the ninth rib to the caudal flank and from the dorsal to the ventral midline on the right side. The insertion site is draped.

3. If tranquilization is used instead of general anesthesia, approximately 0.5 to 2 ml of the local anesthetic agent

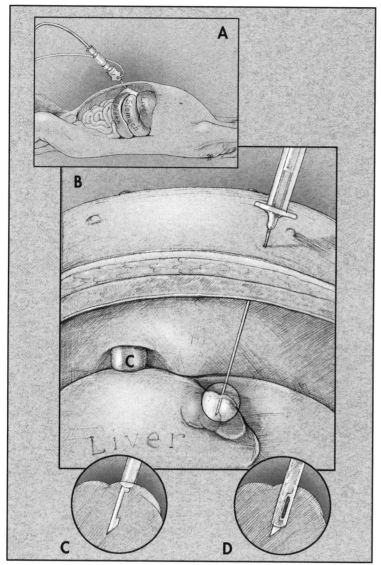

Figure 8-7: *Laparoscopy is ideal for visually characterizing the health and structure of many abdominal organs, including the liver (**A**). In addition, it is effective for directing a biopsy instrument to localized lesions, greatly increasing the diagnostic value of a biopsy sample. After the laparoscope is in place in the abdomen and the cavity is insufflated, a biopsy needle is introduced from a tangential direction (**B**). The needle is placed at an area of interest on the liver, and the inner stylet of the biopsy instrument is advanced into the tissue (**C**). The outer cannula is closed over the stylet (**D**), and the sample is removed.*

lidocaine is injected in and around the site where the laparoscope and any biopsy needles are to be introduced. The 2% lidocaine will sting less upon injection if it is diluted 50:50 with 8.4% bicarbonate.

4. A Verres needle is inserted into the right side, below the lateral spinous processes of the lumbar vertebrae and caudal to the last rib, into the peritoneal cavity. After it is determined that the needle is not in a hollow viscous or blood vessel, carbon dioxide or nitrous oxide is used to insufflate the abdomen to 10 mmHg. Injecting saline and aspirating material through the needle looking for

blood, bowel contents, or urine can check the placement of the Verres needle. Extreme care should be taken to make sure that the cat is breathing properly.

5. A small incision (0.5 to 1 cm) is made ventral to the lumbar muscles and caudal to the costal arch on the right side. The trocar and cannula assembly is then pushed into the gas-filled abdomen through the incision. The Verres needle is removed. The trocar is removed, and the laparoscope that is attached to the carbon dioxide or nitrous oxide insufflator and light source are advanced through the cannula to visualize the liver and other abdominal organs. If blood or other material obscures visualization, the laparoscope (but not the outer cannula) is removed and cleaned in a bowl of saline.

6. A biopsy needle is advanced through the laparoscope or through a separate puncture site nearby. The alligator or needle biopsy instrument is directed to the sites of interest by direct visualization. Five to six biopsy specimens are taken; at least one is submitted for bacterial culture and sensitivity and another for copper stains, if indicated.

7. After the biopsy sites are observed for several minutes for excessive bleeding, the carbon dioxide is evacuated, the instrument is removed from the abdominal cavity, and the small incision is sutured with simple interrupted absorbable s utures.

Supportive Care: Oral or parenteral analgesics.

REFERENCES

1. Ogilvie GK, Moore AS: Digestive System Biopsy, in *Managing the Veterinary Cancer Patient: A Practice Manual.* Trenton, NJ, Veterinary Learning Systems, 1995, pp 29–36.

2. Lightdale CJ: Liver biopsy, in Wittes RE (ed): *Manual of Oncologic Therapeutics 1991/1992.* Philadelphia, JB Lippincott, 1991, pp 20–22.

3. Jones BD, Hitt M, Hurst T: Hepatic biopsy. *Vet Clin North Am Small Anim Pract* 15:39–64, 1985.

4. Withrow SJ: Biopsy principles, in Withrow SJ, MacEwen EG (eds): *Clinical Veterinary Oncology.* Philadelphia, JB Lippincott, 1989, pp 53–57.

5. Lightdale CJ: Upper gastrointestinal endoscopy, in Wittes RE (ed): *Manual of Oncologic Therapeutics 1991/1992.* Philadelphia, JB Lippincott, 1991, pp 14–15.

6. Penninck DG, Nyland TG, Kerr LY, Fisher PE: Ultrasonographic evaluation of gastrointestinal diseases in small animals. *Vet Radiol* 31:134–141, 1990.

7. Penninck DG, Crystal MA, Matz ME, Pearson SH: The technique of percutaneous ultrasound guided fine-needle aspiration biopsy and automated micro-core biopsy in small animal gastrointestinal diseases. *Vet Radiol Ultrasound* 34:433–436, 1993.

8. Crystal MA, Penninck DG, Matz ME, et al: Use of ultrasound-guided fine-needle aspiration biopsy and automated core biopsy for the diagnosis of gastrointestinal diseases in small animals. *Vet Radiol* 34:438–444, 1993.

9. Münster M: Effizienz der Endoskopie bei Magen-Darm-Erkrankungen von Hund und Katze. *Praktische Tierarzt* 4:309–312, 1993.

BIOPSY

CLINICAL CYTOLOGY AND NEOPLASIA

9

Gregory K. Ogilvie and Antony S. Moore

C L I N I C A L B R I E F I N G	
Methods	*Benefits*
Fine-needle aspiration cytology	
"Needle-on" Technique	Cheap, easy, rapid.
"Needle-off" Technique	Lack of negative pressure reduces chance for dilution of cells of interest with blood or fluid; ideal for vascular and very small lesions.
Impression smears	Increased chance for obtaining many representative cells and may indirectly reveal architecture and associated cells of mass.
Tissue scrapings	Potentially therapeutic and diagnostic.
Needle core biopsy	Ideal for sarcomas and other tissues that exfoliate poorly.

Cytology is a practical, cost-effective, minimally invasive diagnostic tool for making a tentative diagnosis and directing the initial management and staging of the cat with cancer. It is also helpful to provide information and a tentative prognosis. Aspiration cytology is a rapid screening test that gives the power of information quickly to the clinician, the team, and the caregiver. A histopathologic diagnosis also is important for the evaluation of a cat with cancer but is often interpreted with increased accuracy if the results are combined with the findings of cytology:

- First, a representative sample must be obtained by the attending clinician. Virtually every part of the body can be sampled.
- Next, the sample must be adequately prepared.
- Finally, the sample must be accurately interpreted. Tentative diagnosis may be attempted by the attending clinician, but it is always advisable to obtain the interpretation of a board-certified veterinary cytopathologist.

FINE-NEEDLE ASPIRATION

This method is used to acquire tissue or fluid quickly from almost any part of the body with minimal risk.

Fine-Needle Aspiration of Solid Tissues[1-3]

Indication: Any condition suspected as being benign or malignant.

Contraindications: Coagulopathies (rarely); any abscessed or neoplastic tissue that may rupture, spill into, and contaminate a body cavity.

Benefits: Aspiration can be selectively performed to acquire cells to analyze cellularity and cell morphology, with or without the direction of imaging modalities such as ultrasonography or fluoroscopy; in most cases, the procedure can be done on an outpatient basis without any anesthesia; if there are any concerns about the cat's ability to lie quietly while a deep abdominal organ is being sampled, general anesthesia (Table 8-2) should be performed.

Limitation: Small samples may not be representative of the entire tissue of interest.

Equipment: A 3, 6, or 12 ml syringe; a 22 ga needle with sufficient length to sample the tissue of interest; microscope slides; proper staining materials; a microscope.

Technique:
1. The mass to be sampled is identified and immobilized.
2. The skin is then cleaned with surgical soap and alcohol if an abdominal cavity is to be entered. Superficial skin lesions can be cleaned solely with alcohol.
3. The needle is advanced into the tissue and partially withdrawn several times, with or without the syringe attached (Figure 9-1), in several different directions through the same entry point in the skin.
   —The "*needle-off*" *technique* is ideal for vascular tissues such as thyroid tumors to avoid diluting the sample

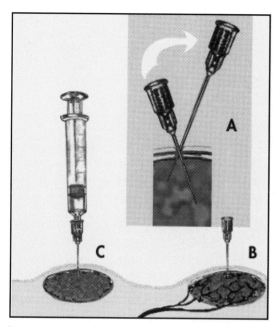

*Figure 9-1: Fine-needle aspiration is performed by advancing the needle into the tissue and partially withdrawing it several times (**A**), with or without the syringe attached, in several different directions through the same entry point in the skin. The "needle-off" method (**B**) is ideal for vascular tissues, whereas the "needle-on" technique (**C**) is ideal for tissues that do not exfoliate well, such as soft tissue sarcomas. When using the needle attached to the syringe ("needle on"), suction is applied as the needle is advanced through the tissue in several different directions. All negative pressure is then released before the needle is withdrawn from the tissue. The objective is to fill the needle with cells. The sampling is discontinued if blood or other tissue is noted in the hub of the needle or in the syringe. With both methods, the syringe is filled with air before the needle filled with cells is attached, and the cellular contents of the needle are forcefully expelled onto clean glass slides.*

with blood and results in a higher probability of a diagnostic sample.

—The *"needle-on" technique* is ideal for tissues that do not exfoliate well, such as soft tissue sarcomas, because of the presence of negative pressure. Suction is applied as the needle is advanced through the tissue in several different directions. All negative pressure is released before the needle is withdrawn from the tissue. The objective is to fill only the needle with cells; therefore if blood or other tissue is noted in the hub of the needle or in the syringe, sampling should be discontinued.

4. The needle is removed from the syringe. The syringe is filled with air before it is reattached, and the cellular contents of the needle are forcefully expelled onto clean glass slides.

5. A "squash-prep" is made by placing two slides on top of each other in a perpendicular orientation so that only the weight of the upper slide "squashes" the cells as they are pulled apart. The result is a smear of fluid or tissue on both slides.

—Alternatively, slides also can be made by spreading a drop of fluid in the same manner as preparing a blood smear. That is, the drop of fluid is spread across the primary slide by placing a second slide at a 45 degree angle to it. The slide that is at an angle is then backed into the sample so that the acute angle is facing it. The angled slide is then firmly and smoothly pushed along the other slide until the entire sample is distributed. The best smears can be obtained when the volume of the sample is relatively small; this prevents making a thick smear.

Supportive Care: Short-term oral analgesics may be helpful but are usually not necessary.

Abdominal Paracentesis[1]

Indication: Evaluation of any fluid within the abdominal cavity.

Contraindications: Coagulopathies; any abscessed or neoplastic tissue that may rupture, spill into, and contaminate a body cavity; fluid may leak into subcutaneous sites or completely through the skin following the aspiration procedure; injury to the bowel or other organs is rare but possible.

KEY POINT

The "needle-off" technique is ideal for vascular tissues because it avoids dilution of the sample with aspirated blood.

Benefits: Aspiration of the abdominal cavity can be selectively performed to acquire fluid but is best used with the direction of imaging modalities such as ultrasonography or fluoroscopy (which will also reduce the risk of penetration into organs such as the spleen); in most cases, the procedure can be done on an outpatient basis, with or without local anesthesia.

Limitations: Fluid analysis may not be diagnostic for an underlying malignancy.

Equipment: A 12 ml syringe; 22 ga needle; microscope slides; proper staining materials; a microscope.

Technique:

1. To reduce the possibility of accidentally aspirating the spleen, abdominal paracentesis should be performed at a site 3 to 5 cm caudal to the umbilicus and to the right of midline. The area is clipped and prepared following aseptic techniques.

2. Local anesthesia or tranquilization (Table 3-1) is preferred.

3. The syringe is filled with 1.5 ml of air. The needle on the syringe is then advanced slowly into the abdominal cav-

ity. Negative pressure is gently applied after the abdominal wall is penetrated. If no fluid is acquired, 0.5 ml of air is injected into the abdomen to clear the needle of any blockage. Negative pressure is applied once more. The procedure is repeated with the needle in different positions or depths within the abdominal cavity.

Supportive Care: Oral analgesics may be helpful for short-term discomfort.

Thoracentesis[1-3]

Indication: Evaluation of any fluid within the thoracic cavity.

Contraindications: Coagulopathies; any abscessed or neoplastic tissue that may rupture, spill into, and contaminate a body cavity.

Complications: Fluid may leak into subcutaneous sites or completely through the skin; alternatively, a pneumothorax may develop; injury to the lung or heart is rare but possible.

Benefits: Aspiration of the abdominal cavity can be selectively performed to acquire fluid with or without the direction of imaging modalities such as ultrasonography or fluoroscopy; in most cases, the procedure can be done on an outpatient basis, with or without local anesthesia.

Limitations: Fluid analysis may not be diagnostic for an underlying malignancy.

Equipment: A 12 to 60 ml syringe; a three-way stopcock; a 22 ga needle; microscope slides (cleaned and prepared before the procedure); proper staining materials; a microscope.

Technique:

1. Ideally, the cat should be standing and quiet. The administration of analgesics and/or tranquilizers is preferred; however, many of these drugs can depress respiration and can place cats with minimal respiratory reserve at risk. Local anesthesia is recommended in addition to analgesia and tranquilizers. To reduce the sting associated with the injection of 2% lidocaine, this drug can be diluted with equal parts of 8.4% bicarbonate. The site for thoracentesis varies depending on the site of the fluid but is commonly around the seventh or eighth intercostal space. The area is clipped and prepared with surgical scrub and alcohol.

2. The needle on the syringe is advanced slowly into the thoracic cavity just cranial to the nearby rib to prevent hitting the intercostal arteries, which are located just caudal to the ribs. The bevel should face the pleural lining. Negative pressure is gently applied after the pleural space is entered. The three-way stopcock can be used to prevent air from leaking into the chest while syringes are changed to drain the chest.

3. Once a sample is acquired, it is put into EDTA and a culturette for bacterial culture and sensitivity, if indicat-

ed. Slides also can be made directly, or the fluid can be centrifuged to concentrate the cells for subsequent analysis.

IMPRESSIONS AND SCRAPING TECHNIQUES[1-3]

Once tissue has been removed from the cat, cells can be acquired from masses or biopsy specimens by doing impressions of the tissue or by actually scraping cells from that tissue. Impression smears are ideal for lymph nodes, whereas scrapings are optimal for tissues that do not exfoliate easily, such as soft tissue sarcomas.

Indications: Almost any potentially abnormally tissue that has been removed from the cat; occasionally, an ulcerated mass on the cat can be sampled by making an impression or by scraping cells directly from its surface.

Contraindications: None known.

Benefits: An impression is ideal for indirectly acquiring information about the cell types involved as well as providing some idea of cellular architecture within the mass itself; if done correctly, the cells may be less traumatized than when aspirates and "squash preps" are made.

Limitation: Small samples may not be representative of the entire tissue of interest.

Equipment: A surgical blade; Brown-Adson forceps; microscope slides; proper staining materials; a microscope.

Technique:

Impressions

1. A freshly removed piece of tissue is blot-dried before it is transected in half to obtain a flat surface for performing the impressions. The surface should be smaller than the slide to allow multiple impressions.

2. The cut surface is then blotted on an absorbent surface such as a paper towel.

3. Several impressions are made on each slide.

Scrapings

1. The tissue is blotted dry to allow any blood or fluid to be removed. The surface of the tissue is then gently scraped with a new surgical blade, and the cells on the blade are gently smeared across the slide.

Supportive Care: Oral or parenteral analgesics may be needed.

SLIDE PREPARATION

At least one slide from every site should be saved for submission to a clinical pathologist. In each case, slides should be prepared with the utmost care. Tumor cells often are very fragile and easily disrupted. After the slides are made, one representative slide should be stained and examined to ensure that it is likely to be diagnostic. The most frequently used stains in the clinic or laboratory are Wright's-Giemsa, new methylene blue, and Papanicolaou stains. An adaptation of the Wright's stain (Diff-Quik®) is commonly used in feline practice; it can be performed in a 15 second, three step procedure. In addition, the stain is very effective in providing good cytoplasmic detail. The new methylene blue stain also is easy to perform and provides good nuclear detail. The Papanicolaou stain is more labor-intensive and generally is used only in a clinical pathology laboratory but provides excellent cellular morphology.

KEY POINT

The practitioner should call upon the expertise of a clinical pathologist to confirm pivotal diagnoses and to help make subtle diagnoses.

GENERAL CYTOLOGIC INTERPRETATION[1-3]

Detailed interpretation of cytology requires considerable experience and knowledge of normal cellular morphology. The practitioner should call upon the expertise of a clinical pathologist to confirm diagnoses. With practice, the clinician can determine whether a sample is likely to have adequate cellularity for subsequent diagnosis by an expert in the field. In addition, with experience, inflammation can be differentiated from neoplasia, which can be of great value for directing other diagnostic tests. In any case, the cytology should be interpreted in combination with other clinical information to make an appropriate diagnosis.

Once all the slides are reviewed, representative clusters of cells are evaluated at 100× (oil immersion). The cells are then assessed to determine whether they represent normal tissue (Plate 1), an inflammatory process (Plate 2), hyperplasia, or neoplasia (Plates 3 to 14). (Color plate section begins on page 49; captions appear on page 52.)

An inflammatory process (Table 9-1) can be divided somewhat arbitrarily into acute, chronic active, or chronic or granulomatous based on the presence or absence of neutrophils, monocytes, plasma cells, eosinophils, and differentiated macrophages.

Acute inflammation can be diagnosed when greater than 70% of the inflammatory cells are neutrophils. The neutrophils can be well preserved, hypersegmented, toxic, or lysed. Chronic active inflammation can be diagnosed when 30% to 50% of the inflammatory cell population is composed of plasma cells and monocytes. Chronic inflammatory responses are those in which mononuclear inflammatory cells and macrophages predominate. If epithelial or inflammatory giant cells are present, the condition is considered to be granulomatous.

It is important to differentiate hyperplasia from neoplasia. Hyperplasia principally differs from normal tissue in that hyperplastic cells exhibit the features of cytoplasmic activity and are cytologically immature. Therefore reactive or hyperplastic cells may have more basophilic cytoplasm and the nuclei may be larger than in normal cells. One key differentiating feature is that hyperplastic cells have a fairly constant nuclear:cytoplasmic ratio, whereas neoplastic tissue does not.

The diagnosis of neoplasia is made on the cytologic characteristics (see Box on next page) of nuclear, cytoplasmic, and structural features. In brief, the criteria for diagnosing malignancy include[1-3]:

- **Nuclear changes and appearance**
  (Plates 3B, 6B, 7B, 10B, 11B, 14B)
  —Marked variation in nuclear size
  —Marked variation in nuclear:cytoplasmic ratio
  —Irregular nuclear membrane
  —Variably sized, irregular nucleoli
  —Irregular chromatin that clumps
  —Abnormal mitotic figures

- **Cytoplasmic changes and appearance**
  (Plates 6B, 7B, 10B, 11B, 14B)
  —Vacuolization
  —Basophilia with Wright's stain
  —Irregular and indistinct cytoplasmic boundaries
  —Variable cytoplasmic amount from cell to cell

- **Structural changes and appearance**
  Discrete Cell Neoplasms: Round Cell Tumors
  (Plates 3 to 10)
  —Round to oval cells
  —Easy exfoliation of individual cells
  —Well-defined cytoplasmic margins

TABLE 9-1
Inflammatory Processes

Type of Inflammation	Characterization
Acute	>70% of the inflammatory cells are neutrophils; the neutrophils can be well preserved, hypersegmented, toxic, or lysed
Chronic active	Approximately 30%–50% of the inflammatory cell population are plasma cells and monocytes; neutrophils are also present in significant numbers
Chronic or granulomatous	Mononuclear inflammatory cells and macrophages predominate

Immunohistochemistry

The accuracy of histologic diagnosis can be improved by the use of immunohistochemical staining for various cell-specific antigens or structural elements. A brief synopsis of the concepts of immunohistochemistry are noted below:

- *Intermediate filaments* are intracellular structural proteins that can be identified by staining in order to distinguish between epithelial tumors (such as carcinomas) and mesenchymal tumors (sarcomas). These structures also differ between types of mesenchymal cells. Stains to document the presence of intermediate filaments are most useful in distinguishing the histogenesis of poorly differentiated tumors. For example, an oral tumor may be so poorly differentiated that the pathologist cannot tell if it is an adenocarcinoma, a fibrosarcoma, or a melanoma. Overfixation of tissue (longer than a few days) in formalin may make it impossible to perform these stains.

- *Cytokeratins* are found in a variety of epithelial tumors and are therefore a marker for carcinomas. There are different cytokeratins used for cat tissues, but they cannot easily distinguish between different *sorts* of carcinomas.

- *Vimentin* is found in all mesenchymal cells and is therefore a marker for sarcomas.

- *Desmin* is found in tissues of muscle derivation and may therefore be used to distinguish a rhabdomyosarcoma or a leiomyosarcoma from other *vimentin-positive* sarcomas.

- *Glial fibrillary acidic protein (GFAP)* is a marker of neuroectodermal tissue and may distinguish tumors of that histogenesis.

- *S-100* is a structural protein that is seen in some tissues of neuroectodermal origin as well as in melanomas and is therefore a good marker for poorly differentiated melanomas.

- *Melan A* is a more sensitive marker for melanoma cells than S-100.

- *Factor VIII* may be used to distinguish tumors with vascular endothelial derivation, such as hemangiosarcomas.

- Lymphomas can be distinguished from other tumors and subclassified into two groups by stains for antigens that distinguish B and T lymphocytes from each other. A common T-cell marker is *CD-3*. Histiocytic cells may be distinguished using a *CD-68* stain.

Carcinomas: Epithelial Cell Tumors
(Plates 11 and 12)

—Easy exfoliation of cells in clusters, clumps, or sheets
—Oval to round cells
—Arranged in ductular or acinar pattern around a central lumen
—Cytoplasm may contain a secretory product

Sarcomas: Connective Tissue Tumors
(Plates 13 and 14)
—Difficult to exfoliate
—Individual cells or disorganized clusters
—Spindle-shaped cells
—Cytoplasmic extensions with ill-defined cytoplasmic borders

KEY POINT

Hyperplasia is difficult to differentiate from neoplasia in many cases. When there is a question, a biopsy should be performed.

CYTOLOGY OF SPECIFIC NEOPLASMS

Once a neoplastic process is suspected using the criteria above, the cells are examined and categorized into the following:

- Benign or malignant
- Carcinomas, sarcomas, or discrete cell tumors
- Specific cell type
- Degree of differentiation

The references noted at the end of this section are excellent resources to further understand clinical veterinary cytology.[1-3] A brief description of some of the more common tumors diagnosed cytologically in veterinary medicine follows. In each case, a biopsy should be done to confirm the cytologic diagnosis.

Discrete Cell Neoplasms: Round Cell Tumors (Plates 2 to 10)

Round cell tumors, commonly seen in feline medicine, have unique distinguishing cytologic features. Upon cytologic evaluation the cells are all round, have well-defined cytoplasmic borders, and are easily exfoliated into single cells because of their lack of cell-to-cell attachments. The following is a brief description of some distinguishing features of specific types of round cell tumors:

- **Lymphomas** (Plates 3 to 5) are usually found in the gastrointestinal tract, lymph nodes, liver, spleen, bone marrow, and extranodal sites such as the skin. The cells are made up of a monotonous population of small to large, poorly differentiated lymphoid cells with scant blue cytoplasm, dense nuclear margins, and round to slightly irregularly shaped nuclei, with generally at least one nucleolus. Some lymphoma cells may have azurophilic granules upon staining. Lymphoma cells usually resemble lymphoblasts, although in many cases they can be very well differentiated and resemble normal lymphocytes; therefore a biopsy and histologic confirmation are required to confirm the diagnosis prior to initiation of therapy. In each case, lymphoma must be differentiated from lymphoid hyperplasia, which is characterized by the presence of lymphocytes in all stages of differentiation; however, immature cells such as lymphoblasts and lymphocytes are increased in numbers when compared to those in a normal lymph node. Mitotic figures may be increased in number in hyperplastic lymph nodes, but the appearance of mitotic figures is normal within a lymph node.

- **Plasma cell tumors** (Plate 6) contain cells that are oval to round with round nuclei and coarse, clumped chromatin. A single, relatively small nucleolus may be identified within each nucleus. The mitotic activity of these cells is generally low due to the benign nature of this condition. The amount of basophilic cytoplasm in these cells varies. Plasma cell tumors from cats with multiple myeloma appear cytologically similar to immature plasma cells (Plates 6A and B). The more mature cells may have an eccentric nucleus and a round to oval cytoplasm, which may have a perinuclear halo consistent with active production of immunoglobulin.
- **Mast cell tumors** (Plates 7 to 9) are found in the skin, spleen, liver, lymph node, and bone marrow of affected cats. Mast cell tumors may contain eosinophils and fibroblasts. They are round and vary in size from 10 to 40 μm in diameter. Staining reveals eccentric round to oval nuclei that may be hidden by variable numbers of fine to coarse blue-black to reddish-purple granules. Diff-Quik® may not stain the granules effectively; leaving the slide in the methanol fixative for at least 2 minutes may stain the granules more completely. Normal mast cells can be seen in a variety of inflammatory conditions; however, they are usually accompanied by neutrophils and macrophages in these cases.
- **Melanomas** (Plate 10) are rare but considered by some to be a discrete/round cell tumor. Others believe the tumor has characteristics of both epithelial and mesenchymal cells. This neoplastic process is uncommon in cats. The lesion may be pigmented or amelanotic. As expected, pigmented lesions are almost black in color, whereas amelanotic lesions may be pink or white. Because melanomas often have intracytoplasmic granules, they must be differentiated from mast cell tumors and pigmented basal cell tumors. With most stains, the granules are black or brown and irregular in shape and size. The granules are often noted extracellularly because they are released from some cells. The melanoma can be composed of round, epithelioid, or spindle-shaped cells; sometimes, there are cells of different shapes within the same tumor. Malignant melanomas must be differentiated from mast cell tumors, pigment-

ed basal cell tumors, and macrophages that contain hemosiderin; this is best done by combining a cytologic suspicion with tissue biopsied for histopathologic evaluation.

Carcinomas: Epithelial Cell Tumors (Plates 11 and 12)

Epithelial cell tumors are found throughout the body. Regardless of whether they originate from the lung, the intestine, or the mammary gland, they all have similar characteristics, including easy exfoliation of cells in clusters, clumps, or sheets; oval to round cells; ductular or acinar arrangement around a central lumen; and cytoplasm that may contain a secretory product. This secretory product may induce a "signet ring" appearance because the nucleus is eccentrically located within the cytoplasm. A clinical pathologist may be able to determine the cell of origin. The following are some characteristics of epithelial cell tumors commonly seen in feline practice:

- Cytologic interpretation of the cells from a **mammary adenocarcinoma** (Plate 11) is classic for any adenocarcinoma. The cells often are arranged in clusters and exhibit cytoplasmic basophilia and variable nuclear:cytoplasmic ratios. Mitotic figures are common; some cells may be distended with a cytoplasmic product, forming a "signet ring" appearance.
- **Squamous cell carcinomas** (Plate 12) occur throughout the body in cats and often have a different biologic behavior depending on the location of the tumor. They may be ulcerated, with an inflammatory component mixed with a bacterial infection. Squamous cell carcinomas often exfoliate into clusters; however, they are just as likely to be individual cells. The cells of this tumor may vary morphologically depending on the degree of differentiation. The more anaplastic cells are small and round with a basophilic cytoplasm, which often contains hyperchromatic nuclei. Cells in an intermediate stage of differentiation are larger, with more abundant, paler cytoplasm. The nuclei generally are large and have marked clumps of chromatin. More mature cells actually show signs of forming keratin, which may be seen in the extracellular space. The more mature cells may have cytoplasmic borders that appear quite angular due to keratinization. An inflammatory response is often seen in conjunction with the tumor cells. As with all aspirates, a histologic sample is essential to confirm the diagnosis.

Sarcomas: Connective Tissue Tumors (Plates 13 and 14)

Connective tissue tumors exfoliate poorly and therefore may be difficult to diagnose cytologically. Cytologic diagnosis of a sarcoma is reasonably straightforward; however, specifically distinguishing connective tissue tumors may not be possible. Types include:

- **Soft tissue sarcomas** (Plates 13 and 14) may occur anywhere on the cat's body. Injection (vaccine)-associated sarcomas are a widely recognized entity. In general, soft tissue sarcomas have a relatively low probability for metastasis and are locally invasive. The cells exfoliate poorly and usually are seen alone or in disorganized clusters. The cytoplasm often is indistinct and spindle shaped. Biopsy is required to distinguish fibrosarcomas, neurofibrosarcomas, fibromas, schwannomas, myxosarcomas, and myxomas from each other.
- **Osteosarcomas** may have sufficient distinguishable cytologic characteristics to allow the practitioner to make a tentative diagnosis based on fine-needle aspiration cytology, especially when combined with the history, physical examination, and radiographs. These tumors often occur in the metaphyses of long bones or in the axillary skeleton. Cytologically, the tumor may be composed primarily of osteoblasts that vary dramatically in size, but they usually are quite large. The cells are often spindle shaped and have abundant foamy basophilic cytoplasm that surrounds a variably sized nucleus, with coarse chromatin and variable numbers of nuclei. Some of these cells have an eosinophilic substance within the cytoplasm that occasionally may be noted extracellularly as an osteoid matrix. Normal osteoblasts may be seen in conjunction with the malignant cells.

REFERENCES

1. Rebar AH: *Handbook of Veterinary Cytology.* St Louis, Ralston Purina, 1977.
2. Wellman ML: The cytologic diagnosis of neoplasia. *Vet Clin North Am Small Anim Pract* 20:919–938, 1990.
3. MacWilliams PS: Cytologic techniques in cancer diagnosis, in Withrow SJ, MacEwen EG (eds): *Clinical Veterinary Oncology.* Philadelphia, JB Lippincott, 1989, pp 41–52.

COLOR PLATES *See captions on page 52.*

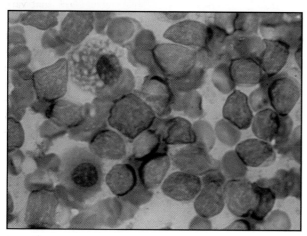

Plate 1: *Normal lymph node.*

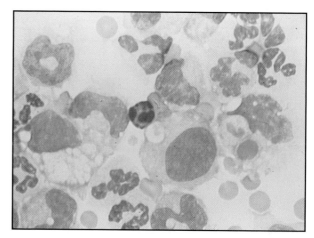

Plate 2: *An inflammatory process.*

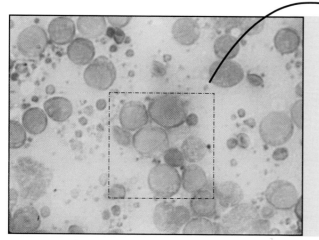

Plate 3A: *Discrete cell tumor/cutaneous lymphoma.*

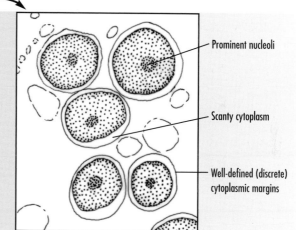

Prominent nucleoli

Scanty cytoplasm

Well-defined (discrete) cytoplasmic margins

Plate 3B: *Discrete cell tumor/cutaneous lymphoma.*

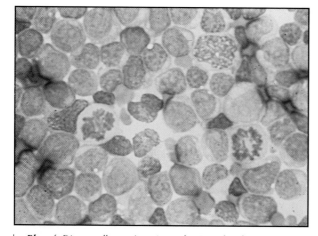

Plate 4: *Discrete cell tumor/anterior mediastinum lymphoma.*

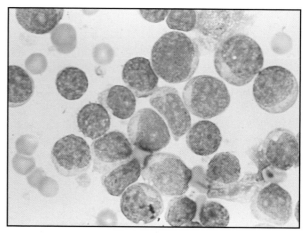

Plate 5: *Discrete cell tumor/lymphoma.*

COLOR PLATES   *See captions on page 52.*

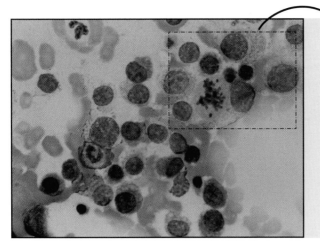

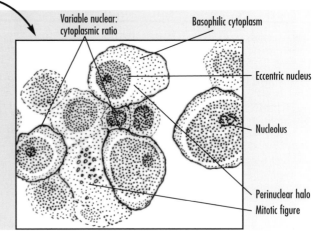

Plate 6A: *Plasma cell tumor/multiple myeloma.*   **Plate 6B:** *Plasma cell tumor/multiple myeloma.*

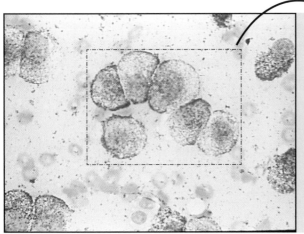

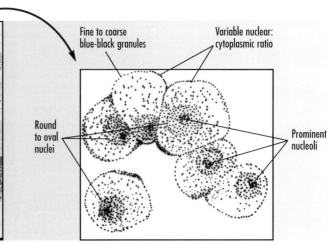

Plate 7A: *Mast cell tumor.*   **Plate 7B:** *Mast cell tumor.*

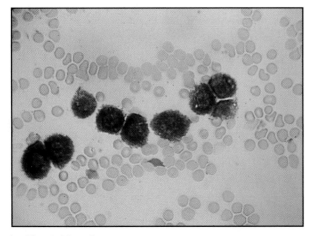

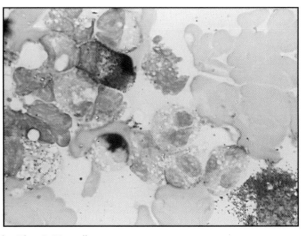

Plate 8: *Mast cell tumor.*   **Plate 9:** *Mast cell tumor.*

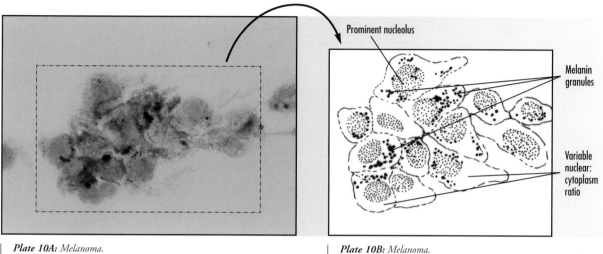

Plate 10A: *Melanoma.*

Plate 10B: *Melanoma.*

Prominent nucleolus

Melanin granules

Variable nuclear: cytoplasm ratio

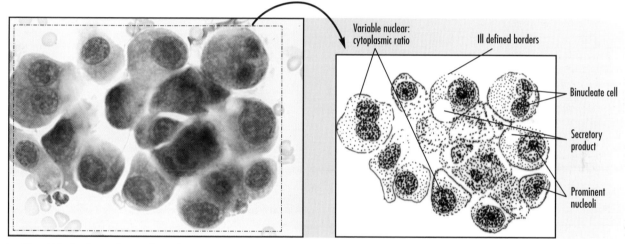

Plate 11A: *Carcinoma (intestinal tumor).*

Plate 11B: *Carcinoma (intestinal tumor).*

Variable nuclear: cytoplasmic ratio

Ill defined borders

Binucleate cell

Secretory product

Prominent nucleoli

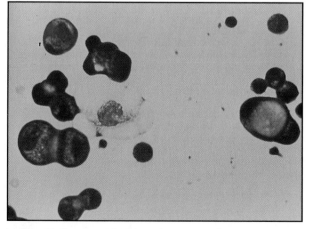

Plate 12: *Squamous cell carcinoma/mammmary adenocarcinoma.*

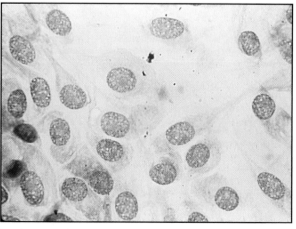

Plate 13: *Soft tissue sarcoma/oral fibrosarcoma.*

COLOR PLATES

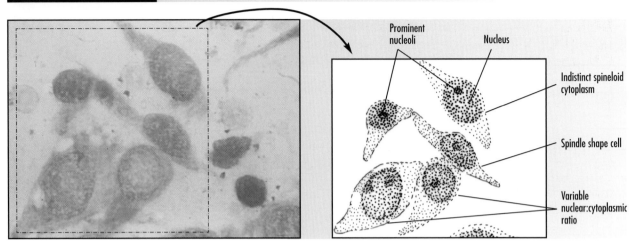

Prominent nucleoli

Nucleus

Indistinct spineloid cytoplasm

Spindle shape cell

Variable nuclear:cytoplasmic ratio

Plate 14A: *Soft tissue sarcoma/oral fibrosarcoma.*

Plate 14B: *Soft tissue sarcoma/oral fibrosarcoma.*

COLOR PLATE CAPTIONS

Plate 1: *Cytology from a normal lymph node. Lymph nodes—even reactive lymph nodes—have an orderly maturation of lymphocytes; however, small lymphocytes usually predominate.*

Plate 2: *Nondegenerate neutrophils, macrophages, and erythrocytes predominate in this lymph node aspirate that is diagnostic for an inflammatory condition. It is important to differentiate hyperplasia or inflammation from neoplasia. Hyperplasia principally differs from normal tissue in that hyperplastic cells exhibit the features of cytoplasmic activity and are cytologically immature. Therefore reactive or hyperplastic cells may have more basophilic cytoplasm and the nuclei may be larger than in normal cells. One key differentiating feature is that hyperplastic cells have a fairly constant nuclear:cytoplasmic ratio, whereas neoplastic tissue does not.*

Plates 3–10: *Round cell or discrete cell tumors have round to oval cells with well-defined cytoplasmic borders. They include lymphoma, mast cell tumors, and plasma cell tumors.*

Plate 3–5: *These photomicrographs are representative of lymphoma. Note the mitotic figures and the prominent nucleoli that are characteristic features of malignancy. The cells are characterized as being made up of a monotonous population of large, poorly differentiated lymphoid cells with scanty blue cytoplasm, dense nuclear margins, and round to slightly irregularly shaped nuclei, generally with at least one nucleolus. Some cells may have azurophilic granules. Lymphoma cells usually resemble lymphoblasts, although in a few rare cases they can be very well differentiated and resemble normal lymphocytes. A biopsy is required to confirm the diagnosis of each case of lymphoma, especially small cell or well-differentiated lymphoma. Plates 3A and 3B depict malignant lymphocytes with prominent nucleoli, a scanty rim of cytoplasm, well-defined or discrete borders, and a variable nuclear:cytoplasmic ratio.*

Plate 6: *This is the cytology from the bone marrow of a cat with a monoclonal gammopathy in the serum, Bence Jones proteins in the urine, and hypercalcemia consistent with a diagnosis of a plasma cell tumor, also known as multiple myeloma. Note the round cell tumor cells with eccentric nuclei. The cytoplasm of plasma cells often contains a perinuclear halo that is actually immunoglobulin prior to release from the cell. The cytologic features noted in Plate 6B outline characteristics of a malignant plasma cell tumor, including eccentric nucleus, perinuclear halo, and variable nuclear:cytoplasmic ratios.*

Plates 7–9: *Mast cell tumors. Mast cells are round and vary in size from 10 to 40 μm in diameter. They have eccentric round to oval nuclei that may be hidden by variable numbers of fine to coarse blue-black to*

reddish-purple granules. The line drawing of Plate 7B points out the features of a typical mast cell tumor, including fine to coarse granules, variable nuclear:cytoplasmic ratio, prominent nucleoli, and discrete borders.

Plate 10: *Melanomas are rare in cats but are considered by some to be a discrete cell tumor. Others believe the tumor has characteristics of both epithelial and mesenchymal cells. Because melanomas often have intracytoplasmic granules, they must be differentiated from mast cell tumors. With most stains, the granules are black or brown and irregular in shape and size. They are usually small and appear dustlike. The granules are often noted extracellularly because they are released from some cells. The features depicted in Plate 10B show typical prominent nucleoli, melanin granules, and the variable nuclear:cytoplasmic ratio.*

Plates 11 and 12: *Epithelial cell tumors easily exfoliate in clusters, clumps, or sheets of oval to round cells. The cells may arrange into a ductular or acinar pattern around a central lumen, and the cytoplasm may contain a secretory product.*

Plate 11: *Carcinoma from a cat with an intestinal tumor. Note the round cells, some with multiple nuclei, multinucleated cells, variable nuclear:cytoplasmic ratios, and other indications of malignancy. The characteristics depicted in 11B show the ill-defined borders, binucleate cells, secretory product, prominent nucleoli, and variable nuclear:cytoplasmic ratio.*

Plate 12: *Cytology from a mammary mass confirmed histologically as a mammary adenocarcinoma. Note the secretory product within some cells and the attempt of some cells at maintaining a ductlike arrangement. The secretory contents often make the cells resemble "signet rings," which is characteristic of many carcinomas.*

Plates 13 and 14: *Sarcomas or mesenchymal tumors exfoliate with difficulty. They have individual cells or disorganized clusters. The cells are recognized as being spindle shaped and have cytoplasmic extensions with ill-defined cytoplasmic borders. The cytologic features of variable nuclear:cytoplasmic ratio, spindeloid cytoplasm, and prominent nucleoli are characteristic of sarcomas of many types.*

Plate 13: *Fine-needle aspiration of an oral mass from a cat with an oral fibrosarcoma.*

Plate 14: *Fine-needle aspiration of a submandibular lymph node from the same cat.*

DRUG HANDLING AND ADMINISTRATION

Gregory K. Ogilvie and Antony S. Moore

10

CLINICAL BRIEFING

Risk	Recommendation
Absorption via skin or mucous membranes	Wear latex gloves, protective eyewear, and a disposable gown with long, cuffed sleeves; wash hands frequently; do not allow food in work area.
Inhalation	Wear a respirator-type or high-dust mask.
Aerosol formation during reconstitution	Use a hydrophobic filter (chemotherapy "pin") for removing liquid chemotherapeutic agents.
Metabolites or drug (e.g., carboplatin) in urine	Wear latex gloves when handling waste.
Self-inoculation when recapping needles	Do not recap needles.

The health and well-being of the veterinary health care team—as well as that of the client and patient—must be a high priority regardless of whether one is dealing with anesthetic agents, antibiotics, or chemotherapeutic agents. Like all drugs, chemotherapeutic agents have potential risks if they are handled improperly. As the benefits of anticancer drugs become more apparent, their use is rapidly expanding, which in turn puts the veterinary health care team at increased risk of exposure during drug preparation and administration. All chemotherapeutic agents are potentially toxic, most are mutagenic or teratogenic, and at least some are carcinogenic. Reliable information regarding the amount of drug exposure needed for any of these effects is difficult to obtain; however, some toxicities have been seen in caregivers who prepare and administer chemotherapy for human patients.[1,2]

Exposure to cytotoxic agents can occur in four ways:

- Inhalation due to aerosolization during mixing and/or administration of the drug
- Absorption of the drug through the skin
- Ingestion through contact with contaminated food or cigarettes
- Accidental inoculation

Common clinical examples of situations in which exposure may occur include:

- Withdrawal of a needle from a pressurized drug vial (the "pssst" as the needle is withdrawn)
- Transfer of drugs between containers
- Opening of glass ampules
- Expulsion of air bubbles from drug-filled syringes
- Failure or improper setup of equipment
- Exposure to excreta from patients treated with certain cytotoxic drugs
- Crushing or breaking of tablets

Safe drug handling is possible in feline practice. Because of the relatively small doses of chemotherapy delivered by most practitioners, the risk of exposure is low. However, everyone who prepares or administers antineoplastic drugs should have routine health examinations. Women of childbearing age should exercise extreme caution when handling cytotoxic agents, and pregnant women should not handle antineoplastic drugs at all. Procedures for handling chemotherapeutic agents must meet or exceed the guidelines outlined by the Occupational Safety and Health Administration (OSHA) and any state or local regulations.

Antineoplastic agents should be stored according to the manufacturers' directions. Drugs that require refrigeration should be kept in a separate refrigerator away from other medications and foodstuffs. If a reconstituted drug is stored, the vial should be placed in a sealable plastic bag labeled with the date of reconstitution.

The ideal way to prepare cytotoxic agents is in a biologic safety cabinet (hood)—specifically, a Class II, type A vertical laminar air flow cabinet exhausted outside the facility. Many pharmacies will prepare chemotherapeutic agents for a fee. Practitioners should take advantage of this option when possible. Although it is impractical for most veterinary practices to own such a hood, many of the safety principles involved in drug handling and reconstitution are the same regardless of whether a hood is used.

If a hood is not available, other pieces of equipment can help provide a safe environment in which to prepare chemotherapeutic agents. All drugs should be prepared in a low-traffic area away from doorways, windows, or any drafts. Eating, drinking, and smoking should not take place in the drug preparation area. A disposable, absorbent, plastic-backed pad or liner should be used. Gloves and a gown should be worn, as should a dust-and-mist respirator and goggles. Using chemotherapy dispensing pins ("chemo-pins") with hydrophobic filters further reduces the risk of exposure to injectable drugs during preparation.

The following information is provided for people involved in the day-to-day technical aspects of chemotherapy preparation and administration (see Box at left). The reader is advised to review this section and all OSHA guidelines for information that can reduce the risks inherent in handling these drugs.

PREPARING CHEMOTHERAPEUTIC AGENTS

The biologic safety cabinet or hood is the preferred site for mixing chemotherapeutic agents and is essential for practices that handle large volumes of these drugs. Howev-

---

Guidelines for Handling Chemotherapeutic Agents

Mixing Chemotherapeutic Agents

– Wear a disposable, closed, moisture-barrier gown with elastic or knit cuffs, latex gloves, safety glasses, and mask.
– Use a vertical laminar flow hood if possible.
– Mix agents in a quiet area.
– Use absorbent plastic-backed liners to collect spills.
– Use hydrophobic filters (chemo-pins) to air vent vials.
– Use Luer-lok® syringes.
– Have a pharmacy prepare injectable agents when possible.

Handling Accidental Spills

– Have a commercially available spill kit on site.
– Wear two pairs of nonpowdered latex gloves.
– Wash skin with soap and water on contact with drug.
– Clean minor spills with 70% isopropyl alcohol or chlorine bleach.
– Decontaminate large spills with a neutralizing agent or high pH soap.

Administering Chemotherapy

– Wear disposable nonpowdered latex gloves.
– Use absorbent plastic-backed liners to catch spills.

Disposal

– Properly dispose of contaminated needles and syringes in appropriate container.
– Place other cytotoxic waste into chemotherapy disposal system.

First 48 Hours after Chemotherapy

– Wear latex gloves and a closed, moisture-barrier gown when handling blood, vomitus, and litterboxes.

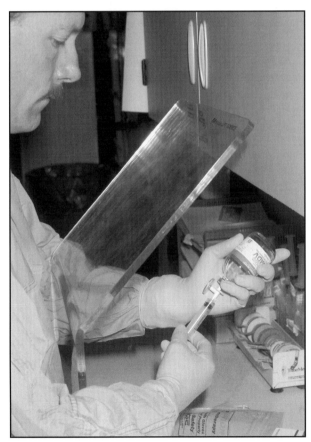

Figure 10-1: *A biologic safety cabinet should be used when possible. Latex gloves and a nonpermeable gown should be worn when preparing chemotherapeutic agents. When a safety cabinet is not available, a plastic shield can provide some protection while mixing chemotherapeutic agents.*

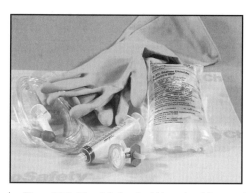

Figure 10-2: Materials that should be on hand for preparing or handling chemotherapeutic agents include latex gloves, chemotherapy dispensing pins to prevent contamination of the bottle or exposure to the handler, Luer-loc® syringes, and prefilled IV drip sets.

er, because most practices handle small volumes of these drugs, this section is designed for those situations. Even when a biologic safety cabinet is being used, the following handling guidelines should be followed.

When chemotherapeutic agents are mixed, certain materials should always be available in the quiet, low-traffic drug preparation area. Plastic shields can be used as a barrier between drugs and the handler (Figure 10-1). Materials that should be kept readily available in the mixing area include a plastic-backed absorbent liner to absorb any leaks and spills (the liner should be changed if it becomes contaminated with any drug and when the area is cleaned), heavy-duty latex gloves, hydrophobic filters (chemo-pins), IV lines prefilled with NaCl (if appropriate), a stack of gauze squares, and alcohol-soaked cotton balls or swabs (Figure 10-2). A large, sealable plastic bag should be available for chemotherapy waste, and a puncture-proof container is needed for all contaminated sharps.

All materials needed for drug preparation should be placed in the area before starting any work. Outer packages should be discarded to prevent accumulation of debris. Before reconstituting a drug, recommendations for the diluent should be verified. For most chemotherapy drugs, 0.9% NaCl or sterile water is used; however, for some drugs (e.g., carboplatin), a solution of 5% dextrose in water is required.

When preparing cytotoxic agents, a gown with long sleeves, closed cuffs, and a closed front should be worn. The gown should be made of a disposable fabric with low permeability. Latex gloves should be pulled over the cuffs of the gown to protect the skin from drug exposure (Figure 10-3). Vinyl gloves should not be used—they are more permeable and thus more likely to allow skin contamination. Goggles and a mask are necessary. The use of a dust-and-mist respirator or a mask with a filter to prevent inhalation of aerosolized drugs is recommended. A conventional surgery mask does not provide adequate protection.

Chemo-pins prevent aerosolization of the drug and pres-

sure from building in the vials when reconstituting drugs and are thus recommended when preparing injectable drugs (Figure 10-3). Luer-lok® syringes (Figure 10-4) are recommended because they prevent the syringe from separating from the chemo-pin or needle.

To prepare injectable drugs, the first step is removing the plastic lid from the vial and aseptically wiping the top of the vial with an alcohol swab. The chemo-pin is then inserted into the vial. The vial is kept upright while the syringe is attached to the chemo-pin and twisted tight. When reconstituting a drug, diluent is slowly pushed into the vial, and the bottle is gently rolled or shaken. A Luer-lok® syringe can remain attached while mixing. Next, the vial is turned upside down, and the drug is aspirated into the syringe slowly to avoid excess air bubbles. When the correct amount has been retrieved, any air or excess drug should be pushed into the vial. The vial should then be turned upright and put

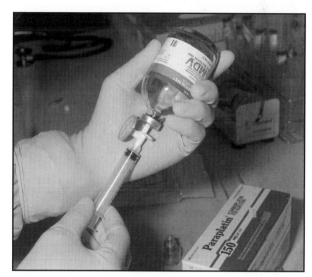

Figure 10-3: Chemotherapeutic agents can be safely mixed if the handler wears latex gloves and uses hydrophobic filters (chemo-pins; essential to prevent aerosolization of cytotoxic agents during preparation). Note that the side vent is filtered for protection from the accidental escape of the drug.

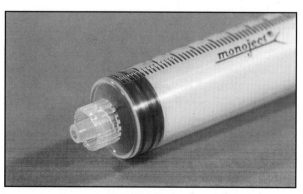

Figure 10-4: Luer-loc® syringes should be used whenever possible because their screw-on end allows a secure connection with the needle.

down. An alcohol-moistened gauze square is wrapped around the top of the pin and syringe, and the syringe is gently pulled from the pin. The gauze will trap any drug that leaks or aerosolizes. A covered needle should be placed on the syringe and the chemo-pin capped after clearing the filter with an air-filled syringe. The labeled syringe should then be put into a sealable plastic bag (Figure 10-5). If the remaining drug is to be stored, the chemo-pin is left attached to the vial to allow access for multiple doses.

If chemo-pins are not available, the diluent must be slowly added to the drug directly through the needle and the displaced air allowed to escape back into the syringe to avoid excess pressure in the vial. Once the drug has been reconstituted and the correct dose retrieved, an alcohol-moistened gauze square should be wrapped around the top of the vial and the needle. The needle should then be slowly pulled out of the vial. Any air bubbles that are present should be injected into an alcohol-soaked cotton ball and discarded in the appropriate waste container. The cap should be carefully placed on the needle and the syringe put into a sealable plastic bag and labeled. As a general rule, needles should not be recapped, although sometimes this is not possible.

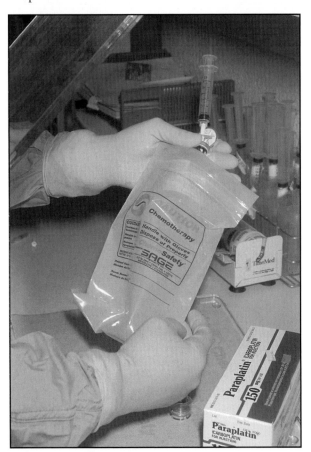

Figure 10-5: *Drugs and syringes should be placed in plastic bags to contain any inadvertent spills during transportation in the hospital.*

It is extremely important to label all chemotherapeutic drugs. All syringes, fluid bags, pill bottles, and so forth must have a chemotherapy label listing the drug name and dose. The drug vial should be put into a sealable plastic bag to be stored in a refrigerator or discarded according to storage instructions. Every drug has a package insert that states the expiration date and storage conditions.

All nonsharp materials used in drug preparation should be placed into a large sealable plastic bag, and all sharps must be placed in a puncture-proof container. Once everything is discarded and all vials and syringes are inside sealable plastic bags, gloves should be removed by rolling them off the hands; they can then be placed in the plastic bag with the rest of the items. Care must be taken to avoid touching the outside of the gloves.

Bags containing the drugs should be sealed before protective gear is removed. If protective garments are contaminated during drug preparation, they should be discarded and replaced immediately. Thorough hand washing following drug preparation is strongly recommended to remove any potential drug residues. A large, clearly labeled barrel or chemotherapy waste container should be kept in the drug preparation area for full waste bags (containing contaminated gauze squares, cotton balls, and the like) and all contaminated safety gear (e.g., gowns, gloves, masks).

When preparing a drug to be delivered by IV drip infusion, it is a good idea to prime the administration set by filling the fluid lines with diluent from the bag before the chemotherapeutic agent is added (Figure 10-2). This reduces the risk of exposure when connecting the drip set to the patient. Once reconstituted, the drug should be slowly injected into the bag. A gauze square wrapped around the injection port as the needle is withdrawn helps prevent aerosolization of the drug. The fluid that contains the drug should be stored in a labeled, sealable bag until it is administered. Again, materials should be discarded appropriately.

Some chemotherapy agents are prepared for oral administration. When preparing or administering pills, nonporous latex gloves are strongly recommended. Cytotoxic powder has been found as far as 12 inches away from where tablets are crushed or split; therefore drugs are best dispensed in whole tablets only. When small quantities of some orally administered drugs are needed, they may be prepared from the injectable formulation for use as an elixir (rather than splitting tablets). When crushing or splitting of pills cannot be avoided—and especially if a safety hood is not available—gown, goggles, and respirator mask are mandatory, and the preparation surface must be well cleaned afterward. Oral medications that are to be dispensed to owners for home administration should be placed in clearly labeled containers with a warning label. Owners should wear latex gloves when administering oral agents to their pets and should return empty vials to the veterinarian for proper disposal. Detailed information about how owners should administer and dispose of these medications should accompany each prescription. Latex gloves should be worn when handling bodily fluids or stool (including disposal of litter) from patients that have received chemotherapeutic agents. Caution should be employed to reduce aersolization of bodily waste.

KEY POINT

Caregivers should be empowered with information about the disease and decisions regarding the treatment. They should be considered as the most important members of the veterinary health care team.

Intralesional injections consisting of a cytotoxic agent mixed with a vehicle (e.g., bovine collagen matrix, sterile sesame oil, or some other biodegradable polymer or material that acts to slowly release the the drug into the tumor) have been recommended for some localized cancers. These mixtures are prepared in the biologic safety cabinet, but two Luer-lok® syringes, one containing the cytotoxic agent and one containing the vehicle, should be prepared. Each agent should be placed into a syringe with sufficient capacity to contain both liquids when combined. The syringes are attached to a three-way stopcock, and the two liquids can then be rapidly mixed between the syringes to create an oily emulsion. The syringe that now contains all of the mixture should be detached after covering the attachment with an alcohol-moistened gauze swab to prevent aerosolization, and a needle is attached. The remaining syringe and stopcock should be discarded as contaminated waste.

It is preferable to mix multiple small volumes of drug in this way rather than a single large volume because separation of drug from vehicle may occur rapidly, thereby reducing the efficacy of the treatment. Likewise, the drug-vehicle mixture should be administered soon after preparation. If a delay is encountered, the drug can be remixed with its vehicle using a new syringe and three-way stopcock; gloves, mask, goggles, and a gown must be worn. It may be wise to mix inside a sealable plastic bag. The needles on used syringes should not be recapped. All materials should be disposed of as contaminated waste.

When chemotherapeutic agents are spilled, the contaminated area should be closed and traffic rerouted. Commercially available "spill kits" should be used when possible. The following recommendations should be followed: Wear two pairs of nonpowdered latex gloves, wash skin with soap and water upon contact with the drug, clean minor spills with 70% isopropyl alcohol, and decontaminate large spills with a neutralizing agent or high pH soap. Protective clothing should be worn when cleaning up fecal matter and urine for approximately 48 hours after the administration of chemotherapeutic agents.

THE HEALTH CARE TEAM

Cancer chemotherapy requires a team approach; team members include the veterinarian, who listens, diagnoses, and prescribes therapy, the animal health technicians or nurses, who provide care, information, and technical expertise, and the receptionist, who informs, coordinates, and enables the caregiver and the health care team. The team approach also involves extended team members, such as the attending or consulting oncologist or internist, pharmacist, and radiologist; these members are a vital link in the advanced care of the cancer patient, especially when it comes to chemotherapy. Yet the most important members of the team are the caregivers/clients. When the caregiver is recognized, enabled, and empowered with information and the ability to extend care to his or her best friend, compassionate care can really be delivered. This empowering process involves giving detailed oral and written information about the cancer and chemotherapy, providing ongoing intellectual and emotional support via the entire team, and assuring that the caregiver understands and is able to provide continual and seamless care at home. The following information summarizes the technical procedures associated with the administration of chemotherapy, yet the most important aspects of providing this type of care are dependent on the ability of the health care team to extend compassionate care to the patient and the caregiver.

ADMINISTERING CHEMOTHERAPEUTIC AGENTS

Chemotherapeutic agents can be administered via several routes: intravenous, intramuscular, intracavitary, subcutaneous, intralesional (with a vehicle to slow absorption),

TABLE 10-1
Methods of Administration

Method of Administration	Sample Drugs
Intracavitary	Carboplatin, mitoxantrone
Intralesional	Carboplatin, cisplatin, bleomycin
Intramuscular	L-Asparaginase
Intravenous	
Butterfly catheter	Vincristine, vinblastine
Over-the-needle or indwelling catheter	Doxorubicin, mitoxantrone
Oral	Cyclophosphamide, chlorambucil, melphalan
Subcutaneous	Bleomycin

and oral (Table 10-1). Intrathecal and intraarterial administration are used less commonly in feline medicine. Regardless of the route of administration or who is administering the drugs, latex gloves should be worn when handling cytotoxic agents. Wearing a gown, goggles, and mask minimizes the risk of exposure.

KEY POINT

Doses should always be double-checked. Care should be taken with drugs for which milligrams do not equal milliliters (e.g., doxorubicin, which is 2 mg/ml). Chemotherapeutic drugs can be toxic enough at the correct dose! If there is a question about anything, stop! Do not proceed until all questions are answered. It is impossible to be too careful when dealing with chemotherapeutic agents.

Dosing

The dosing of chemotherapy also requires a team approach. Because many of the drugs used to treat cancer can have serious, potentially life-threatening side effects and the margin of safety is not as great as with other medications, team members must constantly check and recheck dosages, labels, and administration procedures. The safety of the patient, caregiver, and the veterinary health care team must be paramount.

There has recently been discussion in the literature about the validity of dosing chemotherapeutic agents using body surface area (BSA) in square meters (m²).[3-6] These studies have shown that this dosing method may not be ideal for all veterinary patients, especially smaller animals such as cats, in which increased toxicity may be observed.[6] The best known example is doxorubicin: The standard dose of 30 mg/m² may be too high, and a dose of 1 to 1.1 mg/kg (or 20 to 25 mg/m²) is more routinely used in feline medicine. Until a better dosing scheme is developed, many chemotherapeutic agents will continue to be dosed on a square meter basis.

General Concepts in Calculating and Administering Doses

1. Convert weight in pounds (lb) to kilograms (kg) by dividing by 2.2. An 11 lb cat weighs 5 kg (11 ÷ 2.2 = 5).
2. Weight in kilograms can then be found on a weight to BSA conversion table (Table 10-2).
3. Determine the dose of a drug (in this example, vincristine) by multiplying the dosage (0.5 to 0.75 mg/m²) by the patient's body surface area (m²).
4. Before the quantity of drug is drawn up or obtained, the

TABLE 10-2
Converting kg to m² in Cats

kg	m²
2.0	0.159
2.5	0.184
3.0	0.208
3.5	0.231
4.0	0.252
4.5	0.273
5.0	0.292
5.5	0.311
6.0	0.330
6.5	0.348
7.0	0.366
7.5	0.383
8.0	0.400
8.5	0.416
9.0	0.432
9.5	0.449
10.0	0.464

concentration (mg/ml or mg/pill or capsule) of the chemotherapeutic agent is checked. For example, doxorubicin (and some other drugs) has a concentration of 2 mg/ml, so it is necessary to divide the milligrams by 2 to determine how many milliliters to administer. If the drug is in pill or capsule form, the amount to be administered is rounded down to the next whole tablet. Chemotherapy pills or capsules must never be split, crushed, reformulated, or repackaged to prevent inadvertent exposure of the handler to cytotoxic drugs and/or overdose of the patient.

KEY POINT

If the neutrophil count is below 3,000/μl, the drug should not be given and the CBC should be checked again in 3 to 4 days. A CBC should also be performed 7 to 10 days after administration of any drug that has the potential to cause myelosuppression to ensure the neutrophil count is above 1,500/μl.

5. Before the drug is administered, the dose and results of the CBC are double-checked. If the neutrophil count is below 3,000/μl, administration of myelosuppressive drugs (e.g., doxorubicin, cyclophosphamide) should be postponed and the CBC rechecked in 3 to 4 days.
6. A CBC is sometimes obtained 7 days after administering the first dose of any potentially myelosuppressive drug (7 days is the neutrophil nadir for most drugs; refer to drug tables in Chapter 11 for individual varia-

tion). If the neutrophil count is below 1,500/μl 7 days after treatment, the drug dose may be reduced by 25%, especially if the cat demonstrates clinical signs relating to neutropenia. The new dose can be administered subsequently, assuming the patient does well with the reduced dose. Doses can then be increased by increments of 10% until the originally calculated "full" dose is reached, provided the patient continues to tolerate the lower doses.

7. Anorexia is a common side effect of many chemotherapeutic agents in cats. If severe or accompanied by more than 10% loss of body weight, a dose reduction should be considered. A good rule of thumb is 25%, although the dose may subsequently be increased by increments of 10% if no further anorexia is observed.

Intravenous Administration

Many chemotherapeutic agents are administered IV. Because some of these agents are vesicants or irritants, every attempt must be made to ensure that the veins are cared for and that catheters are placed as cleanly and atraumatically as possible. As a general rule, peripheral veins should never be used for venipuncture to collect blood samples to ensure that the veins are preserved for catheter placement only. Chemotherapeutic agents are usually administered by butterfly catheter, over-the-needle catheter, or a through-the-needle intracatheter (such as used for central venous access).

Peripheral vessels are preferred for IV drug administration because of the ease of monitoring for drug extravasation. Regardless of the type of catheter used, certain preparatory steps should be taken. The leg to be used should be clipped at the site of injection and prepared using aseptic technique. When a drug is known to be a vesicant, an indwelling catheter should be placed, particularly if the drug is not being administered as a bolus.

Drugs should never be administered when venipuncture is less than perfect (i.e., when the vein is entered more than once); another leg should be used instead. If another leg is unavailable, the first venipuncture site should be allowed to clot before another attempt is made proximal to that site. A second venipuncture should never be attempted distal to the site of a failed attempt. It is a good idea to alternate and record the veins being used to allow them to recover between administrations.

The catheter should be flushed with nonheparinized 0.9% NaCl (minimum, 10 ml) before and after each drug administration to determine patency. When multiple drugs are being given, the catheter should be flushed between agents. Nonheparinized 0.9% NaCl is recommended because heparin causes precipitates to form when mixed with some drugs (e.g., doxorubicin).

The catheter and leg should be monitored constantly during drug administration to detect any extravasation. If the catheter is to be secured, use only one piece of tape and ensure that visualization of the injection site, the area surrounding the site, and the leg proximal to the site is not obscured.

It is important to check whether there is a specific rate at which a drug should be administered to minimize toxicity. For example, undiluted doxorubicin should be given at a maximum rate of 1 ml/minute whereas vincristine can be given as a bolus. Alternatively, doxorubicin can be placed in 35 ml of 0.9% NaCl and administered over 10 to 15 minutes. The drug should be injected slowly and evenly to prevent excessive pressure to the vein and leakage of the drug around the needle or catheter.

After the drug has been administered and the catheter flushed, a piece of gauze or an alcohol-soaked cotton ball should be placed (with a gloved hand) over the needle as it is withdrawn from the injection port or over the catheter as it is removed from the vein; this minimizes drug aerosolization. All of the drug should be flushed through the catheter without reaspirating the catheter, as reaspirating at this time allows diluted drug to remain in the catheter. A cotton ball can be taped over the insertion site after the catheter is removed, and pressure is applied for several minutes.

All materials should be discarded into appropriate chemotherapy waste containers. Syringes and needles should be placed in a puncture- and leak-proof container that is clearly marked as containing hazardous or chemotherapeutic waste. Even though latex gloves are always worn, it is important to wash hands thoroughly after every drug administration.

Butterfly Catheter (Figure 10-6)

A butterfly catheter is generally recommended when administering a small amount (3 ml or less) of drug as a bolus. When using a butterfly catheter, all materials should be organized and readily available (within arm's reach) before starting. Equipment needed includes two or three 3 to 5 ml

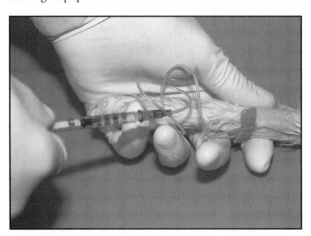

Figure 10-6: *Butterfly catheters are ideal for IV administration of small volumes of drugs (e.g., vincristine). Care should be taken to ensure that the catheter is patent to prevent extravasation.*

syringes of nonheparinized 0.9% NaCl for flushing the catheter, the labeled drug, an alcohol swab, the butterfly catheter, and a pressure bandage. Place the labeled syringes on a pad or a plastic bag and line them up in order of use. The needles should be removed (or the caps loosened) to help the administration proceed swiftly and smoothly.

When all of the drug has been delivered, the syringe should be detached and a saline flush attached quickly to prevent any drug from leaking out. When very small doses are administered (e.g., vincristine), a small amount of leakage can result in loss of a substantial portion of the dose. The following methods can be used to reduce leakage:

- Produce an air bubble at the bottom of the syringe containing the drug (i.e., at the end farthest from the needle) so that air, rather than drug, leaks out.
- Clamp or kink the catheter while changing syringes; however, this technique is cumbersome and may dislodge the catheter.
- Use a three-way stopcock.
- Use an injection port at the end of the butterfly catheter so that detaching syringes during administration is unneccesary.

Intravenous Over-the-Needle Catheter (Figure 10-7)

Generally, drugs that are to be given as a bolus (but over a period of minutes) or in a volume greater than 3 ml are given through IV over-the-needle catheters (e.g., Abbotcath®-T). Over-the-needle catheters should be used for doxorubicin administration, for which a slow rate of delivery is important to prevent an allergic reaction. It is preferable to place the catheter while wearing latex gloves, but it may be placed before drugs are prepared as long as pa-

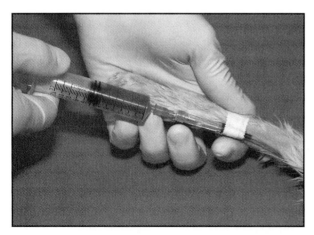

Figure 10-7: Intravenous over-the-needle catheters are ideal for IV administration of slow bolus infusions of drugs (e.g., doxorubicin). The area of the injection site, the injection port, and the leg above the injection site should be clearly visible to the person administering the drug so that any extravasation or leakage can be attended to promptly.

tency is reconfirmed before drug administration.

For over-the-needle catheter administration, long, clear, male adapter injection ports allow for better viewing of the flashback of blood and the drug being administered. In addition, these plugs allow the person administering the drug to determine when all of the drug has been flushed out of the catheter at the end of the procedure.

Once the catheter has been placed, a 4 × 4 inch gauze square should be folded in half and slipped under the injection cap to absorb any drug that may leak out of the injection cap during administration. Needles should be inserted as far as possible into the injection port to allow for easier flushing of residual drug after injection.

Continuous Intravenous Infusion

An indwelling catheter should be used when drugs (e.g., cytosine arabinoside, ifosfamide) are to be administered over a long period (6 to 48 hours).[6] The catheter site and all connections in the IV line should be monitored frequently for patency and leakage. The patient must be prevented from chewing or disconnecting the IV line.

During long periods of drug administration, disposal of contaminated waste, particularly urine, becomes important. When the patient or any waste is handled, latex gloves, a gown, goggles, and a mask should be worn to reduce the risk of exposure to excreted active metabolites. Cages or excreta should not be hosed, because this aerosolizes the drug and distributes it more widely. All waste, including litter material, should be discarded as contaminated material.

Intramuscular, Subcutaneous, or Intralesional Administration

IM injections are administered in the normal fashion, but latex gloves should be worn. Because L-asparaginase can cause an anaphylactic reaction when given IV, the syringe must be checked for blood to ensure that a vessel has not been inadvertently entered before injecting the drug IM. Preferred sites of injection include well-muscled areas such as the caudal thigh region or lumbar musculature. Intralesional chemotherapy is always administered as a suspension in oil or other vehicle, not as pure drug. Latex gloves, goggles, and a protective gown should be worn when administering intralesional chemotherapy, and it is important to watch the area carefully for any leakage of the chemotherapeutic agent. If leakage occurs, the area should be swabbed and cleaned with soap and water and the cleaning materials disposed of as hazardous waste.

Oral Administration

Wearing latex gloves is necessary when administering pills. The patient is given the pills in the normal fashion. It is important to assure oneself that the patient has indeed swallowed the pill; it may be helpful to follow pill administration with water given via syringe. If owners are to administer oral chemotherapy, they must be instructed to wear disposable protective latex gloves and wash their hands immediately after administration.

Intracavitary Administration

Some chemotherapeutic agents (e.g., carboplatin) can be administered into body cavities (thorax or abdomen).[1,4] Both the person administering the drug and the one restraining the animal should wear gloves. As with IV administration, the IV line needs to be primed *before* the drug is added to the bag. The diluent should be warmed to body temperature before the drug is added and the solution administered.

For thoracic administration, the patient is placed in lateral recumbency and the injection site is aseptically prepared. The right side is preferred, and the area of the cardiac notch provides the least risk of lung puncture. The area is infiltrated with lidocaine, and an 18 ga rigid plastic IV cannula is inserted between the ribs and flushed with a minimum of 12 ml of warm saline to ensure a patent pathway. If there is resistance to the flush or if the cat appears uncomfortable or coughs, the cannula should be removed and a new one inserted.

For abdominal administration, the patient is placed in dorsal recumbency and a midline site caudal to the umbilicus is used. The site chosen should be caudal enough to avoid the spleen. Allowing the patient to urinate before administration reduces the risk of bladder puncture. The site is aseptically prepared, and the catheter should be placed as described for thoracic administration.

Once the patency is determined, the fluid line is attached and the drug is administered. A maximum volume of 60 ml should be infused into the thoracic cavity and 250 ml into the abdominal cavity. The fluid should flow fairly easily into the cavity. If the fluid drip slows or is intermittent, the cannula can be adjusted slightly. The area should be monitored constantly to make sure the fluid is not being administered SQ. Once the bag is empty, the IV line should be turned off; a piece of gauze should be wrapped around the cannula and the cannula slowly removed. At this point, the person restraining the animal should hold an alcohol-moistened gauze square over the site and apply pressure to stop any bleeding and/or leakage that may occur. Finally, the patient should be allowed to move around for a few minutes to allow the drug to distribute through the entire cavity. All materials must be discarded as contaminated waste.

REFERENCES

1. *OSHA Work Practice Guidelines for Personnel: Dealing with Cytotoxic Drugs.* OSHA Instructional Publication 8-1.1, Washington DC, Office of Occupational Medicine, 1986.
2. Falck K, Grohn P, Sorsa M, et al: Mutagenicity in urine of nurses handling cytotoxic drugs. *Lancet* 1:1250–1255, 1979.
3. Chabner BA: Principles of cancer therapy, in Wyngaarden JB, Smith LH (eds): *Cecil Textbook of Medicine.* Philadelphia, WB Saunders, 1982, p 1032.
4. Madewell BR, Theilen GH: Chemotherapy, in Theilen GH, Madewell BR (eds): *Veterinary Cancer Medicine.* Philadelphia, Lea & Febiger, 1979, pp 157–183.
5. Madewell BR: Adverse effects of chemotherapy, in Kirk RW (ed): *Current Veterinary Therapy IIX.* Philadelphia, WB Saunders, 1983, p 419.
6. Ogilvie GK: Principles of oncology, in Morgan RV (ed): *Handbook of Small Animal Internal Medicine.* Philadelphia, Churchill & Livingston, 1992, pp 799–812.

THERAPEUTIC & SUPPORTIVE PROCEDURES

CHEMOTHERAPY—PROPERTIES, USES, AND PATIENT MANAGEMENT

11

Gregory K. Ogilvie and Antony S. Moore

Common Drugs	Potential Toxicoses	Reported Indications
Alkylating Agents		
CCNU	BA; hepatotoxicity; thrombocytopenia	Lymphoma; mast cell tumor
Chlorambucil	BAG; cerebellar toxicity	Chronic lymphocytic leukemia; lymphoma
Cyclophosphamide	BAG; rarely, sterile hemorrhagic cystitis	Lymphoma; sarcoma; mammary adenocarcinoma
Ifosfamide	BAG	Soft tissue sarcoma; lymphoma
Melphalan	BAG	Multiple myeloma
Mustargen	BAG	Lymphoma
Procarbazine	BAG	Lymphoma
Thiotepa	BAG	Transitional cell carcinoma
Antimetabolites		
Cytosine arabinoside	BAG	Lymphoma; leukemia
Methotrexate	BAG	Lymphoma
Antibiotics		
Actinomycin D	BAG; perivascular slough	Lymphoma
Doxorubicin	BAG; perivascular slough; allergic reaction during administration; anorexia and weight loss; rarely, renal failure; cardiomyopathy	Lymphoma; sarcoma, including hemangiosarcoma; thyroid carcinoma; mammary adenocarcinoma
Mitoxantrone	BAG	Lymphoma; mammary adenocarcinoma; squamous cell carcinoma
Enzymes		
L-Asparaginase	Anaphylaxis; DIC pancreatitis; pain on injection	Lymphoma
Vinca Alkaloids		
Vinblastine	BAG; peripheral neuropathy; perivascular slough	Lymphoma; mast cell tumor
Vincristine	BAG[a]; peripheral neuropathy; perivascular slough	Lymphoma; sarcoma; mast cell tumor; thrombocytopenia
Hormones		
Prednisone	Iatrogenic Cushing's syndrome	Lymphoma; mast cell tumor

Common Drugs	Potential Toxicoses	Reported Indications
Miscellaneous Agents		
Carboplatin	BAG; nephrotoxicity; rarely, emesis	Squamous cell carcinoma; germinal cell tumors; transitional cell carcinoma
Cisplatin	Death (with IV administration); local swelling, necrosis, and edema (with intralesional administration)	Squamous cell carcinoma
Paclitaxel	BAG; diluent Cremophor® EL causes acute allergic reaction on administration	Mammary adenocarcinoma
Piroxicam	GI ulceration and nephrotoxicity	Transitional cell carcinoma; squamous cell carcinoma; pain relief

aBone marrow suppression is dose dependent.
BAG = **B**one marrow suppression, **A**lopecia, and **G**astrointestinal toxicity (anorexia and weight loss are the most common GI toxicities in cats).

Advances in the use of chemotherapy to treat tumors in animals are continually being made. Before anticancer drugs are used, practitioners must understand the principles and properties of chemotherapeutic agents and the subsequent management of animals treated with these drugs.

GENERAL PRINCIPLES OF CANCER THERAPY

Before a therapeutic strategy can be defined and instituted, the patient should be fully evaluated and stabilized and the tumor identified histologically and staged to determine the extent of the disease. In addition, both the client and veterinarian need to be aware of:

- The potential benefits and toxicoses associated with the administration of chemotherapeutic agents—Both parties should be committed to preventing toxicosis from developing and promptly resolving it if it does occur.
- The need to follow the treatment protocol.
- The expenses associated with chemotherapy (fortunately, many chemotherapeutic agents are becoming available as generic products at a fraction of the cost of the patented parent drug).

Chemotherapeutic agents are used to induce remission and for intensification, consolidation, and maintenance therapy. A patient is considered to be in *remission* when all clinical evidence of a tumor has disappeared. *Intensification,* which is introduced after remission has been attained, involves the administration of a chemotherapeutic agent with a different mechanism of action in an attempt to kill any resistant tumor cells. *Consolidation,* which also takes place after a patient is in remission, is the phase of treatment in which different drugs are administered to improve clinical response by reducing the microscopic tumor burden.

Maintenance therapy refers to the drugs used to keep the patient in remission. Consolidation and maintenance therapies are more important in the treatment of hematopoietic tumors than solid tumors. Chemotherapeutic agents also can be used as *adjuvant therapy* following another treatment modality to delay recurrence and increase survival time. *Neoadjuvant therapy* is used to decrease the bulk of primary tumors with chemotherapy before surgery or radiation.

The beneficial effects of chemotherapy are inversely proportional to tumor size; therefore whenever anticancer drugs are not being used as adjuvants, the tumor should be reduced to its smallest volume and number of cells with surgery or radiation therapy before chemotherapy is initiated. To use chemotherapeutic agents to their fullest advantage, clinicians should be knowledgeable about a drug's indications for use, doses, timing of administration, resistance, and toxicity. Chemotherapy should be considered for patients with such malignancies as leukemia, lymphoma, multiple myeloma, and other hematopoietic tumors or with highly malignant tumors that metastasize rapidly.

KEY POINT

The most effective dose of chemotherapeutic agents is often very close to the toxic dose, and thus careful client education and vigilant medical monitoring and care are essential.

DRUGS

Compared with multiple drug regimens, single drug regimens are less toxic, less expensive, and require less time for clients and the veterinary health care team. Conversely, multiple drug protocols are believed to be more effective—

especially for lymphoid malignancies—furthermore, because a combination of drugs is used, resistance develops more slowly. Currently in veterinary medicine, however, few multiple drug protocols have been shown to be more effective than single agent protocols for the treatment of nonlymphoid malignancies.

Doses

The objective in determining doses of chemotherapeutic agents is to minimize toxicity while maximizing effectiveness. The most effective dose of chemotherapeutic agents is often very close to the toxic dose. In addition, a given dose of a drug kills a constant fraction of cells regardless of the number of cells present at the start of therapy. Doses of chemotherapeutic agents are often given on the basis of body surface area (BSA) in square meters (m^2). One notable exception is doxorubicin; because this drug is neither excreted nor metabolized in a complex fashion, recent recommendations are to dose it on a mg/kg basis. All other antineoplastic agents seem to be metabolized or excreted in a complex fashion and thus should be dosed on a m^2 basis. Table 10-2 provides a chart for converting weight in kilograms to BSA.

KEY POINT

The response to chemotherapy is inversely proportional to the amount of tumor present. In addition, the success of therapy is directly related to appropriate drug selection, dosages, and timing of therapy.

Dosing can depend on many factors, including an animal's ability to metabolize and eliminate chemotherapeutic agents. Table 11-1 reviews conditions in which doses may need to be changed depending on the way the drug is metabolized.

Timing

The timing of administration of antitumor drugs is critical. Unlike many tumor cells, normal cells have repair mechanisms that are able to correct cellular damage. Therefore cytotoxic drugs must be given at proper intervals to allow the tumor cells to die while normal cells recover. An improper administration schedule results in either excess toxicity or a lack of antitumor activity.

Resistance

In contrast to normal cells, most tumor cells develop resistance to antitumor medicine. Resistance is one of the limiting factors in tumor chemotherapy. This resistance results from an acquired or induced phenomenon known as *multiple drug resistance* (MDR), which is caused by a cell membrane protein that literally pumps out cellular toxins, such as chemotherapeutic agents. Certain anticancer drugs (e.g., doxorubicin, paclitaxel) are eliminated from the cell by this mechanism even though they have different molecular structures, but there seems to be little cross-resistance among alkylating agents (e.g., cyclophosphamide, chlorambucil, melphalan). Resistance to other drugs, such as the enzyme L-asparaginase, is induced when antibodies are formed against the drug, thereby causing a rapid destruction of the substance after administration.

Toxicity (Table 11-2)

Several chemotherapeutic agents and their toxicities are noted in the Clinical Briefing at the beginning of this chapter. Most of these agents kill or damage rapidly dividing cells. The most clinically important toxicoses include **B**one marrow suppression, **A**lopecia, and **G**astrointestinal toxicity (BAG). Methods of identifying and treating some of the more common side effects are discussed beginning on page 66.

TABLE 11-1
Possible Effect of Organ Dysfunction on Dosing of Select Chemotherapeutic Agents

Drug	Critical Organ	Dose Modifications
Bleomycin	Kidney	Decrease initial dose by as much as 50%–75% if creatinine clearance is <25 ml/min/m^2 or directly related to the severity of renal disease
Carboplatin	Kidney	Dose reduction is directly proportional to creatinine clearance
Cyclophosphamide	Kidney, liver	Decrease initial dose by as much as 50%–75% if creatinine clearance is <25 ml/min/m^2 or directly related to the severity of renal disease; because the liver is necessary to activate the drug, liver disease may warrant dose modification
Doxorubicin	Liver	Decrease initial dose by as much as 50% when bilirubin is >2 mg/dl
Methotrexate	Kidney	Dose reduction is directly proportional to creatinine clearance or directly related to the severity of renal disease

TABLE 11-2
Toxicities Associated with Some Commercially Available Anticancer Drugs and Hormones

Drug	Acute Toxicity	Delayed Toxicity
L-Asparaginase	Anaphylaxis or hypersensitivity (less likely if given IM), nausea and vomiting, fever, chills, abdominal pain, and hyperglycemia leading to coma	CNS depression or hyperexcitability, acute hemorrhagic pancreatitis, coagulation defects, thrombosis, renal damage, and hepatic damage (not reported but seen in other species)
Bleomycin	Nausea and vomiting, fever, anaphylaxis, and other allergic reactions	Pneumonitis and pulmonary fibrosis, rash, and alopecia
Busulfan	Nausea and vomiting; rarely, diarrhea	Bone marrow suppression, pulmonary infiltrates and fibrosis, hyperpigmentation, alopecia, and leukemia
Cisplatin[a]	Death if given IV; give only intralesionally	Death if given IV
Carmustine[b]	Nausea and vomiting and local phlebitis	Leukopenia and thrombocytopenia (may be prolonged), pulmonary fibrosis (may be irreversible), renal damage, and reversible liver damage
Chlorambucil	Bone marrow suppression, pulmonary infiltrates and fibrosis, leukemia, hepatic toxicity, and hallucinations	Bone marrow suppression
Cyclophosphamide	Nausea and vomiting and Type I (anaphylactoid) hypersensitivity	Bone marrow suppression, hemorrhagic cystitis, bladder fibrosis and cancer, sterility (may be temporary), pulmonary infiltrates and fibrosis, hyponatremia, and leukemia
Cytarabine HCl	Nausea and vomiting, diarrhea, and anaphylaxis	Bone marrow suppression, oral ulceration, hepatic damage, and fever (not reported but seen in other species)
Dacarbazine[c]	Nausea and vomiting, diarrhea, anaphylaxis, and pain on administration	Bone marrow suppression, renal impairment, hepatic necrosis, photosensitivity, and alopecia
Dactinomycin	Nausea and vomiting, diarrhea, local reaction and phlebitis, and anaphylactoid reaction	Stomatitis, oral ulceration, bone marrow suppression, alopecia, folliculitis, and dermatitis in previously irradiated areas
Daunorubicin	Nausea and vomiting, diarrhea, severe local tissue damage and necrosis on extravasation, transient ECG changes, and anaphylactoid reaction	Bone marrow suppression, cardiotoxicity (may be irreversible), alopecia, anorexia, diarrhea, and fever and chills
Doxorubicin	Nausea and vomiting, severe local tissue damage and necrosis on extravasation, diarrhea and colitis, transient ECG changes, ventricular arrhythmia, anaphylactoid reaction, and urticaria and pruritus after one injection	Bone marrow suppression, renal damage, cardiotoxicity, stomatitis, anorexia, diarrhea, fever, and alopecia
Etoposide VP16-213[b]	Nausea and vomiting, profound hypotension, anaphylaxis, cutaneous reactions, diarrhea, and fever	Bone marrow suppression, peripheral neuropathy, allergic reactions, hepatic damage, and alopecia
Fluorouracil[a]	Contraindicated: Death	Death
Hydroxyurea[c]	Nausea and vomiting	Bone marrow suppression, stomatitis, dysuria, and alopecia
Lomustine	Nausea and vomiting	Delayed leukopenia and thrombocytopenia (may be prolonged), transient elevation of transaminase activity, neurologic reactions, and pulmonary fibrosis
Mechlorethamine[c]	Nausea and vomiting, local reaction, and phlebitis	Bone marrow suppression, diarrhea, oral ulcers, pulmonary infiltrates and fibrosis, leukemia, and alopecia
Melphalan	Mild nausea and hypersensitivity reactions	Bone marrow suppression (especially platelets), pulmonary infiltrates and fibrosis, and leukemia
Methotrexate	Nausea and vomiting, diarrhea, fever, and anaphylaxis	Oral and GI ulcers, bone marrow suppression, hepatic toxicity (including cirrhosis)
6-Mercaptopurine	Nausea and vomiting and diarrhea	Bone marrow suppression and cholestasis, hepatic necrosis (rare), oral and intestinal ulcers, and pancreatitis
Mitotane	Nausea and vomiting and diarrhea	Adrenal insufficiency, CNS depression, rash, albuminuria, and hypertension
Mitoxantrone	Nausea and vomiting	Bone marrow suppression

(continued)

TABLE 11-2 (continued)

Drug	Acute Toxicity	Delayed Toxicity
Thiotepa	Nausea and vomiting; local pain and perivascular slough with extravasation	Bone marrow suppression, pulmonary infiltrates and fibrosis, and leukemia
Vinblastine	Nausea and vomiting; local reaction and phlebitis with extravasation	Bone marrow suppression, stomatitis, loss of deep tendon reflexes, jaw pain, muscle pain, paralytic ileus, inappropriate ADH secretion, and alopecia
Vincristine	Local slough with extravasation	Peripheral neuropathy, mild bone marrow suppression, constipation, paralytic ileus, inappropriate ADH secretion, hepatic damage, jaw pain, seizures, and alopecia

ADH = antidiuretic hormone; CNS = central nervous system; ECG = electrocardiogram.
Adapted from Ogilvie GK: Principles of oncology, in Morgan RV (ed): *Handbook of Small Animal Internal Medicine.* Philadelphia, Churchill Livingston, 1992, pp 799–812.
[a]Not recommended in cats.
[b]Not reported to be used in cats.
[c]Still investigational in cats.

Bone Marrow Toxicity (Table 11-3)

Many antitumor drugs cause a decrease in the number of blood cells days to weeks after administration. Neutropenia and thrombocytopenia are the early signs of bone marrow suppression. Anemia may develop later because RBCs have a longer life span. Clinical signs may include those related to sepsis, petechial and ecchymotic hemorrhages, pallor, and weakness. Many animals are physically normal despite low WBC and platelet counts, so only patients exhibiting clinical signs should be treated. The treatment of clinically significant bone marrow toxicity includes using aseptic techniques when placing indwelling devices (e.g., catheters), minimizing trauma, and controlling any bleeding with prolonged application of direct pressure or cold packs.

If an animal develops a fever or becomes septic, urine, blood, and, if indicated, material obtained via transtracheal aspiration should be cultured. The affected animal should be treated with broad-spectrum bactericidal antibiotics (e.g., cephalosporins, trimethoprim-sulfa) until results of culture and sensitivity testing are available. Do not delay antibiotic treatment while awaiting culture results. In addition, the patient should be supported with fluids, warmth, and nutritional therapy and given transfusions of fresh whole blood (collected in plastic containers) or specific cell lines as needed.

The availability of recombinant human granulocyte colony-stimulating factor now makes it possible to treat

KEY POINT

Resistance of the tumor to chemotherapy is a consistent and ever-present threat. Use chemotherapeutic agents at appropriate doses and schedules from the outset to minimize resistance.

TABLE 11-3
Myelosuppressive Potential of Some Commonly Used Chemotherapeutic Agents in Veterinary Medicine

Highly Myelosuppressive	Moderately Myelosuppressive	Mildly Myelosuppressive
Paclitaxel	Methotrexate	Corticosteroids
Doxorubicin	Melphalan	L-Asparaginase[a]
Vinblastine	Procarbazine	Vincristine[a]
Cyclophosphamide		Bleomycin
Actinomycin D		Chlorambucil
Busulfan		
Hydroxyurea		
Mitoxantrone		
Carboplatin		
Mustargen		
CCNU		
Ifosfamide		

[a]Myelosuppression can occur if L-asparaginase and vincristine are administered concurrently.

bone marrow toxicity by boosting endogenous production of neutrophils. Recombinant human erythropoietin is useful in treating cats with nonregenerative anemia secondary to chemotherapy or the underlying malignancy. Caution is advised when using recombinant human products because antibodies to these foreign proteins can develop in approximately 3 to 6 weeks and occasionally may react with the patient's own hematopoietic growth factors. The drug(s) that induced the bone marrow suppression should be discontinued until blood counts have recovered; subsequent doses of that myelosuppressive drug should be reduced (e.g., decrease cyclophosphamide doses by 25%).

Alopecia

Alopecia is an uncommon complication of chemotherapy but is often a major concern for caregivers. Cats can lose their whiskers, but the development of generalized alopecia is extremely rare. Coat color changes, however, are common during prolonged courses of chemotherapy.

Gastrointestinal Toxicity

The clinical signs of this relatively common side effect include vomiting, anorexia, and diarrhea. The treatment includes antiemetics (e.g., metoclopramide, chlorpromazine), protectants and absorbents (e.g., Kaopectate®), and broad-spectrum antibiotics, if indicated. In addition, support with fluids, warmth, and nutritional therapy should be provided. As a preventative measure, some clinicians dispense metoclopramide to the client to initiate therapy at home when a medication with the potential to cause nausea is administered. Clients may be instructed to give metoclopramide even if nausea and vomiting are not noted, both as a preventative measure and because nausea may be difficult for caregivers to accurately assess. Metoclopramide is preferred because of its overall efficacy and lack of systemic side effects; chlorpromazine may induce the clinically worrisome side effect of sedation.

Anorexia in cats can often be resolved with antiemetics, adequate hydration, pain relief, and administration of the appetite-stimulating drugs cyproheptadine and megestrol acetate. Subsequent doses of that specific chemotherapeutic agent should be reduced by 25%.

Allergic Reactions

Signs of L-asparaginase hypersensitivity include urticaria, vomiting, diarrhea, hypotension, and loss of consciousness soon after administration. These signs can essentially be eliminated by administering the medication IM. Doxorubicin- or paclitaxel-induced allergic reactions include cutaneous hyperemia, intense pruritus, head shaking, and vomiting during administration. These reactions can be reduced substantially by slowing the infusion rate (e.g., give the entire dose over approximately 20 to 30 minutes). Other drugs

that can induce allergic reactions include bleomycin, cytosine arabinoside, and procarbazine. Both etoposide and paclitaxel induce dramatic cutaneous reactions and hypotension during administration, not because of the medication itself but rather the vehicle that keeps each drug in solution.

Treatment for allergic reactions includes immediately discontinuing drug administration and giving epinephrine, diphenhydramine, and glucocorticoids for acute allergic reactions. Premedication with diphenhydramine, cimetidine, and glucocorticoids may prevent or reduce allergic reactions to doxorubicin, paclitaxel, or etoposide; for doxorubicin, simply slowing the infusion rate is sufficient to prevent allergic reactions during administration.

Cardiac Toxicity

Unlike the situation in dogs, doxorubicin has not been shown to induce dose-dependent dilated (congestive) cardiomyopathy and transient dysrhythmias during administration in cats. Until more is known, some oncologists limit the cumulative dose of doxorubicin to 180 to 240 mg/m^2 (six to eight treatments) during a cat's lifetime. While the relative prevalence of doxorubicin-induced cardiotoxicity in cats is unknown, routine echocardiograms and electrocardiograms should be performed on cats given more than 180 mg/m^2 (6–8 mg/kg) of doxorubicin.

Cystitis

Cyclophosphamide has not been reported to induce sterile chemical cystitis in cats, but this has been noted as a rare clinical syndrome (Figure 11-1). Clinical signs include

> **KEY POINT**
>
> *Anaphylaxis caused by the administration of L-asparaginase can be reduced substantially if the drug is administered intramuscularly rather than intravenously or intraperitoneally.*

stranguria, hematuria, and dysuria. Treatment includes replacing cyclophosphamide with another alkylating agent (e.g., chlorambucil) to prevent exacerbation of the condition. Secondary infections are common, so urine should be collected for culture and sensitivity testing anytime cystitis is suspected. Appropriate antibiotics must be administered if cystitis becomes septic. If renal function is normal, piroxicam (0.3 mg/kg PO every other day) may be helpful in reducing adverse effects. The risk of developing cystitis can be decreased by administering cyclophosphamide in the morning (thereby allowing the animal maximum opportunity to urinate during the day), encouraging fluid intake (e.g., salting food) and, if a combination protocol that includes pred-

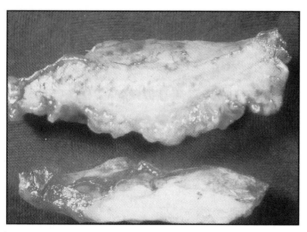

Figure 11-1: *Sterile hemorrhagic cystitis is a rare consequence of cyclophosphamide therapy. The thickened bladder wall secondary to this adverse effect can last for several weeks to months and precludes further administration of this drug.*

nisone is being used, giving cyclophosphamide at the same time as the glucocorticoid (steroids tend to induce polydipsia and secondary polyuria).

KEY POINT

Doxorubicin may cause cardiomyopathy, but whether this is a common problem in the cat is unknown. Until more is known, cats with preexisting cardiac disease should be treated with extreme caution.

Nephrotoxicity

Doxorubicin and carboplatin have been associated with the development of nephrotoxicity in cats, especially those with preexisting renal disease. Identifying animals with evidence of kidney disease and ensuring adequate hydration are essential to limit this problem.

Neurotoxicity

Vincristine, vinblastine, and 5-fluorouracil are reported to cause neurotoxicity in animals. Peripheral neuropathy is associated with vincristine and vinblastine; 5-fluorouracil has been shown to cause severe seizures and disorientation in cats and thus is contraindicated in this species.

KEY POINT

Any chemotherapeutic agent administered IV should be given through a "first stick" patent catheter to prevent drug extravasation.

Local Dermatologic Toxicity

Doxorubicin, actinomycin D, vincristine, and vinblastine have been known to cause severe localized cellulitis if they are extravasated. These reactions and their prevention are discussed in detail in Chapter 29. Treatment includes stopping the injection, aspirating the drug and 5 ml of blood back into the syringe, and then withdrawing the syringe. For perivascular injections of vincristine and vinblastine, infiltrating the area with 4 to 6 ml saline and approximately 8 mg of dexamethasone and then applying warm compresses may be helpful (cold packs should be applied to areas of doxorubicin extravasation). Aggressive surgical debridement and skin grafts may be necessary for deep ulcerative lesions.

Pulmonary Toxicity

Bleomycin and cisplatin have been associated with the development of pulmonary toxicoses. Bleomycin can induce severe pulmonary fibrosis. Even when very low doses are used, cisplatin may induce severe, often fatal, pulmonary edema and pleural effusion in cats; therefore cisplatin is contraindicated in Felidae except for intralesional use.

SPECIFIC DRUGS USED IN VETERINARY CHEMOTHERAPY

Chemotherapeutic drugs can be classified as alkylating agents, antimetabolites, antibiotics, enzymes, vinca alkaloids, nitrosoureas, and synthetic anticancer drugs.

ALKYLATING AGENTS

Alkylating agents are cell-cycle nonspecific drugs that act by cross-linking DNA.

CYCLOPHOSPHAMIDE

How supplied: 25 and 50 mg tablets; 100, 200, and 500 mg and 1 and 2 g vials.

Dosage: 50 mg/m^2 PO daily in the morning on days 3, 4, 5, and 6 after doxorubicin therapy or 250 mg/m^2 PO every 3 weeks. Adjust actual dose based on tablet size. For example, a calculated total dosage of 62 mg may result in a dosing regimen of approximately 25 mg PO q24–48h for two doses.

Route of administration: PO in morning. May be mixed with any volume of saline for IV administration: Shake well, allow to stand for 10 to 15 minutes so that crystals dissolve completely, administer over 20 to 30 minutes.

Storage: Vials of unreconstituted drug can be stored at

room temperature; reconstituted solution should be used within 24 hours if stored at room temperature or 6 days if refrigerated.

Mechanism of action: Alkylating agent; prevents cell division by cross-linking strands of DNA.

Metabolism: Requires in vivo activation by enzymes (phosphamidase) in the liver and serum. Cyclophosphamide and its metabolites are excreted by the kidneys. Dosage should be reduced if serum creatinine levels are elevated and may require modification in the presence of liver disease.

Toxicity: Anorexia and vomiting occur frequently with IV administration and usually begin 6 hours after drug administration. Oral administration may reduce the incidence of vomiting. Alopecia (whisker loss) may be noted. Leukopenia (nadir, 7 to 14 days) may be the dose-limiting toxicity; recovery occurs 7 to 10 days after the nadir. Thrombocytopenia is usually not a problem. Sterile chemical cystitis may occur in some cats treated with IV and oral cyclophosphamide as a result of chemical irritation of the bladder by cyclophosphamide metabolites; chemical irritation has been associated with development of bladder tumors in dogs and humans. The risk of this complication can be reduced by maintaining high fluid intake, frequent urination, morning administration, and concurrent use of corticosteroids. If cyclophosphamide-induced hemorrhagic cystitis occurs, the drug should be discontinued indefinitely and chlorambucil (6–8 mg/m² PO daily, which is equivalent to 2 mg/cat given every other day) should be considered.

Note: Cyclophosphamide is one of the most common and effective antineoplastic agents used in veterinary medicine. It is effective for the treatment of lymphoma, soft tissue sarcomas (when combined with vincristine and/or doxorubicin), feline mammary neoplasia (when combined with doxorubicin), and other sarcomas.

CHLORAMBUCIL

How supplied: 2 mg coated tablets.

Dosage: 0.1 mg/kg daily; 6–8 mg/m² daily (in cats, this usually translates to a 2 mg tablet being given every 2–3 days because tablets should never be broken).

Route of administration: PO.

Storage: Store at room temperature.

Mechanism of action: Alkylating agent similar to mechlorethamine.

Metabolism: Well absorbed from the GI tract, but information on metabolism is incomplete.

Toxicity: BAG (alopecia primarily seen as whisker loss).

Note: Chlorambucil is used for treatment of lymphoma (especially when substituted for cyclophosphamide in patients with induced sterile hemorrhagic cystitis) and chronic lymphocytic leukemia. Remission exceeding 1 year has often been reported in patients with chronic lymphocytic leukemia treated with chlorambucil.

MELPHALAN

How supplied: Scored 2 mg tablets; 500 mg vials.

Dosage: 0.1 mg/kg/day for 10 days, then 0.05 mg/kg/day; 2 mg/m² daily for 7 to 10 days, then no therapy for 2 to 3 weeks (Note: Because of the tablet size, it may be necessary to have the drug compounded to an appropriate dosage size or give total dose less frequently; e.g., 2 mg tablet given q48–72h).

Route of administration: PO, IV.

Storage: Store at room temperature; injectable solution must be used within 60 minutes of reconstitution.

Mechanism of action: Alkylating agent; cytotoxic action produced by cross-linking of DNA.

Metabolism: Absorption from GI tract; erratic metabolism.

Toxicity: Myelosuppression can be marked. Recovery may take up to 4 weeks. IV product may cause severe slough if injected perivascularly. Alopecia and GI signs may also be noted.

Note: Melphalan has been used for several years to treat multiple myeloma (also known as plasma cell myeloma). Remissions exceeding 1 year have frequently been reported.

THIOTEPA

How supplied: 15 mg vials.

Dosage: Maximum systemic dosage is largely unknown but is thought to be 9 mg/m². Bladder instillation: 30 mg/m² every 3–4 weeks; remove after 1 hour.

Route of administration: For intravesicular administration into bladder, dilute 5 to 10 mg powder in 30 ml 0.9% NaCl. For systemic administration, give IM or SQ. Drug may be administered into the pleural or abdominal cavity.

Storage: Keep refrigerated. The reconstituted solution is stable at 4°C for 5 days.

Mechanism of action: Alkylating agent; multiple cross-linking of DNA.

Metabolism: Unknown; 20% of the dose introduced into the bladder is absorbed systemically.

Toxicity: Myelosuppression is the dose-limiting toxicity; leukopenia and thrombocytopenia reach their nadir at 7 to 28 days; alopecia and GI signs may also be seen.

Note: This drug has been used intravesicularly to treat transitional cell carcinoma of the bladder and intracavitarily for malignant pleural or peritoneal effusions; however, such use has not been published.

BUSULFAN

How supplied: 2 mg tablets.

Dosage: 2 mg/m² daily. (Note: Due to tablet size, administering at 2 mg q48–72h may be necessary.)

Route of administration: PO.

Storage: Store at room temperature.

Mechanism of action: Alkylating agent.

Metabolism: Well absorbed orally; metabolites are excreted in urine.

Toxicity: Myelosuppression is the major toxicity; thrombocytopenia may be particularly dangerous. Prolonged bone marrow suppression may occur. Pulmonary fibrosis has been reported in humans.

Note: Busulfan has been reported to be effective for the treatment of chronic myelogenous leukemia and polycythemia.

HYDROXYUREA

How supplied: 500 mg capsules.

Dosage: 80 mg/kg every 3 days. Because methemoglobinemia can occur following large single doses, it may be prudent to start even the largest cat at a dosage of no more than 125 mg/cat every 2 days for 2 weeks, followed by 250 mg/cat twice weekly for 2 weeks, and then as needed to maintain a normal hematocrit level. Capsule can be mixed in water and administered immediately if the patient is unable to swallow whole capsules. Rather than splitting capsules to meet dosing requirements, this drug may be prepared at a compounding pharmacy.

Route of administration: PO.

Storage: Store at room temperature.

Mechanism of action: Inhibits DNA synthesis.

Metabolism: Rapidly absorbed from the GI tract and excreted in urine.

Toxicity: Myelosuppression is often rapid and marked; thus frequent monitoring of the WBC count is required and doses may need to be adjusted. This drug can cause anemia in cats.

Note: Hydroxyurea has been used to treat chronic myelogenous leukemia and polycythemia (primary erythrocytosis).

CCNU

How supplied: 10, 40, and 100 mg capsules.

Dosage: 50–60 mg/m^2 every 6 weeks.

Route of administration: PO.

Storage: Store at room temperature.

Mechanism of action: Alkylating agent.

Metabolism: Rapidly absorbed from the GI tract and metabolized by the liver.

Toxicity: Myelosuppression (neutropenia) can be rapid and marked (nadir, approximately 1 week but often 2–5 weeks). This drug can cause a cumulative thrombocytopenia in dogs and may also do so in cats. Hepatic and renal toxicities are rare in dogs but may occur in cats.

Note: CCNU has shown efficacy in the treatment of lymphoma and mast cell tumors in cats. Because it is lipophilic, it has been effective in treating brain tumors in dogs and the same may be true for cats.

MECHLORETHAMINE

How supplied: 10 mg vials.

Dosage: 3 mg/m^2 as per protocol (usually MOPP protocol; see Chapter 36).

Route of administration: Slow IV push. (Note: This is a strong vesicant when administered extravascularly). Reconstitute vial with 10 ml 0.9% NaCl to concentration of 1 mg/ml.

Storage: Store unopened vials at room temperature; discard unused reconstituted material.

Mechanism of action: Nitrosourea alkylating agent.

Metabolism: Rapidly metabolized through spontaneous hydrolysis.

Toxicity: Myelosuppression (neutropenia) can be rapid and marked (nadir, 1 week). Nausea and vomiting may occur 30 minutes to 2 hours after administration and last for up to 8 hours. This drug is a strong vesicant and can cause tissue necrosis and sloughing if extravasated.

Note: This agent has shown efficacy against lymphoma in cats when used in combination protocols (e.g., MOPP).

PROCARBAZINE

How supplied: 50 mg capsules (10 mg capsules can be reformulated by a compounding pharmacy).

Dosage: 50 mg/m^2 daily for 14 days.

Route of administration: PO.

Storage: Store at room temperature.

Mechanism of action: Nonclassic alkylating agent.

Metabolism: Rapidly absorbed from the GI tract and metabolized by the liver.

Toxicity: Myelosuppression (neutropenia) is seen in other species, but whether this occurs in cats is uncertain as the drug is usually given concurrently with mechlorethamine. Nausea and vomiting occur commonly and can be dose limiting; diarrhea and anorexia also occur frequently. If these side effects are noted, cease drug administration and reinstitute when resolved with antinausea medications and/or at an every other day schedule; use prophylactic antinausea medications for future administration.

Note: Procarbazine has shown efficacy against lymphoma in cats when used in combination protocols (e.g., MOPP).

IFOSFAMIDE

How supplied: 1 and 3 g vials (mesna is included in the package).

Dosage: 500–900 mg/m^2 every 3 weeks (investigational).

1 g vial: Reconstitute with 20 ml 0.9% NaCl = 50 mg/ml. 3 g vial: Reconstitute with 30 ml 0.9% NaCl = 100 mg/ml.

Route of administration: IV as continuous infusion diluted in 0.9% NaCl and given over 30 minutes. Must be preceded (for 30 minutes) and followed (for 5 hours) by fluid diuresis (with 0.9% NaCl) at a rate of 18.3 ml/kg/hr. To help prevent hemorrhagic cystitis, the drug mesna should be administered in three doses, each equal to 20% of the ifosfamide dose. Mesna is given as an IV bolus at the start of pretreatment diuresis and 2 and 5 hours after ifosfamide infusion.

Storage: Store unopened vials at room temperature. Reconstituted solution is chemically stable for 7 days at room temperature and 6 weeks refrigerated.

Mechanism of action: Alkylating agent.

Metabolism: Hepatic metabolism to active form (as for cyclophosphamide).

Toxicity: Myelosuppression (neutropenia; nadir, 1 week). Monitor serum creatinine and urinalysis before each treatment as hemorrhagic cystitis may occur; renal toxicity has been seen in humans.

Note: Ifosfamide has shown efficacy against soft tissue sarcomas and lymphoma in cats.

ANTIMETABOLITES

Antimetabolites interfere with biosynthesis of nucleic acids by substituting them for normal metabolites and inhibiting normal enzymatic reactions. The dosing of each drug varies by protocol.

METHOTREXATE

How supplied: 2.5 mg tablets; 5, 20, 50, 100, 200, and 250 mg and 1 g vials for injection.

Dosage: 2.5 mg/m^2 daily.

Route of administration: PO, IV, IM, SQ.

Storage: Store at room temperature. The drug must be protected from light. Vials may be frozen.

Mechanism of action: Antimetabolite; inhibits conversion of folic acid to tetrahydrofolic acid by binding to the enzyme dihydrofolate reductase, which inhibits synthesis of thymidine and purines essential for DNA synthesis.

Metabolism: A large percentage of the drug is excreted unchanged in the urine. The drug is bound to serum albumin, so simultaneous administration of drugs that displace the methotrexate from the plasma protein (e.g., sulfa drugs, aspirin, metoclopramide, chloramphenicol, phenytoin, tetracycline) should be avoided to prevent excessive toxicity. Daily dose should be reduced if serum creatinine level is elevated.

Toxicity: Anorexia and vomiting occur frequently but may be prevented by premedication with antiemetics. The nadir of myelosuppression is 6 to 9 days in some species

but has not been documented in cats. Alopecia (whisker loss) may also be seen.

Note: Methotrexate has been used in combination with other drugs to treat lymphoma. It is a folic acid inhibitor and can be given at a very high dose and then reversed ("rescued") with leucovorin to prevent potentially fatal toxicities.

6-MERCAPTOPURINE

how supplied: 50 mg tablets.

Dosage: 50 mg/m^2 daily. (Note: Because of the tablet size, may need to be dosed at 50 mg q48–72h.)

Route of administration: PO.

Storage: Store at room temperature.

Mechanism of action: Purine antimetabolite; inhibits nucleotide synthesis required for RNA and DNA synthesis.

Metabolism: Metabolized by the liver and degraded by the enzyme xanthine oxidase. Xanthine oxidase is inhibited by allopurinol, so concurrent use of other drugs that use this enzyme necessitates a 75% dosage reduction.

Toxicity: Myelosuppression.

Note: 6-Mercaptopurine has been suggested as a treatment for leukemia and lymphoma; results are varied.

5-FLUOROURACIL

CONTRAINDICATED IN CATS due to fatal neurotoxicity.

CYTOSINE ARABINOSIDE, CYTARABINE

How supplied: 100 and 500 mg and 1 and 2 g vials.

Dosage: 100 mg/m^2 daily IV continuous infusion for 4 days; if no toxicity, increase to 150 mg/m^2 daily for 4 days or 10 mg/m^2 SQ once or twice daily. Can be administered intrathecally.

Route of administration: IV, SQ. If administered IV, infuse via a Buretrol® over 10 to 20 minutes or as continuous infusion.

Storage: Store at room temperature. Reconstituted solution is stable at room temperature for 48 hours. Discard solution if a slight haze develops.

Mechanism of action: Antimetabolite; pyrimidine analogue; inhibits DNA synthesis.

Metabolism: The drug is activated and inactivated by liver enzymes.

Toxicity: Myelosuppression is the major toxicity. Leukopenia and thrombocytopenia (nadir, 7 to 14 days in dogs) frequently occur and apparently are related to the dose and frequency of administration. Fever and thrombophlebitis are rarely seen. Alopecia (whisker loss) may be seen.

Note: This drug has been used alone or in combination with other agents to treat lymphoreticular neoplasms and myeloproliferative disorders. It has been administered intrathecally to cats to treat CNS lymphoma.

ANTIBIOTICS

Antibiotics form stable complexes (intercalate) with DNA and therefore inhibit DNA or RNA synthesis.

DOXORUBICIN

How supplied: 10, 20, 50, 150, and 200 mg vials.

Dosage: 25 mg/m^2 or 1 mg/kg IV every 3 weeks; total cumulative dose of up to 180 to 240 mg/m^2.

Route of administration: Dilute with 30 ml of 0.9% NaCl and administer IV over 15 to 30 minutes or give undiluted drug IV at a rate of 1 ml/min. (Do not heparinize as this will cause precipitation.)

Storage: Store at room temperature. Reconstituted solution is stable for months if refrigerated. Avoid storing with aluminum-hubbed needles.

Mechanism of action: Antitumor antibiotic; inhibits DNA and RNA synthesis.

Metabolism: Metabolized predominantly by the liver. Approximately 50% of the drug is excreted in bile. In animals with bilirubin levels above 2 mg/dl, the dose should be decreased by 50% to reduce toxicity. The drug is also excreted in urine and causes a red color in urine for up to 2 days after administration.

Toxicity: Leukopenia and thrombocytopenia (nadir, 7 to 10 days). The cumulative dose that is likely to cause cardiotoxicity in cats has not been clearly elicited, but some oncologists limit this agent to 180 to 240 mg/m^2. Extravasation causes severe tissue necrosis. Immediately apply ice or cold compresses to the area of extravasation and continue for 6 to 10 hours. The drug has been reported to cause renal toxicity in cats. Allergic reactions occur occasionally but may be eliminated by slowing the infusion or by pretreating the cat with antihistamines. Alopecia (whisker loss) may be seen in some cats.

Note: Doxorubicin is used to treat lymphoma, thyroid carcinomas, sarcomas, and mammary carcinoma. This antineoplastic agent seems to have a broad spectrum of activity against a variety of tumors.

MITOXANTRONE

How supplied: 20, 25, and 30 mg multidose vials.

Dosage: 6.5 mg/m^2 IV (administered over at least 3 minutes) every 3 weeks.

Route of administration: IV.

Storage: Store at room temperature. The drug is incompatible with heparin. Do not freeze.

Mechanism of action: Intercalates DNA; inhibits DNA and RNA synthesis.

Metabolism: Liver.

Toxicity: Unlike doxorubicin, this drug does not readily cause allergic reactions, cardiomyopathy, cardiac arrhythmias, or severe tissue damage at the site of extravasation. It is more myelosuppressive than doxorubicin and can cause alopecia (predominately whisker loss) and GI disturbances.

Note: Mitoxantrone is moderately effective for the treatment of lymphoma, squamous cell carcinoma, transitional cell carcinoma, mammary gland tumors, and a number of other neoplastic conditions.

IDARUBICIN

How supplied: 2 mg capsules; 5 and 10 mg vials.

Dosage: 2 mg/cat every 3 weeks.

Route of administration: PO, IV; limited availability worldwide.

Storage: Store at room temperature. Reconstituted injectable form is stable for 7 days if refrigerated. Incompatible with heparin.

Mechanism of action: Antitumor antibiotic; inhibits DNA and RNA synthesis.

Metabolism: Metabolized predominantly by the liver.

Toxicity: Bone marrow suppression, GI disturbances, and whisker loss in cats.

Note: Orally administered idarubicin has been shown to be effective for the treatment of lymphoma in cats.

BLEOMYCIN

How supplied: 15 U vials (1 U = 1 mg).

Dosage: 0.3–0.5 U/kg weekly IM, IV, or SQ to an accumulated dose of 125–200 mg/m^2. IV push over at least 10 minutes.

Route of administration: IM, SQ; may be used intralesionally. May cause pain at injection site. IV administration should be slow (1 U/min).

Storage: Can be stored for 24 hours at room temperature, 1 to 2 months if refrigerated, and 2 years if frozen. It should not be used with heparin.

Mechanism of action: Antitumor antibiotic; inhibits DNA synthesis and, to a lesser extent, RNA and protein synthesis.

Metabolism: Rapidly excreted by the kidneys. Dose should be decreased if serum creatinine level is elevated because of renal disease.

Toxicity: Pulmonary fibrosis has been reported in some species and seems to be dose related. A maximum cumulative dose of 200 mg/m^2 is recommended. In addition, allergic reactions (fever) have been reported.

Note: Bleomycin has been suggested as a treatment for squamous cell carcinoma.

ACTINOMYCIN D

How supplied: 0.5 mg vials.

Dosage: 0.5–0.9 mg/m^2 slow IV infusion every 3 weeks.

Route of administration: Slow IV (over a minimum of 20 minutes); may cause pain at injection site.

Storage: Use within 24 hours of reconstitution because of the absence of preservatives.

Mechanism of action: Antitumor antibiotic that inhibits DNA synthesis and, to a lesser extent, RNA and protein synthesis.

Metabolism: Excreted by the liver.

Toxicity: Bone marrow suppression, GI toxicity, alopecia, and extravasation reactions can occur with this drug.

Note: This drug has been used to treat lymphoma.

ENZYMES

The most commonly used enzyme in veterinary and human medicine is L-asparaginase.

L-ASPARAGINASE

How supplied: 10,000 U vials.

Dosage: 10,000–20,000 U/m² or 400 U/kg weekly or less frequently.

Route of administration: IM.

Storage: Refrigerate. Reconstituted drug may be active for up to 7 days. Do not use if cloudy.

Mechanism of action: Enzyme; inhibits protein synthesis by depriving tumor cells of the amino acid asparagine.

Metabolism: Not completely understood.

Toxicity: Allergic and anaphylactic reactions are seen, especially after several doses have been given. The incidence of anaphylaxis is minimal when administered IM. If administered IV, the potential for inducing an acute anaphylactic reaction is high. Pretreatment with antihistamines and steroids may reduce risk of reactions. If anaphylaxis occurs, L-asparaginase should be discontinued indefinitely. Other toxicities include fever and vomiting shortly after administration. The drug has been associated with acute pancreatitis in dogs and humans. Myelosuppression may occur if this drug is administered concurrently with vincristine.

Note: The drug is used to treat lymphoma and lymphoblastic leukemia and may be combined with other antineoplastic agents. L-Asparaginase does not induce a sustained remission when used alone in the treatment of lymphoma.

VINCA ALKALOIDS

Vinca (plant) alkaloids bind to the microtubules to prevent the normal formation and function of the mitotic spindle, thus arresting the cell division in metaphase.

VINCRISTINE

How supplied: 1, 2, and 5 mg vials; hyporets (1 and 2 mg/ml disposable syringes).

Dosage: 0.5–0.75 mg/m² weekly.

Route of administration: Administer through a patent IV catheter; follow with adequate saline flush (10 ml).

Storage: Refrigerate. Protect from light until immediately before injection.

Mechanism of action: Plant alkaloid. Causes metaphase arrest by binding to microtubular protein used in formation of mitotic spindle.

Metabolism: Rapidly cleared from plasma and excreted in bile. Decrease dose by 50% in animals with bilirubin levels above 2 mg/dl.

Toxicity: Can cause neurotoxicity and resultant paresthesia, constipation, and paralytic ileus. Anorexia in treated cats may be due to ileus. This drug is a potent irritant that can cause severe tissue irritation and necrosis if extravasated; if extravasation occurs, apply warm compresses immediately and infiltrate with saline and 8 mg dexamethasone. Myelosuppression is dose related and uncommon unless drug is given in combination with L-asparaginase. Vincristine causes a marked increase in peripheral platelet count in animals with adequate megakaryocytes.

Note: Vincristine is most commonly used to treat lymphoma, sarcomas, thrombocytopenia, and mast cell tumors.

VINBLASTINE

How supplied: 10 mg vials.

Dosage: 2 mg/m² every 3 weeks.

Route of administration: Potent irritant, avoid extravasation. Administer through a patent IV catheter; follow with adequate saline flush (10 ml).

Storage: Refrigerated reconstituted drug is stable for 30 days. Protect from light.

Mechanism of action: Plant alkaloid. Causes metaphase arrest by binding to microtubular protein used in the formation of mitotic spindle.

Metabolism: Rapidly cleared from plasma; excreted in bile. A 50% decrease in dose is recommended in animals with bilirubin levels above 2 mg/dl.

Toxicity: Unlike vincristine, vinblastine may cause severe bone marrow suppression (WBC nadir, 4 to 7 days after administration). Neurotoxicity and mild peripheral neuropathies occur but are less severe than with vincristine. Extravasation can cause severe tissue irritation and necrosis. If extravasation occurs, immediately pack with warm compresses and infiltrate the area with saline and 8 mg dexamethasone.

Note: Vinblastine is used to treat lymphoma and mastocytoma.

HORMONES

Hormones are believed to interfere with the cellular receptors that stimulate growth. The most common examples of hormones used to treat cancer are the corticosteroids used to treat lymphoma and mast cell tumors.

THERAPEUTIC & SUPPORTIVE PROCEDURES

PREDNISONE

How supplied: 5, 10, 20, and 50 mg tablets; 1 mg/ml syrup; injectable solution.

Dosage: 30 to 40 mg/m^2 daily or every other day or 1 mg/kg daily for 4 weeks; 1 mg/kg every other day thereafter as long as the tumor is in remission and the patient is doing well.

Route of administration: PO, IV.

Storage: Store at room temperature.

Mechanism of action: Binds to cytoplasmic receptor sites, which then interact with DNA and prevent cell division.

Metabolism: Metabolized by the liver and excreted in the urine. Prednisone is activated by the liver to its active form, prednisolone; severe liver disease, however, does not significantly affect activation.

Toxicity: Polydipsia and polyuria are the major side effects. Long-term use may be associated with development of alopecia and other signs of iatrogenic Cushing's syndrome.

Note: Active in treatment of lymphoma and mast cell tumors. Prednisone does not induce a sustained remission when used alone in the treatment of lymphoma.

MISCELLANEOUS AGENTS

CISPLATIN
(*CIS*-DIAMMINEDICHLOROPLATINUM II)

How supplied: 10, 50, and 100 mg vials.

Dosage: IV USE CONTRAINDICATED IN CATS due to fatal pulmonary edema. Intralesional administration ONLY as a suspension in oil or collagen matrix at 1.5 mg/cm^3 of tumor and surrounding normal tissue. Because aluminum causes precipitation, do not use aluminum needles.

Route of administration: IV use is contraindicated; intralesional administration as a suspension in oil or collagen matrix only.

Storage: Dry powder is stable at room temperature for 2 years. Reconstituted solution is stable at room temperature for 20 hours. The reconstituted solution should not be refrigerated because a precipitate will form.

Mechanism of action: Similar to alkylating agents and other heavy metals. Binds to DNA and causes cross-linkage.

Metabolism: When given IV to dogs, cisplatin is rapidly distributed to the liver, intestine, and kidneys; less than 10% is in plasma after 1 hour, and 50% of the administered dose is excreted in urine in 24 to 48 hours.

Toxicity: IV use in the cat is associated with fatal pleural effusions and pulmonary edema. Intralesional administration as a suspension in oil or collagen matrix is rarely associated with significant systemic absorption. Local reactions include necrosis, swelling, and inflammation.

Note: Cisplatin is effective for the intralesional treatment of squamous cell carcinoma and soft tissue sarcomas.

CARBOPLATIN

How supplied: 50, 150, and 450 mg vials.

Dosage: 200–220 mg/m^2 every 4 weeks (investigational).

Route of administration: IV; must be diluted with 5% dextrose in water. Intralesional administration as a suspension in oil or collagen matrix. Intracavitary.

Storage: Dry powder is stable at room temperature for 2 years. Reconstituted solution is stable at room temperature for 8 hours.

Mechanism of action: Similar to alkylating agents and other heavy metals. Binds to DNA and causes cross-linkage.

Metabolism: Metabolized by the liver and kidneys. Dose should be reduced if serum creatinine level is increased because of renal disease.

Toxicity: Myelosuppression is the most significant toxicity (neutrophil nadir, 17 to 21 days and may be prolonged). Carboplatin should not be administered without the current neutrophil count being known. Unlike with cisplatin, nephrotoxicity and emesis are rare.

Note: Carboplatin is used in treatment of squamous cell carcinoma and possibly other carcinomas and sarcomas.

PACLITAXEL

How supplied: 50 mg/5 ml vials.

Dosage: 5 mg/kg every 3 weeks (investigational).

Route of administration: IV. Must dilute with 0.9% NaCl to a concentration of 0.6 to 0.7 mg/ml. Prepare in a glass container; administer through a 0.22 μm inline filter using non-PVC tubing. Pretreat with corticosteroids, diphenhydramine, and H$_2$ receptor antagonists.

Storage: Refrigerate vials before use. Reconstituted solution is stable at room temperature for 24 hours.

Mechanism of action: Inhibits microtubule disassembly.

Metabolism: Metabolized by the liver and kidneys.

Toxicity: Myelosuppression and anaphylactoid reactions (due to the diluent Cremophor EL) are the most significant toxicities.

Note: Paclitaxel is a relatively new chemotherapeutic agent. Studies are underway to define its usefulness in veterinary medicine.

PIROXICAM

How supplied: 10 and 20 mg capsules.

Dosage: 0.3 mg/kg PO q48h; may need to be reformulated by a compounding pharmacy.

Route of administration: PO. Avoid other GI irritants and nephrotoxins.

Storage: Store at room temperature.

Mechanism of action: Unknown; possible biologic response modifier.

Metabolism: Metabolized by the liver and kidneys.

Toxicity: Nephrotoxicity and GI irritation.

Note: This nonsteroidal antiinflammatory agent has been shown to cause measurable regression in transitional cell carcinoma of the urinary bladder and squamous cell carcinoma in dogs and may therefore be of value in cats.

ETOPOSIDE

Has not been studied in cats, but the diluent causes an allergic reaction in dogs when administered IV. Not currently recommended for use in cats.

APPLIED CHEMOTHERAPY (TABLE 11-4)

As noted previously, there are many benefits to multiple drug treatment protocols. Tumor resistance generally develops more slowly than with single drug regimens, and multiple drug protocols are more effective, especially with lymphoid tumors. Disadvantages associated with the use of multiple antineoplastic agents include increased cost and potential for toxicity. Cures attributable to chemotherapy were not seen in human medicine until effective combinations were employed. Whenever drugs are used in combination, several important points must be kept in mind:

- Each drug must be effective when used alone to treat a specific malignancy.
- Combinations of drugs with overlapping toxicities should be avoided unless they are arranged in a protocol to prevent superimposition of toxicoses.

TABLE 11-4
Examples of Commonly Used Combination Protocols for Neoplastic Conditions in Veterinary Medicine

Neoplasia	Therapy	No. of Cats	Overall Response (%)	Complete/ Partial Responses (%)	Median Remission Duration (months)	Overall Median Survival (months)	Reference	Comments
Lymphoma (see Chapter 36)	D	19	64	32/32	12	N/A	3	
	VCM, L	103	82	62/20		7	5	
	CVP +CVP +D	38 (11) (7)		47/NA	2.8 8.6		7 7 7	Of the 47%, 11 remained on CVP and 7 were switched to D.
	CVP	38 12 7 5 4	94	79/15 92/NA 86/NA 80/NA 100/NA	5 6 4.5 28 5		8 8 8 8 8	All cats Mediastinal only Alimentary tract Peripheral nodes Multicentric
	CVP, I	18			6.1		18	
	VLCMPD	21	95	38/57	5	8	4	Alimentary
	CVP	28		32	7.6 (mean, 18.2)	1.6 (mean, 8)	9	Alimentary
	CVP P only	9 3	100 67	67/33 0/67	3.5 2		6 6	Spinal (CVP + laminectomy in 1 cat = MRD of 62 wk)
	VCML + Ca	28		61/NA	4.3		10	Renal
Nasal Planum SCC (see Chapter 50)	Intratumoral carboplatin	15		73.3/NA		55% 1 year survival	11	
Oral SCC (see Chapter 41)	Carboplatin + radiation	9	100	44/56		5.4	12	Systemic carboplatin + 30 Gy
	Mitoxantrone + radiation	7		6		30% 1 year survival	13	60 Gy

(continued)

TABLE 11-4 *continued*

Neoplasia	Therapy	No. of Cats	Overall Response (%)	Complete/ Partial Responses (%)	Median Remission Duration (months)	Overall Median Survival (months)	Reference	Comments
Facial SCC (see Chapter 50)	Intralesional cisplatin	16		50/75			14	
	Intralesional 5-fluorouracil	20	75	30/45			14	
Mammary Adenocarcinoma (see Chapter 45)	D, C	11	64	27/37		9 (CR) 3.7(PR) 1.8 (NR)	16	
	D, C	14		None/50		5 (PR) 2.5 (NR)	17	Advanced mammary ADC; 11 had previous surgery
	Surgery + D	26				9.6 days	15	Previously untreated
		8				5.8 days	15	Prior surgery with local recurrence

ADC = adenocarcinoma; C = cyclophosphamide; Ca = cytosine arabinoside; CR = complete remission; D = doxorubicin; I = idarubicin; L = L-asparaginase; M = methotrexate; MRD = mean remission duration; NR = no remission; P = prednisone; PR = partial remission; SCC = squamous cell carcinoma; V = vincristine

- Drugs should be used with an intermittent treatment schedule for maximum efficacy.
- Combined chemotherapeutics are most effective when they have different mechanisms of action and act at different stages of the cell cycle.

REFERENCES

1. Chabner BA: Principles of cancer therapy, in Wyngaarden JB, Smith LH (eds): *Cecil Textbook of Medicine.* Philadelphia, WB Saunders, 1982, p 1032.
2. Ogilvie GK: Principles of oncology, in Morgan RV (ed): *Handbook of Small Animal Internal Medicine.* Philadelphia, Churchill Livingston, 1992, pp 799–812.
3. Peaston AE, Maddison JE: Efficacy of doxorubicin as an induction agent for cats with lymphosarcoma. *Aust Vet J* 77:442–444, 1999.
4. Zwahlen CH, Lucroy MD, Kraegel SA, Madewell BR: Results of chemotherapy for cats with alimentary malignant lymphoma: 21 cases (1993–1997). *JAVMA* 213:1144–1149, 1998.
5. Mooney SC, Hayes AA, MacEwen EG, et al: Treatment and prognostic factors in lymphoma in cats: 103 cases (1977–1981). *JAVMA* 194:696–699, 1989.
6. Spodnick GJ, Berg J, Moore FM, Cotter SM: Spinal lymphoma in cats: 21 cases (1976–1989). *JAVMA* 200:373–376, 1992.
7. Moore AS, Cotter SM, Frimberger AE, et al: A comparison of doxorubicin and COP for maintenance of remission in cats with lymphoma. *J Vet Intern Med* 10:372–375, 1996.
8. Cotter SM: Treatment of lymphoma and leukemia with cyclophosphamide, vincristine, and prednisone. I. Treatment of dogs. II. Treatment of cats. *JAAHA* 19:159–172, 1993.
9. Mahony OM, Moore AS, Cotter SM, et al: Alimentary lymphoma in cats: 28 cases (1988–1993). *JAVMA* 207:1593–1598, 1995.
10. Mooney S, Hayes A, Matus R, MacEwen E: Renal lymphoma in cats: 28 cases (1977–1984). *JAVMA* 191:1473–1477, 1987.
11. Theon AP, VanVechten MK, Madewell BR: Intratumoral administration of carboplatin for treatment of squamous cell carcinomas of the nasal plane in cats. *Am J Vet Res* 57:205–10, 1996.
12. Wood CA: Combination coarse fractionation radiation therapy and carboplatin chemotherapy for treatment of feline oral squamous cell carcinoma: an interim analysis. *Vet Cancer Soc Newsl* 22:1, 4, 1998.
13. LaRue SM, Vail DM, Ogilvie GK, et al: Shrinking-field radiation therapy plus mitoxantrone for the treatment of oral squamous cell carcinoma in the cat. *Vet Cancer Soc Newsl* 15:4, 7, 1991.
14. Kitchell BE, McCabe M, Luck EE, et al: Intralesional sustained-release chemotherapy with cisplatin and 5-fluorouracil therapeutic implants for treatment of feline squamous cell carcinoma (abstract). *Proc 12th Annu Meet Vet Cancer Soc:*55, 1992.
15. Mauldin GE, Mooney SC, Patnaik AK, Mauldin GN: Adjuvant doxorubicin for feline mammary adenocarcinoma. *14th Annu Conf Vet Cancer Soc:*6, 1994.
16. Jeglum KA, deGuzman E, Young KM: Chemotherapy of advanced mammary adenocarcinoma in 14 cats. *JAVMA* 187:157–160, 1985.
17. Mauldin GN, Matus RE, Patnaik AK, et al: Clinical study of 23 cats with malignant nonhematopoietic tumors treated using a protocol of doxorubicin [Adriamycin: Adria Laboratories] and cyclophosphamide [Cytoxan: Bristol Meyers]. *J Vet Intern Med* 2:60–65, 1988.
18. Moore AS, Ruslander D, Cotter SM, et al: Efficacy of, and toxicoses associated with, oral idarubicin administration in cats with neoplasia. *JAVMA* 206:1550–1554, 1995.
19. MacEwen EG, Rosenthal RC: Approach to treatment of cancer patients, in Ettinger SJ (ed): *Textbook of Veterinary Internal Medicine.* Philadelphia, WB Saunders, 1989, pp 527–546.
20. Rosenthal RC: Chemotherapy, in Slatter D (ed): *Textbook of Small Animal Surgery,* ed 2. Philadelphia, WB Saunders, 1993, pp 2067–2074.
21. Moore AS: Recent advances in chemotherapy for nonlymphoid malignant neoplasms. *Compend Contin Educ Pract Vet* 15:1039–1052, 1993.
22. Vail DM: Recent advances in chemotherapy for lymphoma of dogs and cats. *Compend Contin Educ Pract Vet* 15:1031–1037, 1993.

RADIATION THERAPY—PROPERTIES, USES, AND PATIENT MANAGEMENT

12

Gregory K. Ogilvie and Antony S. Moore

C L I N I C A L   B R I E F I N G

Types of Radiation Therapy

Teletherapy	External beam radiation delivered by orthovoltage or megavoltage machines.
Brachytherapy	Placement of radioactive substances within or around malignant tissue.
Systemic Therapy	Administration of radioactive substances that preferentially localize within specific tissues in the body.

Potential Tissue Injuries and Possible Therapy

Skin	Clean with mild soap and water; prevent self-mutilation and secondary infections. Other possible treatments include vitamin E and hydrogen peroxide/saline lavage as well as selected systemic therapy; ear canals can be treated with steroid-containing ear medication.
Oral Cavity, Pharynx	Consider palatable food and esophagostomy or gastrostomy tube feeding early; oral rinses with saline or black tea.
Colon, Rectum	A low-residue diet with a stool softener may alleviate painful defecation; steroid enemas, stool softeners, and a high-fiber diet may be helpful for nonresponsive colitis.
Eye	Artificial tears for keratoconjunctivitis sicca and steroid ophthalmic solution or ointment for selected nonerosive conditions after fluorescein staining.
Bone	Sequestra should be removed.

Selected Indications	Local control of oral tumors, nasal tumors, soft tissue sarcomas, mast cell tumors, brain tumors, thyroid tumors (including thyroid adenomas), and some malignant effusions can be palliative for primary or metastatic bone disease.

Clients, veterinarians, and other health care professionals have preconceived notions about what radiation therapy does and its effect on the cancer patient. Radiation therapy is often shrouded in misconceptions and misperceptions. When thinking of therapeutic radiation therapy, horrible images of the victims of the nuclear bomb attacks of Nagasaki and Hiroshima often fill the minds of clients and veterinary staff alike. However, this treatment modality has been used to help restore the health and well-being of cats with cancer for many years, and it will always be a critical component of comprehensive care for cats with cancer. To ensure that feline patients receive the best care possible, clients and the rest of the veterinary health care team must be made aware of the realities of radiation therapy.

When radiation therapy for a cat with cancer is planned, analgesia, antiemetics, and nutritional support must be considered and a treatment plan outlined prior to the start of therapy. The adverse effects of radiation therapy usually do not arise until the end of the therapy period and continue for weeks after the treatment has concluded; analgesia is required during this period. Eicosanoids and glutamine may be very helpful in minimizing the adverse effects associated with radiation therapy. Antiemetics may be indicated to treat the adverse effects associated with certain anesthetic agents or for GI tract injury related to the radiation therapy. Nutritional support must begin before any evidence of weight loss is identified.

Radiation therapy has been used for decades in veterinary and human oncology. The equipment only recently became readily available to large segments of the veterinary profession, primarily through referral centers. Radiation therapy can effectively control a wide range of tumors in cats. Palliative therapy (i.e., therapy to improve quality but not necessarily length of life) can be delivered in one to six treatments for a total dose of 6 to 30 Gy. Curative intent dosages range from 30 to 60 Gy, delivered in 9 to 40 treatments over 3 to 6 weeks.[1-22] This treatment modality is used alone or in combination with other cancer therapies, including surgery and chemotherapy. Radiation therapy is usually a local treatment, and thus extreme care should be taken to ensure that the cat's cancer has been properly staged to delineate the extent of the neoplastic process. Consultation with an oncologist is essential to determine whether a cat with a malignancy is likely to benefit from radiation therapy. Before a practitioner can understand the potential benefits and risks of radiation therapy, a brief review of the properties and uses of radiation therapy is warranted.

TYPES OF RADIATION THERAPY

Teletherapy

The delivery of radiation therapy from a machine to the patient is called *teletherapy* or *external beam radiation therapy*. In feline medicine, external beam radiation therapy is primarily delivered by linear accelerators, radioactive cobalt (^{60}Co) or cesium (^{137}Cs) source units, or orthovoltage radiation therapy machines.

Megavoltage radiation produced by either a linear accelerator or a ^{60}Co or ^{137}Cs source machine is preferred for the treatment of many neoplastic conditions (Figure 12-1). Megavoltage radiation has excellent penetrating capability and is able to reach deep-seated tumors while minimizing injury to overlying tissues. If megavoltage radiation therapy is used to treat superficial tumors, the energy must be slowed by using a sheet of tissue-equivalent material called *bolus*, which is placed over the tumor. This allows most of

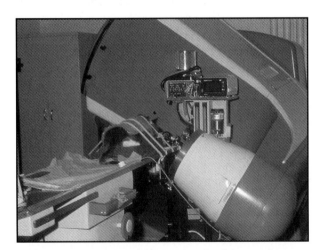

Figure 12-1: *Megavoltage radiation is the preferred treatment for many neoplastic conditions. This linear accelerator, like all other megavoltage radiation therapy units, has excellent penetrating capability and is able to reach deep-seated tumors while minimizing injury to overlying tissues when photon radiation is used. Some linear accelerators can produce electrons instead of photons; electrons are very effectively used for superficial tumors.*

the energy to be deposited more superficially on the tumor itself. Alternatively, electron beams produced by a linear accelerator can be used to treat superficial tumors because electrons do not penetrate to deep tissues.

The radiation produced in orthovoltage therapy does not effectively penetrate more than a few centimeters and thus is not suitable for tumors situated deep within the body. Orthovoltage is valuable, however, for treating superficial tumors and tumors within air-filled cavities, such as nasal tumors. Orthovoltage radiation therapy units deposit maximum doses to the skin surface, which can result in injury to those tissues.

Brachytherapy

Radiation therapy can also be administered via radiation sources implanted within or around the tumor itself *(brachytherapy)*. Brachytherapy is performed by delivering very high doses of radiation to very localized sites within the body. One technique involves implanting "seeds" or "straws" of radioactive materials within the tumor. Radioactive sources also can be administered into body cavities; sources vary depending on the tissue to be implanted (e.g., cesium or radium for intracavitary placement, iridium for interstitial implants). Interstitial brachytherapy sources often are implanted in a removable package (e.g., Silastic® tubing) and then removed once the calculated dose has been delivered. Brachytherapy is very effective for specific delivery of extremely high radiation doses to a local site, and normal tissue damage is usually restricted to the immediately surrounding tissues; radiation particles typically do not penetrate very far into tissues in this type of therapy. The amount of normal tissue injured is directly proportional to the energy of the radiation implanted or delivered to a specific site. A strontium 90 source may be used to deliver radiation therapy to a localized, superficial area, such as early facial squamous cell carcinoma.

Systemic Therapy

Systemically injected radioactive materials (i.e., radioiodine [^{131}I]; Figure 12-2) are very useful for treating hyperthyroidism in cats. The radioactive material is designed to be selectively taken up by or incorporated in the tissue to be treated. Many oncology centers around the world use this form of therapy. Radioactive material has recently been linked to monoclonal antibodies that "seek out" specific tumor tissues.

TREATMENT METHODS

Specifically delivering the proper doses of radiation therapy to a tumor while minimizing damage to normal tissue requires the skills of highly trained individuals. In addition, precise imaging is required to delineate the extent of the tumor. Radiation planning, which is usually done in combination with computerized tomography (CT), uses computer technology and lead "wedges" to distribute the dose

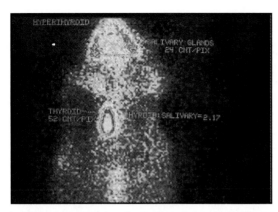

Figure 12-2: Hyperthyroidism is effectively treated with ^{131}I administered IV or PO. Prior to ^{131}I therapy, another radioactive material, technetium-99m, is used to determine the extent of disease. In hyperthyroid cats, technetium-99m is taken up by the abnormal thyroid gland to a much greater extent than the salivary gland.

evenly throughout the tumor while minimizing normal tissue injury and maximizing tumor control. Whenever external beam radiation therapy is delivered, the adverse effects of radiation therapy can be minimized by expanding the time over which the radiation dosage is delivered (i.e., 6 versus 3 weeks), increasing the number of doses delivered to the patient, and delivering the radiation through several different portals while using lead wedges to distribute the energy evenly. Delivering radiation therapy daily (Monday through Friday) for 4 weeks is generally less toxic to normal tissues than delivering the same total dose on a twice-weekly basis over the same period.

Treatment planning precisely prescribes the best way to administer radiation therapy to control the tumor and minimize unnecessary morbidity to the patient. After the treatment plan has been devised, a dosage is prescribed and the least toxic method of administration is determined. The dosage generally is limited by the tolerance of nearby normal tissues. The goal is to have less than a 5% probability that a patient's tissues will experience significant toxicity. External beam radiation therapy is frequently delivered over several weeks, and the cat must be placed in the exact same position for each treatment or "fraction." The skin can be tattooed or other methods may be used to ensure that the patient's position is the same for each session. Because of the number of treatments, short-acting induction agents (e.g., propofol) are preferred prior to endotracheal intubation and isoflurane or other inhalant anesthesia.

FACTORS INFLUENCING TUMOR CONTROL

The beneficial effect of radiation therapy depends on the modulation of at least four factors affecting irradiated cells: repair, repopulation, redistribution, and reoxygenation. These are discussed very briefly to help in the clinical reasoning of dosing and scheduling of radiation to benefit the cat with cancer.

Repair

Both normal and tumor cells repair themselves within a few hours of irradiation, and repair from radiation injury apparently is approximately equal in normal and malignant cells. Inhibiting this repair mechanism can enhance the beneficial effects of radiation therapy on the tumor, which is why radiation therapy is usually administered frequently.

Repopulation

Repopulation involves the replacement of cells killed by radiation therapy with the progeny of surviving cells through cell multiplication. Both normal and malignant tissues are capable of recovering from radiation therapy in this way. The repopulation of cells differs depending on the tissue from which they originate, thereby explaining why some tissues are more sensitive to radiation than others. Drugs or other methods to reduce repopulation can enhance tumor control.

Redistribution

Redistribution of cells throughout all phases of the cell cycle (e.g., M, S, G_1, G_2, G_0) occurs after a dose of radiation therapy. Because radiation therapy is most effective in G_1 and G_2 phases, the beneficial effects of radiation therapy can be enhanced by administering treatments when the majority of cells are in these phases. Fractionation of radiation therapy takes advantage of this phenomenon.

Reoxygenation

During reoxygenation, the tumor and normal tissues reestablish an oxygen source. This is very important because hypoxic tumor cells are known to be radioresistant. Therefore any method that enhances oxygenation of the tumor cells, such as the use of certain drugs, can heighten the effect of radiation therapy.

ADVERSE EFFECTS AND PATIENT MANAGEMENT[21,23]

Because radiation therapy is a local treatment, side effects are confined to the area being treated. The only exception to this is when the entire body is irradiated, as for bone marrow transplantation, although this procedure is uncommon in feline medicine. It is important to educate clients about this localized effect, the ways in which different tissues will respond to radiation therapy, and the timing of the appearance of adverse effects.

Skin

The skin is often injured in external beam radiation therapy, particularly with orthovoltage radiation or sources of low-energy electrons. Interestingly, skin toxicities are usually milder in cats than in dogs given an equivalent radiation dose. Acute reactions that generally appear toward the end of radiation therapy include erythema, dry desquamation with pruritus, and moist desquamation. The best treatment for these cutaneous injuries is unknown. Most cats will keep the area clean until the skin becomes very tender. Some advocate cleansing affected areas with mild soap and water. A Water-Pic® or hydropulsion with a 60 ml syringe may be used to help clean the lesion. If self-mutilation is a problem, an Elizabethan collar or (less commonly) bandages may be employed. Non–petroleum-based vitamin E ointments have been used.

Although controversial, some suggest that cats with severe pruritus or moist desquamation may benefit from cleansing the area with a 1:1 solution of hydrogen peroxide and normal saline and possibly treating with a topical or oral corticosteroid. If a topical corticosteroid is used, a non–petroleum-based spray product is recommended. Combining cleansing with a wetting solution such as Cara-klenz® and subsequent application of aloe vera gel extract (Carrington Dermal Wound Gel®) has been suggested. Extreme caution should be employed to prevent consumption of these ointments as toxicoses are possible. Telfa® pads should be used whenever the area needs to be covered.

Patients may occasionally develop a pruritic rash originating from the area of treatment and spreading to areas outside the treatment field. Systemic antihistamines, such as diphenhydramine, or topical corticosteroids may be indicated for these patients. Other adverse effects that can occur with higher radiation doses include hyper- or hypopigmentation, telangiectasia, ulceration, and fibrosis, which can be quite painful if extensive (Figures 12-3 and 12-4). Debilitating late skin changes, which are extremely rare, can be repaired with reconstructive techniques using well-vascularized tissue.

Oral Cavity and Pharynx

Damage to the oral cavity and pharynx is very common in cats receiving radiation therapy for nasal and oral tumors. This area can be very frustrating to treat because radiation-induced oral mucositis may result in anorexia and secondary debilitation. Placing an esophagostomy or gastrostomy tube before initiating radiation therapy is recommended unless the tube placement site would be in the radiation field. The tube should be placed before the cat declines beyond a good plane of nutrition and any time that the oral cavity is to be included in the radiation field (e.g., oral squamous cell carcinoma in older cats).

A secondary benefit of placing an assisted feeding tube is that medication and/or supplements can easily be given. Supplementing with glutamine and omega or n-3 fatty acids may be helpful in minimizing the adverse effects associated with radiation damage. Oral mucositis and anorexia are common in the acute phase of radiation therapy,

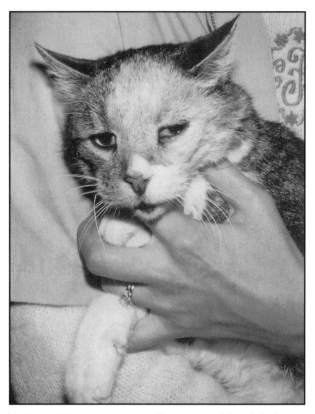

Figure 12-3: Acute reactions generally appear toward the end of radiation therapy and may include erythema, dry desquamation with pruritus, and moist desquamation. Hair and skin color change are commonly seen weeks to months later, as in this cat treated for a nasal tumor. Note the lighter color of the hair overlying two thirds of the face and loss of the dark pigment of the nasal planum. This cat was treated with megavoltage radiation therapy for a nasal tumor 2 years before this photograph was taken. Clients should be informed that radiation can result in ocular changes that may impair vision, although cats do not exhibit associated clinical signs.

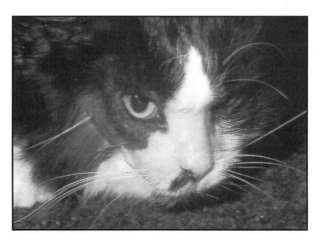

Figure 12-4: A nasal squamous cell carcinoma was successfully treated with electron beam radiation therapy (generated from a linear accelerator) 2 years before this photograph was taken. Note the loss of hair growth, which can be a transient or permanent consequence of radiation therapy. Also note the depigmentation of the nose.

whereas xerostomia and dental caries may be seen in the chronic phase. Bone necrosis of the mandible or maxilla is extremely rare but has been noted as a late injury. Care should be taken to ensure that all necessary dental work is completed prior to the start of radiation therapy.

During treatment, owners may want to rinse their cat's mouth with a solution of salt and water (1 teaspoon salt in 1 quart of water). Some recommend adding Maalox® to this saltwater solution to coat the mouth. Cool tea solutions can be used to lavage the mouth three to six times per day and may reduce oral discomfort and freshen the breath. Because oral and nasal damage from radiation therapy may reduce taste and smell sensations, more palatable and warmed aromatic foods should be prescribed. Increasing the amount of liquids given may help overcome xerostomia brought on by salivary gland radiation. Artificial saliva preparations, such as a mixture of sorbitol, sodium, carboxymethyl cellulose, and methylparaben (Salivart®), may be beneficial in these patients. Mucositis usually resolves within 30 days after radiation therapy is completed.

KEY POINT

Generally, the acute effects of radiation therapy start toward the end of the treatment period, may actually worsen substantially 1 to 3 weeks after treatment is discontinued, and may last for several weeks. Late effects may occur 6 months to years after the end of treatment.

Colon and Rectum

Occasionally, the colon and rectum are in the area of radiation. Irritation to these tissues manifests as bleeding, tenesmus, and pain. A low-residue diet and a stool softener may provide relief. Steroid enemas (e.g., Proctofoam®) may be beneficial in select cats. Whenever the anus and perianal area are injured by radiation therapy, the area should be kept clean using soap and water and dried thoroughly.

Eye

The eye is often in the radiation field in cats with nasal tumors (Figure 12-3). The lens of the eye is considered sensitive to relatively low doses of radiation, which can result in cataract formation months to years after radiation therapy is complete. In addition, retinal hemorrhages may result in blindness. Conjunctivitis or keratoconjunctivitis sicca may occur acutely, and it is important to monitor tear production in animals during and after therapy. Artificial tear preparations are necessary for cats with keratoconjunctivitis sicca. It is important to confirm that no corneal ulcers are present before prescribing steroid-containing ophthalmic ointments.

Hematology

Bone marrow suppression may occur when significant amounts of bone marrow are included in the radiation field. In addition, all lymphocytes that pass through the radiation field are lysed. This often results in a leukopenia that can be dramatic if concurrent chemotherapy is used.

Bone

If bone is included in the radiation field, bone sequestrum due to necrosis may result. This is a late effect that occurs many months to years after therapy. Removal of the sequestrum is indicated. Whenever brachytherapy is used to deliver radiotherapy to very localized areas, the radiation can damage surrounding structures, including bone.

Miscellaneous Sites

Other areas that can be damaged include the esophagus, stomach, small intestine, and liver. The endocrine system, including the pituitary gland and thyroid, may be injured when radiation therapy involves the head and neck. Relatively low doses of lung radiation can result in radiation pneumonitis, which can cause decreased respiratory tidal volume. When the heart is included in the radiation field, pericarditis and resultant pericardial effusion may be identified 4 to 6 months after therapy is complete. A pericardectomy may be necessary to treat these cats.

When the urinary bladder is subjected to single high doses of radiation, such as those used in intraoperative radiation therapy, severe fibrosis and lack of elasticity can develop. Fibrosis may also occur as a late effect of fractionated external beam radiation therapy. In humans, cranial radiation therapy occasionally results in headache, nausea, vomiting, and papilledema. Steroid therapy generally is indicated for these patients and should be considered during and after treatment. The most severe effect of radiation therapy to the brain or spinal cord is localized necrosis, which can result in severe neurologic problems.

CLINICAL USE OF RADIATION THERAPY TO CONTROL MALIGNANT DISEASE (TABLE 12-1[8,16,22,24-36])

Radiation therapy is effective for the treatment of oral, nasal, rectal, perianal, and anal tumors, soft tissue sarcomas, lymphoproliferative disorders, and CNS tumors in feline patients. The variability in response to radiation therapy of these various tumor types is related to the amount of radiation delivered, the method by which it is given, and the course and scheduling of the therapy. With the increased availability of megavoltage radiation therapy, computerized treatment planning, and delineation of the extent of the

TABLE 12-1
Select Beneficial Effects of Radiation Therapy for Various Feline Malignancies

Tumor Type	No. of Cats	DFI or Progression-Free Survivial (days)	Survival (%)	Median/ Mean Survival (days)	Reference	Comments
Oral SCC	52		N/A	96/60	24	
	7		30% 1 yr	180/NA	27	Mitoxantrone used with radiation (59–61Gy)
	6			87/NA	28	54 Gy
	11			107/NA	28	63 Gy
	11			102/NA	28	63 Gy combined with hyperthermia
	11	119 (median), 137 (mean)		161/170	25	Carboplatin with 30 Gy
	11			132/NA	26	52 Gy with etanidazole (a hypoxic cell sensitizer)
Mandibular SCC	7		57% 1 yr	420/450	8	Radiation following mandibulectomy
Nasal Plenum or Pinnae SCC	13		61.5% 1 yr 23% 2 yr 15% 3 yr	365/531	31	
	25	1,020	89% 1 yr 82% 5 yr		30	Brachytherapy with ^{90}Sr (plesiotherapy)
	11	361		383/NA	29	46 Gy average
	90	495	60.1% 1 yr 10.3% 5 yr		33	40 Gy
Intra- or Paranasal Sinus Tumor						
Carcinoma	3			330/357	31	Surgery and radiation (2 cats) or radiation alone (1 cat)
Carcinoma (10 cats) or Sarcoma (6 cats)	16		44.3% 1 yr 16.6% 2 yr	30–1,000+	32	48 Gy
Carcinoma or Sarcoma	9		66.7% 1 yr 44% 2 yr 33% 3 yr	624/837	16	25–50 Gy
Ceruminous Gland Carcinoma	9	1,185	56% 1 yr		34	48 Gy
Fibrosarcoma						
	33	398 700 112		600/NA	35	Radiation (48 Gy) followed by surgery (26 negative tumor margin; 5 positive tumor margin)
	5	356 (median)/ 214 (mean)		372/240	36	Acemannan immunostimulant with surgery and radiation
Localized Lymphoma	10	500+			22	Photo radiotherapy (2.5–4 Gy fractions for nasal, retrobulbar, mediastinal, and maxillary tumors) or electron radiation (3.6 and 5 Gy for subcutaneous and mandible tumors, respectively)

DFI = disease-free interval; SCC = squamous cell carcinoma.

disease by CT and MRI, the beneficial effects of radiation therapy are bound to increase substantially. The future of radiation therapy will be tied to the use of radiobiologic and tumor biology information to enhance its beneficial effects. In addition, the combination of radiation therapy with surgery, hyperthermia, and chemotherapy may result in substantial improvement in the efficacy of this treatment modality.

> ## KEY POINT
>
> *The best tumor control for all malignancies is achieved when radiation is used early in the course of disease. In some cases, such as large vaccine-associated sarcomas, radiation can be used preoperatively to improve tumor control.*

Oral Tumors

Squamous cell carcinomas and fibrosarcomas are the most common oral tumors in cats. Feline oral squamous cell carcinomas are generally considered resistant to the effects of radiation therapy. Control rates of 10% to 20% at 1 year have been reported by one investigator.[7] Radiation following mandibulectomy for mandibular squamous cell carcinoma resulted in a median survival time of 14 months and a 1 year survival rate of 57%.[24] Other researchers have shown improved results by treating oral squamous cell carcinomas with a combination of radiation therapy (nearly 60 Gy) and mitoxantrone chemotherapy (median survival time, 6 months versus 2 months with any other treatment modality).[9]

Non-Oral Squamous Cell Carcinoma

Seventy percent of cats with dermal squamous cell carcinomas have been reported to respond to radiation therapy.[7]

Nasal Tumors

Although nasal tumors are much less common in cats than in dogs, they apparently respond better to radiation therapy. In a recent study, nine cats with nasal tumors were treated with surgery prior to receiving radiation therapy and subsequent orthovoltage treatment; mean and median survival times were 27.9 and 20.8 months, respectively.[16] Radiation therapy of intranasal lymphoma in cats can result in control times exceeding 500 days.[16] One year survival rates exceeded 60% for squamous cell carcinoma of the nasal planum treated with radiation therapy.[10,13] While the response to therapy for nasal tumors depends on the histologic type of the tumor, nasal tumors can be effectively treated with radiation therapy.

Soft Tissue Sarcomas

Soft tissue sarcomas are challenging neoplastic conditions that frequently recur after incomplete surgical excision. In part, this is because these tumors have many "fingers" that extend into surrounding tissues. Such tumors are often excised only around the palpable area, which ensures that disease will recur. Radiation therapy is frequently used to prevent recurrence of incompletely excised tumors. Radiation therapy also seems to be effective for treating gross evidence of malignant soft tissue sarcomas (Figure 12-5). When complete excision cannot be attained, debulking to the level of microscopic disease followed by radiation therapy is the current recommended treatment for all soft tissue sarcomas. In one study of the treatment of non-oral fibrosarcomas, radiation therapy (48 Gy) followed by excisional surgery resulted in a median disease-free interval of over a year and an overall median survival of almost 2 years.[31] Current protocols involve treating the patient once or twice daily for 6 weeks.

Other Tumors

Thyroid adenoma or adenomatous hyperplasia is treated effectively with ^{131}I with a high probability (>80%) of permanent control. Rectal, colonic, bladder, and prostate tumors have been successfully treated with radiation therapy. In each case, the extent of the disease must be clearly defined and the tumor appropriately staged using at least abdominal radiography or ultrasonography, hemogram, biochemical profile, and urinalysis. When radiation therapy is delivered to these particular sites, such problems as dysuria,

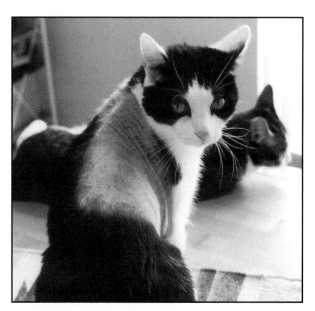

Figure 12-5: *Vaccine-associated sarcomas are commonly treated with radiation therapy. Large radiation fields are used pre- or postoperatively. Note the thinning of the hair coat and leukotrichia 4 months after radiation therapy was completed.*

colitis, and prostatitis must be expected. When possible, radiation therapy should be combined with other treatment modalities to enhance the beneficial effects.

Palliative Therapy

Radiation therapy can be given to alleviate pain and discomfort associated with a wide variety of malignancies, especially those involving bone. Palliative radiation therapy of oral tumors is a logical and often effective mode of improving quality of life for patients in which surgical removal or amputation is not an option.

REFERENCES

1. Dewhirst MW, Sim DA, Saparateo S, et al: Importance of minimum tumor temperature in determining early and long term response of spontaneous canine and feline tumors to heat and radiation. *Cancer Res* 44:43–50, 1984.
2. Gillette EL, McChesney SL, Dewhirst MS, et al: Response of canine oral carcinomas to heat and radiation. *Int J Radiol Oncol Biol Phys* 13:1861–1867, 1987.
3. Evans SM, Shofer F: Canine oral nontonsillar squamous cell carcinoma. Prognostic factors for recurrence and survival following orthovoltage radiation therapy. *Vet Radiol* 29:133–137, 1988.
4. McChesney SL, Withrow SJ, Gillette EL, et al: Radiotherapy of soft tissue sarcomas in dogs. *JAVMA* 194:60–63, 1989.
5. Overgaard J, Vondermaase H, Overgaard M, et al: A randomized study comparing two high dose per fraction radiation schedules in recurrent or metastatic malignant melanoma. *Int J Radiol Oncol Biol Phys* 11:1837–1839, 1985.
6. Thrall DE: Orthovoltage radiotherapy of acanthomatous epulides in 39 dogs. *JAVMA* 184:826–829, 1984.
7. Turrel JM: Radiation and hyperthermia, in Holzworth J (ed): *Diseases of the Cat: Medicine and Surgery.* Philadelphia, WB Saunders, 1987, pp 606–619.
8. Hutson CA, Willamer CC, Walder EJ, et al: Treatment of mandibular squamous cell carcinoma in cats by use of mandibulectomy and radiotherapy: Seven cases (1987–1989). *JAVMA* 201:777–781, 1992.
9. Ogilvie GK, Moore AS, Obradovich JE, et al: Toxicoses and efficacy associated with the administration of mitoxantrone to cats with malignant tumors. *JAVMA* 11:1839–1844, 1993.
10. Brooks WMB, Matus RE, Leifer CE, et al: Chemotherapy vs chemotherapy post-radiotherapy in the treatment of tonsillar squamous cell carcinoma in the dog. *J Vet Intern Med* 2:206–211, 1988.
11. MacMillan R, Withrow SJ, Gillette EL: Surgery and regional irradiation for treatment of canine tonsillar squamous cell carcinoma: Retrospective review of eight cases. *JAAHA* 18:311–314, 1982.
12. Thrall DE, Adams WM: Radiotherapy of squamous cell carcinoma of the canine nasal plane. *Vet Radiol* 23:193–196, 1982.
13. Thrall DE, Harvey CE: Radiotherapy of malignant nasal tumors in 21 dogs. *JAVMA* 183:663–666, 1983.
14. McEntee MC, Thrall DE, Page RL, et al: A retrospective study of 27 dogs with intranasal neoplasms treated with radiation therapy. *Vet Radiol* 32:135–139, 1991.
15. Evans SM, Goldschmidt M, McKee LJ, et al: Prognostic factors in survival after radiotherapy for intranasal neoplasms in dogs—70 cases (1974–1985). *JAVMA* 194:1460–1463, 1989.
16. Evans SM, Hendrick M: Radiotherapy of feline nasal tumors: A retrospective study of 9 cats. *Vet Radiol* 30:128–132, 1989.
17. McChesney SL, Gillette EL, Dewhirst MW, et al: Influence of WR 2721 on radiation responsive canine soft tissue sarcomas. *Int J Radiol Oncol Biol Phys* 12:1957–1963, 1986.
18. Evans SM: Canine hemangiopericytoma: A retrospective analysis of response to surgery and orthovoltage radiation. *Vet Radiol* 28:13–16, 1987.
19. Atwater SW, LaRue SM, Powers BE: Adjuvant radiotherapy of soft tissue sarcomas in dogs. *Proc 12ᵗʰ Annu Vet Canc Soc:*41–42, 1992.
20. Turrel JM, Kitchell BE, Miller LM, et al: Prognostic factors for radiation treatment of mast cell tumors in 85 dogs. *JAVMA* 193:936–940, 1988.
21. LaRue SM, Gillette EL: Recent advances in radiation oncology. *Compend Contin Educ Pract Vet* 15:795–805, 1993.
22. Elmslie RE, Ogilvie GK, LaRue, et al: Radiotherapy with and without chemotherapy for localized lymphoma in 10 cats. *Vet Radiol* 32:277–280, 1991.
23. Savage DE: Principles of radiation oncology, in Rosenthal S, Casignan JR, Smith BD (eds): *Medical Care of the Cancer Patient*, ed 2. Philadelphia, WB Saunders, 1989, pp 27–39.
24. Postorino-Reeves NC, Turrel JM, Withrow SJ, et al: Oral squamous cell carcinoma in the cat. *JAAHA* 29:438-441, 1993.
25. Wood CA: Combination coarse fractionation radiation therapy and carboplatin chemotherapy for treatment of feline oral squamous cell carcinoma: An interim analysis. *Vet Cancer Soc Newsl* 22:1, 4, 1998.
26. Evans SM, LaCreta F, Helfand S, et al: Techniques, pharmacokinetics, toxicity, and efficacy of intratumoral etanidazole and radiotherapy for treatment of spontaneous feline oral squamous cell carcinoma. *Int J Radiat Oncol* 20:703–708, 1991.
27. LaRue SM, Vail DM, Ogilvie GK, et al: Shrinking field radiation therapy in combination with mitoxantrone chemotherapy for the treatment of oral squamous cell carcinoma in the cat. *Proc 11ᵗʰ Annu Conf Vet Cancer Soc:*99, 1991.
28. Mauldin GN, Mauldin GE, Meleo KA: Treatment of feline oral squamous cell carcinoma with radiation therapy alone or radiation therapy and hyperthermia. *Vet Cancer Soc Newsl* 16:4-5, 1992.
29. Lana SE, Ogilvie GK, Withrow SJ, et al: Feline cutaneous squamous cell carcinoma of the nasal planum and the pinnae: 61 cases. *JAAHA* 33:329–332, 1997.
30. Van Vechten MK, Theon AP: Strontium-90 plesiotherapy for treatment of early squamous cell carcinomas of the nasal planum in 25 cats. *Proc 13ᵗʰ Annu Conf Vet Cancer Soc:*107–108, 1993.
31. Cox NR, Brawner WR Jr, Powers RD, Wright JC: Tumors of the nose and paranasal sinuses in cats: 32 cases with comparison to a national database (1977 through 1987). *JAAHA* 27:339–347, 1991.
32. Theon AP, Peaston AE, Madewell BR, Dungworth DL: Irradiation of nonlymphoproliferative neoplasms of the nasal cavity and paranasal sinuses in 16 cats. *JAVMA* 204:78–83, 1994.
33. Theon AP, Madewell BR, Shearn VI, Moulton JE: Prognostic factors associated with radiotherapy of squamous cell carcinoma of the nasal plane in cats. *JAVMA* 206:991, 1995.
34. Theon AP, Barthez PY, Madewell BR, Griffey SM: Radiation therapy of ceruminous gland carcinomas in dogs and cats. *JAVMA* 205:566–569, 1994.
35. Cronin K, Page RL, Spodnick G, et al: Radiation therapy and surgery for fibrosarcoma in 33 cats. *Vet Radiol Ultrasound* 39:51–56, 1998.
36. King GK, Yates KM, Greenlee PG, et al: The effect of Acemannan Immunostimulant in combination with surgery and radiation therapy on spontaneous canine and feline fibrosarcomas. *JAAHA* 31:439–447, 1995.

BIOLOGIC RESPONSE MODIFIERS—PROPERTIES, USES, AND PATIENT MANAGEMENT

Gregory K. Ogilvie and Antony S. Moore

13

CLINICAL BRIEFING

Definition	Agents that reconstitute or enhance the immune system to fight a malignancy using endogenous biologic processes.
Categories	BCG, L-MTP-PE, acemannan, levamisole, cimetidine, TNF, IL-2, monoclonal antibodies, and gene therapy.
Efficacy	Lymphoma, mammary adenocarcinoma, and soft tissue sarcomas (including fibrosarcoma).

Biologic response modifiers (BRMs) are rapidly becoming an important modality for the treatment of cancer in humans and cats. In this type of therapy, the immune system is reconstituted or enhanced to fight a malignancy using endogenous biologic processes. This can be done with a wide variety of substances, including biologic products, chemicals, lymphokines, cytokines, hematopoietic growth factors, antibodies, and vaccines[1-3] (Table 13-1). The attractiveness of using BRMs is obvious; however, this approach has not been documented to be effective as a single agent for the treatment of any malignant disease in cats.

KEY POINT

BRMs have not been documented to be effective as a single agent for the treatment of any malignant disease in the cat. They appear to be most effective when combined with other modalities.

This chapter focuses on agents that are likely to be of clinical use (or at least the focus of discussion by veterinary practitioners) now or in the near future. These include bacillus Calmette-Guerin (BCG), liposome-encapsulated muramyl tripeptide-phosphatidylethanolamine (L-MTP-PE), acemannan, levamisole, cimetidine, tumor necrosis factor (TNF), interleukin-2 (IL-2), monoclonal antibodies, and gene therapy. Hematopoietic growth factors, considered as BRMs by some, are discussed in Chapter 21, and the use of herbal products is covered in Chapter 16.

NONSPECIFIC IMMUNOMODULATORS

Biologic agents (e.g., BCG, L-MTP-PE) and chemical immunopotentiators (e.g., levamisole, cimetidine) are categorized as active nonspecific immunotherapeutic agents. They actively stimulate the immune system to respond to a wide variety of substances that may harm the body, including cancer.[1-3]

BCG has been evaluated extensively in a variety of neoplastic diseases in humans and cats.[1-3] The active subunit of BCG is muramyl dipeptide, a potent macrophage activator that has also been used therapeutically.[4] BCG has recently been described as an effective agent for the treatment of some early cases of transitional cell carcinomas of the bladder in humans. The therapeutic utility of this substance in feline medicine is being investigated.

L-MTP-PE is a nonspecific activator of monocytes and macrophages with anticancer effects. Studies are underway to determine whether L-MTP-PE is effective for the treatment of neoplastic disorders in cats. Postsurgical administration of L-MTP-PE has been shown to improve the survival of dogs with various tumors through targeted macrophage activation; however, there was no improvement in survival of cats with mammary carcinoma treated with adjuvant L-MTP-PE.[4]

Acemannan, an extract from the aloe vera plant, is a nonspecific immunostimulator that has been shown to be taken up by macrophages, thereby enhancing the release of interferon, interleukin-1, TNF, and prostaglandin E_2.[1] It has direct immunostimulatory effects and, apparently, direct antiviral activity against HIV-1. The commercially available product has been reported to delay the develop-

TABLE 13-1
Substances Used as Biologic Response Modifiers

General Category	Biologic Response Modifier
Nonspecific Immunomodulators	BCG
	C. parvum
	Staphage lysate
	L-MTP-PE
	Levamisole
	Cimetidine
	Acemannan
Lymphokines/ Monokines	IL-1
	IL-2
	Interferon
	TNF
Adoptive Cellular Therapy	Lymphokine-activated killer cells
	Tumor-infiltrating lymphocytes
Antibody Therapy	Antibody directed against lymphoma cells
Growth Factors	Granulocyte colony-stimulating factor
	Granulocyte-macrophage colony-stimulating factor
	Macrophage colony-stimulating factor

ment of clinical signs in cats infected with FeLV.[6] Acemannan has been promoted as having antitumor properties against fibrosarcoma in cats,[5,7] but there is some controversy about this effect. Four cats with fibrosarcomas were injected with acemannan (2 mg/kg intralesionally weekly for 6 weeks) before receiving surgery and megavoltage radiation therapy (60 Gy); the cats then received 1 mg/kg intraperitoneally weekly for 6 weeks and monthly thereafter for as long as they responded to therapy. One cat experienced tumor recurrence 8 months after surgery, but the other three had no recurrence between 14 and 19 months after surgery.[5] Since long survivals are seen following surgery and radiation therapy alone, the true contribution of acemannan to survival in these cats is difficult to evaluate. Acemannan is the only polymer BRM approved for commercial use as an antitumor agent in the treatment of solid tumors in feline medicine. Its efficacy has not been clearly determined.

Levamisole is an imidazole compound that has immunorestorative properties.[8] Several veterinary studies involving this agent have been performed. In one study evaluating 73 cases of feline mammary tumors, cats were randomized after surgery to receive levamisole or a place-

bo.[8] No significant difference in survival time between the two groups was found. Additional feline studies exploring the potential benefit of this agent are needed.

Postsurgical immunotherapy with *Corynebacterium parvum* or a cocktail of *Streptococcus pyogenes* and *Serratia marcescens*[1,3] did not significantly improve recurrence rate or survival time compared with surgery alone for cats with mammary carcinomas.

Cimetidine is an H_2-receptor antagonist that potentiates the immune system.[1] As a single agent, it has been shown to alter the activity level of suppressor cells. Some studies have shown that cimetidine is synergistic with interferon in the treatment of oral malignant melanoma in humans. The therapeutic value of this drug in small animal medicine has not been defined.

CYTOKINES

Cytokines are soluble mediators secreted by a variety of cell types regulating several aspects of the immune system.[1-3] Biotechnology has resulted in the development of production methods to provide health care professionals with large quantities of cytokines for therapeutic uses. TNF and IL-2 are two such therapeutic cytokines.

TNF is secreted from macrophages in response to a number of substances, including lipopolysaccharides. TNF release results in the death of tumor cells through a variety of mechanisms, including inhibition of protein and RNA synthesis and development of cytopathic pores in the tumor cell membrane. IL-2 may also be effective used alone or with cytokines other than TNF to treat specific malignancies.

SPECIFIC MONOCLONAL ANTIBODIES

Specific monoclonal antibodies developed against tumor-specific or tumor-associated transformation antigens may prove to be an important therapeutic modality.[1] These monoclonal antibodies can be used for therapeutics and diagnostics. Using hybridomas, large quantities of monoclonal antibodies against a wide variety of malignant cells may be developed. These antibodies can be used to mediate antitumor cytotoxicity through either complement-mediated cytotoxicity or antibody-dependent cellular cytotoxicity. In addition, antibodies can be "tagged" with a radioactive material to identify the presence of malignancies within the body.

GENE THERAPY

Gene therapy is the process of inserting genes (or gene-containing cells) that code for certain proteins or cytokines to benefit the patient. These genes can be inserted into the tumor or injected into the blood or lymphatic system. Gene therapy is just beginning to be explored as a cancer treatment in cats. For example, in a study of fibrosarcoma treatment in cats, xenogeneic cells (Vero hIL-2) that secrete human recombinant IL-2 (hrIL-2) were infiltrated around the tumor at the time of surgical resection and implantation of ^{192}Ir seeds for brachytherapy.[9] This infiltration was repeated 5 days later and another five times over the next 2 months. Of 16 cats treated by this protocol, 2 had local recurrence and 3 had metastases for an overall median survival of 16 months. In comparison, 11 of 16 cats that did not receive Vero hIL-2 cells had tumor recurrence and a median survival of 8 months. Antibodies to the cells were detected after 5 days of treatment, and most cats had a local inflammatory reaction to the injection. One cat developed anaphylaxis.[9]

Gene therapy will likely become a viable tool in the treatment of a wide variety of diseases in feline medicine. Regulatory issues to ensure that this approach is safe for the health care team, patient, and client have yet to be determined.

REFERENCES

1. MacEwen EG, Helfand SC: Recent advances in the biologic therapy of cancer. *Compend Contin Educ Pract Vet* 15:909–922, 1993.
2. Elmslie RE, Dow SW, Ogilvie GK: Interleukins: Biological properties and therapeutic potential. *J Vet Intern Med* 5:283–293, 1991.
3. MacEwen EG: Approaches to cancer therapy using biological response modifiers. *Vet Clin North Am Small Anim Pract* 15:667–688, 1985.
4. Fox LE, MacEwen EG, Kurzman ID, et al: L-MTP-PE treatment of feline mammary adenocarcinoma. *Proc 14th Annu Conf Vet Cancer Soc*:107–108, 1994.
5. King GK, Yates KM, Greenlee PG, et al: The effect of acemannan immunostimulant in combination with surgery and radiation therapy on spontaneous canine and feline fibrosarcomas. *JAAHA* 31:439–447, 1995.
6. Sheets MA, Unger BA, Giggleman GF, et al: Studies of the effect of acemannan on retrovirus infections: Clinical stabilization of feline leukemia virus-infected cats. *Mol Biother* 3:41–45, 1991.
7. Harris C, Pierce K, King G, et al: Efficacy of acemannan in treatment of canine and feline spontaneous neoplasms. *Mol Biother* 3:207–213, 1991.
8. MacEwen EG, Hayes AA, Mooney S, et al: Evaluation of effect of levamisole on feline mammary cancer. *J Biol Response Mod* 5:541–546, 1984.
9. Quintin-Colonna F, Devauchelle P, Fradelizi D, et al: Gene therapy of spontaneous canine melanoma and feline fibrosarcoma by intratumoral administration of histoincompatible cells expressing human interleukin-2. *Gene Ther* 3:1104–1112, 1996.

THERAPEUTIC & SUPPORTIVE PROCEDURES

SURGICAL ONCOLOGY—PROPERTIES, USES, AND PATIENT MANAGEMENT

14

Gregory K. Ogilvie and Antony S. Moore

CLINICAL BRIEFING

Cancer Prevention	Education and preventive surgery (e.g., ovariohysterectomy).
Diagnosis	Carefully premeditated biopsy procedures, including aspiration, punch, needle core, incisional, and excisional biopsy, performed in close consultation with the surgeon who will perform the definitive surgery.
Definitive Treatment	Therapy for the primary tumor and, if indicated, residual and metastatic disease.
Palliation	Therapy to relieve pain and other symptoms.
Rehabilitation	Reconstructive techniques for rapid return to normal function.
Supportive Care	Analgesia and nutritional support.

Surgery, the oldest form of cancer therapy in human and feline medicine, has been responsible for the cure of more patients than any other treatment modality. This great success is mainly related to the development of new surgical techniques and a greater understanding of the biologic behavior of malignancies.[1-4] Development of new adjunctive treatments, such as chemotherapy, radiation therapy, and biologic response modifiers, has enhanced the control of microscopic disease and prompted surgeons to reassess the type of surgery necessary. Despite advances in these fields, surgeons have an important role in the prevention, diagnosis, definitive treatment, palliation, and rehabilitation of feline cancer patients. Surgeons who treat cancer must have an understanding of the biologic behavior of individual malignancies and must have a strong command of the principles of surgical oncology as well as the aforementioned modalities.

While surgery is a critical step in the treatment of most feline malignancies, the surgical procedure can both empower and frighten clients: It can empower them with the knowledge that they have done something important to help their pets and to reach a diagnosis, thereby improving their understanding of the likely outcome and options ahead. This procedure can be frightening, however, because of the perceived and actual risks associated with surgery and anesthesia and the potential consequences for the patient. Many clients are concerned that cancer surgery will inevitably be disfiguring or unduly decrease a pet's quality of life.

Providing oral and written information about the risks and benefits of surgery is essential to empowering clients with the facts while dispelling the myths associated with cancer and oncologic surgery. Additional tools include photographs of patients taken before and at different times after the same type of surgery. In many practices, former clients will agree to be contacted to give their perspective of the surgery. Education and a comprehensive, coordinated approach should be presented by the entire veterinary health care team to ensure that the client can be more confident and comfortable with this difficult decision-making process.

ROLES OF SURGERY IN CANCER PATIENTS

Prevention

Preventing cancer through ovariohysterectomy and orchiectomy is not as well defined in cats as in dogs. These surgical procedures can be critical in preventing both malignant disease (uterine and ovarian neoplasia) and nonneoplastic conditions (pregnancy, pyometra, behavioral problems). Although helpful, early spaying does not completely eliminate the risk of mammary carcinoma in cats.[5] In one study, the relative risk of a spayed female developing mammary carcinoma was approximately half that of an intact cat.[6] Therefore surgery is important for reducing the risk of cancer development in feline patients.

Diagnosis

The veterinarian who performs the surgery plays an important role in staging and determining the extent of malignant disease in feline cancer patients.[1-4] A surgical biopsy is always required to make a definitive diagnosis. Methods to diagnose the malignant condition or the extent of the disease include aspiration, needle core, punch, incisional, and excisional biopsies.[1-4] It is exceedingly important to know the histologic diagnosis of a neoplasia before performing most definitive procedures. For example, knowing whether a tumor is a benign basal cell tumor or a malignant vaccine-associated sarcoma is extremely important: Even though they may have the same outward appearance, the latter requires extensive surgical resection and additional diagnostic procedures (i.e., abdominal and thoracic radiographs, lymph node aspiration/biopsy) to determine the extent of disease. In contrast, a benign basal cell tumor may need only a simple resection.

Because tumors in cats have a higher likelihood of being malignant compared with other species, the following principles should be kept in mind when a surgical biopsy is performed[1-4] (refer to the Biopsy section for further details):

- Needle tracts or biopsy incisions should be made with careful thought so that the entire biopsy tract (i.e., tissue in contact with and/or disturbed by the biopsy instrument) can be removed when the definitive surgical procedure is performed. Veterinarians who are unlikely to perform the definitive procedure should consult with the oncologic surgeon before collecting biopsy samples.
- Extreme care should be taken to not spread cancer cells to surrounding tissues or through tissue planes during the biopsy procedure. For example, care must be taken to avoid the formation of a hematoma or a seroma, which might spread cancer cells as it dissects between fascial planes, thereby necessitating more extensive definitive resection. When multiple biopsy specimens are taken from different sites, care should be taken to change instruments so that tumor cells are not transplanted from site to site by the surgeon.
- Biopsy techniques should be carefully selected to allow acquisition of sufficient tissue to make a histopathologic diagnosis. In addition, tissues should be prepared in a manner that allows adequate evaluation by different procedures, such as immunohistochemistry. Collecting multiple biopsy specimens increases the likelihood of obtaining an accurate diagnosis as long as an excisional biopsy is not planned.
- The biopsy specimen should be handled with extreme care to prevent crushing, artifacts, or alteration of the orientation of the tissue specimen. The recent increased use of laser surgery has introduced a new variable—this methodology can significantly alter tissue, which can prevent an adequate diagnosis. Specimens should be sufficiently small and placed in enough preservative to allow complete fixation (a good rule is 1 part tissue to 10 parts formalin); however, prolonged fixation or storage in formalin may reduce the chances for future successful immunohistochemical staining. Using ink or sutures to mark tissue margins may give pathologists information regarding orientation of biopsy tissue within the body. Check with your pathologist to determine his or her preferred tissue-marking method.
- Surgeons should have an acute awareness of the biologic behavior of malignant conditions to ensure that all possible sites of metastasis are evaluated before a definitive procedure is performed.

Treatment

Surgical treatment of cancer can be divided into six areas:

- Definitive surgical treatment for primary cancer
- Surgery to reduce the bulk of residual disease
- Surgical resection of metastatic disease
- Surgery to treat emergencies
- Surgery for palliation
- Surgery for reconstruction and rehabilitation

Definitive Surgery for Primary Cancer (Figure 14-1)

Because tumors are more likely to be malignant in cats than in other species, proper execution of the surgical procedure is very important. Definitive surgery for primary cancer is the most common use of surgery in veterinary cancer patients. Before such surgery can be performed, the patient must be completely staged to determine the extent of the cancer.

Surgeons should be well aware of the biologic behavior of malignant conditions to ensure that all possible sites of metastasis are evaluated and must consider all options and alternatives when planning a definitive procedure. For example, a relatively conservative surgical procedure may result in a 90% cure rate for a basal cell tumor.[4] A soft tissue sarcoma, however, must be treated with a wide surgical excision that should extend at least one fascial layer below the detectable margins of the tumor. Therefore it is important to know the specific tumor type being treated and its biologic behavior so that clients can be educated about the prognosis and amount of surgery needed for a satisfactory outcome.

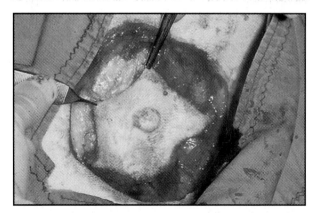

Figure 14-1: Before definitive surgery, the tumor should be identified by a preoperative biopsy, the cancer must be completely staged, and the surgeon should be acutely aware of the cat's health and the biologic behavior of malignant conditions.

It is equally vital that surgeons know their limits and abilities. For example, an invasive soft tissue sarcoma may best be referred to a boarded specialist for appropriate therapy and the best chance for a positive outcome. Finally, other options such as radiation therapy should be considered and offered to clients instead of or as an adjunct to surgery as appropriate.

Important recent advances in cancer surgery in cats include:

- Craniotomy to remove feline meningiomas
- Hemipelvectomy to remove pelvic or proximal femoral lesions
- Mandibulectomy or maxillectomy to remove oral tumors
- Orbitectomy to remove tumors of the ocular area and surrounding structures
- Tracheotomy to remove tracheal tumors
- Chest wall resection to remove rib or other chest wall tumors
- Scapulectomy to remove tumors of the scapula or surrounding structures
- Rhinectomy to remove squamous cell carcinoma of the nasal planum
- Plastic surgery techniques to repair soft tissue defects

KEY POINT

Whenever considering surgery for a neoplastic process, the following questions should be asked[a]:

1. *What am I treating?*
2. *What is the biologic behavior?*
3. *Is a cure possible?*
4. *What "surgical dose" should be used?*
5. *What are my alternatives?*

Surgery for Residual Disease

The first surgery is the best opportunity for curing a cat with malignant disease; however, tumors are sometimes incompletely resected during the first surgery, and subsequent therapy is therefore needed. In many cases, surgery is unable to adequately treat the remaining disease, and thus other treatment modalities, such as radiation therapy and chemotherapy, are indicated.[1-3] For example, resection of a soft tissue sarcoma in the distal extremity may result in significant morbidity if the tumor is completely resected; if, however, the tumor is removed until only microscopic disease remains and the surgical field is irradiated postoperatively, morbidity is usually minimal and the probability for long-term control is very good. "Debulking" (cytoreductive) surgery alone is rarely an acceptable form of therapy and should not be used inappropriately to reduce tumor bulk without anticipating the need for additional therapy

[a]Courtesy of S.J. Withrow.

to control residual disease.[1] Except in cases of palliative surgery, there is no role for cytoreductive surgery when other effective therapies for the treatment of that malignant disease are available.

Surgery for Metastatic Disease

Resection of metastases should be considered in select cases when it is obvious that the malignant disease is not progressing rapidly and the metastatic disease is restricted to a single site or a few sites that are amenable to surgical excision. This is especially true when surgery for the metastatic disease will improve quality of life or serve as a diagnostic tool for the management of the case. In most instances, however, once a tumor has metastasized, surgery has little use except to provide palliation of bulky disease.

Surgery for Oncologic Emergencies

The most common applications for oncologic surgery in an emergency setting include the treatment of hemorrhage, perforation, or obstruction of organs or the drainage of abscesses.[1-3] An example is an intestinal resection and anastomosis to treat a perforated malignancy of the GI tract.

Surgery for Palliation

When a tumor or its metastasis results in significant discomfort for the veterinary cancer patient, surgery can improve or maintain the animal's quality of life.[1-4] In these situations, surgery should be used only if the owner is clearly aware that this procedure will not be curative. An example may be a mastectomy in a cat with a bleeding, abscessed mammary adenocarcinoma that also has pulmonary metastatic disease. The mastectomy may improve quality of life by reducing pain, even though the overall survival time may not be substantially increased by the procedure.

Surgery for Reconstruction and Rehabilitation

Very wide resection of a malignancy is now possible because of the development of plastic surgery techniques, including free flap and microvascular anastomotic methods. These techniques can be used to rehabilitate areas that have been irradiated or where substantial tissue injury is noted.

REFERENCES

1. Rosenberg SA: Principles of surgical oncology, in DeVita VT, Helman S, Rosenberg SA (eds): *Cancer Principles and Practice of Oncology*, ed 4. Philadelphia, JB Lippincott, 1993, pp 238–247.
2. Merrick HW: Principles of surgery in cancer management, in Skeel RT (ed): *Handbook of Cancer Chemotherapy*, ed 3. Boston, Little, Brown & Co, 1991, pp 27–31.
3. Langmuir VK, Schwartz SI, Patterson WB: Principles of surgical oncology, in Rubin P (ed): *Clinical Oncology: A Multidisciplinary Approach for Physicians and Students*, ed 7. Philadelphia, WB Saunders, 1993, pp 41– 50.
4. Withrow SJ: Surgical oncology, in Withrow SJ, MacEwen EG (eds): *Clinical Veterinary Oncology*, ed 2. Philadelphia, JB Lippincott, 1995, pp 58–62.
5. Hayes AA, Mooney S: Feline mammary tumors. *Vet Clin North Am Small Anim Pract* 15:513–520, 1985.
6. Hayes HM Jr, Milne KL, Mandell CP: Epidemiological features of feline mammary carcinoma. *Vet Rec* 108:476-479, 1981.

HYPERTHERMIA, CRYOTHERAPY, AND PHOTODYNAMIC THERAPY— PROPERTIES, USES, AND PATIENT MANAGEMENT

Gregory K. Ogilvie and Antony S. Moore

15

CLINICAL BRIEFING

Equipment

Local Hyperthermia	Local hyperthermia is generally applied with a handheld radiofrequency device.
Cryotherapy	Liquid nitrogen is applied via probes or spray applicators; nitrous oxide is applied via probes.
Photodynamic Therapy	Required equipment includes a laser to produce a specific wavelength of light (usually infrared), a fiberoptic delivery system, and a photosensitizing agent.

Indications

Local Hyperthermia	Most effective for the treatment of localized tumors in combination with radiation therapy or chemotherapy; handheld hyperthermia devices are effective for the treatment of small (<1.0 cm in diameter) benign and malignant superficial tumors, such as basal cell tumors and squamous cell carcinoma.
Cryotherapy	Used in the treatment of small (<1.0 cm in diameter) benign and malignant superficial tumors (e.g., basal cell tumors, squamous cell carcinoma) of such areas as the eyelid, nose, oral cavity, or skin.
Photodynamic Therapy	Same indications as for local hyperthermia and cryotherapy; in addition, photodynamic therapy may be useful in treating esophageal or bladder tumors.

Supportive Care	Analgesics are essential during and several days after these procedures; patients receiving photodynamic therapy should be kept away from direct sunlight for some time after therapy as certain photosensitizers make cats susceptible to sunburn.

Hyperthermia and cryotherapy have been used to treat neoplastic conditions in feline medicine for decades. Whole body hyperthermia units raise the cat's overall body temperature to approximately 42°C[1,2]; local hyperthermia techniques, which are more practical in private practice, kill tumor cells by increasing the temperature of regional tissue and have a minimal chance of causing burns. Hyperthermia is most effective when used in combination with chemotherapy and radiation therapy; it is of limited efficacy when used alone.

Cryotherapy involves the use of very cold temperatures to kill tumor cells. This technique was initially used to treat a variety of types and sizes of malignant and nonmalignant tumors but is currently used most effectively to treat select, very small tumors. Because this treatment modality is fast, relatively inexpensive, and can be employed with local and systemic anesthesia, it remains a standard treatment for a variety of localized small malignancies in feline medicine.

Photodynamic therapy (PDT) involves the administration of a tumor-localizing photosensitizing agent, which may require metabolic synthesis (i.e., a prodrug), followed by activation of the agent using a specific wavelength of light (usually generated by a laser). This therapy results in a sequence of photochemical and photobiologic processes that irreversibly damage tumor tissues. Results from preclinical and clinical studies conducted worldwide over a 25 year period in human and feline medicine have established PDT as a useful treatment approach for some cancers. The most common application in feline medicine has been in the treatment of cutaneous squamous cell carcinoma. Because of the significant equipment costs and the limited application of this treatment modality, PDT is available in only a few—usually academic—sites around the world.

HYPERTHERMIA

Equipment

Whole body hyperthermia can be achieved by using various energy sources, including a radiant heat device, or extracorporeal heating techniques to raise a patient's core body temperature to 41.8°C to 42.0°C.[1,2] Although whole body hyperthermia is available only in specific research institutions, it generally results in a more uniform temperature increase within tumor tissues compared to local treatment techniques, in which areas of both extreme heat and relatively normal temperatures may reduce the efficacy of hyperthermia.

Local hyperthermia techniques involve the use of external or internal heating sources.[1,2] External hyperthermia uses microwaves, ultrasound, or radiofrequency energy sources to deposit energy within the tissue from an external applicator. Microwaves and radiofrequency methods deposit adequate energy approximately 3 to 4 cm in depth, whereas ultrasound energy can penetrate to a depth of 6 to 14 cm. Radiofrequency and microwave energy sources can also be inserted directly into the targeted tissues to produce interstitial hyperthermia.

General Technique[1,2]

Whole body hyperthermia is a complicated technique involving intensive measurement of a wide variety of physiologic parameters during treatment. Very few academic centers use whole body hyperthermia because of the cost and the need for extensive, labor-intensive monitoring.

Handheld radiofrequency hyperthermia units are used in some small animal practices.

1. Ideally, the lesion to be treated should be smaller than 1 cm in diameter.
2. The cat is placed under general anesthesia, and a systemic analgesic is administered to minimize discomfort. Local anesthesia (0.25–0.5 ml of 2% lidocaine mixed 50:50 with sodium bicarbonate) is injected around the lesion.
3. After a biopsy specimen is obtained, radiofrequency tips are placed on either side of the lesion. If the lesion is suspected to extend more than 0.2 cm below the skin surface, invasive radiofrequency tips are placed through the skin and down to the level of the deepest portion of the tumor.
4. The lesion is heated at least twice; if nearby tissue is to be treated, the applicator probes are repositioned as needed. It is important to remember that both the tumor and a surrounding "cuff" of normal tissue should reach therapeutic temperatures (>42°C).
5. The heated area will become indurated and be somewhat painful for the first 24 to 48 hours after therapy. A scab may form and later fall off, revealing a bed of gran-

ulation tissue. The lesion gradually shrinks, leaving a small, hairless area or an area where the hair and skin are a different color.
6. Postoperative oral or transdermal analgesics are recommended for several days.

Clinical Application

Hyperthermia alone provides only marginal control of local disease. In combination with radiation therapy or chemotherapy, however, the synergy enhances tumor control and subsequent survival. In actuality, local hyperthermia is not a commonly used modality.

CRYOTHERAPY[3]

Equipment (Figure 15-1)

Cryotherapy is a valuable tool in the treatment of a number of superficial dermal and oral lesions. It is ideal for cutaneous squamous cell carcinoma in such locations as the eyelids, nose, and mouth and is helpful in treating other tumors, including basal cell tumors and sebaceous adenomas. Liquid nitrogen and nitrous oxide are the cryogens used most often in cryotherapy. Liquid nitrogen evaporates slowly and requires careful monitoring; nitrous oxide tanks are the same as those used for anesthetic purposes, and the gas does not evaporate between uses. Costs are similar regardless of which cryogen is used. Nitrous oxide has limited depth of penetration but is effective for lesions smaller than

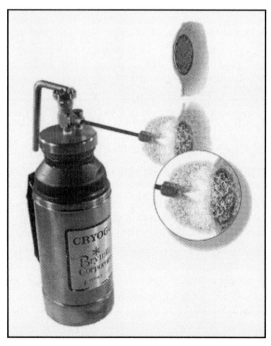

Figure 15-1: *This cryotherapy apparatus has a small thermal container for liquid mitrogen and several contact probes or spray nozzles to treat superficial tumors <1 cm in diamter.*

1 cm in diameter; it cannot be used in spray applicators. Liquid nitrogen is much more effective for larger lesions or lesions with a rich blood supply that need to be frozen faster or that would be better treated with a spray applicator. Regardless of the cryogen used, temperature monitoring devices (e.g., thermocouple needles) should be used to ensure that the tumor is frozen to critical temperatures (< −20°C).

General Technique (Figure 15-2)

1. Cryotherapy should be restricted to small tumors (<1.0 cm in diameter) of the skin and other external areas.
2. The cat is placed under general anesthesia, a systemic analgesic is administered, and local anesthesia (0.25–1 ml of 2% lidocaine mixed 50:50 with sodium bicarbonate) is injected around the area to be frozen.
3. The surrounding hair is parted or minimally clipped and cleaned.
4. The tumor is debrided, and the tissue is submitted for histopathology.
5. The tissue can be coagulated with silver nitrate or a caustic agent or a pursestring suture can be applied to reduce bleeding at the site to be frozen. Blood flow should be restricted when possible to increase the rate of freezing and decrease the rate of warming.
6. Each tumor should be rapidly frozen and slowly thawed at least twice. When a probe is used, it should be approximately the same size as the lesion. Warm probes are applied to a warm, moist tumor surface. When freezing is initiated, the tumor freezes to the applicator and is maintained in that position throughout the process,

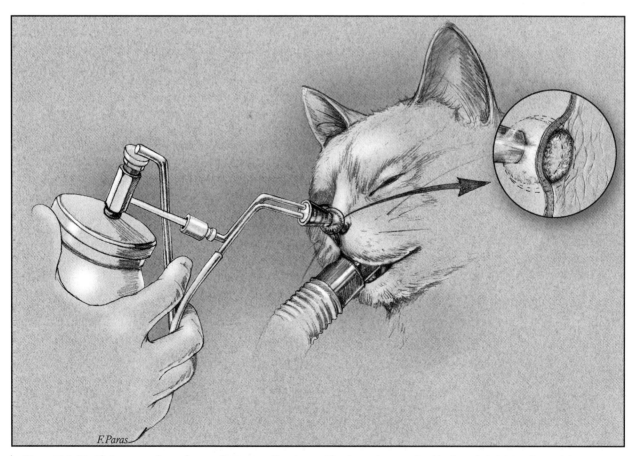

Figure 15-2: Liquid nitrogen cryotherapy for a nasal squamous cell carcinoma. After the area is prepared and local anesthesia is injected around the treatment area, the tumor is debrided and the tissue is submitted for histopathology. Each tumor should be rapidly frozen and slowly thawed at least twice. In this figure, liquid nitrogen is applied with a contact probe directly to the tumor to form an iceball. Adequate temperatures (< −20°C) are reached at the peripheral margins of the tissue surrounding the tumor. Once the freezing is discontinued, the entire lesion is allowed to thaw; the target tissue is then frozen and allowed to thaw a second (and possibly a third) time. Tumors <1 cm in diameter are ideal for this type of therapy.

THERAPEUTIC & SUPPORTIVE PROCEDURES

which can last from seconds to several minutes.

7. Once the first iceball forms and adequate temperatures (–20°C or less) are reached at the peripheral margins of the tissue surrounding the tumor, freezing is discontinued and the probe is allowed to thaw until it detaches from the lesion. The entire lesion is then allowed to thaw, at which point a second (and possibly a third) freezing is initiated. Liquid nitrogen can be used as a spray, especially for larger tumors.

8. Owners should be warned that a scab will form at the site of freezing and then fall off in approximately 10 to 21 days, exposing a pink bed of epithelium or granulation tissue. This area will contract and epithelialize, leaving a small hairless area. The surrounding hair may change color, which must be mentioned to the owner. If bone is frozen, it may need to be debrided 2 to 3 months after cryotherapy. General hygiene is all that is required for the freezing site.

9. If the cat appears to be uncomfortable, oral or transdermal analgesics are recommended several days postoperatively.

Clinical Application

Cryotherapy has been successfully used for decades to control localized tumors in humans and cats. Best results occur with small (<1.0 cm diameter), localized, benign tumors.

Eyelid Tumors

Benign tumors of the eyelid, such as meibomian gland adenomas, papillomas, and melanomas, generally are treated very effectively with cryotherapy. Biopsy samples of the tumor should be submitted for histopathology prior to freezing. Recurrence rates are less than 5% if the tumor is smaller than 1 cm in diameter and adequately frozen.

Oral Tumors

Cryotherapy is effective in treating very small lesions of the oral cavity that invade bone, especially such benign lesions as epulides. The tissue sloughs rapidly after freezing as a result of abrasion within the oral cavity. A superficial area of dead bone may be exposed and become necrotic. If a sequestrum forms, it must be removed.[4]

Skin Tumors

Small skin tumors are commonly treated with cryotherapy.[5] For example, basal cell tumors, squamous cell carcinomas, and papillomas smaller than 1 cm in diameter can be frozen with excellent response. Squamous cell carcinomas are probably the only malignant tumor for which cryotherapy should be offered. As a general rule, tumors larger than 1 cm in diameter should be treated by other therapeutic modalities.

PHOTODYNAMIC THERAPY

Equipment

The equipment required for PDT includes a laser to produce a specific wavelength of light (usually infrared), a fiberoptic delivery system, and a photosensitizing agent. Because the wavelength of laser light currently in use cannot pass through more than 2 cm of tissue, PDT is mainly used to treat tumors on or just under the skin or on the lining of internal organs. A photosensitizing agent is injected into the bloodstream and absorbed by cells throughout the body; the agent remains in cancer cells longer than in normal cells. When the treated cancer cells are exposed to laser light, the photosensitizing agent absorbs the light and produces an active form of oxygen that destroys the cancer cells. An advantage of PDT is that it causes minimal damage to healthy tissue. This treatment modality is available in only a few institutions in the United States, Europe, and Japan.

General Technique (Figure 15-3)

1. PDT should be restricted to small tumors (<1.0 cm in diameter) of the skin or on the lining of internal organs.
2. The photosensitizing agent is administered 6 to 48 hours (depending on the agent used) prior to PDT.
3. The cat is placed under general anesthesia, its eyes are cov-

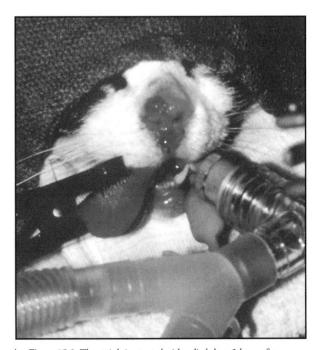

Figure 15-3: *The cat is being treated with a diode laser 3 hours after infusion of EtNBS (a benzophenothiazine photosensitizer). The eyes are covered with dark cloth to reduce risk of photosensitization reaction, and the tumor and a surrounding "cuff" of normal tissue are exposed to the light. Eschar formation after treatment is common, but the normal tissue heals quickly due to lower accumulation of the drug. (Courtesy of A.E. Frimberger)*

ered, a systemic analgesic is administered, and local anesthesia (0.25–1 ml 2% lidocaine mixed 50:50 with sodium bicarbonate) is injected around the treatment site.

4. The surrounding hair is parted or minimally clipped and cleaned.

5. The tumor is debrided and the tissue submitted for histopathology.

6. Laser light is directed through a fiberoptic conduit (a very thin glass strand) that has been positioned close to the cancerous lesion. If indicated, the conduit can be passed through a bronchoscope into the lungs or through an endoscope into the esophagus to treat lung or esophageal cancer, respectively.

7. Light exposure must be timed carefully so that it occurs when most of the photosensitizing agent has left healthy cells but is still present in cancer cells.

8. PDT makes the skin and eyes sensitive to light for 6 weeks or longer after treatment. Cats should be kept indoors and out of direct sunlight and bright indoor light until they are less photosensitive (at least 6 weeks for most drugs).

9. If the cat appears to be uncomfortable, oral or transdermal analgesics are recommended several days postoperatively.

REFERENCES

1. Dewhirst MW, Page RL, Thrall DE: Hyperthermia, in Withrow SJ, MacEwen EG (eds): *Clinical Veterinary Oncology.* Philadelphia, JB Lippincott, 1989, pp 113–123.

2. Theon AP, Madewell BR, Moore AS, et al: Localized thermo-cisplatin therapy. A pilot study in spontaneous canine and feline tumors. *Int J Hyperthermia* 7:881–892, 1991.

3. Withrow SJ: Cryosurgery, in Withrow SJ, MacEwen EG (eds): *Clinical Veterinary Oncology.* Philadelphia, JB Lippincott, 1989, pp 106–112.

4. Harvey HJ: Cryosurgery of oral tumors in dogs and cats. *Vet Clin North Am Small Anim Pract* 10:821–830, 1980.

5. Krahwinkel Jr DJ: Cryosurgical treatment of skin diseases. *Vet Clin North Am Small Anim Pract* 10:787–801, 1980.

THERAPEUTIC & SUPPORTIVE PROCEDURES

COMPLEMENTARY AND ALTERNATIVE MEDICINE—PROPERTIES, USES, AND PATIENT MANAGEMENT

16

Gregory K. Ogilvie and Antony S. Moore

CLINICAL BRIEFING

Acupuncture	Stimulation of specific anatomic points on the body for therapeutic purposes using needles, heat, pressure, friction, suction, or impulses of electromagnetic energy.
Chiropractic Science	Method that concerns itself with the relationship between biomechanics, structure, and function or impulses of electromagnetic energy in the body.
Massage Therapy	Manipulation of soft body parts to a state of normalcy.
Biofield Therapy	Ancient art of the laying on of hands.
Homeopathic Medicine	Treatment with extreme dilutions of remedies made of naturally occurring substances from plants, animals, and minerals.
Pharmacologic/ Biologic Therapy	Treatment with drugs and vaccines that are not currently accepted by mainstream medicine and surgery.
Herbal/Botanical Medicine	Treatment with herbs and other plants.
Nutritional Therapy	Treatment with nutrients to prevent and treat cancer and a wide variety of other diseases as well as to support individuals in the face of disease.

More and more clients are using complementary therapies for their cats and themselves despite limited data on efficacy and toxicity. People around the world use the words "complementary," "alternative," "integrative," or "holistic" interchangeably to mean non-Western style therapies. While many Westerners remain skeptical about some of these therapies, it is useful to keep in mind that approximately 4 billion people—80% of the world population—use at least one form of complementary medicine, and many of these people seek this type of care for their pets when they become ill. Conservative estimates indicate that one third of all Americans routinely use alternative and complementary therapies, especially as a supplement to conventional health care methods. In fact, Americans visit alternative practitioners more often than their physicians, at a cost of more than $14 billion per year.[1] Americans spend yet another $4 billion annually on alternative products such as vitamins and herbs.

> **KEY POINT**
>
> *Complementary therapy has never been shown to cure cancer when used alone; its potential place is to support the patient.*

This same trend is occurring in veterinary health care. Anyone who has practiced during the past 5 years can appreciate clients' growing demand for complementary medical treatments for their pets. This is true especially in the treatment of cancer patients for whom traditional options are limited and potentially toxic. Because traditional veterinary medicine has been regarded as the standard of care for cancer treatment, there have been few Western-style studies to document the efficacy of complementary medicine as a useful adjunct. This has changed somewhat recently, as scientists have undertaken and published studies using traditional research methods to discover the efficacy of certain treatments. With the results of each new study, our comfort level in using some of these treatments grows. Despite the increased use of complementary or alternative medical treatments, none have ever been documented to cure a cancer patient. Their potential place in feline oncology and medicine is to support the patient. The practitioner should first be aware of the definition of these alternative modalities so as to be at least conversant with interested clients. Second, clinicians should know that while almost nothing is known about the efficacy and toxicity of complementary therapies in feline medicine, there are some documented efficacies and toxicities in other species. We have noted some of these studies, particularly those that are relevant to cancer treatment.

KEY POINT

While almost nothing is known about the efficacy and toxicity of complementary therapies in feline medicine, there are some documented efficacies and toxicities in other species.

The feline veterinary health care team should understand that confrontation over or complete rejection of complementary therapy may alienate some clients and prevent their pets from receiving appropriate and comprehensive care. On the other hand, the team and the client must clearly understand the strengths and the limitations of this care. Few can disagree that complementary medicine is becoming an important aspect of palliative and supportive cancer care, but there is not a single complementary intervention that has been demonstrated to constitute an effective cure for cancer. Therefore it seems prudent to state that it is unethical to promote complementary medicine as a cancer cure in feline medicine. False promotion of complementary medicine can misguide clients into giving up effective conventional treatments; it can raise false hopes of clients and caregivers alike; and it can financially exploit caring people who seek any help for their cat with cancer.

Despite the limitations of complementary medicine and the scarcity of data on this type of care, there is little doubt that patients can be helped in the palliative setting. Complementary medicine in palliative care aims at providing comfort and increasing the quality of life of cats with cancer. Goals include, but are not limited to, promoting relaxation, decreasing fear, anxiety, and stress, relieving pain and nausea, enhancing appetite, and improving sleep. The end goal is improving quality of life through comprehensive, compassionate care.

The objectives of this chapter are simply to introduce and define some complementary therapeutics that have been used in the treatment of cancer and other diseases in animals and humans. Due to space limitations, the reader is encouraged to seek additional information in the references provided. Entire books have been written on each of the subjects introduced below.

ACUPUNCTURE

Definition

Acupuncture involves the stimulation of specific anatomic points on the body for therapeutic purposes with needles, heat, pressure, friction, suction, or impulses of electromagnetic energy (Figure 16-1).[2-24] This ancient healing art is generally well accepted and widely used by human and veterinary health care professionals to treat a wide variety of ailments.

Mechanism of Action

Acupuncture is used to normalize or correct the flow of *Qi* (pronounced "chee," which refers to the body's life-giving force) to restore health. Acupuncture points are very specific areas that can be stimulated by needles, laser, heat, beads, etc., to result in an effect, often at a distant site. Many of these points are related or linked via "meridians." The acupuncture points of cats have been defined, but not as extensively as in humans. Sound scientific data have shown that the stimulation of specific points in the body alters the chemical neurotransmitters in the body. Acupuncture is one of the most commonly used complementary therapies in human and veterinary medicine.

Indications

Well-designed studies in humans show efficacy of acupuncture for the treatment of osteoarthritis, chemotherapy-induced nausea, asthma, back pain, and headache,

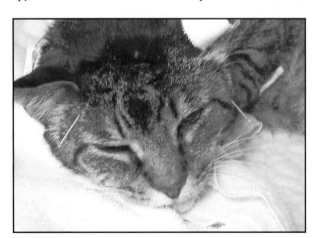

Figure 16-1: *Acupuncture involves the stimulation of specific anatomic points on the body for therapeutic purposes with needles, heat, pressure, friction, suction, or impulses of electromagnetic energy. In this case, copper acupuncture needles are placed at specific sites along meridians or linear anatomic locations between defined sets of acupuncture points. This often results in a state of relaxation, as exhibited in this cat during therapy. This ancient healing art is generally well accepted and widely used by human and veterinary health care professionals to treat a wide variety of ailments.*

THERAPEUTIC & SUPPORTIVE PROCEDURES

among other conditions. The most dramatic reports on the efficacy of acupuncture have been its use in surgical analgesia.[2] In 1973, up to 25% of all surgeries in mainland China were performed using acupuncture analgesia with efficacy reported in up to 90% of the cases.[2,3] These numbers are anticipated to be at least as high today. Acupuncture surgical anesthesia is not widely utilized in the United States in human or feline medicine. This modality obviously has the potential for benefiting feline cancer patients where surgery is the mainstay of therapy.[4,5] Acupuncture is commonly used at the Animal Cancer Center at Colorado State University (CSU) and elsewhere to prevent and reduce postsurgical and radiation-induced discomfort and to enhance well being of feline patients receiving cancer care of all types. In addition, chemotherapy-induced nausea is commonly treated with acupuncture.

KEY POINT

Acupuncture has been documented in a number of peer-reviewed journals to be effective for preventing and treating pain and nausea in some species.

To become minimally qualified in veterinary acupuncture, a veterinarian should take specific courses offered by groups such as that at CSU and by the International Veterinary Acupuncture Society. Certification by the latter group is one mark of training for minimal competence.

CHIROPRACTIC SCIENCE

Definition

Chiropractic science is a healing method that concerns itself with the relationship between structure and function.[1,23,24] The structure of the spine and function of the nervous system are the primary areas of interest to those practitioners who subscribe to its theories.

Mechanism of Action

Healing occurs via manipulative procedures and interventions, not surgical or chemotherapeutic treatments. The orthopedic structures in question are altered or aligned into a normal relationship with the rest of the body to restore health and wellness. In some cases, this will result in spinal alignment and alleviate nerve compression. Chiropractic care involves integration of the disciplines of radiology, sports medicine, neurology, osteopathy, and orthopedics.

Indications

Research on the beneficial effect of chiropractic therapy within the veterinary profession is still very much in its infancy. Little data exist concerning the efficacy of this treatment discipline in feline medicine. Studied areas of efficacy in humans include back and other orthopedic pain and somatovisceral disorders such as hypertension. Chiropractic care for the feline cancer patient primarily seeks to improve general comfort, lameness, and mobility, especially in areas of orthopedic or neurologic disorders. Veterinarians who wish to become minimally qualified to perform chiropractic procedures should take a set of manipulative courses such as those offered by CSU. A certification course will be available in the near future.

MASSAGE THERAPY

Definition

Massage therapy is the manipulation of soft body parts to a state of normalcy.[1,23–26]

Mechanism of Action

This modality incorporates the use of fixed or movable pressure, rubbing, stroking, tapping, or kneading the body with a view toward treating physical or emotional conditions. This ancient healing art affects the musculoskeletal, circulatory, lymphatic, and nervous systems. Healing by touch in massage therapy involves *vis medicatrix naturae* (helping the body heal itself). When massage therapy is performed by a highly trained and experienced therapist, there is no doubt that the procedure results in intensive and pleasant relaxation to the body and mind (as reflected in improved attitude, appetite, and actions in the case of a cat). Techniques include Swedish massage, deep-tissue massage, neuromuscular massage, manual lymphatic massage, reflexology, zone therapy, tuina, acupressure, Rolfing, Trager®, the Feldenkrais® method, and the Alexander technique. Various adaptations of these techniques in human medicine are being used in veterinary medicine, although few data exist documenting efficacy in cats.

Indications

Trials in humans have shown efficacy in acute and chronic pain, acute and chronic inflammation, chronic lymphedema, nausea, muscle spasm, various soft tissue dysfunctions, grand mal epileptic seizures, anxiety, and depression.[24] Massage has also been shown to stimulate the body's ability to control pain naturally by producing endorphins.[25] Some suggest that massage therapy is contraindicated in the cancer patient because increased blood flow may result in increased metastases, but this has never been convincingly documented. Applications of massage therapy for the feline cancer patient may revolve around relieving pain and discomfort and maintaining function. Some oncology centers combine massage with acupuncture or use it alone to relieve lameness or discomfort not exclusively due to orthopedic disease. For example, massage therapy can be used to prevent or reduce deterioration of the use of a limb being treated with radiation or surgery for a soft tissue sarcoma of the extremity. Special training in manipulative techniques is available for veterinarians to become minimally qualified to practice in this area.

BIOFIELD THERAPY

Definition

Biofield therapy or spiritual healing is the ancient art of the laying on of hands. The earliest records of this healing method date between 2,500 and 5,000 years ago.[1,23,24]

Mechanism of Action

Healing is said to come from two sources. The first is from a source other than the therapist, such as God, the cosmos, or another supernatural entity. A second source is from a practitioner of the modality, who modifies or amplifies the patient's biofield. During this type of healing, the therapist places his or her hands on or near the patient's body to improve general health or a disease condition. Practitioners of this therapy note that a biofield emanates for a distance beyond the physical body and that the strength, distance, and color of the field depend on the health and emotional state of the individual. Three forms of biofield therapeutics are used[1,23,24]: healing touch (Reiki), therapeutic touch, and SHEN therapy. Reiki originated from Japan in the 1800s and has a theoretical basis in channeling energy from an external source (e.g., God) through the healer to the patient to enhance well-being. In Reiki, the spiritual body is healed and is then expected to heal the physical body. In SHEN therapy, healing is reported to occur through a biofield conforming to the natural laws of physics with a discernible pattern throughout the body. Therapeutic touch involves a practitioner who restores the correct vibrational component to the patient's universal, unitary field.

Indications

One review of 23 placebo-controlled studies showed that 57% of these studies arrived at a positive conclusion of these treatments.[24] There are no good studies documenting the efficacy of biofield therapy in feline medicine. Until further data are known, this treatment approach should be used with caution and obviously never in place of a modality known to be effective.

HOMEOPATHIC MEDICINE

Definition

Homeopathic medicine is the use of extreme dilutions of substances to treat diseases or disorders. It is practiced worldwide, especially in Europe, Latin America, and Asia.[1,23,24] Homeopathic remedies are made of naturally occurring substances from plants, animals, and minerals that are diluted to as low as 10^{-30} to $10^{-20,000}$. These homeopathic substances are recognized and regulated by the Food and Drug Administration; however, this regulation does not suggest endorsement of the efficacy of homeopathic remedies.

Mechanism of Action

Diseases or disorders are treated with extreme dilutions of "like" substances. For example, radiation illness could be treated with extreme dilutions of radium. Critics of homeopathy suggest that such extreme dilutions of compounds preclude any probability for efficacy. Scientists that have not rejected the potential benefits of homeopathy suggest that the efficacy can be explained by quantum physics where the electromagnetic energy of these remedies may interact with the body for beneficial purposes. A phenomenon known as the "memory of water" is used to explain how extreme dilutions can result in retained efficacy. In this theory, the structure of a water and alcohol solution is altered during the procedure of making the remedies so that the structure of the molecule is retained even after none of the actual substance remains.

Indications

The *British Medical Journal* published a meta-analysis on 96 published reports of 107 controlled trials.[27] Trials were scored using a predefined system, and 22 were designated as well-designed clinical trials involving homeopathy. Fifteen of 22 showed positive results. These rarely included any cancer patients. The types of human patients that were improved included those with allergic diseases, arthritis, and the like. Therefore homeopathy may be of benefit for supporting a cancer patient, but little data exist to suggest that it can be used to directly treat or prevent a malignant process. The issue of vaccine-associated sarcomas in cats has led many homeopathic practitioners to suggest that homeopathic remedies should be used instead of traditional vaccines. This may have great appeal; however, efficacy data are not available for feline patients. These homeopathic remedies are often available in grocery stores and are therefore easily obtained and frequently used by clients.

PHARMACOLOGIC AND BIOLOGIC TREATMENTS

Definitions

Pharmacologic and biologic treatments utilize a wide variety of drugs and vaccines that are not yet accepted by mainstream medicine and surgery. There are no data published documenting the efficacy of these agents in feline medicine. Some of the more common agents being used in human and veterinary medicine include the following[1,23-34]:

- **Antineoplastons,** peptide fractions originally derived from blood and urine, are being used to treat a wide variety of malignancies in humans. This controversial treatment is being evaluated in a National Institutes of Health (NIH) funded study. Early studies showed efficacy in a number of tumors.[29,30]

- **Cartilage products,** especially those from sharks and cattle, are very popular at this time. Cartilage has been shown to have antiangiogenic properties. In addition, it contains tissue inhibitors of metalloproteinases (TIMPs) that inhibit tumor metastasis. Shark cartilage has become very popular because of reports of studies in Mexico and Cuba suggesting that this product resulted in the effective treatment of cancer in humans. These original studies were soundly criticized because of faulty study design, lack of controls, and failure to confirm that patients had a malignancy. Despite the fact that 50,000 Americans use cartilage products and spend $7,000 per year per person on this product, little exists to document its efficacy. One reported abstract failed to confirm the efficacy of shark cartilage for the treatment of cancer in veterinary patients.[32] No clinical study reported to date has shown efficacy associated with shark cartilage therapy.

KEY POINT

To date, there have been no well-controlled clinical trials documenting the efficacy of shark cartilage as an anticancer agent for any species, including the cat.

- **Ethylene diamine tetraacetic acid (EDTA) chelation therapy** has been used to treat a number of conditions; however, the mechanism for treating cancer has not been clearly stated. It is interesting that metalloproteinases, especially those of gelatinase capability, are indeed inhibited by EDTA. Metalloproteinases 2 and 9 are critical for tumor growth and invasion. Therefore there may be a reasonable explanation for the potential value of this type of therapy.
- **Immunoaugmentive therapy** is an experimental form of cancer therapy consisting of treatment with substances that enhance the immune system. Work done in dogs with osteosarcoma suggests that specific immunoaugmentive therapy with BCG derivatives improves disease-free intervals and survival.[33,34] Similarly, dogs that have limb-sparing surgery for osteosarcoma and get an infected allograft (a nonspecific immune enhancing effect from an unwanted complication of surgery) have a significantly longer disease-free interval than those that do not have infected allografts. Other studies suggest efficacy by administering derivatives of aloe vera to enhance various aspects of the immune system.[34] Therefore there may be some basis in logic for this type of therapy or preferably a more focused approach to provide directed immunoaugmentive therapy to result in maximal benefit and minimal toxicity.

HERBAL AND BOTANICAL MEDICINE

Definition

Eighty percent of the world's population, or approximately 4 billion people, use herbal and botanical medicine.[1,23,24] Almost every system of native medicine around the world uses herbal treatments. Despite this widespread use, acceptance differs throughout the world. In the United States, herbal remedies are considered to be without efficacy by many in regulatory bodies, although many drugs we use routinely today are derived from plants. European governments, especially in Germany and France, have formally approved herbs for therapeutic purposes. Indeed, some of the best studies on the efficacy of these herbs have been done in Europe.

Mechanisms of Action

The mechanism of action depends on the active ingredient of the individual herb or botanical agent. In many cases, the mechanism is unknown. Agents used in China include sesquiterpenes, diterpenes, triterpenes, quinones, podophyllotoxins, paclitaxel, alkaloids, and others.[35,36] Many of these have been adapted for Western-style cancer therapy, such as paclitaxel, vincristine, and etoposide.

Indications

In China and elsewhere in the world, herbs and other plant derivatives have been used to treat a number of disorders, including cancer, chemotherapy-induced nausea, and depression associated with the diagnosis of cancer. The number of herbs and other plant-based materials used therapeutically is beyond the scope of this introduction. As an example of the potential benefit of these agents, in 1981, the U.S. Department of Agriculture, in conjunction with the National Cancer Institute, concluded a 25 year study of plants with anticancer properties. The work includes 365 folk medicinal species and identifies more than 1,000 pharmacologically active phytochemicals.[37] Few data clearly define the therapeutic benefit of most herbs for the treatment of cancer. These substances can have an impact on the pharmacokinetics of other prescription drugs in the cat. Similarly, because cats have a unique metabolism compared with dogs and humans, extreme care should be taken when extrapolating dosage and efficacy of these substances to feline medicine.

Postgraduate courses do exist in the field of herbal and botanical medicine. The use of these substances is akin to using pharmaceutical agents. Extreme care should be taken when considering their dosage, toxicity, efficacy, and drug interactions. When these data do not exist, as often occurs in the cat, caution should be employed and the patient should be carefully monitored.

NUTRITIONAL THERAPY

Definition

Nutritional therapy revolves around the notion that nutrients other than those noted above can be used to prevent, support, and treat humans and animals with cancer and a wide variety of other diseases.[1,23,24] See Chapter 19 for additional details.

Garlic

Epidemiologic studies have suggested a correlation between high garlic consumption and reduced risk of cancer development.[39] Garlic extract and several thioalkyl compounds from garlic have been shown to inhibit the activation of carcinogens and the bonding of polyarene thiol epoxide to DNA bases, which causes DNA lesions and initiates chemically-induced carcinogenic process. Garlic and the thioalkyl compounds inhibit carcinogen-induced aberrations in the cell nucleus. In addition, garlic extracts have an antipromotion effect in animals exposed to carcinogens. Also, garlic exerts direct cytolytic effects against cancer-cultured human breast cancer cells and human melanoma cells. Concentrations of garlic used in these studies arrested cancer cell growth, with no effect on normal cells. Pretreatment of rodents with garlic protects against subsequent induction of tumors by a variety of carcinogens. There are no studies demonstrating the safety and efficacy of garlic for the prevention or treatment of cancer in people or in veterinary medicine.

Tea

Although it may be a while before cats acquire a taste for tea, there are compelling data that suggest that green and black teas may have anticancer properties.[40–42] Many clients ask about the potential efficacy of teas or tea extracts for their pets. Green tea extracts contain catechin, and black tea contains fermentation products, thioflavine, and theorubigins. These active agents inhibit cancer-promoting agents, protect against oxidative damage, and enhance antioxidant enzymes. Black tea seems to have soothing properties to reduce the discomfort associated with radiation-induced oral mucositis. The tannic acid and other ingredients act as an astringent and a local anesthetic when the oral cavity of affected cats is lavaged two to three times a day.

CONCLUSION

Caution needs to be employed when assessing the efficacy of complementary therapies; however, existing data suggest that some of these modalities may be helpful in treating the feline cancer patient. Well-controlled studies must be encouraged and performed as they are essential to docu-

ment efficacy and toxicity. The expanding postgraduate opportunities for practicing veterinarians and the incorporation of didactic and clinical programs at key leading veterinary schools are important steps toward the logical use of complementary medicine in veterinary medicine. As mentioned earlier, the biggest concern for veterinary practitioners may be that unproven therapies may be used instead of known treatments. Therefore the client should be informed of all the benefits and risks of "traditional" and "nontraditional" therapies alike.

REFERENCES

1. Eisenberg DM, Kessler RC, Foster C, et al: Unconventional medicine in the United States. Prevalence, costs, and patterns of use. *N Engl J Med* 328:246–252, 1993.

2. Helms JM: *Acupuncture Energetics: A Clinical Approach for Physicians.* Berkeley, CA, Medical Acupuncture Publishers, 1995, pp 42–57.

3. Diamond EG: Acupuncture analgesia: Western medicine and Chinese traditional medicine. *J Am Med Assoc* 218:1558–1561, 1971.

4. Report of the medical delegation to the People's Republic of China, June 15–July 6, 1973. Washington DC, National Academy of Sciences, Institute of Medicine, 1973, p 79.

5. Lee MHM: Acupuncture analgesia in dentistry. A clinical investigation. *N Y State Dental J* 39:288–301, 1973.

6. Filshie J, Redman D: Acupuncture and malignant pain problems. *Eur J Surg Oncol* 11:389–394, 1985.

7. Filshie J: Acupuncture for malignant pain. *Br Med J* 8:38–39, 1990.

8. Dundee JW: Reduction in the emetic effects of opioid preanesthetic medication by acupuncture. *Br Med J* 22:583–584, 1986.

9. Dundee JW: Traditional Chinese acupuncture: A potentially useful antiemetic. *Br Med J* 293:583–584, 1986.

10. Ghally RG: Antiemetic studies with traditional Chinese acupuncture: A comparison of manual needling with electrical stimulation and commonly used antiemetics. *Br J Anesth* 42:1108–1113, 1987.

11. Ghally RG: Acupuncture also reduces the emetic effects of pethidine. *Br J Anesth* 59:135–137, 1987.

12. Yang LC: Comparison of P6 acupoint injection with 50% glucose in water and intravenous droperidol for the prevention of vomiting after gynecological laparoscopy. *Acta Anaesthesiol Scand* 37:192–194, 1993.

13. Dundee JW: Acupuncture prophylaxis of chemotherapy-induced sickness. *J Royal Soc Med* 82:268–271, 1989.

14. Sato T, Yu Y, Guo SY, et al: Acupuncture stimulation enhances splenic natural killer cell cytotoxicity in rats. *Jap J Physiol* 46:131–136, 1996.

15. Jianguo Y, Rongxing Z, Mingsheng Z, Qimei G: Effect of acupuncture on peripheral T lymphocytes and their subgroups in patients with malignant tumors. *Int J Clin Acupun* 4:53–58, 1993.

16. Xunshi W, Zhaolin Z, Chenrang S, et al: Clinical study on the use of second metacarpal holographic acupoints for re-establishing gastrointestinal motility in patients following abdominal surgery. *Am J Acupun* 22:353–356, 1994.

17. Aglietti L: A pilot study of metoclopramide, dexamethasone, diphenhydramine and acupuncture in women treated with cisplatin. *Cancer Chemother Pharmacol* 26:239–240, 1990.

18. Lewis, GB: An alternative approach to premedication: Comparing diazepam with auriculotherapy and a relaxation method. *Am J Acupun* 15:205–214, 1987.

19. Muxeneder R: Die konservative Behandlung chronischer Hautveränderungen des Pferdes durch Laserpunktur. *Der praktische Tierarzt* 69:12–21, 1988.

20. Liaw M, Wong AM, Cheng P: Therapeutic trial of acupuncture in phantom limb pain of amputees. *Am J Acupun* 22:205–213, 1994.

21. Blom M, Davidson I, Fernberg JO, et al: Acupuncture treatment of patients with radiation-induced xerostomia. *Oral Oncol Eur J Cancer* 32B:182–190, 1996.

22. Filshie J, Penn K, Ashley S, Davis CL: Acupuncture for the relief of cancer-related breathlessness. *Pal Med* 10:145–150, 1996.

23. Alternative Medicine: Expanding Medical Horizons, A report to the National Institutes of Health on Alternative Medical Systems and Practices in the United States. 1994.

24. Astin JA, Harkins E, Ernest E: The efficacy of "distant healing": A systemic review of randomized trials. *Ann Intern Med* 132:903–910, 2000.

25. Kaarda B, Tosteinbo O: Increase of plasma beta endorphins in connective tissue massage. *Gen Pharmacol* 20:487–489, 1989.

26. Sharma HM, Dwvedi C, Satter HA, et al: Antineoplastic properties of Maharishi 4 against DMBA-induced mammary tumors in rats. *J Pharm Biochem Behav* 35:767–773, 1990.

27. Kleijnen J, Knipschild P, Reir GT: Clinical trials of homeopathy. *Br Med J* 302:316–323, 1991.

28. Arnold JT, Korytynski EA, Wilkinson BP, et al: Chemopreventative activity of Maharishi Amrit Kalash and related agents in rat tracheal epithelial and human tumor cells. *J Proc Am Assoc Cancer Res* 32:128–151, 1991.

29. Bertelli A, Mathe G: Antineoplastons (1). *Drugs Exp Clin Res* 12(Suppl 1): 23–37, 1985.

30. Bertelli A, Mathe G: Antineoplastons (2). *Drugs Exp Clin Res* 13(Suppl 1): 433–440, 1987.

31. Simone C: Presentation at a hearing on alternative medicine before a subcommittee of the Committee on Appropriations, US Senate, 103rd Congress, June 24, 1993.

32. Meyer JA, Dueland RT, et al: Canine osteogenic sarcoma treated by amputation and MER. *Cancer* 49:1613–1616, 1982.

33. MacEwen EG, Kurzman ID, Rosenthal RC, et al: Therapy for osteosarcoma in dogs with intravenous injection of liposome-encapsulated muramyl tripeptide. *J Natl Cancer Inst* 81:935–938, 1989.

34. Harris C, Pierce K, King G, et al: Efficacy of acemannan in treatment of canine and feline spontaneous neoplasms. *Molec Biother* 3:207–213, 1991.

35. Lin JH, Rogers PA, Yamada H: Chinese herbal medicine: Pharmacological basis, in Schoen AM, Wynn SG (eds): *Complementary and Alternative Veterinary Medicine.* St. Louis, Mosby, pp 379–404, 1998.

36. Lien EJ, Li WY: *Structure Activity Relationship Analysis of Chinese Anticancer Drugs and Related Plants.* Taiwan, Oriental Healing Arts Institute, 1985, pp 1–140.

37. Duke JA, Ayensu ES: *Handbook of Medicinal Herbs.* Boca Raton, FL, CRC Press, Inc., 1985.

38. Weisburg JH: Interactions of nutrients in oncogenesis. *Am J Clin Nutr* 53:2265, 1991.

39. National Academy of Sciences: *Diet, Nutrition and Cancer.* National Academy Press, Washington DC, 1982.

40. Wang ZY, Agarwal R, Khan WA, Mukhtar H: Protection against benzo(a)pyrene and N-nitrosodiethylamine-induced lung and forestomach tumorigenesis in A/J mice by water extracts of green tea and licorice. *Carcinogenesis* 13:1491–1496, 1992.

41. Khan SG, Kartiyar SK, Agarwal R, Mukhtar H: Enhancement of antioxidant and phase II enzymes by oral feeding of green tea polyphenols in drinking water to SKH-1 hairless mice: Possible role in cancer prevention. *Cancer Res* 52:4050-4056, 1992.

42. Wang ZY, Hong JY, Huang MT, et al: Inhibition of N-nitrosodiethylamine and 4-(methylnitrosamino)-1-(3-pyridyl)-1-butanone-induced tumorigenesis in A.J mice by green tea and black tea. *Cancer Res* 52:1943–1954, 1992.

TREATMENT OF PAIN

Gregory K. Ogilvie and Antony S. Moore

CLINICAL BRIEFING

General Concepts of Pain Management	For maximum benefit, analgesics should be used preventatively; to minimize discomfort, compassionate care, gentle handling, and a comfortable environment should be accompanied by local and systemic analgesics.
Mild Pain	NSAIDs, α_2-adrenergic agonists, opioid agonists, agonist-antagonists.
Moderate Pain	NSAIDs with or without opiate analgesics, α_2-adrenergic agonists, local anesthetics; changing the route of administration (e.g., oral to IV, SQ, or IM) may be beneficial.
Severe Pain	Opiate analgesics should be combined (if needed) with local analgesia (local, regional, intracavitary, or epidural analgesia), sustained-release patches, and palliative procedures (e.g., radiation therapy, surgery); maximize blood levels of analgesics with systemic administration.

Compassionate care is the watchword of feline oncology, and pain control is the cornerstone of the caring process. Sadly, pain control in cats has sometimes been ignored and is only recently being investigated seriously. Feline pain management can be difficult; cats tend to be secretive, which precludes identifying pain early when it is easiest to treat. The key to compassionate pain control is timely intervention with analgesics, optimally before pain receptors ever identify discomfort.

MECHANISMS OF CANCER PAIN

The most common mechanism of cancer pain is associated with tumor invasion and subsequent tissue damage that causes activation of pain receptors.[1-6] Some forms of therapy can induce pain as well. For example, surgery and radiation therapy may ultimately relieve pain and suffering but can cause significant short-term discomfort from tissue and nerve damage. Similarly, although chemotherapy can help control the underlying malignant process, these drugs can cause discomfort. Vincristine and vinblastine have caused painful polyneuropathy in a small number of human cancer patients. This adverse effect is suspected to occur in a very small number of cats and can decrease the patient's quality of life.

While very little is known about feline pain, a basic understanding of the types of discomfort may help increase awareness of how cats with cancer can be managed compassionately. The types of pain associated with cancer include visceral pain, inflammatory and somatic pain, neuritis, and neuropathic pain.[1-6]

Visceral Pain

Humans describe this type of pain as a dull, deep, constant aching pain. Visceral pain is poorly defined; humans with significant visceral pain often respond best to narcotic and/or nonnarcotic analgesics. It is suspected that this type of pain results in decreased activity, anorexia, and behavioral changes in cats.

Inflammatory and Somatic Pain

Frequently described in human medicine but rarely in feline medicine, this pain is well localized, constant, and aching.[6] Common sources of this type of pain include bone metastasis, tissue damage, and musculoskeletal, dental, and integumental pain. Cats may lick or bite at an area or may exhibit signs of discomfort in subtle ways, such as by decreasing their activity or limping (if an extremity is affected).

Neuritic Pain

Inflammation of nerves or nerve roots causes neuritic pain and can present as part of a paraneoplastic syndrome or as a direct effect of tumor compression. Humans describe it as a constant, dull, aching pain that may have periods of burning "shock-like" sensations. In cats, these shock-like sensations can result in sudden, unexplained behavioral changes, such as aggression or scratching and biting at an area, often to the point of self-mutilation.

Neuropathic Pain

This type of pain occurs when a segment of the nervous system that normally transmits pain stimuli is damaged. It arises from metabolic, immunologic, or direct physical effects on the nervous system. Neuropathic pain is difficult to control with standard analgesics.

RECOGNIZING PAIN

Cats instinctively hide most outward and measurable manifestations of pain and rarely exhibit signs until discomfort is quite advanced. Indeed, the only clinical indicator of pain and discomfort may be increased systolic blood pressure. Experienced practitioners and caregivers watch for subtle changes in activity level, appetite, and movement. Vocalization, while not a specific indicator of pain, is noted in some cats, especially when discomfort is significant. Some cats become more reclusive whereas others, especially younger animals, pace and may thrash around. Tachypnea, tachycardia, and dilated pupils can be used to assess pain in cats, even when they are stuporous.

The best feline practitioners anticipate and intervene early rather than waiting for clinical signs associated with discomfort. Caregivers need to be aware of which procedures are likely to cause discomfort, and preemptive analgesia should be practiced when possible.

Comprehensive management of pain involves careful evaluation and treatment of each cat.[1-6] To maximize quality of life, response to therapy, and survival time for feline patients, adequate pain control must be the highest goal for the veterinary practitioner. Pain control in feline medicine has only recently come to the forefront of attention, primarily because of the inappropriate attitudes of clinicians, lack of knowledge about analgesic medications, and lack of skill in assessing pain and appropriate therapeutic methods.[2,3] In many cases, analgesics have been withheld because of fear of associated adverse side effects and because research demonstrating the beneficial effects of pain relief in cats is scanty. Client demand has been an important force in bringing pain control to the forefront of compassionate care. Despite our lack of understanding, we must respond to our patients' needs and our clients' concerns by making pain relief and compassionate care a priority.

GENERAL CONCEPTS OF PAIN THERAPY (TABLE 17-1)

Recent research has demonstrated that once pain is elicited, the pain response is magnified. Preventative therapy is therefore preferable to suppression of established pain. Premeditated, judicious use of analgesics is likely to increase cat comfort, decrease the need for hospitalization (and the associated costs), and reduce the amount of pain medication needed to achieve the same level of comfort.[3,6]

The management of pain begins with high-quality, compassionate care by every member of the veterinary health care team. Careful nursing, gentle handling, and provision of a comfortable and relaxing environment are of great ben-

TABLE 17-1
General Approach to Pain Management

Degree of Pain	Clinical Approach[a]
Mild	NSAIDs[b] ± acupuncture
Mild-Moderate	NSAIDs[b] ± acupuncture + opioids
Moderate	NSAIDs[b] ± acupuncture + opioids (dose escalation) ± anxiolytics
Moderate-Severe	NSAIDs[b] ± acupuncture + opioids (dose escalation, different route of administration) ± anxiolytics
Severe	NSAIDs[b] ± acupuncture + opioids (dose escalation, different route of administration) ± anxiolytics + other palliative procedures (e.g., radiation, surgery)

[a]Treat the underlying disease.
[b]Use with caution in patients with renal disease.

efit to cats. Local anesthesia should be employed to alleviate discomfort, and systemic analgesia should be used when local analgesia may be insufficient.

Mild Pain[1,3,6]

The treatment of mild pain must begin with general compassionate care that includes a comfortable environment, appropriate bedding, and effective bandaging if indicated. Social cats will respond well to petting and talking. This is often followed with regular doses of one of the following:

- Nonsteroidal antiinflammatory drugs (NSAIDs) such as aspirin, piroxicam, or ketoprofen, provided renal function is normal and there is no evidence of gastric inflammation
- Local nerve blocks or acupuncture
- α_2-Adrenergic agonists such as xylazine or medetomidine
- Opioid agonists such as morphine, oxymorphone, or fentanyl
- Opioid agonist-antagonists such as butorphanol or buprenorphine

These agents are generally given individually, and NSAIDs are usually administered first. The NSAID carprofen is widely used in cats in Europe and is expected to be approved in the United States in the near future. If NSAIDs are ineffective, an agent from one of the other categories is selected based on what works best in that patient. Only oral NSAIDS and oral butorphanol can be given at home.

Moderate and Severe Pain

Moderate and severe pain can be treated with compassionate care, local analgesia when possible (including acupuncture), or NSAIDs (e.g., carprofen, which has not been approved for use in the cat worldwide and thus should be used with caution; ketoprofen) in judicious combination with drugs from one of the following categories:

- α_2-Adrenergic agonists
- Opioid agonists
- Opioid agonist-antagonists

When drugs are combined, additive toxicity must be monitored. As much as possible, therapy for the malignancy itself must be a high priority. For example, radiation therapy at sites of bone pain may be profoundly beneficial. In addition, using another route of administration for analgesics (e.g., switching from subcutaneous to intravenous administration) may be effective. In some cases, sustained-release fentanyl patches, which are applied to the skin and slowly release the analgesic over 72 hours, may be helpful.

ANALGESIC AGENTS (TABLES 17-2 AND 17-3)

Nonsteroidal Antiinflammatory Agents

Phenylbutazone, acetaminophen, and ibuprofen are generally not used in cats because of the potential for severe toxicity.

Aspirin

Aspirin can be used with extreme caution at 10 mg/kg PO q48–72h. Aspirin has a variable duration of action and is indicated for mild somatic pain and inflammation. Serum half-life is much longer in cats because they lack adequate glucuronyl transferase for hepatic metabolism of salicylates. Because of the recent availability of safer NSAIDS, aspirin is rarely used for the treatment of pain in cats.

TABLE 17-2
Selected Analgesics in Cats[2-5]

Drug	Dose (mg/kg)	Route	Dosing Interval (hr)
NSAIDs			
Ketoprofen	1–2	IV, IM, SQ	24
	1	PO	24
Piroxicam	0.3	PO	48
Carprofen	0.5–2	PO	8–12
α_2-Adrenergic Agonists			
Xylazine	0.5	IV, IM, SQ	0.5–2
Medetomidine	0.001–0.01	IV, IM, SQ	0.5–2
Local Anesthetics			
Lidocaine HCl	1.5	Intrapleural prior to bupivacaine	0.3
Bupivacaine HCl	1–2 mg/4.5 kg	Local nerve block(s) Intrapleural administration prn	
Opioid Agonists			
Morphine	0.1–0.5	IM, SQ	2–6
	0.05–0.2	IV	1–4
Oxymorphone	0.02–0.05	IV	2–4
	0.05–0.2	IM, SQ	2–6
Fentanyl	0.0002–0.05	IV bolus prior to CRI	2–6
	0.001–0.004	CRI	Duration of infusion
	2.5 mg (25 µg/hr) patch	Dermal application	Replace every 3–5 days
Opioid Agonist-Antagonists			
Buprenorphine	0.005–0.01	IV, IM, SQ	4–8
Butorphanol	0.1–0.4	IV, IM, SQ	1–4
Tranquilizers and Anxiolytics			
Xylazine	0.05–0.2	IV, IM	15–30 min
Ketamine	0.5–1	IM	30 min

CRI = constant rate infusion.

TABLE 17-3
Example Protocols for Sedation, Anesthesia, and Analgesia in Stable, Uncomplicated Cases[a]

Procedure/ Pain Level	Sedative or Preemptive Medication Options	Anesthesia Options	Perioperative Analgesia Options	Postoperative Analgesia Options
Minor Procedure/ No Pain	• Medetomidine (5–20 µg/kg IM) or xylazine (0.5–1 mg/kg IM) + butorphanol (0.2 mg/kg IM) • Acepromazine (0.025–0.05 mg/kg IM or SQ) + butorphanol (0.2–0.4 mg/kg IM or SQ) • Diazepam (0.2 mg/kg IV) + butorphanol (0.2 mg/kg IV) • Propofol (2–6 mg/kg IV) • Ketamine (5 mg/kg IV) + diazepam (0.2 mg/kg IV)	• Usually not necessary	• Usually not necessary	• Usually not necessary
Minor Surgery/ Minor Pain	• Medetomidine (10–15 µg/kg IM) + butorphanol (0.2 mg/kg IM) • Acepromazine (0.025–0.05 mg/kg IM or SQ) + butorphanol (0.2–0.4 mg/kg IM or SQ) • Butorphanol (0.2–0.4 mg/kg IV) + ketamine (5 mg/kg IV) + diazepam (0.2 mg/kg IV) • Butorphanol (0.2–0.4 mg/kg IM) + tiletamine-zolazepam (3–5 mg/kg IM) • Butorphanol (0.2–0.4 mg/kg IV) + propofol (3–6 mg/kg IV to effect)	• Thiopental (2–10 mg/kg IV to effect) • Propofol (1–3 mg/kg IV to effect) • Ketamine (1–4 mg/kg IV to effect) • Tiletamine-zolazepam (1–2 mg/kg IV to effect) • Mask or chamber induction	Topical or local blocks with lidocaine (<0.5 mg/kg) or bupivacaine (1–2 mg/4.5 kg) such as: • Mandibular nerve block for dental surgery and mandibulectomy • Median and ulnar nerve blocks for digital amputations, etc. • Postoperative analgesia as needed • Acupuncture	• NSAIDs, alone or in combination with opioid agonist-antagonist drugs • Acupuncture
Moderate Surgery/ Moderate Pain	• Medetomidine (10–15 µg/kg IM) + butorphanol (0.2 mg/kg IM) • Acepromazine (0.025–0.05 mg/kg IM) + butorphanol (0.2–0.4 mg/kg IM) • Tiletamine-zolazepam (2–4 mg/kg IV or IM) • Tiletamine-zolazepam/ketamine/xylazine mixture[b] (0.1 ml/5 kg IM) • Ketamine (5–10 mg/kg IM) + medetomidine (30–50 µg/kg IM) • Ketamine (5–10 mg/kg IM) + xylazine (1 mg/kg IM)	• Same as for minor surgery/minor pain	• Same as for minor surgery/minor pain	• NSAIDs • Oral opioid agonist preparations • Butorphanol syrup (1 ml of 1% butorphanol in 1 oz of Pet-Tinic™ syrup or fish flavored base; dose at 1 ml/4.5 kg) • Opioid-NSAID combinations • Acupuncture
Major Surgery/ Major Pain	• Placement of transdermal fentanyl patch (2.5 mg [25 µg/hr] patch) 12–24 hours prior to induction • Fentanyl (1–5 µg/kg/hr IV) + concurrent application of 2.5 mg [25 µg/hr] transdermal fentanyl patch • Local IV anesthetics	• Same as for minor surgery/minor pain	• Epidural lidocaine (1 ml/4.5 kg) or morphine (0.1–0.2 mg/kg as needed with saline to 1 ml/4.5 kg) • Intraarticular morphine (0.2 mg/kg) or bupivacaine (1–2 ml of a 0.5% solution) • Fentanyl (1–5 µg/kg/hr) or morphine (0.2 mg/kg/hr) IV infusion during and after surgery • Protective bandaging • Postoperative opioid suppositories	• NSAIDs plus opioids • Oral opioid agonist preparations • Fentanyl patch • Acupuncture

[a]Adapted from Tranquilli W, Grimm K, Flaggella A, et al: *A Roundtable Discussion: Rethinking Your Approach to Sedation, Anesthesia, and Analgesia* [monograph]. Lenexa, KS, Veterinary Medicine Publishing, 1997.

[b]Mixture of 1 ml 10% xylazine and 4 ml ketamine as a diluent in a vial of tiletamine-zolazepam.

Aspirin should be used with extreme caution in cats because the half-life is substantially prolonged in this species, especially in young and old cats.

Ketoprofen

Ketoprofen is a relatively new NSAID. A single postsurgical dose (1–2 mg/kg IV, IM, or SQ) can be given. Gastric ulceration and renal tubular damage are possible, albeit rare, adverse effects.

Piroxicam

Piroxicam is a relatively new and potent NSAID and is probably more effective than ketoprofen. The most common adverse effects associated with piroxicam therapy include gastric ulceration and renal tubular damage. The dosage for cats is 0.3 mg/kg daily for 4 days and 0.3 mg/kg every other day thereafter. Piroxicam is best dispensed by compounding the drug in a tasty, flavored base (e.g., fish) and administering as an oral liquid; the compounded medication must be used immediately due to its short shelf life.

Local Anesthetics

Local anesthetics and analgesics are effective for temporary relief of mild to moderate pain. Lidocaine and bupivacaine are used most commonly and can be administered locally, within a cavity (e.g., chest cavity), or epidurally.

Local Administration

Local anesthetics, such as 2% lidocaine, are administered to effect near an incision and provide regional analgesia for about 1 hour. Bupivacaine (0.75%) can be given to effect to provide 6 to 10 hours of regional analgesia for peri-incisional pain. Lidocaine can be administered at or near intercostal nerves proximal to a thoracotomy incision to reduce postsurgical pain. This agent is also frequently administered into the pleural cavity prior to bupivacaine administration to decrease discomfort associated with thoracotomy. Lidocaine or bupivacaine can be used as a maxillary or mandibular nerve block for oral surgery.

Epidural Administration

Hindlimb pain can be controlled by epidural administration of preservative-free 2% lidocaine (0.5 ml/kg) or 0.75% bupivacaine (1 mg/4.5 kg); duration of anesthesia is 60 to 90 minutes with lidocaine and 4 to 6 hours with bupivacaine. Fentanyl (4 µg/kg) or medetomidine (10 µg/kg) in 1 ml saline can be injected epidurally for analgesia of the hindlimb (both drugs) or forelimb (medetomidine only). Fentanyl is much less toxic than medetomidine when used in this manner.

Opioid Agonists

Morphine

Morphine is a natural opioid agonist. On rare occasions, it may produce initial excitement manifested by panting, salivation, nausea, vomiting, urination, defecation, and hypotension when administered to cats. These reactions arise from activation of the chemoreceptor trigger zone, vagal stimulation, and histamine release. Initial excitement may be followed by central nervous system (CNS) depression, constipation, urine retention, bradycardia, respiratory depression, and hypothermia. Cats are more resistant than dogs to stimulation of the chemoreceptor trigger zone. Analgesia and CNS depression are noted in cats when morphine doses of 0.1 to 0.5 mg/kg every 2 to 6 hours are used[2,3,6]; doses approaching 1 mg/kg can induce marked hyperexcitability, aggression, and stimulation of the chemoreceptor trigger zone.

Meperidine

At a dose of 2.0 to 5.0 mg/kg IM or SQ, meperidine results in sedation and analgesia, but the effects last only 1 hour in cats.

Oxymorphone

Oxymorphone is a semisynthetic opioid agonist with analgesic properties that are approximately 10 times more potent than those of morphine; its adverse effects on the respiratory, cardiovascular, and gastrointestinal systems are less pronounced. Oxymorphone (0.05–0.2 mg/kg SQ or IM) lasts 2 to 5 hours and is indicated for moderate to severe visceral or somatic pain. Lower doses are used for IV administration. When used alone, however, oxymorphone may result in excitement or hyperalgesia.[2,3,6] Diazepam (0.1–0.2 mg/kg IV or IM) given concurrently with oxymorphone may help reduce these side effects.

Fentanyl

Fentanyl is an effective analgesic that can be given IM, SQ, or IV as a preanesthetic. It can be administered via an IV bolus (0.2–0 µg/kg q2–6h), constant rate infusion (1–4 µg/kg/hr), or transdermal patch. Fentanyl can cause respiratory depression, bradycardia, and somnolence at higher dosages. It can also prolong return to normal body temperature during recovery from anesthesia.

Fentanyl-impregnated transdermal patches reliably release a controlled amount of fentanyl over a 72 hour period (Figure 17-1); depending on the severity of the discomfort, 2.5 mg (25 µg/hr) patches are adequate for treating a 4 to 5 kg cat. The patches maintain adequate blood levels of fentanyl for 72 hours, but therapeutic levels are not attained for 12 to 24 hours; thus patches may be most effective when used in conjunction with other analgesics or in addition to constant rate fentanyl infusion during surgery or other painful procedures.

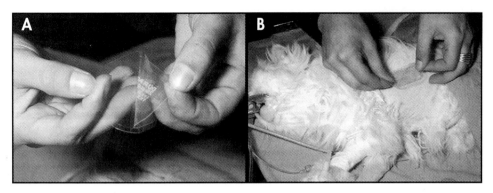

Figure 17-1: Use of the fentanyl patch. The backing of the transdermal fentanyl patch is removed (**A**), and the patch is placed on a flat, hairless area of skin where it is unlikely to be removed by the cat (**B**). Ideally latex rubber gloves should be worn when these patches are handled. The patches are capable of delivering the analgesic over a 72 hour period.

Opioid Agonist-Antagonists

Butorphanol

Butorphanol is a synthetic opioid agonist-antagonist that has five times the analgesic potency of morphine and a duration of analgesia of approximately 1 to 4 hours. Adverse effects such as nausea and vomiting are rare, but the drug can induce sedation in cats. At 0.1 to 0.4 mg/kg IV, IM, or SQ, butorphanol provides 1 to 4 hours of visceral analgesia; a higher dose (0.8 mg/kg IV) is needed for somatic pain, and analgesia lasts only about 2 hours. IV butorphanol may result in transient hypotension or bradycardia.[2,3,6] Butorphanol possesses antagonist properties and reverses the effects of narcotics. Therefore butorphanol must not be given within 12 hours of any pre- or intraoperatively administered narcotics.

KEY POINT

A transdermal analgesic patch system provides constant pain relief throughout the dosing period and obviates the need for constant reevaluation of schedules and dosing.

Buprenorphine

Buprenorphine HCl, an agonist-antagonist, can reverse opioid-induced respiratory depression while maintaining analgesia. Buprenorphine can be given at 0.005 to 0.01 mg/kg IV, IM, or SQ and lasts 4 to 12 hours.

Acupuncture

Acupuncture is the ancient art of inducing a physiologic effect, in this case analgesia, in response to the insertion of a needle into a specific point along a meridian of the body. This analgesic method has been used for centuries and has been proven effective in humans via well-controlled clinical studies. The exact mechanism of action is not completely understood, but the procedure works in part by releasing endorphins and enkephalins. Acupressure produces similar results by applying physical pressure to specific areas.

Tranquilizers and Anxiolytics

In some cases, a cat's anxiety may preclude adequate pain management. Therapeutic trials of tranquilizers (e.g., acepromazine, diazepam, medetomidine, ketamine, xylazine) to relax the patient may be of substantial benefit. Xylazine can be used as an anxiolytic (0.05–0.2 mg/kg IV or IM) or sedative (0.5–2 mg/kg IV, IM, or SQ) to provide 15 to 30 minutes of relief from visceral pain. At the very low dose of 0.5 to 1.0 mg/kg IM, ketamine relieves anxiety for 30 minutes; at higher doses (1.0–4.0 mg/kg IV) the agent lasts approximately 30 minutes and is helpful for short, painful procedures, such as wound and burn care. It may also be indicated during surgical procedures (e.g., amputation of tumor-associated fractures) or radiation therapy at sites of bone pain due to a malignant disease. Ketamine does not depend on renal excretion and thus can be used safely in cats with diminished renal function.

REFERENCES

1. Patt RB, Loughner JE: Management of pain in the cancer patient, in Rosenthal S, Carignan JR, Smith BD (eds): *Medical Care of the Cancer Patient*, ed 2. Philadelphia, WB Saunders, 1993, pp 255–264.
2. Pascoe PJ: Patient aftercare, in Slatter D (ed): *Textbook of Small Animal Surgery*, ed 2. Philadelphia, WB Saunders, 1993, pp 230–240.
3. Hansen B: Analgesics in cardiac, surgical, and intensive care patients, in Kirk RW, Bonagura JD (eds): *Current Veterinary Therapy XI: Small Animal Practice*. Philadelphia, WB Saunders, 1992, pp 82–87.
4. Hellyer PW, Gaynor JS: Acute postsurgical pain in dogs and cats. *Compend Contin Educ Pract Vet* 20:140–153, 1998.
5. Pollet R, Ralph Claxton C, Raffe M: Using butorphanol tartrate to manage pain in cats. *Vet Med* 93:146–155, 1998.
6. Scherk-Nixon M: A study of the use of a transdermal fentanyl patch in cats. *JAAHA* 32:19–24, 1996.

TREATMENT OF NAUSEA AND VOMITING

18

Gregory K. Ogilvie and Antony S. Moore

CLINICAL BRIEFING

Emetic Potential	Nausea and vomiting are not commonly associated with chemotherapy in cats. If vomiting occurs shortly after administration of chemotherapy, it primarily originates from the chemoreceptor trigger zone and emetic center; delayed nausea and vomiting are often caused by damage to the upper GI tract.
Self-Limiting Vomiting	*Therapy:* Correct underlying cause; do not feed by mouth until nausea and vomiting cease for 12 to 24 hours; administer SQ fluids to maintain hydration; initiate small amounts of water by mouth, then introduce a bland, low-fat diet; monitor hydration status and electrolytes.
Life-Threatening Vomiting	*Therapy:* Same protocol as for self-limiting nausea and vomiting except also administer IV fluids (maintenance needs + hydration deficits + losses) and correct electrolyte and pH abnormalities (e.g., serum potassium); in addition, give parenteral antiemetics (e.g., metoclopramide, butorphanol, ondansetron).
Prevention	Cats at high risk for nausea and vomiting or those receiving drugs that are powerful inducers of emesis may benefit from pretreatment with antiemetics.

Nausea and vomiting can occur for many reasons, such as a mass effect from the primary or metastatic tumor or a secondary consequence of the cancer or treatment.[1-3] Nausea and vomiting may reduce a patient's quality of life by inducing such life-threatening problems as dehydration, anorexia, metabolic imbalance, and wound dehiscence due to increased abdominal pressure.[1-5] In addition, caregivers often get the impression that their pet is experiencing unnecessary toxicities, which may result in abandonment of life-saving treatment and lead to subsequent euthanasia.

In cats, anorexia or hypersalivation is more common than overt vomiting. Management of nausea and vomiting is important to improve the quality of life for the cat and can subsequently enhance response to therapy and increase survival time. Indeed, treatment of nausea and vomiting is part of the overall goal of providing compassionate care. If the underlying cause of the nausea and vomiting cannot be corrected immediately, nausea and vomiting should be relieved as soon as they occur.

Many veterinarians find that encouraging caregivers to be part of the health care team helps improve the patient's quality of life. Clients should be educated that nausea and vomiting may be preventable. When therapy with the potential to induce nausea/vomiting is initiated, preventative antiemetic therapy (e.g., metoclopramide) must also be administered. If this is not possible, caregivers should be instructed to start giving oral antiemetics at home as soon as signs as subtle as anorexia are noted. Similarly, if a cat vomits after receiving chemotherapy, it should be treated prophylactically during subsequent rounds of therapy until the attending clinician is confident that nausea and vomiting are no longer major risks for that patient.

MECHANISM OF NAUSEA AND VOMITING

The presence of a tumor can lead to problems (e.g., physical obstruction of the intestinal tract) that may induce nausea and vomiting. In this example, surgical resection of the tumor is the only solution for the underlying clinical problem. Unlike humans, cats rarely exhibit any evidence of nausea and vomiting in association with the administration of chemotherapeutic drugs[2-5]; anorexia or hypersalivation is more commonly seen than overt vomiting. The emetic potential of any chemotherapeutic drug depends on the patient's sensitivity as well as the route of administration and drug dose. Some commonly used chemotherapeutic agents and their associated potential to induce nausea and vomiting are listed in Table 18-1.

TABLE 18-1
Nausea- or Vomiting-Inducing Potential of Selected Chemotherapeutic Agents

Low	Moderate	High
L-Asparaginase	Carboplatin	Dacarbazine
Bleomycin	Cyclophosphamide	Procarbazine
Chlorambucil	Cytosine arabinoside	Mustargen
Tamoxifen	Daunorubicin	
Vinblastine	Doxorubicin	
Steroids	Etoposide	
Mitoxantrone	Methotrexate	
	Vincristine	

Any drug given IV can stimulate the central receptors responsible for nausea, vomiting, salivation, or anorexia within minutes to hours of administration. Similarly, most chemotherapeutic agents can induce these signs 3 to 5 days after treatment because of damage to the gastrointestinal (GI) tract.

The mechanism of chemotherapy-induced nausea and centrally mediated vomiting is complex (Figure 18-1). The emetic center in the medulla regulates nausea and vomiting and receives input from at least four sources: the chemoreceptor trigger zone (CTZ), peripheral receptors, the cerebral cortex, and the vestibular apparatus. The latter probably does not influence cancer- or chemotherapy-associated nausea and vomiting, and thus drugs such as diphenhydramine are probably of minimal value in cats. The CTZ is located in the fourth ventricle of the medulla. It is activated solely by chemical stimuli and plays an important role in chemotherapy-induced nausea and vomiting. Peripheral re-

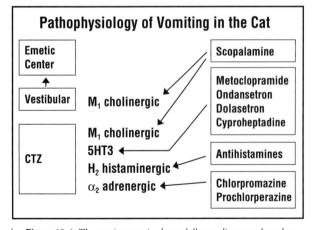

Figure 18-1: *The emetic center in the medulla coordinates and regulates nausea and vomiting and receives input from at least four sources: the chemoreceptor trigger zone (CTZ), peripheral receptors, the cerebral cortex, and the vestibular apparatus. These areas are influenced by cholinergic, serotonin (5HT3), histaminergic, and adrenergic receptors, which are in turn influenced by select drugs.*

ceptors can be triggered directly by chemotherapeutic agents or indirectly by substances released by their effects on other sites; these impulses arrive at the emetic center via the vagus nerve and other autonomic afferent nerves. Input from higher cognitive centers, a common source of nausea and vomiting in humans, is sometimes seen in cats. Indeed, cats will occasionally correlate a car ride or the sight of a hospital or treatment room with a "bad experience" and will salivate profusely and/or develop nausea and vomiting anytime the stimulus is repeated. Pharmacologic intervention targeted at any or all of these pathways is important for eliminating nausea and vomiting in cancer patients.

GENERAL CONCEPTS OF ANTIEMETIC THERAPY

As mentioned, most chemotherapeutic agents rarely induce nausea and vomiting in cats shortly after administration.[2-5] Cats that tend to have "tender tummies" after their first dose of chemotherapy are more likely to experience adverse GI effects following subsequent treatments. They should be treated prophylactically with such antiemetics as metoclopramide or ondansetron/dolasetron just prior to and up to 10 days after chemotherapy is administered.

Self-Limiting Nausea and Vomiting[1-3]

An underlying cause for acute, potentially self-limiting nausea and vomiting should be identified and corrected when possible. Affected animals should be treated as follows:

- Give nothing by mouth until nausea and vomiting have stopped for at least 12 to 24 hours.
- Subsequently, very small amounts of water (e.g., ice cubes) followed by a bland diet can be offered every 2 to 4 hours.
- Once the cat is able to take in food without nausea and vomiting, it can be slowly returned to a normal diet. During this transition period, a soft, low-fat diet is recommended. Fat is a complex nutrient that is difficult to digest and therefore may induce diarrhea; compared to some proteins, fat can delay gastric emptying.
- Cats with minimal dehydration can receive SQ fluids; IV therapy is preferred for significantly dehydrated cats. Many cats improve dramatically shortly after the administration of IV fluids. Potassium chloride (KCl) supplementation should be provided to prevent and/or treat hypokalemia (Table 18-2).

Life-Threatening Nausea and Vomiting[1-3,5]

Cats with severe, life-threatening nausea and vomiting are usually very ill and often obtunded. Treatment is centered around identifying and correcting the underlying cause. Specific treatment includes administration of appropriate fluid therapy to severely dehydrated cats (8% to 12% of normal hydra-

TABLE 18-2
Intravenous Potassium Supplementation to Correct Hypokalemia

Serum Potassium (mEq/L)	KCl (mEq) Added to Each Liter of Fluid	Maximum Rate of Infusion (ml/kg/hr)
<2	80	6
2.1–2.5	60	8
2.6–3.0	40	12
3.1–3.5	28	16

TABLE 18-3
Selected Antiemetics for Use in Cats

Product	Dose
Chlorpromazine	0.5 mg/kg IM or SQ q6–8h
Prochlorperazine	0.1–0.5 mg/kg IM or SQ q6–8h
Diphenhydramine	2.0–4.0 mg/kg PO q8h
Butorphanol	0.1–0.4 mg/kg IM, IV or SQ q1–4h
Dimenhydrinate	8 mg/kg PO q8h
Metoclopramide	1–2 mg/kg CRI IV over 24 hr or 0.2–0.5 mg/kg PO q6–8h
Ondansetron	0.1–0.3 mg/kg IV 15 min before and 12 hr after chemotherapy or PO q12h
Dolasetron	0.6–3 mg/kg IV q24h
Dexamethasone	1–3 mg IV

tion). Deficits in fluid and electrolytes secondary to dehydration should be replaced during the first 24 hours. Up to 44 ml/kg/day of maintenance fluids should be administered. Continued losses, such as from vomiting and diarrhea, should be estimated and replaced. As noted, KCl should be added to fluids to prevent and/or correct hypokalemia, but the administration rate of KCl should not exceed 0.5 mEq/kg/hour because of the risk for cardiac arrest and death. Cats should be monitored for fluid overload by monitoring body weight, capillary refill time, skin turgor, packed cell volume, total solids, and central venous pressure; thoracic auscultation is also indicated.

Antiemetics should be employed anytime nausea and vomiting are noted. Once chemotherapeutic agents cause nausea and vomiting, pretreatment with antiemetics is indicated for all future administrations. For optimum results, antiemetics should be sent home with owners, who should be instructed to administer the drug prophylactically or as soon as nausea or vomiting is suspected.

KEY POINT

Metoclopramide should not be administered if a GI obstruction is identified or suspected.

ANTIEMETIC AGENTS (Table 18-3)

Metoclopramide[1–3]
Metoclopramide is one of the most commonly administered antiemetics in veterinary medicine. It is prescribed to prevent nausea and vomiting and to treat these conditions when they occur at home. Its antiemetic effect is both central and peripheral. Centrally, it is a dopamine antagonist that blocks the CTZ and prevents emesis; peripherally, it increases the tone of the caudal esophageal sphincter and increases gastric antral contractions by relaxing the pylorus and duodenum. This drug should not be administered to cats with GI obstruction. When metoclopramide is used with cimetidine, a small percentage of

cats will develop extrapyramidal side effects that resolve shortly after the metoclopramide is discontinued. Metoclopramide can be given to cats at a dose of 0.2 to 0.5 mg/kg PO q6–8h or 1 to 2 mg/kg constant rate infusion (CRI) over a 24 hour period, preferably through an IV pump.

Phenothiazines[1–3]
Phenothiazines (e.g., chlorpromazine, prochlorperazine) are commonly used as antiemetics for mild chemotherapy-induced nausea; they block the CRT of the emetic center. In human medicine, phenothiazines generally do not effectively reduce efferent GI irritation. Because these drugs can induce vasodilation, they should not be used in dehydrated cats or those with poor cardiac output. In addition, phenothiazines can induce mild depression and make monitoring patients difficult. All phenothiazines can cause seizures in predisposed animals. Chlorpromazine can be administered at 0.5 mg/kg IM or SQ q6–8h; prochlorperazine can be dosed at 0.1 to 0.5 mg/kg IM or SQ q6–8h. A suppository form (Compazine®, SmithKline Beecham) is available for use in select cats that will allow it to be placed

Narcotic Analgesics
Butorphanol (0.1–0.4 mg/kg IM) may help reduce the prevalence of nausea and vomiting in response to chemotherapy. The drug also has mild analgesic properties. For best results, butorphanol should be administered IM shortly after the administration of chemotherapy in cats that tend to become nauseated.

Antihistamines
Antihistamines (e.g., diphenhydramine, dimenhydrinate, trimethobenzamide) block input from the vestibular system

and work against motion-induced nausea and vomiting. Diphenhydramine can be administered at 2 to 4 mg/kg PO q8h; it can cause mild sedation. Although diphenhydramine is rarely beneficial in the treatment of chemotherapy-induced nausea and vomiting, it can be helpful for cats that get "car sick" on the way to and from the hospital or clinic.

KEY POINT

Pretreating cats that are likely to vomit with drugs such as metoclopramide can enhance quality of life.

Dopamine Antagonists and Diphenylbutylpiperidines[1-3]

Haloperidol is a dopamine antagonist that blocks the CRT; at a dose of 110 µg/kg, it can prevent nausea and vomiting for up to 4 days in cats. Pimozide, a long-acting diphenylbutylpiperidine, can protect cats from drug-induced nausea and vomiting for up to 6 days when given at a dose of 100 µg/kg. Clinical experience with these two drugs is minimal.

Serotonin Antagonists[1-3]

Drugs that inhibit the 5-HT-3 (5-hydroxytryptamine) receptor constitute an entirely new and effective class of antiemetics that is being explored for use in human and veterinary cancer patients. Ondansetron (0.1 mg/kg IV), several analogs (dolasetron, 0.6–3 mg/kg IV), and oral preparations are currently available. Serotonin antagonists are very effective for reducing chemotherapy-induced nausea and vomiting. Although these agents are expensive, they are affordable for use in cats because of the small size of the patient. Their cost is expected to decline in the future.

Corticosteroids[1-3]

Dexamethasone has been shown to have antiemetic activity. Its mechanism of action is unknown. Side effects are few except in cats with diabetes or gastric ulcers. Relatively small (1 to 3 mg) IV doses are effective in humans; an appropriate dose for cats is unknown at this time.

REFERENCES

1. Morrow GR: Management of nausea in the cancer patient, in Rosenthal S, Carignan JR, Smith BD (eds): *Medical Care of the Cancer Patient*, ed 2. Philadelphia, WB Saunders, 1993, pp 565–571.

2. Tams TR: Vomiting, regurgitation and dysphagia, in Ettinger SJ (ed): *Textbook of Veterinary Internal Medicine: Diseases of the Dog and Cat*, ed 3. Philadelphia, WB Saunders, 1989, pp 27–32.

3. Leib MS: Acute vomiting: A diagnostic approach and systematic management, in Kirk RW, Bonagura JD (eds): *Current Veterinary Therapy XI*. Philadelphia, WB Saunders, 1992, pp 583–587.

NUTRITIONAL SUPPORT

Gregory K. Ogilvie and Antony S. Moore

19

CLINICAL BRIEFING

Enteral Feeding

General	Enteral routes are preferred whenever possible. Consider diets that are low in simple carbohydrates and moderate in fats; omega-3 fatty acids may be valuable. Diets should provide adequate amounts of highly bioavailable proteins. Adequate fiber is essential for general health. Energy requirements must be determined on an individual basis and may not be higher in a cancer patient than in a normal animal, even during recovery from surgery.
Oral Feeding	Best enteral route. Enhance intake by providing highly palatable, warmed foods. Consider appetite stimulants, such as benzodiazepine derivatives, cyproheptadine, and megestrol acetate. Consider other assisted feeding long before weight loss approaches 10%.
Nasoesophageal or Nasojejunal Tube Feeding	Excellent for short-term feeding. Use liquid nutrient solutions to meet all nutritional needs.
Esophagostomy Tube Feeding	Excellent for short- and long-term feeding as well as oral medication in all but patients with esophageal motility problems or that are vomiting. Feed blenderized foods to meet nutritional needs.
Gastrostomy Tube Feeding	Excellent for long-term feeding and oral medication in patients that are not vomiting and have functional GI tracts. Use blenderized foods to meet nutritional needs.
Jejunostomy Tube Feeding	Excellent choice to bypass the upper GI tract in vomiting patients. Use liquid nutrient solutions. The use of a pump or frequent small feedings by syringe is required.

Parenteral Feeding

General	Excellent choice whenever enteral feeding is not possible. An infusion pump, specially designed nutrients, absolute dedication to aseptic technique, and a separate indwelling catheter are needed.

Recently, a great deal of information has been published on the nutritional management of the veterinary cancer patient.[1-11] The routine use of nutrient delivery systems, such as nasoesophageal, nasojejunal, esophagostomy, gastrostomy, and jejunostomy tubes as well as parenteral feeding techniques, has increased substantially in feline medicine. This has resulted in a better quality of life and better response to therapy for cats that receive this type of care. Research is needed to delineate the impact that cancer has on the metabolism and quality and length of life in cats with cancer. In many species, there is a multitude of profound changes in metabolism associated with the cancer itself. These metabolic derangements occur long before overt weight loss occurs or is detected and has been termed *cancer cachexia*. Cancer cachexia is a complex paraneoplastic syndrome of alterations in metabolism that can eventually result in progressive involuntary weight loss. This occurs even in the face of adequate nutritional intake. The importance of this syndrome cannot be overstated. For example, humans with cancer cachexia have a decreased quality of life, decreased response to treatment, and a shortened survival time compared with patients who have similar diseases but do not exhibit clinical or biochemical signs associated with this condition. Understanding the metabolic alterations in cats with cancer is essential to providing adequate nutritional support to these patients. We must be diligent in treating for this syndrome, even though our patients may not appear clinically "cachectic" and do not exhibit overt symptoms of cachexia until much later in the disease process. We also must never forget that the most consistent quality of life "markers" that caregivers should monitor are appetite and nutrition. Educating caregivers about the metabolic ramifications of cancer and then giving them the tools by which they can affect those ramifications allows the most compassionate care to be delivered.

METABOLIC ALTERATIONS IN CANCER CACHEXIA

Cats are obligate carnivores that not only have unique nutritional needs but also unique metabolic processes that differ from those found in dogs and humans. The abnormalities in carbohydrate, protein, and lipid metabolism associated with cancer in cats are largely unexplored, although at least some are thought to be similar to those found in dogs and humans. The clinical syndrome of cancer cachexia can lead to serious debilitation and death unless addressed by appropriate therapy.[1-2,12-17] The most important concept is that the metabolic alterations associated with cancer cachexia initially are a true metabolic aberration; as such, they occur long before weight loss is observed and persist for weeks, months, and perhaps years after the malignancies are eliminated. Cancer cachexia is an insidious, persistent universal syndrome that, left unchecked, will diminish the potential quality and quantity of our patients' lives; addressing it must become a priority in our treatment plan for compassionate care to result.

Cats have unique needs for specific amino acids such as taurine. In addition, inadequate amounts of cysteine can result in Heinz body anemia that can be of serious consequence to the cancer patient. Arginine has been shown to enhance the immune system in species other than the cat, and glutamine has been documented to be important to the health and well being of the entire GI tract. Cancer cells compete with the host for proteins as energy sources and as building blocks for normal bodily function. Therefore providing a diet that has moderate amounts of highly bioavailable protein may be logical. Ensuring adequate amounts of taurine, cysteine, arginine, and glutamine in a palatable form may be helpful. The clinical value of supplementation to levels above nutritional requirements is unknown.

Abnormalities in lipid metabolism have been linked to a number of clinical problems, including immunosuppression, which correlate with decreased survival in affected humans.[12-17] The clinical impact of the abnormalities in lipid metabolism may be lessened with dietary therapy. In contrast to carbohydrates and proteins, some tumor cells have difficulty using lipid as a fuel source, but host tissues continue to oxidize lipids for energy. This has led to the hypothesis that diets relatively high in fat may be beneficial for cats with cancer compared with diets that are high in simple carbohydrates, assuming that the protein content, caloric density, and palatability remain constant. This hypothesis has not been tested in cats. The kind of fat in the diet, rather than the amount, may be the important factor. For example, omega-3 fatty acids have been shown experimentally to have many beneficial properties[5,15,16]:

- Omega-3 fatty acids, arginine, and RNA improve the immune system, metabolic status, and clinical outcome of human cancer patients.
- When used alone, omega-3 fatty acids improve the immune system and decrease the time for wound healing, duration of hospitalization, and complication rate in humans with GI cancer.
- Omega-3 fatty acids inhibit tumorigenesis and cancer spread in animal models.
- Essential fatty acids that contain omega-3 fatty acids reduce radiation-induced damage to skin. This seems to be specific for normal, not malignant, cells.
- Eicosapentaenoic acid not only has antitumor effects but also anticachectic effects, in part because there is decreased protein degradation without an effect on protein synthesis.

It is essential to determine whether diets supplemented with omega-3 fatty acids improve quality of life and response to therapy in cats with cancer. At the present time, there is some rational clinical information to suggest that the addition of omega-3 fatty acids to a diet already fortified with high fat levels, moderate protein levels, and lower carbohydrate levels may be helpful in supporting feline cancer patients. It is imperative that, regardless of the diet, patients consume adequate nutrients to prevent weight loss.

Nutrient and Water Needs

Our knowledge of the nutrient and water needs of cats is primarily based on work done many years ago or extrapolated from research completed on rodents or humans. The majority of data concerning energy and water requirements in cats may be overestimated.[18] For example, it has been determined that the resting energy expenditure, which is an estimate of the nutrient and water needs of normal cats, is lower than indicated by previously published data.[18] What this means to the practicing veterinarian is that most of the recommendations for the amount to be fed are overestimated for the majority of cats. Caloric requirements differ for each cat, and therefore each cat should be periodically reassessed and individualized in health and disease.

LESS PROVEN NUTRIENT CLAIMS

Many clients come to our doors requesting guidance on the use of nutrients for their cats with cancer and other diseases. Many caregivers are utilizing the Internet and numerous alternative sources for information to help their cats. It is vital that we are able to explain what is known and not known and guide caregivers in their selection of supplements to assure that no harm is done to the patient. The nutritional requirements of cats are unique, and extrapolating from rats, dogs, or humans can be dangerous. The following section is designed to provide a background about some vitamins and other nutrients that have been mentioned in the literature or lay press. Very little information is known about the efficacy of these nutrients in the cat.

Vitamins

Retinoids, beta carotene, and vitamins C, D, and E may influence the growth and metastasis of cancer cells via a variety of mechanisms.[19–28] These vitamins fall into and out of popularity based on the results of select studies and the lay press. The weight of the literature would suggest, however, that many of these vitamins may be of value for some cancer patients. Select examples of the impact of a few vitamins are included below.

Retinoids

Retinoids are not used as a mainstay of cancer therapy; however, there is a growing body of knowledge about their anticancer effect in humans and animals. In humans, 13-*cis* retinoic acid prevents secondary tumors in patients treated for squamous cell carcinoma of the head and neck[19–22] and can reverse the effects of cervical human papillomavirus infection. Retinoic acid, when used in the adjuvant treatment of retino-blastoma (a childhood cancer), leads to translocation of bound receptor vitamin complexes to the nucleus, which results in the regulation of the neuroblastoma gene.[20] Melanoma in mice has been successfully treated with retinoids.[20]

The efficacy of retinoids is not confined to rodents and humans. A study was recently completed to evaluate the synthetic retinoids isotretinoin and etretinate to treat dogs with intracutaneous cornifying epithelioma (ICE), other benign skin neoplasias, and cutaneous lymphoma.[21] This study showed reduction in the size of some tumors and elimination of others. Little is known about the antitumor effect of retinoids in cats, although there is possible anecdotal evidence suggesting some efficacy for the treatment of actinic keratosis (precancer) on the face of light-pigmented cats.

Vitamin C

Vitamin C has been studied continuously over the past several decades as an antioxidant and an agent that can effectively treat conditions such as colds, cardiovascular disease, and cancer. There have been some data suggesting that vitamin C may be of value for the prevention and treatment of certain types of cancers.[15–17] Water-soluble vitamin C has been widely reported to inhibit nitrosation reactions and prevent chemical induction of cancers of the esophagus and stomach.[16–17] Processed foods high in nitrates and nitrites, such as bacon and sausage, are often supplemented with vitamin C to reduce

the carcinogenic capability of the resultant nitrosamines.

A human tissue culture line resistant to vincristine that was established from a small cell lung cancer cell line was pretreated with ascorbic acid, resulting in potentiation of the vincristine effects on resistant but not sensitive cell lines.[15,16] Therefore ascorbic acid may be one therapeutic alternative for overcoming a drug resistance in some cancer cells.

Vitamin E

Lipid-soluble vitamin E, or alpha tocopherol, can also inhibit nitrosation reactions, but in addition, vitamin E has a broad capacity to inhibit mammary tumor and colon carcinogenesis in rodents.[22–24] In addition to its chemopreventative properties, vitamin E may convey potential therapeutic efficacy against certain malignancies.[23–25] This is due to this vitamin's antiproliferative activity. Additional studies, such as those that have been initiated in humans at Harvard School of Public Health, are essential to allow further clarification of the value of these vitamins.

Minerals

Minerals that have been suggested as having chemopreventative or anticancer effects and that are of value as nutrients include selenium, copper, zinc, magnesium, calcium, lead, iron, potassium, sodium, arsenic, iodine, and germanium. Selenium has been one of the most heavily studied minerals associated with the development of cancer.[25–28] Low serum selenium levels have been seen in human patients with prostate and GI cancer.[25] In rodents, dietary supplementation of selenium has been shown to inhibit colon, mammary gland, and stomach carcinogenesis.[26–28] Additional study is essential to determine whether alteration of selenium levels would be of value for the treatment of veterinary or human cancer patients. Selenium may be toxic at high levels and thus should not be supplemented without first seeking advice from a veterinary nutritionist.

Iron transferrin and ferritin have been linked to cancer risk and cancer cell growth.[15] Lung, colon, bladder, and esophageal cancer in humans have been highly correlated with increased serum iron and increased transferrin saturation.[15–16] This may be because many tumor cells require iron for growth.

Therapeutic Enzymes

Enzymes have therapeutic potential but limited approval in the United States. L-Asparaginase is probably the most valuable therapeutic modality for the treatment of lymphoma and leukemia in animals and humans.[29] Oral enzyme preparations are used for the treatment of chronic pancreatic insufficiency and disaccharidase deficiency. Several enzyme preparations are available in Europe for oral adjuvant treatment of cancer and other diseases. Of those, Wobenzyme® and Musal® contain a similar mixture of enzymes. Recent studies report efficacy of therapeutic enzymes in the treatment of cancer patients, the mechanism of which is not precisely known. One hypothesis is that these enzymes eliminate pathogenic immune complexes. Therefore enzymes may indeed be of value for the adjuvant treatment of cancer.

Protease Inhibitors

A great deal of information suggests that soybean-derived Bowman-Birk inhibitor (BBI) can inhibit or suppress carcinogenesis both in vivo and in vitro.[30-34] Extracts of BBI have been shown to inhibit carcinogenesis in several animal model systems, including colon- and liver-induced carcinogenesis in mice, anthracene-induced cheek pouch carcinogenesis in hamsters, lung tumorigenesis in mice, and esophageal carcinogenesis in rats.[30-34] BBI concentration has been shown to inhibit metastasis and weight loss associated with radiation-induced thymic lymphoma in mice.[33] Irradiated rodents treated with dietary BBI concentration have fewer deaths, lower average grade of lymphoma, and larger fat stores compared with controls. Therefore this protease inhibitor from soybeans may be important as an adjunct to cancer chemotherapy protocols and in the prevention of secondary cancers.

NUTRITIONAL SUPPORT FOR CATS WITH CANCER

Theoretically, the ideal way of treating cancer cachexia should be to eliminate the underlying neoplastic condition. Unfortunately, this is not possible for many cats. In addition, in published studies in other species, the metabolic ramifications of cancer cachexia persist even after the patient is rendered free of disease. Therefore dietary therapy has been examined as a modality to reverse or eliminate cancer cachexia. Investigators have raised concerns about the possibility of increasing tumor growth by enhancing the nutritional status of the host. Several studies have failed to show this correlation. The benefits that have been shown with dietary support include weight gain and increased response to and tolerance of radiation, surgery, and chemotherapy. Other factors that have been shown to improve with nutritional support include thymic weight, immune responsiveness, and immunoglobulin and complement levels as well as the phagocytic ability of white blood cells.[1-4]

The single biggest concern in the nutritional support of the feline cancer patient is the prevention and treatment of anorexia. Several steps can be taken, including:

- Provide a variety of fresh aromatic foods that are warmed to just below body temperature. Cats are intermittent eaters, hence they should be provided some food constantly.
- Prevent and treat pain with appropriate analgesia. Cats are stoic and will not commonly exhibit pain in any

way other than through anorexia.
- Prevent and treat nausea. Cats do not commonly vomit when they are nauseated, but like other species, they become anorectic.
- Prevent and treat dehydration. Subclinical dehydration results in anorexia in most species. When in doubt, provide SQ or IV fluids.
- When the above has not worked, consider the addition of appetite stimulants such as cyproheptadine (total oral dose, 2 mg q12–24h) and megesterol acetate (0.25–0.5 mg/kg daily for 3–5 days then q48–72h thereafter). In some cases, a combination can be quite effective. In the hospital, diazepam (0.05–0.1 mg/kg single dose IV) may be used as needed to enhance appetite.
- When oral intake is not possible, assisted tube feeding with esophagostomy, gastrostomy, nasoesophageal, or weighted nasojejunal tube should be considered.

Rodents and humans with cancer that consume diets containing 30% to 50% of nonprotein calories as fat have increased nitrogen and energy balance as well as increased weight gain.[1-4] This type of diet also results in slower tumor growth and decreases in both glucose intolerance and fat loss. Although the ideal dietary formulation for cats is unknown, these facts may serve as guides for future research in this area. Table 19-1 provides a starting point for cats with cancer. The remainder of this section contains general guidelines for dietary therapy of feline cancer patients.

Parenteral Nutrition

Parenteral nutrition should be considered for cats with cancer when enteral feeding is not feasible. Parenteral feeding does require some specialized equipment (e.g., pumps) and strict aseptic technique, but the procedure can safely be carried out in private practice.

Administration and Complications

In feline medicine, parenteral nutrients are preferably administered through a dedicated single-lumen polyurethane catheter or a more expensive multilumen catheter.[1-4] It is essential to ensure that the catheter remains sterile to reduce the incidence of catheter-induced sepsis. Most veterinary centers that administer parenteral nutrients use IV pumps to ensure a constant rate of infusion. The rate of infusion is simplified if lipid is used to provide a percentage of nonprotein calories, because dextrose-containing fluids need to be gradually increased over several days.

With proper technique and patient care, problems associated with the administration of parenteral nutrition are relatively uncommon. Complications can result from destruction or occlusion of the catheter or tubing and pump failure; however, the most serious complication is related to catheter- or solution-related sepsis, which can be avoided

TABLE 19-1
Examples of Commercial Diets for Cats with Cancer

Weight (lb)	5	8	10	12	15
Weight (kg)	2.3	3.6	4.5	5.5	6.8
kcal/day	170	215	250	280	330
Hill's® Prescription Diet® Feline a/d® Canned					
Protein = 45.7, Fat = 28.7, Nitrogen-Free Extract = 16.5[a]					
Arginine (mg/d)	631	798	928	1,039	1,224
Arginine to add (mg)[b]	294	399	432	484	571
Total n-3 (mg/d)	806	1,019	1,185	1,327	1,564
Hill's® Science Diet® Feline Growth® Dry					
Protein = 37.1, Fat = 26.5, Nitrogen-Free Extract = 28.5[a]					
Arginine (mg/d)	755	955	1,110	1,243	1,465
Arginine to add (mg)[b]	170	242	250	280	330
Total n-3 (mg/d)	100	127	148	165	195
Fish oil caps to add[c]	2	3	3.5	4	4.5
Hill's® Science Diet® Feline Adult Seafood Canned					
Protein = 45.1, Fat = 25.4, Nitrogen-Free Extract = 20.1[a]					
Arginine (mg/d)	1,097	1,387	1,613	1,806	2,129
Arginine to add (mg)[b]	0	0	0	0	0
Total n-3 (mg/d)	318	402	468	524	617
Fish oil caps to add[c]	1.5	2	2.5	2.5	3

[a]Nutrients expressed as %DM (dry matter).
[b]Amount of arginine to add to this product (L-arginine is usually available as 500- and 1000-mg tablets).
[c]Number of fish oil capsules to add to this product.
Note: Fish oil capsules should be given with each meal and/or broken open and mixed with food.

by using aseptic technique. Other complications include metabolic and electrolyte abnormalities, including lactic acidosis. Mildly elevated serum urea nitrogen levels and hyperglycemia with glucosuria occasionally occur in cats receiving parenteral nutrient therapy. Hypokalemia is perhaps the most common electrolyte disturbance related to the administration of parenteral nutrition, but it is easily corrected with additional potassium supplementation.

Calculating Contents and Volumes

Although recent research may suggest that cats with cancer do not have increased nutritional requirements, the determination of the amount of parenteral solution for the cat is relatively straightforward.[1-4]

Energy Requirements

- The basal energy requirement (BER, in Kcal/day) is calculated by multiplying 70 by the cat's weight in $kg^{0.75}$. More simplistically, the weight of the cat in kg is multiplied by 30 and then added to 70.
- To get the maintenance energy requirement (MER, in kcal/day) for normal cats that are at rest in a cage, the BER is multiplied by 1 to 1.25. For cats that have undergone recent surgery or that are recovering from trauma or cancer, the BER is multiplied by a factor of 1.25

to 1.5 to determine the illness energy requirement (IER). For cats that are septic or have major burns, the BER is multiplied by 1.7 to 2.0. This may be an overestimate for many patients.
- To calculate the volume of the formula required, divide the MER by the kcal/ml of that formula to get the milliliters of formula per day.

KEY POINT

The energy needs of cats with cancer may not be higher than the needs of normal cats. Similarly, recent research has shown that the energy needs may not increase after major or minor surgery.

Lipid and Carbohydrate Requirements

- Most authors recommend giving 40% to 60% of the nonprotein calories as lipid and the balance of nonprotein calories as dextrose. Therefore because a 20% lipid solution has 2 kcal/ml, 40% to 60% of the IER is divided by 2 kcal/ml to yield the volume of the lipid solution to administer. The rare lipemic cat should not be given lipid-containing solutions.

- To determine the volume of a 50% dextrose solution to be administered (1.7 kcal/ml), divide 40% to 60% of IER by 1.7 kcal/ml. Because the volume of the dextrose-containing fluids should be increased gradually, half of this calculated volume should be administered on the first day and gradually increased to the full amount over the next day or two.

KEY POINT

Although the ideal "cancer diet" is not known, a diet composed of relatively low amounts of simple carbohydrates, moderate amounts of fats (especially omega-3 fatty acids), and adequate amounts of highly bioavailable proteins may be beneficial.

Enteral Nutrition

The standard dogma is that enteral nutrition should be considered for mature cats with functional GI tracts and a history of inadequate nutritional intake for 5 to 7 days or that have lost at least 10% of their body weight over a 1 to 2 week period. Current thinking is that enteral feeding techniques should be employed for all cats long before approaching 10% body weight loss. Indeed, clients should be counseled about the importance of nutritional therapy, including assisted feeding techniques, from the onset. In situations where therapy is likely to be prolonged, the "prophylactic" use of enteral feeding should be considered. In order to optimize appetite, nausea and discomfort should be treated appropriately. In addition, even subclinical dehydration should be treated aggressively. For example, a feline patient will experience loss of appetite at approximately 2% to 3% dehydration, a level far below clinical detection. Thus judicious use of SQ or IV fluid administration may actually be a diagnostic and therapeutic tool in the inappetent patient.

All methods to encourage food consumption should be attempted (Figure 19-1). These include warming the food to just below body temperature, providing a selection of palatable, aromatic foods, and providing comfortable, stress-free surroundings. When these simple procedures fail, such chemical stimulants as benzodiazepine derivatives (e.g., diazepam and oxazepam) and antiserotonin agents (cyproheptadine and pizotifen) can be used. Cyproheptadine (2–4 mg PO daily or twice daily) generally is effective in stimulating appetite in cats, as are megestrol acetate (0.25–0.5 mg/kg daily for 4 days, then every 2–3 days thereafter) and diazepam (0.05–0.5 mg/kg IV). Cats may have improved appetite when metoclopramide is given orally to decrease nausea associated with chemotherapy or surgery. When all the aforementioned fails, enteral nutri-

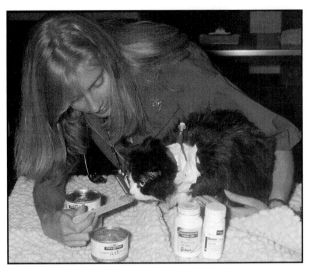

Figure 19-1: *All methods to encourage food consumption, including feeding a variety of highly palatable aromatic foods, warming the food to just below body temperature, and administering chemical stimulants, should be tried before starting enteral support. The optimum pharmacologic agent for use in the veterinary cancer patient is unknown; however, megestrol acetate has been shown to result in substantial weight gain in humans with cancer. Cyproheptadine is especially effective in the cat for enhancing appetite.*

tional support, designed to deliver nutrients to the GI tract by various methods, should be considered because it is practical, cost-effective, physiologic, and safe.[1–4]

Routes of Enteral Feeding

Nasoesophageal Tubes: This is still the most common feeding method used today, although esophagostomy and weighted nasojejunal tubes are becoming more popular.[1–4] The use of small-bore, silastic or polyurethane catheters has minimized complications associated with this delivery system. The procedure is simple to perform (Figure 19-2).

1. Tranquilization is sometimes required during placement of the tube, especially in cats. The swallowing reflex is important to be able to pass the tube into the esophagus and not into the trachea. To decrease any discomfort associated with the initial placement of the catheter, lidocaine is instilled into the nasal cavity with the nose pointed up. Care should be taken not to get any lidocaine into the mouth as it has a bad taste. It may be helpful to place a finger on the septum and push the cat's nose back parallel to the long axis of the head, thereby straightening the nasal passageway.
2. The tube is lubricated and passed to the level of the cat's ninth rib.
3. After the tube has been properly placed, it should be secured. In cats, the tube should be bent dorsally over the bridge of the nose and secured to the frontal region of the head with a permanent adhesive (Superglue®). A su-

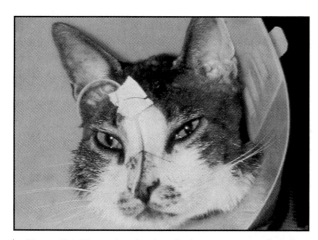

Figure 19-2: Nasoesophageal and weighted nasojejunostomy tube feeding are methods used for short-term nutritional support of cats. Lidocaine is instilled into the nasal cavity, and the tube is lubricated and passed down the esophagus. In the case of the nasoesophageal catheter, it is passed to the level of the ninth rib in cats. Weighted nasojejunostomy tubes are placed into the stomach so that normal peristalsis or the assistance of a fiberoptic endoscope will allow the tube to descend into the duodenum. Permanent adhesive and/or suture should be used to secure the tube to the frontal region of the head.

ture may be used to further secure the tube in place. Care should be taken to prevent any contact with the whiskers.

4. An Elizabethan collar should always be used to prevent the patient from removing the tube.

Weighted Nasojejunal Tubes: Weighted nasojejunal tubes are often preferred over nasogastric tubes because they can bypass the stomach to deliver liquid nutrients into the intestine, which is especially valuable in cats that are vomiting. The use of small-bore, silastic or polyurethane catheters with a flexible weighted tip has minimized complications associated with this delivery system. This system should be considered when short-term enteral nutritional intervention is needed. The procedure is simple to perform (Figure 19-2).

1. Placement of the tube begins as described in step 1 for nasoesophageal tubes. In cats with ileus or poor gastric motility, anesthesia should be employed and an endoscope should be used to bring the weighted tube into the duodenum. Alternatively, if a gastrostomy tube has already been placed, a weighted nasojejunal tube can be advanced into the stomach through the tube. This can be ideal, especially for cats that vomit.

2. The tube is lubricated and passed beyond the level of the ninth rib. Normal esophageal, gastric, and intestinal peristalsis will often sweep the weighted end into the intestine. Alternatively, an endoscope can be used to place the tube into the intestine.

3. The tube is secured as described for nasoesophageal tubes.

Enteral feeding should be used whenever possible—if the gut works, use it!

4. An Elizabethan collar should always be used to prevent the patient from removing the tube.

5. Oddly enough, despite the fact that the tube is essentially a linear foreign body, removal is done by gentle traction. The tubes slip through the intestines and stomach quite easily.

Esophagostomy versus Gastrostomy Tube: Recently, esophagostomy tube feeding has gained great popularity because the tubes can be placed easily without special equipment, removed at any time, and require no waiting time before feeding begins (Figure 19-3). [1-3,5] Fourteen to twenty French (Fr) tubes are used in cats. Esophagostomy tubes can be placed percutaneously with the use of a curved carmault or hemostat. Complications include local cellulitis and oc-

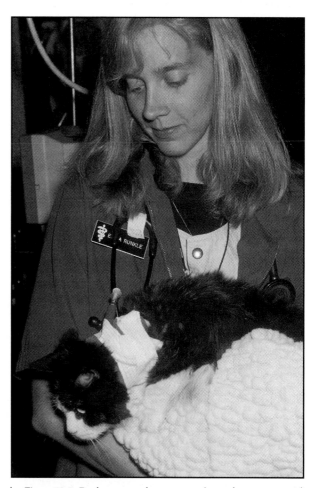

Figure 19-3: Esophagostomy tubes are easy to place and remove compared to most gastrostomy tubes. These tubes are generally well accepted by clients and patients.

casionally a dissecting abscess of the cervical tissues; these complications are rare and heal shortly after the tube is removed and the local reaction treated appropriately.

Many practitioners prefer to place esophagostomy tubes rather than gastrostomy tubes in all cats that have a functional upper GI tract except those that have esophageal motility disorders, such as megaesophagus. The esophagostomy tubes are easier to place, maintain, and remove than gastrostomy tubes. Many caregivers appear to accept esophagostomy tubes over gastrostomy tubes.

Esophagostomy Tube Placement (Figure 19-4)

1. The cat is placed under anesthesia and the left lateral cervical skin is clipped and prepared for surgery. The esophagostomy tube (e.g., red rubber feeding tube or JorVet J-390 14 Fr, 9 inch tube™) is placed in the mid-cervical region between the lateral spinous processes dorsally and the jugular vein and carotid artery ventrally.

2. A curved hemostat is placed down the mouth and into the esophagus, halfway between the angle of the jaw and the thoracic inlet. The curved portion of the instrument should point laterally.

3. The hemostat is then further directed laterally so that it "tents" the esophagus and overlying skin by pushing the tip against the left lateral esophageal wall. A small incision (0.25–0.5 cm) is made over the tip of the hemostat.

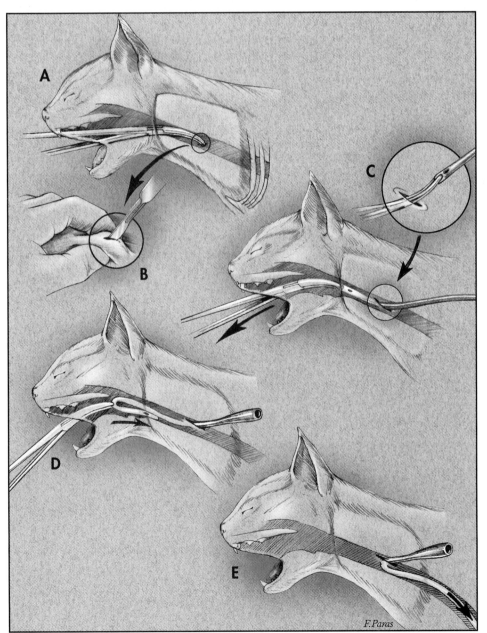

*Figure 19-4: Esophagostomy tube placement. The cat is placed under anesthesia and the left lateral cervical skin is clipped and prepared for surgery. The esophagostomy tube is placed in the mid-cervical region between the lateral spinous processes dorsally and the jugular vein and carotid artery ventrally. A curved hemostat is placed down the mouth and into the esophagus with the curved portion of the instrument pointing laterally, halfway between the angle of the jaw and the thoracic inlet (**A**). The hemostat is then directed laterally so that it "tents" the esophagus and overlying skin by pushing the tip laterally against the left lateral esophageal wall. A small incision (0.25–0.5 cm) is made over the tip of the hemostat. The key is to make a tiny incision through the esophagus just big enough to see the tip of the instrument (**B**). The instrument is pushed through the surgically created hole in the tissue. The jaws of the carmault or hemostat are opened and the tip of the red rubber feeding tube is grasped with the instrument and pulled partially through the skin and out the mouth (**C**). The tube is then pushed aborally down the esophagus with the hemostat to the level of the ninth rib (**D**). The objective is to not allow the tip of the tube to go into the stomach to prevent any vomiting or reflux esophagitis. The esophagostomy tube is then sutured into place and a light wrap is placed over the tube (**E**).*

F. Paras

The key is to make a tiny incision through the esophagus just big enough to see the tip of the instrument. The instrument is pushed through the surgically created hole in the tissue. The jaws of the carmault or hemostat are opened and the tip of the red rubber feeding tube is grasped with the instrument and pulled partially through the skin and out the mouth. The tube is then pushed aborally down the esophagus with the hemostat to the level of the ninth rib. The objective is to not allow the tip of the tube to go into the stomach to prevent any vomiting or reflux esophagitis.

4. The esophagostomy tube is then sutured into place and a light wrap is placed over the tube. Note that a blenderized commercial diet can be fed as soon as the patient can tolerate enteral feeding (Figure 19-5), usually within 24 hours. The amount of kcals provided is generally 25% to 50% of daily need; it is divided, administered every 4 to 8 hours, and then increased daily as fast as the cat can tolerate full feeding. Metoclopramide is often added to enhance normal GI motility.

Gastrostomy tubes are frequently used for cats that need nutritional support for more than 7 days (Figure 19-6).[1-4] These tubes can be placed surgically or with endoscopic guidance. A 5 ml, 18 to 24 Fr balloon-tipped urethral catheter (e.g., Foley catheter) can be placed surgically, as can a mushroom-tipped Pezzer proportionate head urologic catheter. Complications associated with gastrostomy tubes may include local or diffuse peritonitis, bleeding, cramping, vomiting, and diarrhea.

Gastrostomy Tube Placement

1. General anesthesia is required for the placement of a gastrostomy tube. Prior to placement of the tube, the left pericostal area just below the paravertebral epaxial musculature is clipped and prepared for surgery. A 2 to 3 cm incision is made through the skin and subcutaneous tissue just caudal to the last rib to allow blunt dissection through the musculature into the abdominal cavity.

2. The stomach is inflated through a tube that is placed down the esophagus to allow the surgeon to easily locate the stomach through the opening in the abdominal wall. Stay sutures are placed to allow a temporary fixation of the stomach against the abdominal wall; these stay sutures are used later to help close the muscular wall.

3. Two concentric purse-string sutures of 2-0 nonabsorbable nylon suture are then placed deep in the stomach wall; the first purse-string is deep to the second purse-string to allow a two-layered closure.

4. The feeding tube is placed into the lumen of the stomach through a stab incision in the middle of the purse-string sutures. The tip of the catheter generally is clipped off to allow easy introduction of food through the tube and into the stomach.

5. Once the tube is in place, the balloon is inflated with water if the balloon-tipped catheter is used; the Pezzer-tipped catheter has an expanded head that flattens and then returns to its normal shape when a stylet is extended and then removed in the catheter lumen during placement through the stab incision into the stomach.

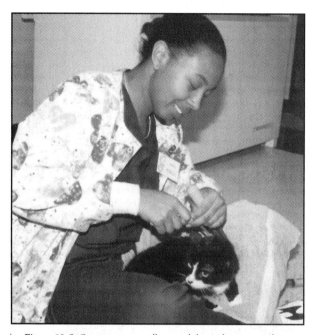

Figure 19-5: *Cats can eat normally around the esophagostomy tube. Feeding can begin immediately and should be gradually increased over several days. Blenderized or "tubeable" food is warmed and placed down the tube and the tube is then subsequently flushed with water to ensure that it does not get plugged. Medication and fluid therapy can also be administered through the tube.*

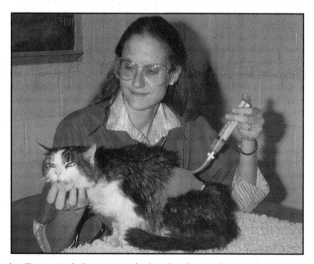

Figure 19-6: *Gastrostomy tubes have long been used to provide nutritional, fluid, and medical support in cats, especially in those with esophageal disorders where esophagostomy tubes are not indicated. The gastrostomy tube must be kept in place for at least 3 weeks in most cancer patients to allow adequate time for a stoma to form along the tube.*

6. With the tube in place, the purse-string sutures are tied to cause the stomach to invert in the region adjacent to the tube. The free ends of the sutures are then used to close the lateral abdominal musculature and subcutaneous tissue.

7. The skin is closed before the tube is secured to the abdominal skin by sutures. To prevent the cat from removing the tube, an abdominal wrap and an Elizabethan collar are recommended.

Feeding can begin 24 hours after the cat has recovered from anesthesia. The tube should be checked daily to ensure proper placement. In addition, the tube should be flushed with warm water after each feeding to maintain patency. After 3 weeks, an adhesion will form, allowing the tube to be removed or replaced as needed. The fistula generally heals within a week after the tube is removed permanently. Closure of the fistula is not needed.

Percutaneous placement of a gastrostomy tube by endoscopic guidance is quick, safe, and effective.[1-4] In this procedure (Figure 19-7), a specialized 20 Fr tube (e.g., Dubhoff PEG, Bard Urological Catheter) is used in all but the smallest cats. Low-profile gastrostomy tubes are available.

1. General anesthesia is also required for percutaneous placement of gastrostomy tubes. Clip and surgically prepare the area of skin outlined previously (left lateral abdomen), and then distend the stomach with air from an endoscope placed into the stomach.

2. Once the stomach is distended to the point that it is in apposition with the body wall, a finger is used to depress an area just caudal to the last left rib below the transverse processes of the lumbar vertebrae. This area of depression is then located by the person viewing the stomach lining by endoscopy.

3. A polyvinyl chloride (PVC) over-the-needle IV catheter is placed through the skin and into the stomach in the area previously located by the endoscopist. The stylet is removed to allow the introduction of the first portion of a 5 foot long piece of 8 lb test weight nylon filament or suture.

4. The piece of nylon is grabbed by a biopsy snare passed

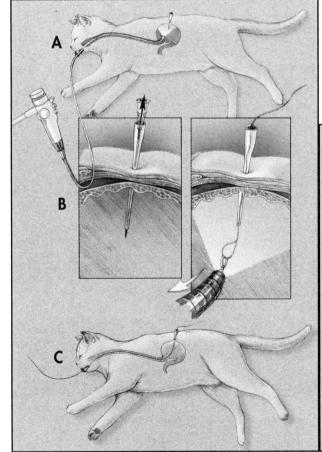

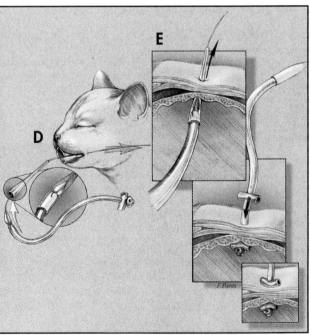

Figure 19-7: *Endoscope-guided percutaneous gastrostomy tube placement. The cat is put in right lateral recumbency (**A**). Note that an endoscope is used to insufflate the stomach so that a catheter can be placed through the skin and into the stomach to facilitate the passage of nylon suture into the stomach (**B**). The endoscope is then used to grasp the suture, which is then pulled through the esophagus and out of the mouth (**B** and **C**). A catheter is then passed over the nylon coming out of the cat's mouth (**C**). The Pezzer-tipped gastrostomy tube is prepared (**D**) by cutting a "V" out of both sides of the open end of the tube. A needle is used to pass the nylon suture coming out of the mouth through the end of the tube, where a knot is securely fastened. The tube is then stretched and forced into the end of the catheter. The catheter-tube combination is pulled with the nylon suture down the esophagus, into the stomach, and through the abdominal wall (**E**), where a "bumper" is placed down the tube and against the body wall.*

through the endoscope. The endoscope and the attached nylon are pulled up the esophagus and out the oral cavity so that the piece of nylon extends through the body wall and out of the mouth of the cat.

5. The end of the gastrostomy tube opposite the mushroom tip is trimmed so that it has a pointed end that will fit inside another PVC catheter, after the stylet is removed and discarded. This second PVC IV catheter is then placed over the nylon suture so that the narrow end points toward the stomach. The free end of the nylon that has just been pulled out of the cat's mouth is sutured to the end of the tube and tied securely.

6. The catheter-tube combination is pulled firmly but slowly from the end of the suture located outside the abdominal wall until the pointed end of the IV catheter comes down the esophagus and out the abdominal wall.

7. The tube is grasped and pulled until the mushroom tip is adjacent to the stomach wall, as viewed by endoscopy.

8. To prevent slippage, the middle of a 3 to 4 inch piece of tubing is pierced completely through both sides and passed over the feeding tube so that it is adjacent to the body wall. This bumper or retainer is then glued or sutured securely in place. The tube is capped and bandaged in place.

An Elizabethan collar is almost always required to prevent the cat from removing the tube. To remove the tube once it has been in place for 3 weeks, the tube just below the bumper is severed to allow the "mushroom" tip to fall into the stomach. This piece should be removed by an endoscope. Some commercially available "low profile" gastrostomy tubes are designed to be removed with a stylet that is used to straighten out the tube and balloon for removal.

Needle catheter jejunostomy tubes should be considered for cats that will not tolerate nasogastric or gastrostomy tube feeding but that have a functional lower intestinal tract.[1-4] This method is especially valuable in cancer patients that have had surgery to the upper GI tract. Complications with this method are similar to those seen with gastrostomy tubes. The procedure is as follows (Figure 19-8):

1. The distal duodenum or proximal jejunum is located and isolated by surgery. A purse-string suture of 3-0 nonabsorbable suture is placed in the antimesenteric border of the isolated piece of bowel.

2. A 12 ga needle is placed from the serosa located at the center of the area encircled by the purse-string suture, subserosally 2 to 3 cm through the wall of the intestine, and into the lumen of loop of bowel. Alternatively, a stab incision can be made into the same location of the bowel using a No. 11 surgical blade.

3. A 5 Fr nasogastric infant feeding tube is passed through

the hypodermic needle or the stab incision to an area down the bowel, 20 to 30 cm from the enterostomy site.

4. If a needle was used, it is now removed.

5. The purse-string is tightened and secured around the tube.

6. The free end of the feeding tube is passed from the serosal surface of the abdominal wall out of the skin through a second hypodermic needle.

7. The loop of bowel with the enterostomy site is secured to the abdominal wall with four sutures that are later cut after the tube is removed after 3 weeks, when feeding is complete.

8. An abdominal wrap and Elizabethan collar are recommended to prevent the cat from removing the tube.

Enteral Feeding Methods

The type of nutrients to be used depends largely on the enteral tube used and the status of the patient.[1-4] Blended canned pet foods may be adequate for feeding by gastrostomy tubes, and human enteral feeding products are easily administered through nasogastric and jejunostomy tubes. In any case, feeding usually is not started until 24 hours after the tube is placed. Once feeding is started, the amount of nutrients is gradually increased over several days and is administered frequently in small amounts, which allows the cat to adapt to this method of feeding. Continuous feeding

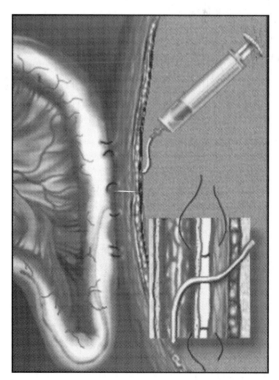

Figure 19-8: *A jejunostomy tube is surgically placed through a stab incision in the antimesenteric side of the jejunum. The other end of the tube is then placed through the abdominal wall, whereupon the jejunum is securely sutured to the abdominal wall. Jejunostomy tubes are ideal for supporting cancer patients with alterations in the upper GI tract.*

TABLE 19-2
Specifics of Diets for the Cancer Patient

Product	Caloric Content (kcal/ml)	Protein Content g/100 kcal (g/ml)	Fat Content (g/100 kcal)	Osmolarity (mOsm/kg)
Hill's Prescription Diet®				
Feline a/d®	1.30	8.06 (0.105)	5.07	N/A
Feline p/d®[a]	0.8	10.89 (0.087)	7.13	N/A
Feline k/d®[b]	0.64	5.62 (0.036)	7.88	N/A
Feline c/d®[b]	0.62	9.02 (0.56)	6.04	N/A
Jevity® (Ross Laboratories)	1.06	4.20 (0.045)	3.48	310
Osmolite® HN (Ross Laboratories)	1.06	4.44 (0.047)	3.68	310
Vital® HN (Ross Laboratories)	1.0	4.17 (0.042)	1.08	460
Clinicare® Feline (Abbot Laboratories Animal Health)	1.0	8.60 (0.086)	5.30	235

[a]Blenderize 0.5 can (225 g) + 0.75 cup (170 ml) water.
[b]Blenderize 0.5 can (225 g) + 1.25 cups (284 ml) water.

may reduce the risk of vomiting caused by overloading the GI tract. Regardless, the tube should be aspirated three to four times a day to ensure there is not excessive residual volume in the GI tract. A column of water should be kept in the tube at all times and the tube should be flushed periodically with warm water to prevent clogging.

Calculating Contents and Volumes

Calculation of the nutritional requirements for enteral feeding is essentially the same as for parenteral feeding noted earlier.[1-4] The energy requirement for the cat with cancer is calculated. It should be kept in mind that some patients have a very high energy expenditure that may exceed those seen in cats that have infections, sepsis, or burns. Other research suggests that the energy needs of most cancer patients do *not* exceed that of healthy cats. Once an IER is determined, it is essential that the patient be monitored for weight gain/loss and adjustments made to maintain optimum weight. Cats with renal or hepatic insufficiency should not be given high protein loads (>4 g/100 kcal). Because most high-quality pet foods can be put through a blender to form a gruel that can be passed through a large feeding tube, the IER of the cat is divided by the caloric density of the canned pet food to determine the amount of food to feed (Table 19-2). The same calculation can be done with human enteral feeding products; the volume fed may need to be increased if the enteral feeding product is diluted to ensure it is approximately iso-osmolar before administration.

REFERENCES

1. Ogilvie GK, Vail DM: Nutrition and cancer: Recent developments. *Vet Clin North Am Small Anim Pract* 20:1–29, 1990.
2. Ogilvie GK: Paraneoplastic syndromes, in Withrow SJ, MacEwen EG (eds): *Clinical Veterinary Oncology.* Philadelphia, JB Lippincott, 1989, pp 29–35.
3. Vail DM, Ogilvie GK, Wheeler SL: Metabolic alterations in patients with cancer cachexia. *Compend Contin Educ Pract Vet* 12:381–395, 1990.
4. Ogilvie GK: Metabolic alterations and nutritional therapy for the veterinary cancer patient. *Compend Contin Educ Pract Vet* 15:925–937, 1993.
5. Ogilvie GK, Vail DM, Wheeler SJ, et al: Effect of chemotherapy and remission on carbohydrate metabolism in dogs with lymphoma. *Cancer Res* 69:233–238, 1992.
6. Vail DM, Ogilvie GK, Fettman MJ, et al: Exacerbation of hyperlactatemia by infusion of lactated Ringer's solution in dogs with lymphoma. *J Vet Intern Med* 4:228–332, 1990.
7. Vail DM, Ogilvie GK, Wheeler SL, et al: Alterations in carbohydrate metabolism in canine lymphoma. *J Vet Intern Med* 4:8–14, 1990.
8. Ogilvie GK, Ford RD, Vail DM: Alterations in lipoprotein profiles in dogs with lymphoma. *J Vet Intern Med* 8:62–66, 1994.
9. Ogilvie GK, Walters LM, Fettman MJ, et al: Energy expenditure in dogs with lymphoma fed two specialized diets. *Cancer* 71:3146–3152, 1993.
10. Ogilvie GK, Fettman MJ, Mallinckrodt CH, et al: Effect of fish oil, arginine, and doxorubicin chemotherapy on remission and survival time for dogs with lymphoma: A double-blind, randomized placebo-controlled study. *Cancer* 88:1916–1928, 2000.
11. Ogilvie GK, Vail DM: Unique metabolic alterations associated with cancer cachexia in the dog, in Kirk RW (ed): *Current Veterinary Therapy. XI.* Philadelphia, WB Saunders, 1992, pp 433–438.
12. Daly JM, Lieberman M, Goldfine J, et al: Enteral nutrition with supplemental arginine, RNA and omega-3 fatty acids: A prospective clinical trial. Abstract, 15th Clinical Congress, American Society for Parenteral and Enteral Nutrition, *J Paren Enteral Nutr* 15:19S–27S, 1991.
13. Lowell JA, Parnes HL, Blackburn GL: Dietary immunomodulation: Beneficial effects on carcinogenesis and tumor growth. *Crit Care Med* 18:S145–S148, 1990.
14. Weisburg JH: Interactions of nutrients in oncogenesis. *Am J Clin Nutr* 53:2265:1991.
15. Quillin P: An overview of the link between nutrition and cancer, in Quillin P, Williams RM: *Adjuvant Nutrition Cancer Treatment.* Arlington Heights, IL, Cancer Treatment Foundation, 1993, pp1–17.
16. National Academy of Sciences: *Diet, Nutrition and Cancer.* National Academy Press, Washington DC, 1982.
17. Boutwell RK: An overview of the role of diet and nutrition in carcinogenesis, in *Nutrition, Growth and Cancer.* New York, Alan R. Liss, Inc, 1988.
18. Fettman MJ, Stanton CA, Banks LL, et al. Effect of neutering on body weight, metabolic rate and glucose tolerance in domestic cats. *Res Vet Sci* 62:131–136, 1997.
19. Chance WT, Balasubramainiam A, Sheriff S, Fischer JE: Possible role of neuropeptide Y in experimental cancer anorexia, in Jacobs MM (ed): *Diet and*

Cancer: Markers, Prevention and Treatment. New York, Plenum Press, 1993, pp 109–134.

20. Niles RM, Loewy BP: Induction of protein kinase C in mouse melanoma cells by retinoic acid. Cancer Res 49:4483–4492, 1989.

21. White SD, Rosychuk RA, Scott KV, et al: Use of isotretinoin and etretinate for the treatment of benign cutaneous neoplasia and cutaneous lymphoma in dogs. JAVMA 202:387–391, 1993.

22. Branda RF: Effects of folic acid deficiency on tumor cell biology, in Jacobs MM (ed): Vitamins and Minerals in the Prevention and Treatment of Cancer. Boca Raton, FL, CRC Press, 1991, pp 167–185.

23. Kline K, Sanders BG: Modulation of immune suppression and enhanced tumorigenesis in retrovirus tumor challenged chickens treated with vitamin E. In Vivo 3:161–185, 1989.

24. Kline K, Cochran GS, Sanders BG: Growth inhibitory effects of vitamin E succinate on retrovirus-transformed tumor cells in vitro. Nutr Cancer 14:27–35, 1990.

25. Shamberger RJ, Rukovena E, Longfield AK, et al: Antioxidants and cancer. I. Selenium in the blood of normals and cancer patients. J Natl Cancer Inst 50:867–887, 1973.

26. Ip C: Factors influencing the anticarcinogenic efficacy of selenium in dimethylbenzanthracene-induced mammary tumorigenesis in rats. Cancer Res 41:2638–2644, 1981.

27. Jacobs MM, Jansson B, Griffin AC: Inhibitory effects of selenium on 1,2-dimethylhydrazine and methylazoxymethanol acetate induction of colon tumors. Cancer Lett 2:133–144, 1977.

28. Jacobs MM, Griffin AC: Effects of selenium on chemical carcinogenesis: Comparative effects on antioxidants. Biol Trace El Res 1:2–21, 1979.

29. Asselin BL, Ryan D, Frantz CN, et al: In vitro and in vivo killing of acute lymphoblastic leukemia cells by L-asparaginase. Cancer Res 49:4363–4369, 1989.

30 Weed H, McGandy RB, Kennedy AR: Protection against dimethylhydrazine induced adenomatous tumors of the mouse colon by the dietary addition of an extract of soybeans containing the Bowman-Birk protease inhibitor. Carcinogenesis 6:1239–1241, 1985.

31. Messadi DV, Billings P, Shklar G, Kennedy AR: Inhibition of oral carcinogenesis by a protease inhibitor. J Natl Cancer Inst 76:447–452, 1986.

32. St. Clair W, Billings P, Carew J, et al: Suppression of DMH-induced carcinogenesis in mice by dietary addition of the Bowman-Birk protease inhibitor. Cancer Res 50:580–586, 1990.

33. Kennedy AR: Effects of protease inhibitors and vitamin E in the prevention of cancer, in Prasad KN, Meyskens FL (eds): Nutrients and Cancer Prevention. Philadelphia, The Humana Press, Inc, 1990, pp 79–98.

34. Witschi H, Kennedy AR: Modulation of lung tumor development in mice with the soybean-derived Bowman-Birk protease inhibitor. Carcinogenesis 10:2275–2277, 1989.

THERAPEUTIC & SUPPORTIVE PROCEDURES

TRANSFUSION SUPPORT

Gregory K. Ogilvie and Antony S. Moore

20

CLINICAL BRIEFING

Blood Donor Characteristics	Most recipients in the United States are Group A and should receive A blood; Group B blood should be given only to recipients known to have that blood type. Group AB blood is rare.
Indications	Clinically significant acute blood loss, hemolytic anemia, nonregenerative anemia, thrombocytopenia, DIC, and hypoproteinemia.
Complications	Hemolysis, hyperthermia, tachycardia, tachypnea, vomiting, collapse, urticaria, angioneurotic edema, and/or CNS alterations may be seen if incompatible blood is given; transfusion should be discontinued.

Cats frequently need transfusions for a variety of problems, including blood loss from the primary tumor, disseminated intravascular coagulation (DIC), clinical syndromes associated with the hypocoagulable state of malignancy, and other hematologic abnormalities.[1-3] In general, transfusions or specific blood components should be given only when specifically indicated.

SEROLOGY[2] (Table 20-1)

Anemia is the most common indication for blood transfusion in cats, and fresh whole blood is typically administered. Recent experimental studies and clinical reports have elucidated the importance of feline blood types in transfusion medicine. Only the AB blood group system is recognized in cats; it consists of three blood types: type A (the most common, especially in the United States), type B (frequently found in certain breeds and in Australia), and type AB (rare). Blood type frequently varies geographically among DSH cats and breeds. Because of the presence of naturally occurring alloantibodies, only AB-matched transfusions are effective and safe. Blood-typing is now readily available, and incompatibilities are easily recognized via blood crossmatching tests. Owing to the general presence of strong anti-A alloantibodies in type B cats, life-threatening acute hemolytic transfusion reactions occur if type A blood is given to a type B cat. Immediately stopping the transfusion and providing supportive care may be lifesaving. Other transfusion reactions, unrelated to AB mismatch, cause only mild and transient signs.

COMPONENT THERAPY

The availability of blood component therapy for cats is extraordinarily limited; with the equipment currently available,

TABLE 20-1
Feline Transfusions[2]

Blood Groups		RBC	Clinical
Recipient	*Donor*	*Half-Life*	*Results*
A	A	32.8 ± 3.1 days	Compatible; no problems
B	B	34.4 ± 2.8 days	Compatible; no problems
A	B	2.1 ± 0.2 days	Not compatible; mild problems
B	A	1.3 ± 2.3 hours	Not compatible; severe problems

the amount of blood required to get adequate amounts of blood components makes this therapy impractical. If blood components are available, they should be administered only to cats that are at risk for showing clinical signs referable to a decrease in the depleted blood component. Whole blood or packed red blood cells (RBCs) may be administered immediately or stored for up to 21 days. Clotting factors in fresh frozen plasma remain adequate for up to 1 year; clotting factors V, VII, and VIII may be diminished in frozen plasma stored for longer than 1 year. In cats, a unit typically is defined as 60 ml, which is the maximum amount that can be safely collected from an average adult cat.

INDICATIONS FOR TRANSFUSION THERAPY[1-3]

Hemorrhage

Although there is a theoretical advantage to transfusing fresh whole blood, packed RBCs can be administered with excellent results. Feline RBCs stored for more than 2 weeks can have a depletion in 2,3 DPG (diphosphoglycerate), which may decrease their oxygen-carrying capacity. In cats with chronic blood loss, transfusions are indicated to keep hematocrit levels above 10%. Regardless of whether blood loss is chronic or acute, patient response to transfusion is just as important a determinant as the hematocrit level or amount to be transfused. Cats with acute blood loss are less tolerant of low hematocrit values, whereas those that have a gradual reduction in RBC count are able to adapt to extremely low RBC numbers.

Oxyglobin®, a commercially available hemoglobin substitute with significant oxygen-carrying capacity, can be used when whole blood or packed RBCs are not available. It has not been completely evaluated in clinical trials involving large numbers of cats with clinical disorders requiring a transfusion, and thus caution is advised when using this product.

Hemolytic Anemia

Immune-mediated hemolytic anemia may require the administration of RBCs, even if this results in lysis of some of the transfused blood. Primary therapy with glucocorticoids, azathioprine, and cyclosporine is often essential to treat the underlying disease. The blood group of cats with hemolytic anemia often cannot be determined adequately because of the presence of antibodies. Frequent evaluation of packed cell volume is essential. While not yet clinically tested, Oxyglobin® may be of value in cats with hemolytic anemia.

Nonregenerative Anemia

Nonregenerative anemia can be relatively mild, and affected patients often do not require transfusion. In some cases, however, nonregenerative anemia can be severe enough to require either whole blood (when platelets are needed) or packed RBCs. Recombinant human erythropoietin may be of value; with prolonged use, however, antibodies directed against human erythropoietin may cross-react with the cat's own erythropoietin.

Thrombocytopenia

Platelet counts above 30,000 to 40,000/µl are rarely associated with bleeding disorders. A very gradual reduction in platelet count can result in cats that appear healthy but have only 2,000 to 3,000 platelets/µl, especially when the platelets are relatively "young," as is seen in patients with immune-mediated thrombocytopenia. Recently released platelets have much greater function than older ones. Platelet transfusion is recommended only for cats that exhibit clinical signs. Platelet-rich plasma may be considered in these patients, although the circulating half-life of platelets may be only minutes, especially when immune-mediated conditions exist. The availability of platelet-rich plasma and platelets is quite limited. Vincristine (0.5 mg/m² IV

as a single dose or every 1–3 weeks) can be administered to induce premature release of platelets from the bone marrow. The platelet count usually increases 3 to 5 days after vincristine administration. This is especially valuable in immune-mediated thrombocytopenia, because vincristine not only directly increases platelet numbers but is also taken up by platelets, where it is cytotoxic to phagocytic cells.

Disseminated Intravascular Coagulation

DIC can result in severe bleeding and consumption of clotting factors and platelets. Fresh frozen plasma, if available, could be given at approximately 0.25 U/5 kg and repeated as needed to maintain prothrombin and partial thromboplastin time at 1 to 1.5 times the normal bleeding time. Heparin use is controversial; if given in conjunction with plasma, however, it may be of benefit. For patients in which all cell lines (RBCs and platelets) are decreased, fresh whole blood can be used (see the Oncologic Emergencies section).

Hypoproteinemia

Plasma transfusions can be valuable in patients that have decreased albumin levels. Increases in plasma proteins after protein administration can be slower than expected because only 40% of body albumin is in the intravascular space whereas 60% resides within the interstitial space. Thus administration of fresh frozen plasma must not only increase albumin within the circulating space but also within interstitial spaces, which may require repeated plasma administration. Obviously, the administration of fresh frozen plasma from various donors can result in the development of antibodies. Although their circulating half-life can be quite short, colloidal solutions, such as dextrans or hetastarch, may be more useful in these patients. Approximately the equivalent of 1 unit of plasma is needed to raise the albumin of a 5 kg cat from 1.8 g/dl to 3 g/dl. While this is theoretically possible, the lack of availability of plasma makes this uncommon.

KEY POINT

Because most feline recipients in the United States have Group A blood, this blood type is the safest to use for transfusions. Group B blood should be given only to recipients known to have that blood type.

BLOOD COLLECTION

The two most common anticoagulants used in collecting blood for transfusion are CPDA-1 (citrate phosphate dextrose adenine) and ACD (acid citrate dextrose). CPDA-1 results in the longest shelf life (approximately 1 month). ACD allows blood to be stored for up to 21 days if the blood is collected in a closed system or 24 hours if collected by syringe. Approximately 1 ml of anticoagulant is used

THERAPEUTIC & SUPPORTIVE PROCEDURES

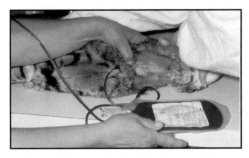

Figure 20-1: Fresh whole blood is collected in a 60 ml syringe containing 7 ml ACD. Long-term storage can be achieved with the use of a standard 450 ml CPDA-1 collection bag by first rolling out all anticoagulant from the collection bag into the satellite bag. The line between the two is clamped, leaving only CPDA-1 in the collection line.

per 7 ml of blood collected from a cat. Note that the accidental IV injection of undiluted citrate anticoagulants may cause cardiac arrest.

The donor cat should be evaluated for general health and to ensure the absence of any diseases. An IV catheter is placed, and fluid therapy and 20 mg ketamine (for sedation) are given IV with or without atropine (Figure 20-1). The jugular is clipped and aseptically prepared. Blood is collected in a 60 ml syringe containing 7 ml ACD. The maximum quantity that can be collected from one cat is 60 ml. This method is used only if fresh whole blood is to be administered within 24 hours.

More long-term storage can be achieved with the use of a standard 450 ml CPDA-1 collection bag. All of the anticoagulant is rolled out of the collection bag into the satellite bag and the line between the two is clamped, leaving only CPDA-1 in the collection line. The volume in the line (8 ml) is enough for 60 ml of feline blood. It is vital that a digital scale be used to weigh collected blood and that collection is stopped at 92 g (60 ml [60 g] blood + 8 ml [8 g] CPDA-1 + collection bag [24 g]).

TRANSFUSION GUIDELINES

Cats with significant acute blood loss should first be treated for shock with crystalloid solutions. Hypertonic saline is useful in select patients. Packed RBCs can be given with crystalloid fluids, or whole blood may be used.

General Rule: Amount (ml) to Transfuse

$$[(2.2 \times wt_{kg}) \times 30] \times \frac{(PCV_{desired} - PCV_{recipient})/}{PCV_{donor}}$$

Note: 2.2 ml of whole blood/kg or 1 ml/kg of packed RBCs raises PCV 1% (transfused whole blood has a PCV of 40%).

General Rule: Maximum Rate of Transfusion

40 ml/30 min with close patient monitoring

COMPLICATIONS[1-3]

Hemolysis, although relatively rare, is probably the most serious adverse effect of transfusion. Signs of an acute hemolytic reaction include elevated temperature, increased heart and respiration rates, and tremors followed by vomiting and collapse. If this occurs, the transfusion should be stopped and the cat's plasma checked for hemoglobinemia. Crystalloid fluids should be initiated and urine output monitored to ensure that it is adequate. Delayed hemolysis may occur in some patients. Fever that develops during transfusion can indicate bacterial contamination of the blood or be associated with leukocyte antigens that elevate endogenous pyrogens. Allergic reactions may manifest as urticaria and angioneurotic edema; if these occur, the transfusion should be discontinued and glucocorticoids administered. Because volume overload can occur when large volumes of blood are administered, the cat's circulating volume should be monitored (e.g., central venous pressure, body weight) and treated appropriately (e.g., fluid restrictions, furosemide). Heparin toxicity is a possible complication of heparinized whole blood transfusion and can cause bleeding. Rarely, blood ammonia levels can rise and cause associated clinical signs, such as mental dullness or seizures, particularly in cats with compromised liver function. This is usually associated with transfusions of packed RBCs that have stored for a prolonged period; treatment is the same as for hepatoencephalopathy.

OXYGEN-CARRYING COLLOID

The only commercially available oxygen-carrying colloid without cellular components is polymerized bovine hemoglobin glutamer-200 (Oxyglobin®). This product is used off-label in cats. Because of the product's vascular expansion properties and lack of cellular components, patient PCV actually decreases during its use. The hemoglobin level and the oxygen-carrying capacity of the blood increase. The product should not be administered at rates faster than 10 ml/kg/hr. Hemoglobinuria is a common observation in treated cats, and these patients develop a jaundice-like color in their sclera and skin due to the by-products present in the product. This makes assessing for icterus more difficult and can be alarming to the caregiver if they are not appropriately educated about this side effect. Indications include acute blood loss, immune-mediated hemolytic anemia, and acetaminophen toxicity.

REFERENCES

1. Stone MS, Cotter SM: Practical guidelines for transfusion therapy, in Kirk RW, Bonagura JD (eds): *Current Veterinary Therapy XI.* Philadelphia, WB Saunders, 1992, pp 479–485.
2. Giger U: The feline AB blood group system and incompatibility reactions, in Kirk RW, Bonagura JD (eds): *Current Veterinary Therapy XI.* Philadelphia, WB Saunders, 1992, pp 470–474.
3. Smith MR: Disorders of hemostasis in transfusion therapy, in Skeel RT (ed): *Handbook of Cancer Chemotherapy,* ed 3. Boston, Little, Brown & Co, 1991, pp 449–458.

HEMATOPOIETIC GROWTH FACTOR SUPPORT

21

Gregory K. Ogilvie and Antony S. Moore

C L I N I C A L   B R I E F I N G

Recombinant Erythropoietin

Indications	Anemia caused by inadequate RBC production despite normal bone marrow; anemia caused by chronic renal failure, chronic malignant disease, chemotherapy, or radiation therapy; especially effective for patients with low endogenous erythropoietin production.
Complications	Erythrocytosis (rare); antibodies can develop to human recombinant erythropoietin, rendering this therapy ineffective.

Recombinant Granulocyte Colony-Stimulating Factor (G-CSF)

Indications	Neutropenia; response is directly proportional to the number of granulocyte precursors present and inversely proportional to the amount of endogenous G-CSF production. Canine recombinant G-CSF is effective for long-term therapy in cats; human recombinant G-CSF may also be helpful in cats receiving chemotherapy.
Contraindications	Neutrophilia can occur but is rarely a clinical problem; antibodies can develop to human recombinant G-CSF, rendering this therapy ineffective.

Recombinant Granulocyte-Macrophage Colony-Stimulating Factor (GM-CSF)

Indications	Same as for G-CSF; response is directly proportional to the number of granulocyte precursors present and inversely proportional to the amount of endogenous GM-CSF production. Canine recombinant GM-CSF is effective for long-term therapy in cats.
Contraindications	Neutrophilia and monocytosis can occur but are rarely clinical problems; antibodies can develop to human recombinant GM-CSF, rendering this therapy ineffective.

Hematopoietic growth factors have the potential for long-term improvement of cat health.[1,2] The most clinically useful growth factors are erythropoietin and granulocyte colony-stimulating factor (G-CSF). Less is known about granulocyte-macrophage colony-stimulating factor (GM-CSF).

ERYTHROPOIETIN

Human recombinant erythropoietin has been used experimentally in cats with chronic renal failure and has produced some beneficial results.[3] Recombinant erythropoietin has been demonstrated to improve quality of life in human cancer patients who have anemia of chronic disease caused by malignancies, chemotherapy, and/or radiation therapy. Similar results have been seen in cats with cancer. Treated cats seem to have improved attitude and quality of life as well as increased numbers of circulating red blood cells (RBCs). Potential secondary effects of human recombinant erythropoietin include systemic hypertension, iron deficiency, hyperkalemia, polycythemia, and the development of antibodies to the recombinant protein in approximately 30% of patients weeks to months after treatment is initiated.

Human recombinant erythropoietin can be administered to cats at a dosage of 75 to 100 U/kg/day SQ for 5 to 7 days; the same dose is then given two to three times a week until the hematocrit approaches the desired level. Erythropoietin can be administered weekly thereafter. Hematocrit levels should be monitored; if antibodies develop and result in a rapid decrease in the number of RBCs, erythropoietin therapy should be discontinued. Results of a study using cats with chronic renal failure showed administration of recombinant erythropoietin increased RBC and reticulocyte counts, hemoglobin concentration, and hematocrit comparably in dogs and cats. Aspects of clinical well-being (e.g., appetite, energy, weight gain, alertness, strength, playfulness) improved variably. Adverse effects, including anemia, anti-erythropoietin antibody production, seizures, systemic hypertension, and iron deficiency, were demonstrated inconsistently in dogs and cats.[4]

GRANULOCYTE COLONY-STIMULATING FACTOR

Recombinant human and canine granulocyte colony-stimulating factors (rhG-CSF and rcG-CSF, respectively) have been produced in large quantities through recombinant technology using *Escherichia coli* bacteria. Most work done with G-CSF has shown that the cytokine is lineage-specific, acting primarily on committed granulocytic precursors to increase neutrophil phagocytosis, superoxide generation, and antibody-dependent cellular cytotoxicity.[1-5]

> ### KEY POINT
>
> *Long-term use of recombinant human hematopoietic growth factors may result in formation of antibodies that can cross-react with the patient's own factors ("auto-antibodies"), although this may not be true in cats receiving chemotherapy.*

We have found that rhG-CSF induces a short-term increase in the number of neutrophils in normal cats.[6] After approximately 14 days, the number of neutrophils and their precursors decreases significantly, presumably because rhG-CSF is sufficiently different from the cat's native G-CSF to induce antibody formation. rcG-CSF increases neutrophils in normal cats to approximately 30,000/µl within 24 hours after initiation of therapy (Figure 21-1).[7] The neutrophil count continues to rise, reaching approximately 67,000/µl on day 14 and then remains within 67,000 to 88,000/µl for 42 days. Once rcG-CSF administration is discontinued, neutrophil counts return to pretreatment lev-

els within 5 days. Occasional irritation at the injection site was the only toxicity noted. Apparently, rcG-CSF is sufficiently homologous to feline G-CSF that antibody formation does not result.[7]

One of the most promising areas of clinical application of G-CSF is in the prevention and treatment of chemotherapy- and radiation-induced cytopenias. Antibodies against rhG-CSF and endogenous G-CSF may not develop in cats that receive chemotherapy. Consequently, rhG-CSF might be useful for ameliorating chemotherapy-induced myelosuppression in small animals, thus permitting more aggressive chemotherapy protocols. Until further studies are completed, veterinarians should avoid administering rhG-CSF within 24 hours before or after chemotherapy. Giving the agent when neutrophil counts are below 1,000 cells/µl is sufficient to decrease the severity of myelosuppression. Short courses (three to six doses) may be sufficient to treat patients with severe myelosuppression. Long-term administration of rhG-CSF to normal cats might lead to the formation of antibodies to endogenous G-CSF.

GRANULOCYTE-MACROPHAGE COLONY-STIMULATING FACTOR

GM-CSF is a glycoprotein produced by a number of different tissues in the body, including T lymphocytes, monocytes, endothelial cells, and fibroblasts. As its name implies, GM-CSF stimulates the production of granulocytes and macrophages and acts in concert with erythropoietin and interleukin-3 (IL-3) to stimulate erythroid precursors. This cytokine also acts with IL-3 to regulate thrombopoiesis. This stimulator of multilineage and committed progenitors also increases the function of mature granulocytes, monocytes, macrophages, and eosinophils. More specifically, the cell-killing activity of neutrophils is enhanced by inhibiting migration of these cells, thereby increasing chemotaxis, adhesion, phagocytosis, and superoxide generation; therefore GM-CSF increases tumoricidal cytotoxicity.

The use of GM-CSF in clinical medicine has the potential to be at least as profound and widespread as that of G-CSF. Recently, canine GM-CSF was shown to effectively increase granulocyte counts in dogs. We have used recombinant human GM-CSF in cats with chemotherapy-induced myelosuppression with variable results. One reason that GM-CSF may not have as profound an effect as G-CSF in cats is because of variable sequence homology between the recombinant products and the native GM-CSF of cats. This has been shown in various species; for example, there is only a 57% sequence homology between human and murine GM-CSF and up to 75% homology between human and murine G-CSF.

Like G-CSF, GM-CSF has been shown to decrease the

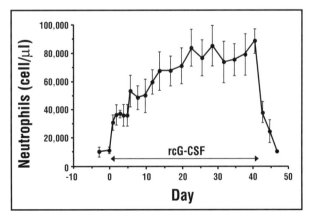

Figure 21-1: *Mean neutrophil counts (± standard deviation) of five normal cats treated with rcG-CSF. Administration of rcG-CSF began on day 0 and ended on day 42 (arrow). Neutrophil counts returned to pretreatment values within 5 days of discontinuing rcG-CSF. (From Obradovich JA, Ogilvie GK, Stadler-Morris S, et al: Effect of recombinant canine granulocyte colony-stimulating factor on peripheral blood neutrophil counts in normal cats. J Vet Intern Med 7:65–69, 1993; with permission.)*

duration and severity of chemotherapy- and radiation-induced neutropenia in humans and laboratory animals. Because GM-CSF affects several cell lines, a variety of disease states can be treated with this growth factor. Diseases linked with leukopenia-associated AIDS, bone marrow failure states (such as myelodysplasia), aplastic anemia, and chronic and acute bacterial infections have been shown to be substantially improved by GM-CSF therapy. GM-CSF may be superior to G-CSF for rapid recovery from bone marrow transplantation. GM-CSF can stimulate some leukemic cells and therefore may be of value in forcing cells into the cell cycle, thus making them more susceptible to cell cycle-specific drugs. Some hypothesize that GM-CSF, like G-CSF, may force leukemic cells to differentiate and die.

REFERENCES

1. Elmslie RE, Dow SW, Ogilvie GK: Interleukins: Biological properties and therapeutic potential. *J Vet Intern Med* 5:283–293, 1991.

2. Obradovich JE, Ogilvie GK: Evaluation of recombinant canine granulocyte colony-stimulating factor as an inducer of granulopoiesis. *J Vet Intern Med* 5:75–79, 1991.

3. Cowgill LD: Clinical experience and use of recombinant human erythropoietin in uremic dogs and cats. *Proc 9th ACVIM Forum*:147–149, 1991.

4. Cowgill LD, James KM, Levy JK, et al: Use of recombinant human erythropoietin for management of anemia in dogs and cats with renal failure. *JAVMA* 212:521–528, 1998.

5. Henry CJ, Buss MS, Lothrop CD Jr: Veterinary uses of recombinant human granulocyte colony-stimulating factor. Part I. Oncology. *Compend Contin Educ Pract Vet* 20:728–735, 1998.

6. Fulton R, Gasper PW, Ogilvie GK, et al: Effect of recombinant human granulocyte colony-stimulating factor on hematopoiesis in normal cats. *Exp Hematol* 19:759–767, 1991.

7. Obradovich JE, Ogilvie GK, Stadler-Morris S, et al: Evaluation of canine recombinant granulocyte colony-stimulating factor in the cat. *J Vet Intern Med* 7:65–69, 1993.

THERAPEUTIC & SUPPORTIVE PROCEDURES

OVERVIEW OF ONCOLOGIC EMERGENCIES

22

Gregory K. Ogilvie and Antony S. Moore

CLINICAL BRIEFING

Types of Emergencies	True life-threatening emergencies.
	Medical problems that are perceived as being life-threatening by well-meaning, concerned clients.
	Emergencies of convenience (i.e., the caregiver wants the cat to be evaluated immediately despite non-life-threatening problems).
Initial Approach	Identify the primary complaint.
	Evaluate vital signs, including airway and breathing ability; heart rate, rhythm, and character; body temperature; and mucous membrane color and capillary refill time.
	Perform a complete physical examination.
	Obtain a complete history, including prior cancer treatment.

Cancer is a word feared throughout the world, regardless of the species affected. A diagnosis of cancer sets in motion feelings of fear and urgency that spur clients to demand rapid response to their concerns by the veterinary health care team. This heightened level of emotion is first witnessed during the initial diagnosis of cancer and decision-making process but is often most apparent in emergency situations. In addition, cats hide their clinical signs until quite late in the disease process and thus are often in a debilitated state by the time cancer therapy begins; therefore speed and decisiveness are key ingredients of successful emergency care.

It is essential that feline oncologic emergencies be handled with extreme medical care but also with understanding. When an emergency or urgent situation is noted, the entire veterinary health care team should be equipped and prepared to provide timely, compassionate care to meet the medical and nonmedical needs of patients and caregivers alike. In some cases, this may mean referring the case to another facility.

There are three types of emergencies[1]:

- True life-threatening emergencies
- Medical problems that are perceived as being life-threatening by well-meaning, concerned clients
- Emergencies of convenience, in which the client wants the cat to be evaluated immediately despite the non-life-threatening nature of the problem in order to accommodate personal needs or schedules

Regardless of the type of emergency, the following steps should be taken[1]:

- Determine the primary complaint
- Evaluate vital signs, including but not limited to:
  —Airway and breathing ability
  —Heart rate, rhythm, and character
  —Body temperature
  —Mucous membrane color and capillary refill time
- Perform a complete physical examination
- Obtain a complete history, including prior cancer treatment

When a cat is presented in an emergency situation, blood and urine samples should be collected and an intravenous catheter placed as soon as possible. Blood and urine can be submitted at any time to determine pretreatment parameters based on a complete blood count, biochemical profile, activated clotting time, and urinalysis. Essential information that is rapidly obtainable and vital for initial decision-making—and that should be obtained on admission—includes urine specific gravity, packed cell volume, white blood cell count, and blood glucose.

As soon as a diagnostic and therapeutic plan is initiated, clients should be made aware of every aspect of the case. Measured, realistic information should be provided as soon as assessments are made and the information is available. It is also important to provide a cost estimate for initial care as well as updates for ongoing supportive care. The team approach to care is vital during emergencies. The client is an integral member of the team and, once empowered with information, is placed in a decision-making role that allows for optimal medical care of the patient while meeting the emotional needs of the caregiver and family. Ongoing communication allows for an open dialogue among team members regarding financial limitations, philosophy for continuing critical care in the face of diminishing hope, and advanced strategies for crisis situations, such as cardiac or respiratory arrest.

Oncologic emergencies, while rare, are potential risks associated with cancer and cancer therapy. Planning for these uncommon and unwanted problems is essential for a positive outcome. It is important to recognize that the true "first step" in handling oncologic emergencies is actually prevention. This step occurs prior to the initiation of treatment and encompasses time spent educating the caregiver about the nature of the disease, the effects of each medication to be administered, and the early and often subtle signs that should be dealt with to prevent a true emergency from ever happening. Similarly, instruc-

tions about what clients can do at home to support their cats are quite helpful. Always remember, the client is perhaps the most important member of the veterinary health care team.

The next step includes educating and empowering the entire team to take an active role in supporting the patient and the client. The words *cancer* and *cancer therapy* often frighten veterinary health care team members as much as they do the clients. There are emergency situations that are likely to be encountered. Developing a treatment strategy or "cookbook" approach to these situations empowers the staff to intervene quickly and efficiently on behalf of the patient. In addition, providing the health care team with information that authorizes them to respond to the emotional component of the emergency on the part of the caregiver is also essential. All members of the team must recognize that it is this emotional component that magnifies the seriousness of almost any health problem.

REFERENCE

1. Wingfield WE: *Veterinary Emergency Medicine Secrets*. Philadelphia, Hanley and Belfus, 2001, pp 1–3.

NEUTROPENIA, SEPSIS, AND THROMBOCYTOPENIA

23

Gregory K. Ogilvie and Antony S. Moore

Emergencies are always frightening to clients/caregivers, but when the emergency is related to cancer or cancer treatment, the intensity of this fear is magnified by the emotional impact imparted by the cancer itself. Therefore the health care team must act swiftly both to provide medical care for the patient and to meet the emotional and nonmedical needs of the client. Sepsis due to chemotherapy and cancer-related neutropenia are two of the more common emergencies handled in feline cancer medicine; bleeding due to thrombocytopenia is much less common. These conditions are usually preventable by judicious monitoring and appropriate supportive care during cancer therapy. In addition, caregivers should be educated about the early clinical signs of sepsis, neutropenia, and thrombocytopenia induced by cancer treatment so that they can seek immediate treatment when these signs occur.

NEUTROPENIA AND SEPSIS

CLINICAL BRIEFING

Diagnosis

History	Anorexia, general malaise, acute decompensation, and collapse, usually occurring 5 to 7 days after receiving myelosuppressive chemotherapy.
Clinical Signs	Depression, poor responsiveness, pyrexia, brick-red mucous membranes, tachycardia, and rapid capillary refill time (hyperdynamic shock), or Pale mucous membranes, evidence of decreased cardiac output (hypodynamic shock), and collapse.
Diagnostics	MDB, including absolute neutrophil count; cultures of blood, urine, stool, pulmonary airways, and/or other tissues as indicated; blood gas analysis; and other diagnostics based on clinical signs.

Therapy

Treat the underlying cause and support the client's nonmedical needs.

Restore tissue perfusion with fluids and stabilize cardiovascular system.

Correct acid-base and electrolyte imbalances and hypoglycemia.

Initiate parenteral bactericidal antibiotic therapy.

Consider hematopoietic growth factor support and/or transfusions of fresh whole blood.

Withhold additional chemotherapy until patient is stabilized; consider reducing the dose the next time the same drug is used.

Sepsis is a common cause of death in human cancer patients, exceeding all other causes combined.[1-7] As the popularity of cats increases and the use of chemotherapy and radiation soars in private practice, this situation is likely to be repeated in feline cancer medicine. Because cats tend to hide their symptoms until late in the disease process, sepsis may be quite advanced when first recognized and thus requires prompt intervention by the health care team.

Neutropenia secondary to malignancy or myelodysplasia or resulting from the myelosuppressive effects of chemotherapy or radiation therapy is a common predisposing factor for the development of sepsis in cats. Septic shock is the state of circulatory collapse that occurs secondary to overwhelming sepsis and/or endotoxemia; this syndrome is frequently fatal (mortality rate, 40% to 90%). The profound systemic effects of septic shock include:

- Vasoconstriction leading to multiple organ failure
- Cardiac dysfunction, in part from lactic acidosis
- Increased vascular permeability, leading to hyperviscos-

ity and hypovolemia
- Liver dysfunction from splanchnic vascular pooling and tissue ischemia
- Acute renal failure
- Worsening neutropenia and thrombocytopenia
- Coagulopathies
- Severe gastrointestinal damage
- Decreased insulin release
- Initial hyperglycemia followed by hypoglycemia

MDB = minimum database; includes CBC, biochemical profile, urinalysis, FeLV/FIV serology, T_4 testing, and thoracic radiographs (three views).

The bacteria that most commonly cause morbidity and mortality in feline cancer patients arise from the patient's own flora.[8] The most important things a clinician can do for the septic feline cancer patient are to quickly identify the source and type of bacterial infection, initiate therapy with broad-spectrum antibiotics, and provide appropriate and aggressive supportive care. Minimizing the chance for exposure to, or the opportunity for development of, resistant strains of bacteria enhances the chance for rapid recovery in response to appropriate antibiotic therapy. Predisposing factors should be avoided or minimized wherever possible.

PREDISPOSING FACTORS[11–14]

- Defects in cellular immunity can cause sepsis in cats with cancer. Cellular immune dysfunction, while extraordinarily difficult to diagnose in cats, may be due to an underlying cause or the result of administration of antineoplastic agents and/or corticosteroids. These defects may lead to various bacterial, mycobacterial, fungal, and viral infections. Humoral immune dysfunction is also associated with an increased prevalence of sepsis in human cancer patients and may cause similar problems in animals. Agammaglobulinemic or hypogammaglobulinemic cats are suspected to be susceptible to infections. Multiple myeloma and chronic lymphocytic leukemia are common neoplasms associated with humoral immune dysfunction in humans and are likely causes in cats as well.
- Neutropenia may be caused by the myelosuppressive effects of chemotherapy, which can be categorized as high, moderate, or mild (Table 23-1). The nadir (lowest part of the white blood cell [WBC] count) varies by drug (Table 23-2).
- Splenectomized cats are susceptible to overwhelming sepsis when they are infected with a strain of encapsulated bacteria against which they have not made antibodies.
- Indwelling vascular or urinary catheters and chest and endotracheal tubes have been associated with an increased prevalence of sepsis. The longer a catheter is present, the higher the probability for infection, especially in neutropenic cats (Figure 23-1).

TABLE 23-1
Myelosuppressive Effects of Chemotherapeutic Agents Used in Feline Medicine

Highly Myelosuppressive	Moderately Myelosuppressive	Mildly Myelosuppressive
Cyclophosphamide	Methotrexate	Bleomycin
Actinomycin D	Melphalan	Corticosteroids
Doxorubicin	Chlorambucil	L-Asparaginase
Vinblastine		Vincristine

TABLE 23-2
Myelosuppressive Drugs Associated with the Development of Pyrexia and Sepsis at Various Times after Treatment

Early Myelosuppression (<7 Days)	Mid-Range Myelosuppression (7–10 Days)	Delayed Myelosuppression (3–4 Weeks)
Paclitaxel	Cyclophosphamide	Carmustine (BCNU)
	Doxorubicin	Lomustine (CCNU)
	Mitoxantrone	Mitomycin C

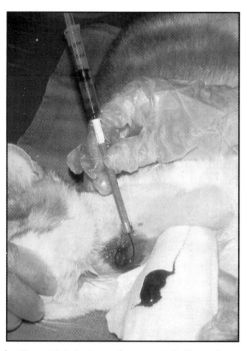

Figure 23-1: *Sepsis secondary to any indwelling catheter, especially one that has been in place for several days, is a serious problem in neutropenic cats. Jugular catheters can be left in place for several days, although the probability of infection is directly related to the number of days the catheter has been in place.*

- Frequent acquisition of blood samples greatly increases the risk of sepsis in cats with cancer.
- Antibiotic administration may lead to increased susceptibility to increasingly resistant strains of organisms.
- Prolonged hospitalization can result in serious consequences, in part because the patient is continually exposed to bacterial strains that are resistant to the antibiotics most commonly used in that facility.
- Malnutrition is a serious cause of debilitation and decreased resistance to bacterial infection, especially in cats with neutropenia.
- Cats with neurologic dysfunction and nonambulatory patients (regardless of cause) are at increased risk for sepsis.

Whenever possible, these risk factors must be avoided or minimized and associated problems recognized and corrected early to reduce the probability of sepsis. The first approach for clinicians and clients is to understand the myelosuppressive effects of various drugs. Clients and the veterinary health care team should be encouraged to be more vigilant for the clinical signs associated with neutropenia and thrombocytopenia around the time of the nadir for the drug being used. By monitoring complete blood counts (CBCs) at the appropriate times, especially early in the course of chemotherapy, veterinarians have a better idea of how low the WBC count is actually dropping. If the count appears too low (<1,000/µl) or the patient becomes even mildly symptomatic, subsequent dose reduction of that drug should be considered.

Additional steps can be taken to minimize the risk of sepsis in cats with cancer. One logical step is to minimize the administration of immunosuppressive drugs, especially corticosteroids. Splenectomized cats being treated for cancer should be watched carefully for complications, including sepsis. The risk of catheter-induced sepsis can be minimized by using aseptic technique and by placing a new catheter in a new site every 2 to 3 days. Strict aseptic procedures should be used, especially with myelosuppressed cats and those with neurologic dysfunction; the latter have a much higher risk for developing sepsis. The use of semipermanent indwelling catheters in patients with cancer may be safe if strict aseptic procedures are followed by caregivers and health care professionals. The duration of hospitalization should be limited as much as possible to limit exposure to resistant bacteria.

DIAGNOSIS

Cats presented with septic shock secondary to neutropenia require immediate intervention and careful client support.[13] Diagnostic and therapeutic interventions must begin concurrently for the patient's benefit. The differential list for neutropenia is quite extensive (Figure 23-2).

The diagnosis of septic shock begins with the physical examination and continues while a catheter is placed and blood samples are acquired. Mucous membrane color can be difficult to ascertain in cats, although brick-red mucous membranes may be noted in some cats with septic shock. The following signs may be identified in cats in the hyperdynamic state of septic shock[1–6]:

- Tachycardia
- Short capillary refill time
- Gastrointestinal signs
- Altered mentation
- Decreased blood pressure

KEY POINT

The incidence of sepsis significantly increases when the neutrophil count drops below 1,000/µl.

End-stage signs reflect a hypodynamic state and include[1–6]:

- Hypothermia
- Mucous membrane pallor
- Marked mental depression
- Bloody diarrhea
- Signs of multiple organ failure

ONCOLOGIC EMERGENCIES

Neutropenia

Mature Neutropenia[a]

1. Marrow hypoplasia[b]
   a. Chemical intoxication
   b. Idiosyncratic drug reactions
   c. Cancer chemotherapy
   d. Viral diseases (FeLV, panleukopenia)

2. Myelophthisis
   a. Myeloproliferative disorders
   b. Lymphoproliferative disorders

3. Increased margination
   a. Endotoxemia
   b. Shock

4. Increased removal
   a. Immune mediated
   b. Hypersplenism

Predominantly Immature Neutrophils

1. Acute overwhelming bacterial infection

2. Viral diseases (FeLV, FIV, panleukopenia)

[a]Bone marrow examination is recommended.
[b]Marrow hypoplasia frequently involves more than one cell line.

Figure 23-2: Differential list for neutropenia in the feline cancer patient.[14]

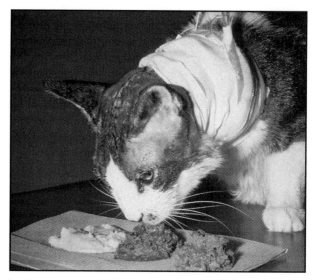

Figure 23-3: Infection from indwelling catheters is not uncommon and is an important risk factor for inducing sepsis. Handling indwelling catheters with aseptic technique is very important. If an infection at the catheter site is suspected, culturing the site and the catheter tip for aerobic and anaerobic bacteria is indicated.

Thrombocytopenia and neutropenia are often identified during the course of septic shock. Hyperglycemia is an early finding and is often followed by hypoglycemia. Metabolic acidosis is common.

KEY POINT

When laboratory and clinical data from a neutropenic cat are evaluated, clinicians must remember that many results may be surprisingly normal despite the presence of overt sepsis.

Blood and urine collected at the time of initial presentation can be very helpful for supporting a diagnosis of septic shock. At a minimum, samples should be obtained for a CBC, biochemical profile, and urinalysis. Other tests may also be indicated.

The absence of circulating neutrophils affects many of the commonly used clinical, laboratory, and radiographic findings that may normally suggest a localized or systemic infection. For example, urinalysis results may not demonstrate pyuria in cats with neutropenia despite the presence of an urinary tract infection. Likewise, without a neutrophilic infiltrate, the presence of which would otherwise

be responsible for many of the radiographic changes associated with pneumonia, thoracic radiographs often appear "normal" even in the presence of significant pneumonia.

Urine and blood cultures should always be obtained, even though they may be negative and results may not be available for a significant amount of time. Appropriate broad-spectrum antibiotics and combinations must be available for immediate parenteral administration. Culture results will guide follow-up oral antibiotic selection.

All suspicious sites should be cultured, including but not necessarily limited to:

- Blood: Two (preferably four) sets of blood cultures (aerobic and anaerobic) should be acquired. However, clinicians must be aware of the total volume of blood collected, including blood for hemograms, biochemical profiles, and other tests, because these cats almost always have some degree of anemia associated with chronic disease. The interval at which samples should be collected is controversial, although sampling every 20 to 30 minutes before antibiotic therapy is initiated may be adequate. At least 2 ml of blood should be injected into appropriate culture containers.
- Catheter: If central venous catheters are present, cultures of the port should be obtained. Ideally, culture bottles containing an antibiotic-binding resin or other antibiotic-binding substance should be used for patients receiving IV antibiotics (Figure 23-3).
- Urine: A urine specimen collected via cystocentesis should be acquired from each patient.
- Cerebrospinal fluid (CSF): When neurologic signs are

present, a sample of CSF should be obtained and cultured appropriately. CSF should be sent for Gram staining, bacterial culture, cell count and differential, and glucose and protein determination. A cryptococcal antigen titer or India ink preparation should be performed in suspect cases. Acid-fast stains and culture are probably not indicated routinely (Figure 23-4).

- Stool: For cats with diarrhea, appropriate cultures should be done for clostridial bacteria, including assays for endotoxin if indicated.
- Lung: Thoracic radiographs and a transendotracheal wash should be obtained, especially from patients showing any signs of respiratory difficulty, such as increased respiratory effort or a cough.

Other diagnostic studies to consider include:

- MDB, including CBC with differential, biochemical profile, urinalysis, and thoracic and abdominal radiographs to detect signs of infection
- Abdominal ultrasonography to evaluate for pancreatitis, abscesses, abdominal effusion, and the like
- Echocardiography to identify the presence of valvular endocarditis
- Bronchoscopy, if pulmonary disease is suspected
- Skin biopsy, if deep cutaneous infection is identified
- Bone marrow aspiration or biopsy to determine the cause and severity of neutropenia
- Percutaneous or laparoscopic-guided liver biopsy or aspiration to evaluate for hepatic infection or abscessation
- Exploratory laparotomy in select cases when other, less invasive tests are unsuccessful yet there is clinical evidence of abdominal disease
- Blood gas analysis

TREATMENT[1-8]

Treatment for septic shock should begin as soon as the condition is suspected, typically when a cat is initially presented for an acute emergency condition. Treatment for septic, neutropenic cats (Figure 23-5) is primarily directed at restoring adequate tissue perfusion, improving metabolic alterations, and controlling systemic infection.

Restoring Adequate Tissue Perfusion

Standard therapy includes administering crystalloid solutions and antibiotics. Although the use of hypertonic solutions for the treatment of shock is being investigated, balanced electrolyte solutions are cited as "the first line of therapy" in most feline texts. The initial infusion rate for critical cats is 40 to 60 ml/kg IV for 1 hour, then 10 to 12 ml/kg/hour thereafter. The administration rate should then be adjusted to meet the needs of each cat as determined by monitoring body weight, heart and respiratory rates, central venous pressure, ongoing losses (e.g., vomiting and diarrhea), and urine output. During that first hour of fluid administration, it is vitally important to monitor for evidence of fluid overload at 15 minute intervals and adjust appropriately.

Improving Metabolic Alterations

When choosing fluid types, some authorities prefer a fluid that does not contain lactate (e.g., Normosol R®, Plasmalyte®; both use acetate and gluconate as buffers); lactate must be metabolized to bicarbonate by a functional liver, but shock and sepsis may impair liver function. Dextrose should be included in fluids when systemic hypoglycemia is identified.

Preventing or Controlling Infection

Asymptomatic cats with fewer than 1,000 neutrophils/µl

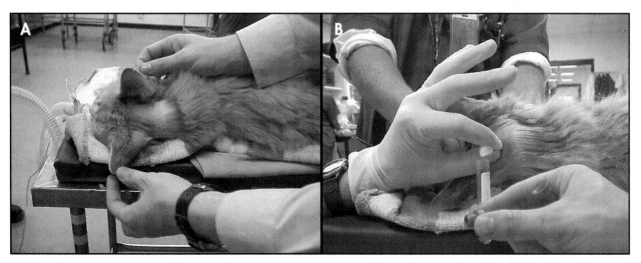

Figure 23-4: Meningitis is a cause of unexplained elevated systemic temperature that may be seen in septic cats. A CSF tap is done by first clipping the hair and preparing the skin as if for surgery (*A*). A 22 ga needle is advanced through the skin into the foramen magnum, and the fluid is allowed to drip into a tube for cytologic analysis and bacterial culture (*B*).

ONCOLOGIC EMERGENCIES

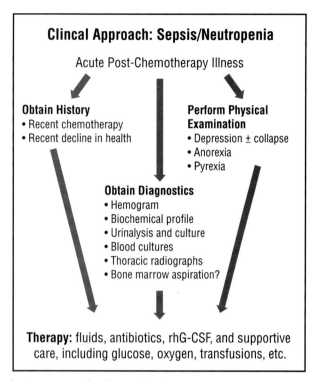

Clincal Approach: Sepsis/Neutropenia

Acute Post-Chemotherapy Illness

Obtain History
• Recent chemotherapy
• Recent decline in health

Perform Physical Examination
• Depression ± collapse
• Anorexia
• Pyrexia

Obtain Diagnostics
• Hemogram
• Biochemical profile
• Urinalysis and culture
• Blood cultures
• Thoracic radiographs
• Bone marrow aspiration?

Therapy: fluids, antibiotics, rhG-CSF, and supportive care, including glucose, oxygen, transfusions, etc.

Figure 23-5: Clinical approach to the septic, neutropenic cat.

MDB = minimum database; includes CBC, biochemical profile, urinalysis, FeLV/FIV serology, T_4 testing, and thoracic radiographs (three views).

TABLE 23-3
Approach to the Febrile, Neutropenic Cat[1-10]

Approach	Action
Identify the site of infection	Perform complete physical examination
	MDB
	Collect two to four blood cultures, urine via cystocentesis for culture and sensitivity, and transtracheal wash for culture and sensitivity
	If indicated, culture and sensitivity testing of CSF, catheters, joint fluid, and feces
Initiate supportive care	Aseptically place indwelling IV catheter and initiate fluid therapy (for patients in shock, administer 40–60 ml/kg for the first hour divided into quarter aliquots administered every 15 min, followed by 10 to 12 ml/kg/hr; monitor patient closely and adjust fluid rate as needed)
	Withhold any additional chemotherapeutic agents
Initiate IV antibiotic therapy	Begin four quadrant (gram-positive, gram-negative, aerobic, and anaerobic) antimicrobial therapy after cultures are obtained: cefoxitin (22 mg/kg tid IV) or ampicillin (22 mg/kg tid IV) and enrofloxacin (5 mg/kg IV slowly daily)
	If aminoglycosides are not contraindicated (i.e., no evidence of dehydration, renal disease, low renal blood flow): cefoxitin (22 mg/kg tid) and gentamicin (2–3 mg/kg over 30 min tid)
	Monitor for nephrotoxicity (urinalysis, evaluate sediment for casts, monitor BUN/creatinine) if aminoglycosides, particularly gentamicin, are administered; consider IV maintenance fluids.
	G-CSF, if available (5 µg/kg/day SQ)
Redefine antibiotic therapy based on culture and sensitivity results	Monitor fever and neutrophil count
Discharge for home care (neutrophils >1,500/µl and afebrile)	Appropriate antibiotic therapy (e.g., trimethoprim-sulfa, 7.5 mg/kg PO bid)
Consider reducing dose (e.g., by 25%) next time the same chemotherapy drug is administered	

should be started on prophylactic antibiotics. Trimethoprim-sulfa (7.5 mg/kg PO bid) is often recommended for prophylactic therapy in asymptomatic neutropenic patients. Neutropenic cats in septic shock should be started on IV fluids and IV antibiotic therapy as soon as samples for bacterial cultures have been acquired (Tables 23-3 and 23-4). Reevaluation of the initial antibiotic regimen is mandatory when the identity and sensitivity patterns of the bacteria become available. For gram-negative infections, a combination of two antibiotics effective against the isolated organism is recommended.

Initially, broad-spectrum antibiotic therapy—often a combination of an aminoglycoside plus penicillin or second-generation cephalosporin (e.g., cefoxitin, cefamandole, cefaclor, cefuroxime, cefonicid, ceforanide, cefotetan, ceftezole)—is commonly used in sepsis. The antibiotics should be changed if the infection does not respond within 24 hours. For gram-negative organisms, aminoglycosides, quinolones, or aztreonam may be used. Extended-spectrum penicillins (e.g., ticarcillin, carbenicillin, azlocillin,

TABLE 23-4
Antibiotics Used to Treat Sepsis in Cats with Cancer

Antibiotic (Dose)	Potential Toxicoses
Gram-Negative Bacteria	
Gentamicin (2.2–4.4 mg/kg IV tid)	Nephrotoxicity, especially with preexisting renal damage; ototoxicity; ensure adequate hydration and check frequently for renal damage during use
Cefazolin (22 mg/kg [10 mg/lb] IV tid)	Phlebitis, muscle pain after IV or IM administration; nephrotoxicity (rare)
Cefoxitin (22 mg/kg IV tid)	Phlebitis; discomfort with rapid IV injection; nephrotoxicity (rare)
Gram-Positive Bacteria	
Na or K penicillin (22,000 units/kg IV qid)	Penicillin allergy can cause anaphylaxis, hives, fever, and pain; neurologic signs may occur with rapid infusion
Cefoxitin (22 mg/kg IV tid)	Penicillin allergy can cause anaphylaxis, hives, fever, and pain; neurologic signs most commonly occur with rapid infusion
Enrofloxacin (5 mg/kg IV sid)	Hives, fever, and pain
Anaerobic Bacteria	
Metronidazole (15 mg/kg IV or IM tid)	Anorexia, vomiting, and neurologic signs
Cefoxitin (22 mg/kg IV tid)	Anorexia, vomiting, and neurologic sign

piperacillin sodium, mezlocillin), third-generation cephalosporins (e.g., cefotaxime, moxalactam, cefoperazone, ceftizoxime, ceftriaxone, ceftazidime, cefixime), and imipenem with cilastatin sodium have sufficiently broad spectrums to be used alone. Cats receiving aminoglycosides, particularly gentamicin, should be monitored for nephrotoxicity via urinalysis (urine sediment should be examined for the presence of casts) and measurement of blood urea nitrogen and creatinine concentrations, and it should be ensured that they are receiving parenteral fluids.

Other treatments include:

- **Corticosteroids:** Steroids remain controversial in the treatment of septic shock. Recommended doses for patients in shock are hydrocortisone at 150 mg/kg, methylprednisolone or prednisone at 10 to 30 mg/kg, or dexamethasone at 4 to 8 mg/kg. Short-term use (i.e., less than 2 days of massive doses) has fewer adverse effects than long-term use.
- **Glucose:** If hypoglycemia is present, glucose can be given at 0.25 g/kg IV bolus, followed by infusions of 2.5% to 10% glucose solutions as needed to maintain normal blood glucose levels.
- **Bicarbonate:** Bicarbonate can be given if severe metabolic acidosis is present. The amount of bicarbonate to administer can be calculated [base deficit × (0.3 × body weight in kg)] or estimated (mild, moderate, or severe acidosis is treated with 1, 3, or 5 mEq bicarbonate/kg IV, respectively). Bicarbonate should be given via slow IV (i.e., over 20 minutes or more).
- **Neutrophil-Rich Transfusions:** These transfusions have not been associated with beneficial responses in controlled trials. In addition, transfusion reactions and allosensitization to specific granulocyte antigens may occur, and increased prevalence of severe pulmonary reactions may be noted.
- **Hematopoietic Growth Factors:** Canine recombinant granulocyte colony-stimulating factor (rcG-CSF; 5 µg/kg/day SQ) and canine recombinant granulocyte-macrophage colony-stimulating factor (rcGM-CSF; 10 µg/kg/day SQ) have been associated with an increased rate of myeloid recovery in dogs and cats with neutropenia. These hematopoietic growth factors increase cell numbers and enhance neutrophil function but are not yet available commercially. Human recombinant G-CSF and GM-CSF are commercially available; however, long-term use may induce antibody formation to the protein. Of the two human recombinant proteins, rhG-CSF induces the most profound increase in canine and feline neutrophil numbers before development of antibodies is noted.
- **Transfusions** of fresh, whole blood.
- **Other Options:** Tumor necrosis factor antiserum, antibody to tumor necrosis factor, interleukin and interferon therapy, pooled immunoglobulin preparations, and monoclonal antibodies to neutralize endotoxin may be future treatments of choice.

ONCOLOGIC EMERGENCIES

THROMBOCYTOPENIA

CLINICAL BRIEFING

Diagnosis

History	Localized or systemic hemorrhage without due cause.
Clinical Signs	Evidence of bleeding, petechial and ecchymotic hemorrhages, hematuria, and hemarthrosis.
Diagnostics	MDB with platelet count and bone marrow aspiration; consider coagulation screening tests (APTT, OSPT, fibrinogen, and FDPs).

Therapy

Treat the underlying cause; support the client's nonmedical needs.

Minimize activity and enforce rest.

Limit heparinized saline flushing of catheter; discontinue aspirin or other nonsteroidal medications.

Correct secondary conditions (e.g., treat DIC and drug-induced myelosuppression).

Consider low-dose vincristine therapy to induce premature release of platelets and transfusion with platelet-rich plasma.

Withhold additional chemotherapy until patient is stabilized; consider reducing the dose the next time the same drug is used.

The most common causes of decreased platelet count are the cytotoxic effects of chemotherapeutic agents, bone marrow infiltration by a malignant process, and feline infectious peritonitis. If a chemotherapeutic agent induces bone marrow suppression resulting in cytopenia, thrombocytopenia usually occurs a few days after neutropenia but before red blood cell numbers decline. Commonly identified abnormalities include a mixed hemostatic defect compatible with disseminated intravascular coagulation (DIC), isolated prolongation of the activated partial thromboplastin time (APTT), and prolongation of both the APTT and one-stage prothrombin time (OSPT).

KEY POINT

Clinical evidence of bleeding is more likely when the platelet count is below 30,000/µl.

PREDISPOSING FACTORS

Thrombocytopenia can occur in any cat with cancer that receives myelosuppressive chemotherapeutic agents (Table 23-1). Drugs such as vincristine, bleomycin, and prednisone do not cause as significant a thrombocytopenia as do some of the more highly myelosuppressive agents (e.g., doxorubicin). Compared to many other myelosuppressive drugs, cyclophosphamide induces less suppression in platelet numbers. Cats with bone marrow infiltration by a malignant process are more sensitive to the cytotoxic effects of chemotherapeutic agents that can result in thrombocytopenia. Other conditions that affect the bone marrow are likely to make it more sensitive to cytotoxic agents. Tumors that are frequently associated with coagulopathies may cause consumptive thrombocytopenia. In addition, hypersplenism and chronic bleeding of any cause can result in a decrease in the number of platelets.

DIAGNOSIS

Because they mask early symptoms of illness, cats are often presented late in the course of clinical disease. This is true for diseases or conditions that result in thrombocytopenia. Clinical signs include, but are not limited to, bleeding diatheses, melena, and weakness. The blood loss can occur from/into any organ and result in multisystemic abnormalities. An acute decline in the number of platelets may result in the development of clinical signs at higher platelet counts than when the decline in platelets is much slower. Therefore if there is any suspicion that thrombocytopenia may be present (gingival hemorrhage, petechial or ecchymotic hemorrhages, or any of the previously mentioned symptoms), proactive interventional and diagnostic measures should be taken after the physical examination is performed. A catheter should be placed and blood obtained with a small gauge needle for routine blood work (CBC with platelet count, biochemical profile, T_4 and FeLV/FIV testing), and a urinalysis should be performed as well to complete the MDB. Diagnosis is confirmed by obtaining platelet counts and by examining bone marrow aspiration or biopsy specimens. Bone marrow evaluation is essential and helps the clinician determine the cause of the thrombocytopenia. Clotting profiles (e.g., APTT, OSPT, and fibrin degradation products [FDPs]) may help determine if the thrombocytopenia is the result of a coagulopathy, such as DIC.

THERAPY

Thrombocytopenia-related clinical signs can be exacerbated when drugs that affect platelet function are administered during the time of overt or impending thrombocytopenia. Therefore aspirin and aspirin-like drugs should be withheld from cats with thrombocytopenia. In addition, the use of heparinized saline for catheter maintenance can be a problem in some patients if multiple catheter "flushes" are performed.

Cats with thrombocytopenia should be kept quiet, and care should be taken during handling. Vincristine (0.5 mg/m² body surface area) can be administered IV to induce premature release of platelets from megakaryocytes.[8] Platelet counts increase 4 days after vincristine is given. Where available, platelet transfusions may be administered to specific cats that are (or have a high likelihood of) bleeding uncontrollably. Administering each unit of platelets with 30 to 60 ml of plasma is recommended. In cats with acute bleeding that is not responsive to other treatments or procedures, hemostatic epsilon aminocaproic acid can be given IV or PO (250 mg/m² q6h).[9] Dose reduction should

occur with the next administration of the same chemotherapeutic agents.

REFERENCES

1. Ogilvie GK: Neutropenia, sepsis and thrombocytopenia, in Wingfield WE (ed): *Veterinary Emergency Medicine Secrets.* Philadelphia, Hanley and Belfus, 2001, pp 235–241.
2. Haskins SC: Shock, in Kirk RW (ed): *Current Veterinary Therapy VIII.* Philadelphia, WB Saunders, 1983, pp 2–27.
3. Kirk RW, Bistner SI: Shock, in *Handbook of Veterinary Procedures Emergency Treatment,* ed 4. Philadelphia, WB Saunders, 1985, pp 59–68.
4. Parker MM, Parrillo JE: Septic shock, hemodynamics and pathogenesis. *JAMA* 250:2324–2230, 1983.
5. Hardie EM, Rawlings CA: Septic shock. *Compend Contin Educ Pract Vet* 5: 369–373, 1983.
6. Wolfsheimer KJ: Fluid therapy in the critically ill patient. *Vet Clin North Am Small Anim Pract* 19:361–378, 1989.
7. Lazarus HM, Creger RJ, Gerson SL: Infectious emergencies in oncology patients. *Semin Oncol* 6:543–560, 1989.
8. Couto CG: Management of complications of cancer chemotherapy. *Vet Clin North Am Small Anim Pract* 4:1037–1053, 1990.
9. Woodlock TJ: Oncologic emergencies, in Rosenthal S, Carignan JR, Smith BD (eds): *Medical Care of the Cancer Patient,* ed 2. Philadelphia, WB Saunders, 1993, pp 236–246.
10. Hughes WT, Armstrong D, Bodey GP, et al: From the Infectious Diseases Society of America: Guidelines for the use of antimicrobial agents in neutropenic patients with unexplained fever. *J Infect Dis* 161:381–396, 1990.
11. Peterson JL, Couto CG, Wellman ML: Hemostatic disorders in cats: A retrospective study and review of the literature. *J Vet Intern Med* 9:298–303, 1995.
12. Quadri TL, Brown AE: Infectious complications in the critically ill patient with cancer. *Semin Oncol* 27:335–346, 2000.
13. Hackner SG: Approach to the diagnosis of bleeding disorders. *Compend Contin Educ Pract Vet* 17:331–349, 1995.
14. Carr AP, Johnson GS: A review of hemostatic abnormalities in dogs and cats. *JAAHA* 30:475–481, 1994.

ONCOLOGIC EMERGENCIES

ACUTE TUMOR LYSIS SYNDROME

24

Gregory K. Ogilvie and Antony S. Moore

CLINICAL BRIEFING

Diagnosis

History | Acute decompensation, anorexia, and collapse within days of receiving chemotherapy for a chemoresponsive tumor.

Clinical Signs | Pale mucous membranes, decreased capillary refill time, evidence of decreased cardiac output (hypodynamic shock), arrhythmias, vomiting, diarrhea, and evidence of tumor lysis.

Diagnostics | MDB may reveal evidence of multiple organ failure, metabolic acidosis, azotemia, and in a few rare cases, hypocalcemia, hyperkalemia, and hyperphosphatemia; hyperkalemia and hyperphosphatemia may have self-corrected if several hours have passed.

Therapy | Prevention (i.e., maintaining adequate hydration) is essential; this condition is rare and the low risk should not be used as grounds for delaying or reducing therapy unless azotemia is identified.

Restore tissue perfusion with fluids and stabilize cardiovascular system.

Correct acid-base and electrolyte imbalances and azotemia.

Withhold additional chemotherapy pending patient recovery.

Acute tumor lysis syndrome (ATLS; Figure 24-1) is an underreported, rare condition characterized by acute collapse—possibly leading to death—soon after administration of a chemotherapeutic agent or radiation therapy for a chemosensitive- or radiation-sensitive tumor.[1-3] ATLS most often occurs shortly after the treatment of lymphoma and lymphoid leukemia or may occur after effective chemotherapy in cats with rapidly growing, bulky, chemosensitive tumors. Cats commonly present with a brief history of acute decompensation, sometimes to the point of imminent death. Rapid diagnosis and therapy are essential to reduce mortality.

PREDISPOSING FACTORS

The actual pathophysiology of ATLS in cats has not been studied and is therefore unknown. In humans, and probably in cats, rapid tumor lysis may cause an acute release of intracellular phosphate and potassium, which leads to hypocalcemia, hyperkalemia, and hyperphosphatemia. Hyperuricemia is also seen in humans who develop ATLS. ATLS is most common in patients with lymphoma or leukemia, partly because the intracellular concentration of phosphorus in human lymphoma and leukemic cells is four to six times higher than in normal cells.[1] Unpublished clinical experience suggests that ATLS is most likely to occur in cats with some degree of volume contraction and a large tumor mass (particularly stage IV or V lymphoma) that rapidly responds to cytolytic therapy. In addition, septic cats and

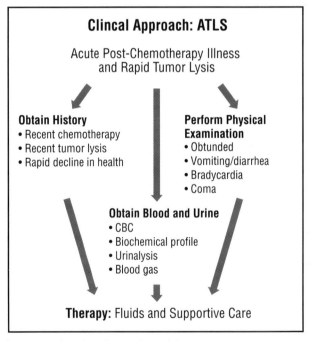

Clincal Approach: ATLS

Acute Post-Chemotherapy Illness and Rapid Tumor Lysis

Obtain History
• Recent chemotherapy
• Recent tumor lysis
• Rapid decline in health

Perform Physical Examination
• Obtunded
• Vomiting/diarrhea
• Bradycardia
• Coma

Obtain Blood and Urine
• CBC
• Biochemical profile
• Urinalysis
• Blood gas

Therapy: Fluids and Supportive Care

Figure 24-1: Clinical approach to ATLS.

those with extensive neoplastic disease that infiltrates the parenchyma of organs are predisposed to ATLS. This condition may be identified within 48 hours after chemotherapy or radiation therapy is first administered.

TABLE 24-1
Therapy for Cats with ATLS

General	Specific
Watch for acute decompensation (hours to days after therapy for a chemoresponsive tumor)	Evaluate the cat. Determine whether the tumor has responded rapidly and dramatically. Perform a complete physical examination to evaluate for systemic disease, hydration status, cardiac output, and so forth. Confirm/eliminate neutropenia, sepsis, radiation coagulopathies, and organ failure via complete blood count, biochemical profile, urinalysis, blood cultures, and other diagnostics as indicated.
Initiate specific support	Treat for shock, provide daily fluid needs, correct dehydration, correct electrolyte abnormalities, and compensate for external fluid losses. Consider non-lactate-containing fluids; in patients with ATLS, 0.9% NaCl may be ideal until hyperkalemia and hyperphosphatemia are corrected. Fluids can be administered during acute shock or shock-like states at a rate of 40–60 ml/kg/hr for the first hour and then 10–12 ml/kg/hr; patients should be monitored closely and fluids adjusted as needed. If hypocalcemia secondary to hyperphosphatemia causes clinically significant signs (rare), exogenous parenteral calcium supplementation may be indicated.
Monitor cat	Monitor hydration, electrolytes, and renal and cardiovascular function. Rate of fluid administration must be "fine-tuned" based on ongoing reevaluation of hydration, cardiovascular, renal, and electrolyte status.
Delay additional chemotherapy pending patient recovery	

KEY POINT

Cats with acute tumor lysis syndrome often present with a history of acute decompensation, sometimes to the point of imminent death (within hours of presentation).[1–3]

DIAGNOSIS

Cats with suspected ATLS present with clinical signs similar to those seen in neutropenic and/or septic cats and are often diagnosed following acute collapse and decompensation hours to days after the administration of chemotherapy. To reduce morbidity and mortality, rapid diagnosis of and therapy for ATLS are essential. Cats with ATLS may have cardiovascular collapse, vomiting, diarrhea, and ensuing shock. Hyperkalemia may result in bradycardia with diminished P wave amplitude and spiked T waves on an electrocardiogram. Biochemical analysis of blood may confirm the presence of hypocalcemia, hyperkalemia, and hyperphosphatemia. If several hours have passed after decompensation, however, hyperkalemia and hyperphosphatemia may have self-corrected. Hyperuricemia is seen in humans with ATLS but has not been identified in cats. In the presence of elevated serum phosphate levels, hypocalcemia develops as a result of calcium and phosphate precipitation. Without effective treatment, cardiovascular collapse, shock, or renal failure may occur in patients with this syndrome; blood urea nitrogen and creatinine concentrations should therefore be monitored closely.

TREATMENT

The best treatment is prevention. Because the kidneys are the main source of electrolyte excretion, metabolic abnormalities may be exacerbated in cats with renal dysfunction. Identification and correction of any volume depletion or azotemia prior to initiation of therapy may reduce the risk of ATLS; chemotherapy should be delayed until metabolic disturbances such as azotemia are corrected. If ATLS is identified, the condition should be treated with aggressive crystalloid fluid therapy (Table 24-1) and careful monitoring of electrolytes and renal parameters. Further chemotherapy should be withheld until the patient is clinically normal and all biochemical parameters have stabilized.

MDB = minimum database; includes CBC, biochemical profile, urinalysis, FeLV/FIV serology, T₄ testing, and thoracic radiographs (three views).

REFERENCES

1. Marcus SL, Einzig AI: Acute tumor lysis syndrome: Prevention and management, in Dutcher JP, Wiernik PH (eds): *Handbook of Hematologic and Oncologic Emergencies.* New York, Plenum Press, 1987, pp 9–15.

2. Woodlock TJ: Oncologic emergencies, in Rosenthal S, Carignan JR, Smith BD (eds): *Medical Care of the Cancer Patient,* ed 2. Philadelphia, WB Saunders, 1993, pp 236–246.

3. Couto CG: Management of complications of cancer chemotherapy. *Vet Clin North Am Small Anim Pract* 4:1037–1053, 1990.

ONCOLOGIC EMERGENCIES

DISSEMINATED INTRAVASCULAR COAGULATION

Gregory K. Ogilvie and Antony S. Moore

25

CLINICAL BRIEFING

Diagnosis

History	Acute decompensation, anorexia, collapse, and inappropriate bleeding from any site.
Clinical Signs	Pale mucous membranes; decreased capillary refill time; evidence of decreased cardiac output due to blood loss or thrombosis; bleeding from any part of the body (including venipuncture sites); dyspnea from blood loss or pulmonary thrombosis.
Diagnostics	MDB with platelet count, blood gas analysis, and coagulation screening tests (PT, APTT, FDPs, ACT, fibrinogen, antithrombin III) may reveal evidence of blood loss, multiple organ failure, coagulopathies, or metabolic acidosis.

Therapy

Treat the underlying cause.

Restore tissue perfusion with fluids; stabilize the cardiovascular system.

Correct acid-base and electrolyte imbalances.

Blood component therapy, including plasma for clotting factors.

Heparin therapy may be of value if thrombosis predominates.

Discontinue chemotherapy, including prednisone, pending patient recovery.

Disorders of hemostasis are an underreported and underrecognized cause of morbidity and mortality in feline and human cancer patients.[1-11] The etiology of this condition is not as clearly defined in cats as in dogs and humans. Until more is known, it may be helpful to characterize hemostatic disorders as follows:

- Disseminated intravascular coagulation (DIC)
- Malignancy-associated fibrinolysis
- Platelet abnormalities
- Hypercoagulable state of malignancy (a clinical syndrome)
- Chemotherapy-associated thromboembolism (e.g., as occurs with L-asparaginase administration)

DIC is a consumptive coagulopathy that often results in a life-threatening condition. DIC has been associated with the parameters listed above and occurs with many malignancies. A malignancy will sometimes induce DIC when clotting factors are activated by tumor-induced procoagulants or when the tumor directly or indirectly stimulates platelet aggregation. The resultant formation of clots in the circulation consumes clotting factors and platelets, which leads to widespread bleeding. In addition, deposition of fibrin throughout the body may result in concurrent microangiopathic hemolytic anemia. To reduce morbidity and mortality, DIC must be identified and treated early.

PREDISPOSING FACTORS

DIC occurs with a wide variety of malignant conditions, including hemangiosarcoma, lymphoma, and mammary adenocarcinoma.[9-11] Treatment with chemotherapeutic agents, surgery, or concurrent infection may induce or exacerbate DIC. Renal failure and loss of low molecular weight coagulation factors through glomeruli may increase the risk of coagulation abnormalities. Thrombosis with or without DIC has been identified in cats with hyperadrenocorticism and in cats that have been treated with high doses of glucocorticoids. The syndrome is more common in dogs than cats.

DIAGNOSIS

Clinical signs supportive of a diagnosis of DIC include oozing from venipuncture sites, nosebleeds, oral bleeding, melena, ecchymoses and petechial hemorrhages anywhere on the body, and hematuria.[1-4] Widespread thrombosis can cause multiple organ failure, which may result in a variety of clinical signs, such as acute renal failure and acute onset of respiratory distress. Laboratory abnormalities associated with DIC vary depending on the organs involved and

TABLE 25-1
Clinical and Laboratory Parameters Used to Diagnose DIC

Tests/Observations	Acute DIC	Chronic DIC
Clinical signs	Clinically evident coagulopathies	Few clinical signs evident
Onset and duration	Rapid onset and quick progression	Insidious and prolonged
PT, APTT, and ACT	Prolonged	Normal to slightly decreased
Platelets	Decreased	Often normal
FDPs	Very high	High
Fibrinogen	Decreased to normal	Normal
AT III	Reduced	Normal
Prognosis	Grave	Good

whether DIC is acute or chronic (Table 25-1); the chronic form of DIC is rarely associated with clinical signs. In addition, alterations in red blood cell morphology (e.g., fragmentation) may result from microangiopathic events associated with DIC. There are many causes for the decreased platelet count and coagulation factor deficiencies seen in patients with DIC. Diagnosis is based on clinical findings and laboratory parameters (Table 25-1), including:

- Increased prothrombin time (PT)
- Increased activated partial thromboplastin time (APTT)
- Thrombocytopenia
- Prolonged activated coagulation time (ACT)
- Decreased antithrombin III (AT-III) concentrations
- Hypofibrinogenemia
- Increased fibrin degradation products (FDPs)

ONCOLOGIC EMERGENCIES

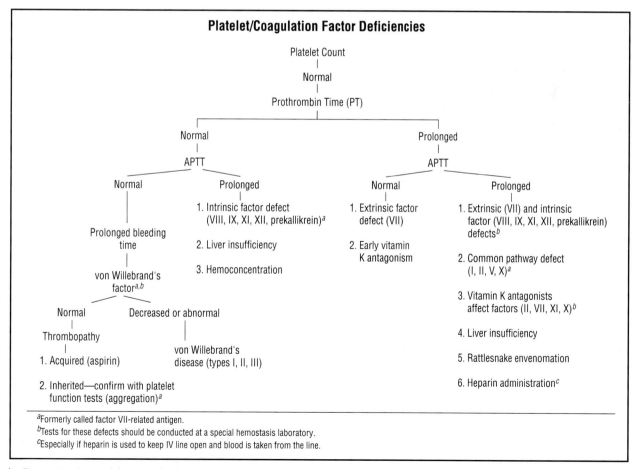

Platelet/Coagulation Factor Deficiencies

Platelet Count
|
Normal
|
Prothrombin Time (PT)

Normal — Prolonged

Normal → APTT:

Normal:
- Prolonged bleeding time
  - von Willebrand's factor[a,b]
    - Normal → Thrombopathy
      1. Acquired (aspirin)
      2. Inherited—confirm with platelet function tests (aggregation)[a]
    - Decreased or abnormal → von Willebrand's disease (types I, II, III)

Prolonged:
1. Intrinsic factor defect (VIII, IX, XI, XII, prekallikrein)[a]
2. Liver insufficiency
3. Hemoconcentration

Prolonged → APTT:

Normal:
1. Extrinsic factor defect (VII)
2. Early vitamin K antagonism

Prolonged:
1. Extrinsic (VII) and intrinsic factor (VIII, IX, XI, XII, prekallikrein) defects[b]
2. Common pathway defect (I, II, V, X)[a]
3. Vitamin K antagonists affect factors (II, VII, XI, X)[b]
4. Liver insufficiency
5. Rattlesnake envenomation
6. Heparin administration[c]

[a]Formerly called factor VII-related antigen.
[b]Tests for these defects should be conducted at a special hemostasis laboratory.
[c]Especially if heparin is used to keep IV line open and blood is taken from the line.

Figure 25-1: Suggested diagnostic plan for cats with hemostatic disorders and normal platelet counts.

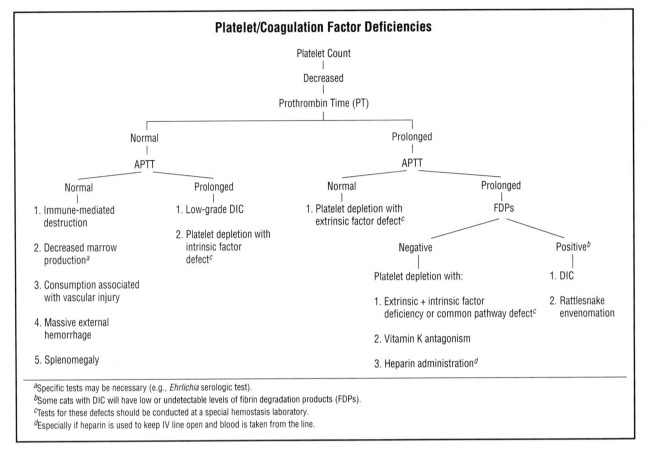

Figure 25-2: *Suggested diagnostic plan for cats with hemostatic disorders and low platelet counts.*

MDB = minimum database; includes CBC, biochemical profile, urinalysis, FeLV/FIV serology, T_4 testing, and thoracic radiographs (three views).

There are many causes for DIC-associated abnormalities (Figures 25-1 and 25-2).[1-11] Decreased platelet counts can be caused by bone marrow failure, increased platelet consumption, or splenic pooling of platelets. Prolonged PT may result from a lack of one or more of clotting factors VII, X, V, II (prothrombin), and I (fibrinogen). Increased APTT may be caused by a deficiency in one or more of clotting factors XII, XI, IX, VIII, X, V, II, and I. Heparin and oral anticoagulant therapy also prolong the APTT. Low fibrinogen levels are associated with decreased production or increased consumption of this protein.

TREATMENT[1-4]

Cats often do not exhibit clinical signs associated with DIC until quite late in the course of the disease. Therefore treatment must begin as soon as possible. Specific treatment for DIC is controversial, but certain procedures are uniformly accepted despite the paucity of data documenting their efficacy. Treatment revolves around:

- **Treating the underlying cause** (the most important therapeutic step).
- **Fluid therapy**, which is essential to correct volume contraction and to reduce the possibility of ensuing renal failure and acid-base abnormalities. The amount of fluid administered, body weight, and urine output must be carefully monitored in all cats. Increases in body weight, heart and respiratory rates, and central venous pressure may suggest volume overload, a condition that is especially threatening in cats that are anuric secondary to acute renal shutdown.
- **Transfusion support**: In cats with severe bleeding diatheses, transfusing fresh blood or plasma with clotting factors and platelets may help replace the blood components that are being consumed.
- **Heparin therapy:** If thrombosis appears to be the most clinically evident problem, heparin therapy may reduce the formation of thrombi. The amount of heparin to be

used is controversial. Methods include administering heparin via intermittent SQ or IV doses or constant-rate infusion (CRI) to prolong APTT by 1.5 to 2 times. Minidose heparin therapy (5–10 IU/kg/hr by CRI or 75 IU/kg SQ q8h) may be helpful in some cases; some practitioners administer 10 IU/kg SQ daily.

KEY POINT

Treatment of the underlying cause and fluid therapy are the two most effective and important treatments for DIC.

- **Discontinuation of chemotherapy:** Chemotherapeutic agents, including prednisone, should be withheld until all evidence of DIC is eliminated and the patient has recovered completely. Dogs that receive glucocorticoid therapy are at major risk for thromboembolic events that can initiate or perpetuate DIC; this is likely true for cats as well.

Because cats with acute DIC have a poor prognosis, identifying patients at high risk and initiating prophylactic treatment are of great value. Routine monitoring of ACTs and platelet counts can identify cats in the early phases of DIC.

REFERENCES

1. Ogilvie GK: Acute tumor lysis syndrome, in Wingfield WE (ed): *Veterinary Emergency Medicine Secrets.* Philadelphia, Hanley and Belfus, 2001, pp 242–243.
2. Smith MR: Disorders of hemostasis and transfusion therapy, in Skeel RT (ed): *Handbook of Cancer Chemotherapy,* ed 3. Boston, Little, Brown & Co, 1991, pp 449–459.
3. Parry BW: Laboratory evaluation of hemorrhagic coagulopathies in small animal practices. *Vet Clin North Am Small Anim Pract* 4:729–742, 1989.
4. Woodlock TJ: Oncologic emergencies, in Rosenthal S, Carignan JR, Smith BD (eds): *Medical Care of the Cancer Patient,* ed 2. Philadelphia, WB Saunders, 1993, pp 236–246.
5. Hackner SG: Approach to the diagnosis of bleeding disorders. *Compend Contin Educ Pract Vet* 17:331–349, 1995.
6. Jordan HL, Grindem CB, Breitschwerdt EB: Thrombocytopenia in cats: A retrospective study of 41 cases. *J Vet Intern Med* 7:261–265, 1993.
7. Matsushiro H, Kato H, Tahara T, et al: Molecular cloning and functional expression of feline thrombopoietin. *Vet Immunol Immunopathol* 66:225–236, 1998.
8. Golden DL, Langston VC: Use of vincristine and vinblastine in dogs and cats. *JAVMA* 193:1114–1117, 1988.
9. Slappendel RJ: Disseminated intravascular coagulation. *Vet Clin North Am Small Anim Pract* 18:169–184, 1988.
10. Couto CG: Disseminated intravascular coagulation in dogs and cats. *Vet Med* 94:547–554, 1999.
11. Lisciandro SC, Hohenhaus A, Brooks M: Coagulation abnormalities in 22 cats with naturally occurring liver disease. *J Vet Intern Med* 12:71–75, 1998.

ONCOLOGIC EMERGENCIES

CENTRAL NERVOUS SYSTEM EMERGENCIES

Gregory K. Ogilvie and Antony S. Moore

26

The most common central nervous system (CNS) emergencies are cerebral herniation, seizures, and epidural spinal cord compression.[1-5] Less common CNS emergencies include bacterial meningitis and other acute infections that may be associated with tumor- or drug-induced neutropenia. Infectious conditions of the CNS are reviewed in Chapter 23.

BRAIN HERNIATION

CLINICAL BRIEFING

Diagnosis	
History	Acute neurologic decompensation.
Clinical Signs	Altered mentation, progressive drowsiness, altered pupil size and function, altered respiration, extensor rigidity, disconjugate eye movements, and arrhythmias.
Diagnostics	MDB, CT, MRI, nuclear imaging of brain, and EEG.
Treatment	Control respiration.
	Decrease intracranial pressure with mannitol, glucocorticoids, and surgical decompression in rare cases.
	Treat the underlying cause.

PREDISPOSING FACTORS

Brain herniation can be caused by a wide variety of primary or secondary malignancies of the brain, intracerebral hemorrhage and intradural hematoma, brain abscess, or acute hydrocephalus. Regardless of the cause, diagnosis must be made swiftly and therapy initiated without hesitation to prevent irreparable neurologic damage or death.

CLINICAL SIGNS

Brain herniation is characterized by any CNS abnormality, including progressive drowsiness, small reactive pupils, periodic respirations (Cheyne-Stokes), and in the most severe cases, bilateral extensor rigidity.[2,4] As the herniation evolves, hyperventilation, disconjugate eye movements, pupillary fixation, and abnormal motor postures can be noted. The "brain-heart syndrome" may be evident if brain stem compression causes cardiac arrhythmias.

DIAGNOSIS

The diagnosis and decision to treat are primarily based on the rapid development of abnormal neurologic signs. Because the decision to withhold therapy may result in death or severe, potentially irreversible neurologic abnormalities, treatment should be initiated immediately or concurrently with diagnostic methods, such as collection of an MDB, computerized tomography (CT), magnetic resonance imaging (MRI), nuclear scans, and, if available, electroencephalography (EEG). A cerebrospinal fluid (CSF) tap at the cisterna magna may actually cause or exacerbate brain herniation and thus should not be used if increased intracranial pressure/herniation is suspected.

TREATMENT

Prognosis is poor. The goals are to prevent further herniation and to treat existing herniation and the underlying cause.[2,4] Intubation and control of respiration may be required as hyperventilation produces cerebral vasoconstriction, decreased blood volume, and decreased intracranial pressure. Mannitol (1–2 g/kg IV slowly qid) can reduce brain water content, reduce brain volume, and decrease intracranial pressure rapidly. Steroids (e.g., dexamethasone NaPO$_4$ [2 mg/kg IV once, followed by 0.25 mg/kg IV qid]) can be administered but may take hours to have full effect. Recent work suggests that hydrocortisone (10–50 mg/kg IV) given at the time of brain trauma may be beneficial.[2,4] In rare cases, surgical decompression may be helpful. Once treatment is underway, plain and contrast CT or MRI may help identify the cause of the herniation.

SEIZURES

C L I N I C A L	**B R I E F I N G**
Diagnosis	
History	Seizure preceded by an aura and followed by a postictal period.
Clinical Signs	Seizures characterized as partial, simple partial, complex partial, generalized, or generalized nonconvulsive.
Diagnostics	Metabolic and traumatic causes should be eliminated immediately; after the patient recovers, other causes should be evaluated via MDB, radiographs, fasting blood glucose, CSF analysis, and brain imaging techniques.
Treatment	Evaluate patient and treat identified metabolic causes (e.g., glucose and calcium).
	Stop the seizures with diazepam or phenobarbital, if indicated.
	Monitor and treat appropriately during recovery.

PREDISPOSING FACTORS

A variety of metastatic and nonmetastatic conditions can cause seizures in feline cancer patients (see Box at right). Vascular disorders, such as intracerebral hemorrhage, subdural hematomas, and thrombosis of the CNS vessels, may be associated with seizures. Hypoglycemia secondary to insulinoma or hepatic tumor may induce CNS abnormalities.[1,2,4,5] Several chemotherapeutic agents and radiosensitizers are reported to cause seizures (e.g., mitoxantrone, L-asparaginase, 5-fluorouracil, vincristine).[3,4]

CLINICAL PRESENTATION

Seizures may appear clinically as partial (focal or local), simple partial (symmetric and rarely associated with loss of consciousness), complex partial (alterations in consciousness plus complex behavior), generalized (involuntary, uncontrolled motor activity), or generalized nonconvulsive (loss of consciousness with lack of spontaneous motor activity and transient collapse) seizures.[1,2] There is generally an aura or period of behavioral change before each type of seizure, followed by ictus or the actual clinical seizure, and finally a postictal period that lasts for approximately 30 minutes, during which time cats exhibit abnormal behavior and possibly even weakness and blindness. If malignancy is associated with the condition, the seizures generally get progressively worse over time because of the enlarging intracranial mass or, in the case of insulin-producing tumors, progressive worsening of hypoglycemia.

DIAGNOSIS

The diagnosis generally is evident from the historical or physical findings. In an emergency situation (often associated with status epilepticus), a definitive diagnosis is made after the cat is stabilized. A diagnosis is generally made with imaging techniques, including skull radiographs, CT, nu-

Causes of Seizures

CNS Metastases

Primary Brain Tumor
- Meningioma
- Glioma
- Astrocytoma
- Choroid plexus papilloma

Metabolic Conditions
- Hyponatremia
- Hypomagnesemia
- Hypoxia
- Hypocalcemia
- Hypoglycemia
- Hyperglycemia

CNS Infarction

CNS Hemorrhage

Infection

Radiation Therapy to Brain
- Early delayed toxicity
- Late delayed toxicity

Chemotherapy
- Methotrexate
- L-Asparaginase
- Vinca alkaloids
- Ifosfamide
- 5-Fluorouracil (fatal)
- Mitoxantrone

Biologic Response Modifiers
- Interleukin-2
- Interferon

clear imaging, or MRI of the brain. If a neoplasm is suspected, a complete staging scheme must be initiated as soon as the patient is stable. Diagnostic testing should include a complete history, complete physical and neurologic examinations, CBC, biochemical profile, urinalysis, thoracic and abdominal radiographs, fasting (more than 24 hours) blood glucose and insulin levels, a CSF tap if the patient is not at risk for brain herniation, and EEG, if available.

TREATMENT

Caution should be used when handling cats during seizure activity (Figure 26-1). The general scheme is noted in Table 26-1; Table 26-2 lists anticonvulsants used in acute situations. If a seizure is in progress, IV diazepam should be administered. Respiration should be monitored and, when necessary, intubation and ventilation should be considered. A loading dose of phenobarbital or pentobarbital can be given if diazepam does not control seizures; phenobarbital is also the drug of choice for long-term seizure control. Phenobarbital therapy may be valuable when a single seizure is expected to continue or if clusters of seizures occur within a short period.

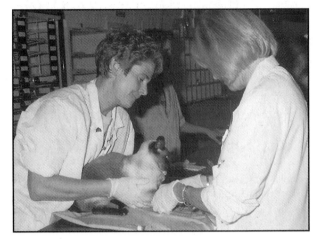

Figure 26-1: Cats can be difficult to handle during seizure activity. Firm yet gentle restraint is used while assessing cats, acquiring venous access, obtaining blood samples before therapy, and administering appropriate therapy.

TABLE 26-1
Emergency Procedures for Status Epilepticus[1-5]

General Principle	Specific Details
Evaluate the cat	Brief history and physical examination
	If possible, place indwelling catheter
	If possible, acquire blood samples; immediately determine glucose and calcium levels while therapy is initiated
Stop the seizures	Administer IV diazepam (2.5–5.0 mg, depending on patient's size)
	Test dosages or definitive therapy for hypoglycemia (e.g., 0.5 g dextrose as a 25% solution given IV over 5 min); if hypocalcemia is present, specific therapy should be initiated (e.g., 1.0–1.5 ml/kg of 10% calcium gluconate solution)
	If necessary, repeat diazepam bolus every 10 min for a total of three doses
	If diazepam is inadequate for seizure control, administer IV phenobarbital or pentobarbital (see Table 26-2); pentobarbital is less effective for controlling seizures but has a more rapid onset of action compared with phenobarbital
	Monitor acid-base status, ability to ventilate, body temperature, electrolyte balance, and hydration status and treat appropriately
Monitor during recovery from seizures	Phenobarbital may be administered (one time loading dose of 6–20 mg/kg IV; then 2 mg/kg PO bid to start maintenance therapy) to reduce seizures; monitor blood levels; when seizures are controlled and the cat is able to swallow, oral phenobarbital therapy should be continued
Initiate definitive diagnostics	CBC, biochemical profile, fasting blood glucose and insulin measurement, urinalysis, CSF tap, CT or MRI of the brain (if indicated), and EEG (if available)

TABLE 26-2
Anticonvulsants Used in an Acute Situation to Treat Seizures in Cats[1,2,4,5]

Anticonvulsant	Recommended Dosages, General Indications, and Precautions
Phenobarbital	2.2–4.4 mg/kg/day divided bid–tid; drug of choice for long-term seizure control; half-life: 40 hr (indicated for grand mal and partial seizures; this drug is most effective in delaying progressive activity known as kindling; monitor for sedation, ataxia, polydipsia, and polyuria; these adverse effects usually abate with time)
Phenytoin	Generally not recommended for emergency therapy
Diazepam	2.5–5 mg tid; half-life: 15–20 hr (indicated for grand mal seizures and status epilepticus; monitor for sedation)

SPINAL CORD COMPRESSION

CLINICAL BRIEFING

Diagnosis	
History	Compatible with acute upper or lower neurologic decompensation.
Clinical Signs	Back pain, root signature, weakness, muscle atrophy, conscious proprioceptive deficits, altered spinal reflexes, and upper or lower motor neuron damage.
Diagnostics	MDB, bone marrow aspiration to rule out lymphoma, myelogram, CT, CSF analysis, spinal decompression, and biopsy.
Treatment	Corticosteroids (but not before diagnostics are completed). Spinal decompression. Treat the underlying cause with chemotherapy, surgery, or radiation therapy.

PREDISPOSING FACTORS

There are many causes of spinal cord disorders in cats. Many malignancy-induced spinal cord compressions in feline cancer patients are extradural.[3,6] This is especially true in cats with posterior paresis, which is often the result of an extradural lymphoma. These cats are almost always young and FeLV-positive and have lymphoma in the bone marrow.[6]

DIAGNOSIS

Clinical signs include back pain, root signature, paresis, or paralysis.[6] Significant spinal cord compression may occur before clinical signs are evident because of slow tumor progression and concurrent compensation of the nervous tissue. In some cases, such as with neurofibrosarcomas, lower motor neuron signs (e.g., muscle atrophy, weakness, lack of spinal reflexes) may precede clinical signs referable to the spinal cord. This is because neurofibrosarcomas originate in peripheral nerves, thus causing lower motor neuron signs, and then progress to involve the spinal canal, resulting in cord compression and upper motor neuron signs.

The importance of early diagnosis cannot be overemphasized. Immediate action must be taken when spinal cord compression is identified to ensure that the underlying cause is specifically diagnosed and treated. Diagnosis is based on clinical findings and results of diagnostic testing, including the MDB, CT or contrast myelogram, and bone scans via scintigraphy. Extradural lymphoma is one of the most common causes of posterior paresis in cats that have no evidence of trauma and good femoral pulses. Most cats with spinal lymphoma can be presumptively diagnosed by determining their FeLV status and coupling this with diagnosis of lymphoma from a bone marrow aspirate. In many cats with spinal cord compression, performing a surgical spinal cord decompression and biopsy can be diagnostic.

TREATMENT[3,4,6]

Cats with lymphoma are effectively treated with chemotherapy (e.g., cyclophosphamide, prednisone, vincristine) and/or radiation therapy to the area of compression (see Chapter 36). Steroids reduce spinal cord edema and may be beneficial when administered before and during radiation treatment. The optimal treatment for epidural spinal cord compression caused by metastatic disease is debated in human medicine. Corticosteroids (i.e., prednisone, 2 mg/kg bid initially) and radiotherapy are the mainstays of therapy for most cats that have solid tumors of the spinal cord. Surgical intervention is indicated if tissue diagnosis is required, the cause of the spinal cord compression is uncertain, relapse occurs in the area of prior irradiation, spinal instability is present, or radiation therapy and steroid treatment fail.

REFERENCES

1. Fenner WR: Seizures, narcolepsy and cataplexy, in Birchard SJ, Sherding RG (eds): *Saunders Manual of Small Animal Practice*. Philadelphia, WB Saunders, 1993, pp 1147–1156.
2. Fenner WR: Diseases of the brain, in Birchard SJ, Sherding RG (eds): *Saunders Manual of Small Animal Practice*. Philadelphia, WB Saunders, 1993, pp 1126–1146.
3. Couto CG: Management of complications of cancer chemotherapy. *Vet Clin North Am Small Anim Pract* 4:1037–1053, 1990.
4. Woodlock TJ: Oncologic emergencies, in Rosenthal S, Carignan JR, Smith BD (eds): *Medical Care of the Cancer Patient*, ed 2. Philadelphia, WB Saunders, 1993, pp 236–246.
5. Bunch SE: Anticonvulsant drug therapy in companion animals, in Kirk RW (ed): *Current Veterinary Therapy IX, Small Animal Practice*. Philadelphia, WB Saunders, 1986, pp 836–844.
6. Luttgen PJ: Spinal cord disorders, in Birchard SJ, Sherding RG (eds): *Saunders Manual of Small Animal Practice*. Philadelphia, WB Saunders, 1993, pp 1157–1164.

KEY POINT

In the "brain–heart syndrome," clinicians may be distracted by the occurrence of bizarre arrhythmias that are actually caused by compression of the cardiac control center and centers of the brain that regulate autonomic control of the heart.

ONCOLOGIC EMERGENCIES

METABOLIC EMERGENCIES— HYPERCALCEMIA, HYPONATREMIA, AND HYPOGLYCEMIA

27

Gregory K. Ogilvie and Antony S. Moore

HYPERCALCEMIA

CLINICAL BRIEFING

Diagnosis

History — Acute history of polyuria, polydipsia, severe dehydration, vomiting secondary to renal failure, coma, and seizures.

Clinical Signs — Vomiting, hyposthenuria, bradycardia, skeletal muscle weakness, depression, stupor, coma, seizures, and death.

Diagnostics — Hypercalcemia and secondary renal damage detected via MDB, ionized calcium concentration, bone marrow aspiration, radiographs, ACTH stimulation, and (if indicated) parathyroid hormone or parathyroid hormone-related peptide concentrations.

Treatment — Reduce hypercalcemia to prevent further renal damage while initiating diagnostics to determine the exact etiology.

Rehydration with saline diuresis is essential to stabilize the patient and decrease serum calcium concentrations; furosemide may be valuable to decrease calcium in well-hydrated cats; consider prednisone only after the underlying cause has been diagnosed.

In refractory cases, consider salmon calcitonin, bisphosphonates, gallium nitrate, and mithramycin.

Hypercalcemia is the most common metabolic emergency in oncology.[1-10] Lymphoma is the leading cause of hypercalcemia in cats, although hypercalcemia occurs much less often in cats with lymphoma than in dogs with lymphoma. Other causes of hypercalcemia in cats include multiple myeloma, squamous cell carcinoma, mammary adenocarcinoma, and primary hyperparathyroidism. Parathyroid carcinomas or adenomas are rare malignancies associated with intractable hypercalcemia caused by elevated parathyroid hormone (PTH) levels. A parathyroid hormone-related peptide (PTH-rp) is most commonly associated with hypercalcemia in dogs and probably in cats as well, although the assay for PTH-rp is not as routinely performed or as reliable in feline medicine as in canine medicine. It has been suggested that bone metastasis can be associated with hypercalcemia, but this is rare in feline medicine.

One recent retrospective study was conducted to characterize the diseases, clinical findings, and clinicopathologic and ultrasonographic findings associated with hypercalcemia (serum calcium concentration >11 mg/dl) in 71 cats.[7] The three most common diagnoses were neoplasia (21 cats), renal failure (18 cats), and urolithiasis (11 cats). Primary hyperparathyroidism was diagnosed in 4 cats. Lymphoma and squamous cell carcinoma were the tumors diagnosed most frequently. Calcium oxalate uroliths were identified in 8 of 11 cats with urolithiasis. Cats with neoplasia had a higher serum calcium concentration (13.5 ± 2.5 mg/dl) than cats with renal failure or urolithiasis and renal failure (11.5 ± 0.4 mg/dl; $p < .03$). Serum phosphorus concentrations were higher in cats with renal failure than in cats with neoplasia ($p < .004$).

CLINICAL PRESENTATION

Emergency malignancy-induced hypercalcemia is characterized by clinical signs associated with a decreased sensitivity to antidiuretic hormone (ADH) by the distal convoluted tubules and collecting ducts and the vasoconstrictive properties of calcium that result in decreased renal blood flow and a reduced glomerular filtration rate.[1-4] The renal epithelium undergoes degenerative changes, necrosis, and calcification. These physiologic and pathologic changes result in progressive renal disease, noted clinically as polyuria and polydipsia followed by vomiting, hyposthenuria, and dehydration. Calcium may also affect the gastrointestinal, cardiovascular, and neurologic systems directly and cause anorexia, vomiting, constipation, bradycardia, hypertension, skeletal muscle weakness, depression, stupor, coma, and seizures.

DIAGNOSIS (FIGURE 27-1)

Other diagnostic differentials that must be considered in cats presented for true hypercalcemia (Ca^{++} >11 mg/dl) include laboratory or interpretation error, hyperproteinemia from dehydration, acute renal failure, vitamin D and calcium toxicosis, granulomatous disorders, nonneoplastic bone disorders, hypoadrenocorticism, and true hyperparathyroidism.[2,5,6]

It is important to interpret calcium levels in relation to serum albumin and blood pH. The following formula takes albumin into account:

$$\text{Adjusted Calcium (mg/dl)} = [\text{Calcium (mg/dl)} - \text{Albumin (g/dl)}] + 3.5$$

Acidosis increases the free, ionized fraction of calcium and can magnify the observed clinical signs associated with hypercalcemia.

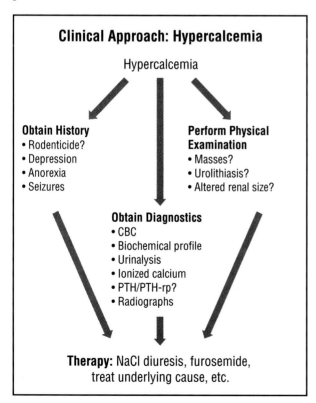

Clinical Approach: Hypercalcemia

Hypercalcemia

Obtain History
• Rodenticide?
• Depression
• Anorexia
• Seizures

Perform Physical Examination
• Masses?
• Urolithiasis?
• Altered renal size?

Obtain Diagnostics
• CBC
• Biochemical profile
• Urinalysis
• Ionized calcium
• PTH/PTH-rp?
• Radiographs

Therapy: NaCl diuresis, furosemide, treat underlying cause, etc.

Figure 27-1: Clinical approach to hypercalcemia in the cat.

MDB = minimum database; includes CBC, biochemical profile, urinalysis, FeLV/FIV serology, T_4 testing, and thoracic radiographs (three views).

Serial serum calcium, electrolytes, blood urea nitrogen (BUN), and creatinine levels should be measured in all hypercalcemic patients. While controversial, a finding of elevated immunoreactive PTH levels in association with hyperphosphatemia may suggest ectopic hormone production. The PTH-rp assay is unreliable in cats but may be helpful in some situations. Cats with multiple myeloma may have elevated calcium levels secondary to abnormal calcium binding to a paraprotein without an elevation in ionized calcium, and malnourished cats with hypoalbuminemia may have symptoms of hypercalcemia despite normal serum calcium levels.

TREATMENT[2,5,6,11–17]

Treatment of a hypercalcemic emergency depends on the severity of the clinical signs and whether renal disease is present. Appropriate management almost always entails the use of IV saline in volumes exceeding daily maintenance (>132 ml/kg$^{0.75}$/day [more than approximately 44–66 ml/kg/day] plus enough to replace exogenous losses from vomiting and diarrhea, plus replacement fluids for dehydration). Potassium depletion should be prevented by adding potassium chloride to fluids based on serum potassium levels (Table 27-1).

The rate of IV potassium should not exceed 0.5 mEq/kg/hour. Cats should be watched carefully for signs consistent with overhydration and congestive heart failure. If hypercalcemia is the result of a malignancy, effective antitumor therapy should be initiated as soon as possible. Thiazide diuretics or vitamins A and D may elevate calcium levels and thus should never be used in these cats.

The most commonly used drugs for managing cats with hypercalcemia include:

- **Furosemide** (1–4 mg/kg IV or PO bid) and IV **bisphosphonates** (e.g., etidronate, disodium pamidronate) may be used in addition to saline diuresis. IV or PO bisphosphonates have rapid hypocalcemic effects due to their inhibition of osteoclast activity.
- **Gallium nitrate** produces concentration-dependent reductions in osteolytic response to parathormone and certain other types of lymphokines that cause hypercalcemia. Gallium nitrate infused at doses of approximately 100 mg/m^2/day for 5 consecutive days successfully reduces high calcium levels in 86% of human patients.[8,9]
- **Mithramycin**, a chemotherapeutic agent that decreases

TABLE 27-1
IV Potassium Supplementation to Correct Hypokalemia

Serum Potassium (mEq/L)	KCl (mEq) to Add to Each L of Fluids	Maximum Rate of Infusion (ml/kg/hr)
<2.0	80	6
2.1–2.5	60	8
2.6–3.0	40	12
3.1–3.5	28	16

bone resorption by reducing osteoclast numbers and activity, also has been shown to be effective in humans. Because mithramycin is a sclerosing agent, it must be given as a bolus (25 µg/kg IV once or twice weekly) through a newly placed line. If extravasation occurs, ulceration and fibrosis will develop. Mithramycin has not been used extensively in dogs or cats; twice-weekly dosing may be required in refractory patients.

- **Salmon calcitonin** (4–8 MRC U/kg SQ) may also be used in refractory patients. Calcitonin inhibits bone resorption and thus causes serum calcium levels to fall within hours of administration. When administered at higher dosages than are clinically applicable (40 MRC U/kg), salmon calcitonin may result in hypocalcemia for several days.
- **Corticosteroids** are effective for treating hypercalcemia. Corticosteroids block bone resorption caused by osteoclast-activating factor, increase urinary calcium excretion, inhibit vitamin D metabolism, and increase calcium absorption after long-term use. To be effective, high doses are generally required for several days. Steroids should not be used until tissue diagnosis is made, primarily because lymphomas are the most common cause of malignancy-associated hypercalcemia and the indiscriminate use of steroids could make diagnosing lymphoma difficult to impossible.

Most cats can be effectively treated with hydration, antitumor therapy, and administration of hypocalcemic-inducing agents, such as mithramycin, calcitonin, or corticosteroids. Serum calcium should be monitored at least twice weekly.

HYPONATREMIA/SYNDROME OF INAPPROPRIATE SECRETION OF ANTIDIURETIC HORMONE

CLINICAL BRIEFING

Diagnosis

History — Anorexia, muscle stiffness progressing to confusion or an unresponsive state, and history of recent administration of a drug that may cause hyponatremia or SIADH.

Clinical Signs — Nausea and neurologic signs progressing to coma and death.

Diagnostics — MDB, fractional excretion of sodium, serum osmolality, and adrenal and thyroid function tests.

Treatment — Treat the underlying cause while initiating supportive, symptomatic therapy.
Judicious water restriction.
Demeclocycline and furosemide.
Lithium carbonate, phenytoin, and hypertonic saline in refractory cases.

The emergency situation caused by the syndrome of inappropriate antidiuretic hormone secretion (SIADH) is a rare and underrecognized, albeit important, cause of true hyponatremia in cancer patients.[6–10] As the name implies, SIADH is the presence of excessive quantities of ADH secondary to a malignancy. Affected cats have a low plasma osmolality despite inappropriately high urine sodium concentrations. Because this situation can also occur in patients with renal disease, hypothyroidism, or adrenal insufficiency, these disorders must be excluded to confirm a diagnosis of SIADH.

PREDISPOSING FACTORS

SIADH may be caused by a malignancy or drug that results in renal activation or enhanced release of ADH. SIADH has been identified in cats with lymphoma. Drugs in feline medicine that can cause this condition include[6–9]:

- Chlorpropamide
- Vincristine
- Vinblastine
- Cyclophosphamide

- Opiates
- Thiazide diuretics
- Barbiturates
- Isoproterenol
- Mannitol
- Morphine
- Other diuretics

The abrupt withdrawal of steroids may also cause SIADH.[6–9]

When hyponatremia develops rapidly or serum sodium falls below 115 mg/dl, cats may develop mental status abnormalities, confusion, or coma. Serum and urine electrolytes, osmolality, and creatinine levels should be measured when SIADH is suspected.

DIAGNOSIS

Clinical signs include anorexia, nausea, and muscle stiffness progressing to confusion, neurologic signs, coma, and death. In patients with SIADH, urine sodium concentration is inappropriately high for the level of hyponatremia. Urine osmolality is therefore greater than plasma osmolality, but the urine specific gravity is never maximally dilute. BUN is usually low because of volume expansion. Hypophosphatemia may be noted. Adrenal and thyroid function should be normal.

TREATMENT

In an emergency setting, initial treatment should be directed at resolution of hyponatremia. Fluids should be restricted to ensure that the cat receives only the amount needed to maintain normal hydration and to keep serum sodium concentration within normal levels. In emergencies, demeclocycline may correct hyponatremia by reducing ADH stimulus for free water reabsorption at the collecting ducts. The most common side effect of demeclocycline is nausea and vomiting. Lithium carbonate and phenytoin have some use in treating SIADH. Hypertonic sodium chloride (3% to 5%) can be used in an emergency but may result in fluid and circulatory overload if not used carefully. Furosemide can be administered concurrently with hypertonic saline to reduce volume overload. It should be noted that rapid correction of hyponatremia may lead to neurologic damage. The following formula may help to determine the approximate amount of sodium needed to correct hyponatremia[10]:

$$Na \text{ for Replacement (mEq)} = \\ (\text{Desired Serum Sodium [mEq/L]} - \\ \text{Observed Serum Sodium [mEq/L]}) \times \\ \text{Body Weight (kg)} \times 0.6$$

HYPOGLYCEMIA

CLINICAL BRIEFING

Diagnosis	
History	Weakness, confusion, seizures, and coma.
Clinical Signs	CNS abnormalities, including weakness, seizures, and coma.
Diagnostics	MDB, fasting blood glucose and insulin levels, radiographs, abdominal ultrasonography, and (when patient is stable) exploratory surgery and biopsy.
Treatment	Treat the underlying cause while initiating supportive, symptomatic therapy.
	Constant rate glucose infusion, prednisone, diazoxide + hydrochlorothiazide.
	Propranolol may be useful in refractory cases.
	Partial pancreatectomy for insulinoma.

PREDISPOSING FACTORS

Fasting hypoglycemia in the face of hyperinsulinemia occurs most commonly with insulinomas, although other tumors of the liver (e.g., hepatomas, carcinomas) have also been associated with this condition.[6–12] Liver disease (including glycogen storage diseases) and sepsis may mimic hypoglycemia of malignancy. In addition, because red blood cells (RBCs) can metabolize glucose rapidly, delay in separating RBCs from serum may lead to artificially reduced serum glucose concentrations.

CLINICAL SIGNS

Before they present with seizures, coma, and impending death, most cats have a history of exhibiting signs of fatigue, weakness, dizziness, and confusion associated with paroxysmal lowering of blood glucose levels. Neurologic signs associated with hypoglycemia may mimic other central nervous system (CNS) abnormalities, such as brain tumors, brain trauma, meningitis, or metabolic encephalopathy.

Insulin-producing tumors can be diagnosed by identifying elevated insulin levels in association with low blood glucose concentrations. In some cases, the identification of malignancy-associated hypoglycemia may require periodic sampling during a 72 hour fast.[11] Diagnosis is confirmed when blood glucose is dramatically reduced while insulin levels are elevated. Although controversial, the amended insulin:glucose ratio has been advocated as a method to help diagnose insulin-producing tumors in domestic cats[12]:

$$\frac{(\text{Serum Insulin } [\mu U/ml] \times 100)}{(\text{Serum Glucose } [mg/dl] - 30)} = \text{Amended Insulin:Glucose Ratio}$$

Values above 30 suggest a diagnosis of insulinoma or other insulin-producing tumor.

KEY POINT

The most common cause of confirmed hypercalcemia in cats is neoplasia (lymphoma and squamous cell carcinoma).

TREATMENT[6–12]

In an emergency situation, medical management is often necessary before, during, and after definitive therapy, especially for insulinomas, which have a high metastatic rate. Glucose-containing fluids (2.5% to 5% dextrose in 0.9% NaCl or another isotonic crystalloid solution) should be administered to meet fluid requirement needs and maintain blood glucose concentrations within acceptable limits. It should be noted, however, that the administration of glucose may trigger the tumor to release more insulin, and thus a constant rate infusion of glucose to maintain normal serum glucose levels is preferred to intermittent administration of high-dose boluses. A cat with hypoglycemia (below 60 mg/dl) and experiencing seizures should be treated with 0.5 g dextrose/kg administered IV slowly over 3 to 5 minutes. Repeat doses may be needed.

Prednisone (0.5–2.0 mg/kg PO divided bid) is often effective in elevating blood glucose levels by inducing hepatic gluconeogenesis and decreasing peripheral utilization of glucose. Diazoxide (10–40 mg/kg PO divided bid) may effectively elevate blood glucose levels by directly inhibiting pancreatic insulin secretion and glucose uptake by tissues, enhancing epinephrine-induced glycogenolysis, and increasing the free fatty acid mobilization rate. The hyperglycemic effects of diazoxide can be potentiated by concurrent administration of hydrochlorothiazide (2–4 mg/kg/day). Propranolol (0.2–1.0 mg/kg PO tid), a β-adrenergic blocking agent, may also be effective in increasing blood glucose levels by inhibition of insulin release through the blockade of β-adrenergic receptors at the level of the pan-

creatic beta cell, inhibition of insulin release by membrane stabilization, and alteration of peripheral insulin receptor affinity. Combined surgical and medical management of pancreatic tumors has been associated with remission periods of 1 or more years. Once the patient is stabilized, surgical extirpation may be the best treatment for a hypoglycemia-causing tumor. Because many tumors (including insulinomas) that induce hypoglycemia as a paraneoplastic syndrome are malignant, surgery often is not curative. A partial pancreatectomy may be indicated for insulinomas; iatrogenic pancreatitis and diabetes mellitus are recognized complications (see Chapter 44).

KEY POINT

When possible, treat clinically significant hypoglycemia with a constant rate infusion of dextrose-containing fluids. A cat with hypoglycemia (less than 60 mg/dl) and experiencing seizures should be treated with 0.5 g dextrose/kg administered IV slowly over 3 to 5 minutes. Repeat doses may be needed.

REFERENCES

1. Ogilvie GK: Metabolic emergencies and the cancer patient, in Wingfield WE (ed): *Veterinary Emergency Medicine Secrets.* Philadelphia, Hanley and Belfus, 2001, pp 247–251.

2. Meuten DJ: Hypercalcemia. *Vet Clin North Am Small Anim Pract* 14:891–899, 1984.

3. Weir EC, Burtis WJ, Morris CA, et al: Isolation of a 16,000-dalton parathyroid hormone-like protein from two tumors causing humoral hypercalcemia of malignancy. *Endocrinology* 123:2744–2755, 1988.

4. Weir EC, Norrdin RW, Matus RE, et al: Humoral hypercalcemia of malignancy in canine lymphosarcoma. *Endocrinology* 122:602–610, 1988.

5. Kruger JM, Osborne CA, Polzin DJ: Treatment of hypercalcemia, in Kirk RW (ed): *Current Veterinary Therapy IX.* Philadelphia, WB Saunders, 1986, pp 75–90.

6. Lowitz BB: Paraneoplastic syndromes, in Haskell CM (ed): *Cancer Treatment,* ed 3. Philadelphia, WB Saunders, 1990, pp 841–849.

7. Savary KC, Price GS, Vaden SL: Hypercalcemia in cats: A retrospective study of 71 cases (1991–1997) *J Vet Intern Med* 14:184–189, 2000.

8. Glover DJ, Glick JH: Oncologic emergencies and special complications, in Calabrese P, Schein PJ, Rosenberg SA (eds): *Medical Oncology: Basic Principles and Clinical Management of Cancer.* New York, MacMillan, 1985, pp 1261–1326.

9. Felds ALA, Jese RG, Bergaagel DE: Metabolic emergencies, in DeVita VT, Hellman S, Rosenberg SA (eds): *Cancer Principles and Practice of Oncology.* Philadelphia, JB Lippincott, 1985, pp 1874–1876.

10. Franco-Saenz R: Endocrine syndromes, in Skeel RT (ed): *Handbook of Cancer Chemotherapy.* Boston, Little, Brown & Co, 1991, pp 379–404.

11. Leifer CE, Peterson ME, Matus RE, Patnaik AK: Hypoglycemia associated with nonislet cell tumors in 13 dogs. *JAVMA* 186:53–62, 1985.

12. Giger U, Gorman NT: Acute complications of cancer and cancer therapy, in Gorman NT (ed): *Oncology.* New York, Churchill Livingstone, 1986, pp 147–168.

13. Sheafor SE, Gamblin RM, Couto CG: Hypercalcemia in two cats with multiple myeloma. *JAAHA* 32:503–508, 1996.

14. McClain HM, Barsanti JA, Bartges JW: Hypercalcemia and calcium oxalate urolithiasis in cats: A report of five cases. *JAAHA* 35:297–301, 1999.

15. Marquez GA, Klausner JS, Osborne CA: Calcium oxalate urolithiasis in a cat with a functional parathyroid adenocarcinoma. *JAVMA* 206:817–819, 1995.

16. Mahoney CP, Cassady C, Weinberger E, et al: Humoral hypercalcemia due to an occult renal adenoma. *Pediatr Nephrol* 11:339–342, 1997.

17. Anderson TE, Legendre AM, McEntee MM: Probable hypercalcemia of malignancy in a cat with bronchogenic adenocarcinoma. *JAAHA* 36:52–55, 2000.

CHEMOTHERAPY-INDUCED ANAPHYLAXIS AND HYPERSENSITIVITY

28

Gregory K. Ogilvie and Antony S. Moore

CLINICAL BRIEFING

Diagnosis

History	Acute decompensation and collapse soon after the administration of a chemotherapeutic agent.
Clinical Signs	Pale or cyanotic mucous membranes, decreased capillary refill time, evidence of decreased cardiac output, alterations in heart rate, thready pulse, and cool extremities; profound pruritus and erythematous reaction are seen in patients with hypersensitivity reactions.
Diagnostics	Eliminate other causes via MDB and cardiac evaluation.

Therapy	Eliminate the underlying cause.
	Ensure a patent airway and adequate cardiac output.
	Establish vascular access.
	Initiate fluid therapy.
	Treat with dexamethasone $NaPO_4$ or hydrocortisone, diphenhydramine, and epinephrine (if indicated).

Although anaphylaxis or an anaphylaxis-like reaction can occur with any drug, these potentially life-threatening reactions usually happen soon after the administration of L-asparaginase. Hypersensitivity reactions can likewise occur with any drug but are most commonly associated with administration of doxorubicin,[1] paclitaxel,[2] and etoposide.[3]

L-Asparaginase is well known for inducing anaphylaxis, hemorrhagic pancreatitis, diabetes mellitus, and coagulopathies in cats, dogs, and humans; 48% of dogs given L-asparaginase intraperitoneally (IP) developed adverse effects,[4] and 30% of these dogs exhibited signs of anaphylaxis. These findings are similar to those in children given L-asparaginase intravenously (IV).[5] The same study showed that intramuscular (IM) administration of the drug completely eliminated signs associated with anaphylaxis without reducing remission rates (Figure 28-1).

L-Asparaginase-induced anaphylaxis and hypersensitivity are common because of enzyme immunogenicity. Anaphylaxis is usually caused by IgE-mediated mast cell degranulation; however, certain substances (e.g., bacterial and fungal cell walls) can trigger anaphylaxis by activating the alternate complement pathway. During the activation of this alternate pathway, complement factors C3a and C5a—known potent anaphylatoxins capable of degranulating mast cells

and basophils[6]—are formed. Although the exact mechanism of L-asparaginase-induced anaphylaxis in cats is largely unexplored, induction of anaphylaxis in children with acute lymphoblastic leukemia is believed to result from complement activation induced by formation of immune complexes of L-asparaginase and specific antibodies.[7] Anaphylaxis usually occurs within seconds to minutes after L-asparaginase administration.

The hypersensitivity reaction secondary to doxorubicin therapy is believed to be related to mast cell degranulation. Cremophor® EL and polysorbate 80, the carriers used in formulations of paclitaxel and etoposide, respectively, are responsible for the hypersensitivity reaction induced by these drugs.

PREDISPOSING FACTORS

One predisposing factor for anaphylaxis secondary to L-asparaginase or other drug therapy is a history of prior exposure to the drug. Because L-asparaginase is a ubiquitous bacterial product in mammals, anaphylaxis is possible after the first administration. In addition, anaphylactic and hypersensitivity reactions are worse in cats with a preexisting condition that results in a buildup of mast cells and eosinophils prior to drug treatment (e.g., atopy). As mentioned, a drug's administration route may be a contributing

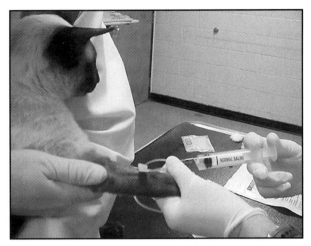

Figure 28-1: *Rapid IV administration of L-asparaginase can result in anaphylaxis; thus L-asparaginase should be administered IM when possible.*

factor to the development of anaphylactic or hypersensitivity reactions.

DIAGNOSIS

The most common clinical signs associated with drug-induced anaphylaxis are acute collapse and cardiovascular failure, which can lead to shock and death. The event usually occurs within minutes after a parenteral injection of the offending drug, although anaphylactic reactions that occur hours to days after drug therapy have been reported. Affected cats are generally pale and weak and usually exhibit such cardiac signs as bradycardia or tachycardia and a rapid, thready pulse. Mucous membranes are typically pale to cyanotic. Peripheral extremities are often cool to the touch, and blood pressure is low. Other causes of acute decompensation and collapse should be ruled out using the results of a minimum database and cardiac work-up.

Hypersensitivity reactions may result in profound pruritus during or after drug administration. Pruritus may result in head shaking, and there may be swelling of the ears, lips, or paws or near the injection site or area being treated. The erythematous reaction usually lasts for the duration of treatment. Occasionally, the edematous and erythematous reaction may last for hours after the treatment is finished.

THERAPY[6,8,9]

Prevention

Hypersensitivity reactions secondary to the administration of doxorubicin can be almost completely eliminated by diluting the drug in 50 ml of 0.9% NaCl and administering over 20 to 40 minutes. With this method, the incidence of hypersensitivity reaction is believed to be reduced to less than 3% in cats.[10] (Even if the possibility of a hypersensi-

tivity reaction is low, some clinicians recommend pretreatment with diphenhydramine and glucocorticoids to further reduce the prevalence of hypersensitivity reactions.

Reactions secondary to the carriers in paclitaxel and etoposide can be reduced by slowing the infusion rate and pretreating with dexamethasone (1–2 mg/kg IV), diphenhydramine (2–4 mg/kg IM), and cimetidine (2–4 mg/kg IV slowly) 1 hour before infusion of the chemotherapeutic agent. If a reaction is noted, the infusion can be discontinued temporarily until the patient is more comfortable and symptoms have abated.

Although L-asparaginase is notorious for inducing anaphylaxis, this is uncommonly reported in the cat. IV or IP administration is far more likely to induce anaphylaxis than IM or SQ administration. Data in dogs suggest that the drug is more effective for inducing remission when given IM instead of SQ.

Treatment

Anaphylaxis is a potentially fatal condition and should be treated immediately with supportive care, fluids, glucocorticoids, H₁ receptor antagonists, and epinephrine (Table 28-1). If anaphylaxis occurs, the responsible drug should not be administered to the patient again. The clinical approach to anaphylaxis in the feline cancer patient is summarized in Figure 28-2.

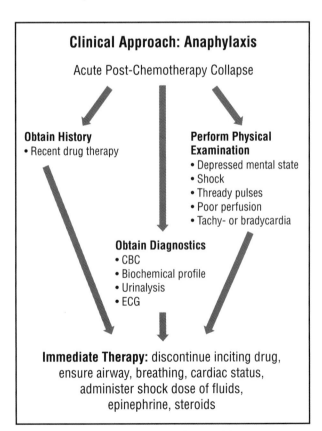

Clinical Approach: Anaphylaxis

Acute Post-Chemotherapy Collapse

Obtain History
• Recent drug therapy

Perform Physical Examination
• Depressed mental state
• Shock
• Thready pulses
• Poor perfusion
• Tachy- or bradycardia

Obtain Diagnostics
• CBC
• Biochemical profile
• Urinalysis
• ECG

Immediate Therapy: discontinue inciting drug, ensure airway, breathing, cardiac status, administer shock dose of fluids, epinephrine, steroids

Figure 28-2: *Clinical approach to anaphylaxis in feline cancer patients.*

TABLE 28-1
General Approach to the Treatment of Cats with Drug-Induced Anaphylaxis

General Principle	Specific Details
Evaluate the cat	Initiate physical examination and ascertain temporal relationship to the drug treatment; discontinue drug infusion or injection immediately if possible, and never repeat that medication
Ensure a patent airway and cardiac output	Initiate CPR if indicated: Establish airway, breathe for the cat after endotracheal intubation, and initiate cardiac compressions and drug therapy
Establish vascular access and initiate fluid and drug therapy	Establish indwelling IV catheter aseptically and initiate fluid therapy For shock: 40–60 ml/kg for the first hr, followed by 10–12 ml/kg/hr; adjust as needed thereafter Initiate drug therapy concurrently: 　Dexamethasone NaPO4 (2 mg/kg IV) 　Diphenhydramine (2–4 mg/kg IM; watch for toxicoses) 　Epinephrine (0.1–0.3 ml of a 1:1000 solution IV or IM for severe reactions)

Hypersensitivity reactions can be treated by terminating drug therapy. Reactions usually subside within minutes. The cat can then be treated with H_1 receptor antagonists (Table 28-1) before reinitiating drug treatment at a much slower rate.

KEY POINT

The risk of L-asparaginase-induced anaphylaxis can be reduced substantially by giving the drug IM rather than IV or IP.

REFERENCES

1. Ogilvie GK, Curtis C, Richardson RC, et al: Acute short term toxicity associated with the administration of doxorubicin to dogs with malignant tumors. *JAVMA* 195:1584–1587, 1989.
2. Ogilvie GK, Walters LM, Powers BE, et al: Organ toxicity of NBT Taxol in the rat and dog: A preclinical study. *Proc 13th Annu Vet Canc Soc Conf*.90–91, 1993.
3. Ogilvie GK, Cockburn CA, Tranquilli WJ, Reschke RW: Hypotension and cutaneous reactions associated with etoposide administration in the dog. *Am J Vet Res* 49:1367–1370, 1988.
4. Teske E, Rutteman GR, van Heerde P, Misdorp W: Polyethylene glycol-L-asparaginase versus native L-asparaginase in canine non-Hodgkin's lymphoma. *Eur J Cancer* 26:891–895, 1990.
5. Nesbit M, Chard R, Evans A, et al: Evaluation of intramuscular versus intravenous administration of L-asparaginase in childhood leukemia. *Am J Pediatr Hematol Oncol* 1:9–13, 1979.
6. Degen MA: Acute hypersensitivity reactions, in Kirk RW (ed): *Current Veterinary Therapy X*. Philadelphia, WB Saunders, 1989, pp 537–542.
7. Fabry U, Korholz D, Jurgens H, et al: Anaphylaxis to L-asparaginase during treatment for acute lymphoblastic leukemia in children. Evidence of a complement-mediated mechanism. *Pediatr Res* 19:400–408, 1985.
8. Ogilvie GK, Atwater SW, Ciekot PA, et al: Prevalence of anaphylaxis associated with the intramuscular administration of L-asparaginase to 81 dogs with cancer: 1989–1991. *JAAHA* 3662–3665, 1994.
9. Ogilvie GK: Chemotherapy induced anaphylaxis, in Wingfield WE (ed): *Veterinary Emergency Medicine Secrets*. Philadelphia, Hanley and Belfus, 2001, pp 257–258.
10. Animal Cancer Center, Colorado State University: Unpublished data.

ONCOLOGIC EMERGENCIES

EXTRAVASATION OF CHEMOTHERAPEUTIC AGENTS

29

Gregory K. Ogilvie and Antony S. Moore

CLINICAL BRIEFING

Diagnosis	
History	Pain or discomfort during infusion and swelling at the injection site.
Clinical Signs	Swelling and discomfort followed by severe tissue necrosis and development of a nonhealing lesion 1 to 4 weeks after infusion.
Therapy	Stop the infusion, leave catheter in place, and aspirate as much fluid and drug as possible from the site.
	Administer antidote:
	For doxorubicin: Apply cold packs; possibly use topical DMSO or infiltrate area with intralesional hydrocortisone.
	For vinca alkaloids: Apply warm compresses, infuse with saline, and instill hyaluronidase; possibly use topical DMSO or infiltrate area with intralesional

---

Many chemotherapeutic agents are known to induce significant tissue injury after extravasation. Some of these agents are severe, irreversible vesicants whereas others induce tissue irritation (see Box, below).

Preventing extravasation is the best "management" method. Atraumatic placement of "true" catheters, appropriate use of butterfly catheters, and adequate patient restraint coupled with monitoring during administration will prevent extravasations and the devastating consequences thereof. Management of extravasations in human and feline medicine is anecdotal and extremely controversial. Despite this controversy, guidelines (Table 29-1) have been established for clinical use.

PREDISPOSING FACTORS

As expected, accurate and secure "first stick" catheter placement is absolutely essential when administering drugs that can cause tissue damage if extravasated perivascularly. Generally, only small-gauge (22 to 23 ga) indwelling intravenous (IV) catheters should be used when treatment volumes exceed 1 ml; 23 to 25 ga butterfly needles can be used for administering small volumes of drugs (e.g., vincristine). Everyone involved in patient care should note when and where blood samples are taken by venipuncture and where catheters have been placed previously. This prevents administration of chemotherapeutic agents through veins that may leak because of previous procedures. Drawing blood samples from peripheral veins should be avoided if at all possible to preserve these veins for catheter access. Only catheters that have been placed very recently should be used for administration of chemotherapeutic agents.

Extreme care should be taken when administering drugs to all cats; however, veins in some patients (e.g., extremely debilitated animals, diabetics, some elderly cats, patients that have been receiving weekly or biweekly therapy for a significant period) are even more fragile. Catheters should be checked for patency by injecting a large volume of saline (e.g., 12–15 ml) before and after drug administration. In addition, it is mandatory that catheters be visually monitored closely and checked for patency throughout drug infusion.

DIAGNOSIS

Usually, there is no doubt whether an extravasation has

Potential Vesicants and Irritants Used in Feline Oncology[1-4]

Actinomycin D	Mechlorethamine
Daunorubicin	Mithramycin
Doxorubicin	Mitoxantrone
Epirubicin	Vinblastine
Etoposide	Vincristine
Idarubicin	

TABLE 29-1
General Treatment Guidelines for Extravasated Drugs[1-4]

General Procedures	Details
Minimize amount of drug at site	Do not remove the catheter or needle
	Use a syringe to immediately withdraw as much drug as possible from the tissue, tubing, and catheter
	Administer appropriate antidote (listed below) or sterile saline to neutralize or dilute the drug

Specific Agents	Antidote
Doxorubicin, daunorubicin, epirubicin, idarubicin, mechlorethamine, and actinomycin D	Apply ice or cold compresses to affected area for 6–10 hr to inhibit vesicant cytotoxicity; *do not apply heat*
	Controversial procedures:
	Topical DMSO
	Infiltrate area with 1 mg/kg hydrocortisone
	Surgical debridement, plastic surgery, or limb amputation may be indicated in rare cases
Vincristine, vinblastine, and etoposide	Infiltrate area with 1 ml of hyaluronidase (150 U/ml) for every milliliter extravasated to enhance absorption and disperse the drug; inject 0.9% NaCl to dilute out drug
	Apply warm compresses to the site for several hours to enhance systemic absorption
	Controversial procedures:
	Topical DMSO
	Infiltrate area with 1 mg/kg hydrocortisone

occurred. Some agents are very caustic when given perivascularly, and cats may vocalize or physically react to pain at the injection site. Treatment for extravasation must begin immediately. Evidence of tissue necrosis generally does not appear for 1 to 10 days after extravasation and may progress for 3 to 4 weeks. The lesions occur early with vinca alkaloids and late with anthracycline antibiotics (e.g., doxorubicin). Lesions may begin as mild erythema and progress to open, draining wounds that will not heal without extensive debridement and plastic surgery; such treatment should not be initiated until all damage is evident (i.e., weeks to months after the perivascular slough begins)

TREATMENT[1-4]

Everyone involved with the administration of chemotherapeutic agents should be aware of procedures for treating extravasation. Such procedures (i.e., immediately aspirating as much drug as possible from the injection site; instilling saline and applying hot compresses if vincristine or vinblastine was administered perivascularly; placing ice packs around the area in question if doxorubicin was administered perivascularly) should be posted in a common area, and all needed materials should be readily available and accessible. Because of their extensive use in feline practice, doxorubicin and the vinca alkaloids are the most common causes of perivascular sloughing. Unfortunately, no method effectively eliminates tissue necrosis. For example,

sodium bicarbonate, corticosteroids, dimethyl sulfoxide (DMSO), α-tocopherol, N-acetylcysteine, glutathione, lidocaine, diphenhydramine, cimetidine, propranolol, and isoproterenol are not effective for treating doxorubicin extravasations.[4]

Once tissue damage is identified, an Elizabethan collar and bandages with nonstick pads are essential to allow the area to heal without self-trauma. Bandages should be changed daily as long as the area is draining or has the potential for infection. If a bacterial infection is noted, culture and sensitivity testing and appropriate administration of antimicrobials are essential. Frequent cleansing and debridement may be necessary. In some cases, reconstructive surgical repair techniques are needed. In the event of doxorubicin extravasations, limb amputation may become necessary.

REFERENCES

1. Ogilvie GK: Extravasation of chemotherapeutic agents, in Wingfield WE (ed): *Veterinary Emergency Medicine Secrets.* Philadelphia, Hanley and Belfus, 2001, pp 259–260.
2. Wittes RE, Hubbard SM: Chemotherapy: The properties and uses of single agents, in Wittes RE (ed): *Manual of Oncologic Therapeutics 1991/1992.* Philadelphia, JB Lippincott, 1991, pp 116–121.
3. Hubbard SM, Jenkins JF: Chemotherapy administration: Practical guidelines, in Chabner BA, Collins JM (eds): *Cancer Chemotherapy: Principals and Practice.* Philadelphia, JB Lippincott, 1990, pp 449–464.
4. Hubbard S, Duffy P, Seipp C: Administration of cancer treatments: Practical guide for physicians and nurses, in DeVita VT Jr, Hellman S, Rosenberg S (eds): *Cancer: Principles and Practice of Oncology,* ed 3. Philadelphia, JB Lippincott, 1989, pp 2369–2402.

ONCOLOGIC EMERGENCIES

CHEMOTHERAPY-INDUCED ACUTE RENAL FAILURE

30

Gregory K. Ogilvie and Antony S. Moore

CLINICAL BRIEFING

Diagnosis	
History	Acute decompensation, anorexia, and vomiting.
Clinical Signs	Oliguria accompanied by increased body weight and increased central venous pressure may be seen following fluid therapy; uremic gastritis, uremic breath.
Diagnostics	MDB, measure central venous pressure, and quantify urine output.
Therapy	Treat or eliminate the underlying cause.
	Correct dehydration.
	Administer fluids to meet daily needs and external losses and induce mild to moderate diuresis.
	Correct acid-base and electrolyte abnormalities.
	Treat oliguria with furosemide, osmotic diuretics, and dopamine in 5% dextrose (if indicated).

Doxorubicin and methotrexate are commonly associated with renal failure in feline patients. Renal failure can also be induced by a variety of malignant conditions (e.g., transitional cell carcinoma, renal lymphoma).

Doxorubicin induces acute and chronic renal failure in cats. One study suggested that renal damage in cats is dose dependent, but this observation has not been repeated. Renal failure in cats has been induced with variable cumulative doses of doxorubicin. Another unrelated drug, methotrexate, is eliminated primarily by the kidneys and has been associated with the development of nephrotoxicity.

Renal failure in cancer patients may also be due to causes unrelated to chemotherapy. Cats with transitional cell carcinoma of the bladder, urethra, or prostate commonly have urethral obstruction that may lead to hydroureter, hydronephrosis, and renal dysfunction. The concurrent septic cystitis seen in most cats with bladder tumors may induce secondary pyelonephritis, which can result in acute and chronic renal failure. Renal lymphoma may cause transient renal insufficiency, which resolves upon successful treatment.

MDB = minimum database; includes CBC, biochemical profile, urinalysis, FeLV/FIV serology, T$_4$ testing, and thoracic radiographs (three views).

PREDISPOSING FACTORS

The most common predisposing factors associated with the development of acute renal failure in feline medicine are cancer and administration of nephrotoxic drugs, including chemotherapeutic agents.[1,2] Therefore when chemotherapeutic agents are used in feline patients, other nephrotoxic drugs, such as aminoglycosides and piroxicam, should be avoided. The vast majority of feline oncology patients are geriatric and thus may have preexisting renal disease. This must always be taken into consideration when designing a therapeutic protocol and selecting and administering medications. Other risk factors associated with the development of acute and chronic renal failure in cats are decreased cardiac output, urinary tract infection, sepsis, dehydration, fever, liver disease, hypokalemia, and hypercalcemia.

DIAGNOSIS

Acute and chronic renal failure are a result of decreased glomerular filtration rate, with or without tubular damage. The parameters used to diagnose these syndromes are related to damage of the glomeruli and tubules. Because at least two thirds of kidney function must be abnormal before renal disease becomes evident, significant renal disease may be present for variable periods before clinical, hematologic, and biochemical abnormalities are identified.

Acute renal failure may be associated with nonoliguria, oliguria, or anuria. Regardless of the amount of urine, it is usually isosthenuric or minimally concentrated with a high sodium content (<40 mEq/L). Glucose, protein, and renal epithelial cells may be detected in urine. Serum urea nitrogen, creatinine, and phosphorus concentrations rise acutely. In oliguric or anuric renal failure, body weight, heart rate, and central venous pressure may increase if fluids are administered before urine flow is reestablished.

THERAPY[2,3]

The best treatment for acute or chronic renal failure is prevention. Substantial data exist to show that chemotherapy-induced nephrotoxicity can be reduced and almost eliminated with adequate hydration. The incidence of doxorubicin- and methotrexate-induced renal failure can be reduced by avoiding these agents in cats with preexisting renal disease and by increasing the duration of administration.

The initial goals for treating drug- and tumor-related acute renal failure in cats are to discontinue all potentially nephrotoxic drugs, document pre- or postrenal abnormalities, and initiate fluid therapy. The primary objectives of fluid therapy are to correct deficits (e.g., dehydration) and excesses (e.g., volume overload) seen in oliguric renal failure, supply maintenance needs, and supplement ongoing losses due to vomiting and diarrhea. Each cat must be assessed carefully, and a treatment plan must be tailored based on the patient's hydration status, cardiovascular performance, and biochemical data. Table 30-1 provides a general approach to cats in renal failure

Maintenance fluid requirements vary from 44 to 110 ml/kg/day; smaller cats require the larger amount. A sim-

TABLE 30-1
General Approach to Cats in Renal Failure

General Procedure	Specifics
Cease administration of nephrotoxins	For example, discontinue methotrexate, doxorubicin, and aminoglycosides; avoid anesthesia
Assess patient status	CBC, urinalysis, and biochemical profile Determine: • Percentage of dehydration • Amount of ongoing losses (e.g., vomiting, diarrhea, blood loss) • Maintenance fluid requirements • Electrolyte and biochemical abnormalities • Cardiovascular performance • Urine output
Select and administer specific fluids	Tailor therapy to the individual needs of each patient: • Administer isotonic polyionic fluid initially, preferably potassium-free (e.g., NaCl) • Correct dehydration over 6–8 hr to prevent further renal ischemia while watching carefully for pathologic oliguria and subsequent volume overload • Meet maintenance requirements (approximately 66 ml/kg/day) • Meet ongoing losses (e.g., due to vomiting and diarrhea) • Induce a mild to moderate diuresis
Monitor urine output and ensure adequate output	Collect urine via a metabolism cage or indwelling catheter For patients with inadequate urine output (<2.0 ml/kg/hr), administer: • Mannitol or 50% dextrose (0.5–1.0 g/kg via slow IV bolus) • Furosemide (2–4 mg/kg IV q1–3h prn) • Dopamine (1–3 µg/kg/min IV [50 mg dopamine in 500 ml of 5% dextrose = 100 µg/ml solution])
Correct acid-base and electrolyte abnormalities	Initiate specific treatment to correct malignancy-induced hypercalcemia, if identified
Provide mild to moderate diuresis	If urine output is 2–5 ml/kg/hr, monitor body weight, heart and respiratory rates, and central venous pressure for signs of overhydration
Consider peritoneal dialysis if not responsive	Temporary or chronic ambulatory peritoneal dialysis with specific dialysate solution may be helpful
Initiate long-term plans	Continue diuresis until BUN and creatinine normalize or until these values stop improving despite aggressive therapy; in the clinically stable patient, gradually taper fluids Control hyperphosphatemia, if indicated Consider cimetidine (2.5 mg/kg PO or IV bid) to correct hyperacidity

ONCOLOGIC EMERGENCIES

pler formula is to use 66 ml/kg/day plus sufficient fluids to replace external losses, such as through vomiting and diarrhea. This amount is needed for daily maintenance. In cats with renal failure, 1.5 to 3 times this amount of fluid is administered daily to achieve diuresis, the success of which can be monitored by documenting adequate urine output (more than 2 ml/kg/hr). In addition to meeting daily needs and replacing ongoing losses, fluid therapy also needs to correct dehydration. The percentage of dehydration should be determined, and approximately 75% of the fluid needed to correct dehydration should be administered during the first 24 hours. Fluid therapy should be altered to correct electrolyte and acid-base abnormalities. Because systemic hyperkalemia often develops in cats with acute renal failure, potassium-containing fluids are generally not advised in these patients. Until more is known about the systemic effects of sepsis, lactate-containing fluids should be avoided—sepsis and cancer are associated with hyperlactatemia, which worsens with the administration of lactate-containing fluids.

If oliguric renal failure is present, a diligent and aggressive effort to increase urine output should be made. This can be done by first increasing glomerular filtration rate and renal blood flow. Additionally, osmotic diuresis can increase urine flow. If urine output is less than 0.5 to 2.0 ml/kg/hour despite aggressive fluid therapy, furosemide should be administered every 1 to 3 hours. Furosemide increases the glomerular filtration rate and enhances diuresis in many cats. If furosemide is ineffective, mannitol or 50% dextrose can be used as an osmotic diuretic to enhance urine production. The advantage of dextrose over mannitol is that dextrose can be detected on a urine glucose test strip. If furosemide and osmotic diuretics are not effective, dopamine in 5% dextrose can be administered via constant rate infusion. Dopamine enhances renal blood flow and increases urine output secondarily.

If the cat does not respond to the preceding therapies, peritoneal dialysis may be necessary. Temporary or chronic ambulatory peritoneal dialysis with specific dialysate solutions may be helpful in this situation.

Cats that are being diuresed should be monitored for signs of volume overload (increased body weight, heart and respiratory rates, and central venous pressure). Blood urea nitrogen (BUN) and creatinine should be monitored and diuresis continued until these values either normalize or at least stabilize. Therapy should then be tapered over several days, and a home treatment plan that includes avoiding nephrotoxic drugs, feeding a high-quality, low-protein diet, maintaining a low-stress environment, and providing fresh, clean water ad libitum should be developed. Treatment for hyperphosphatemia (such as phosphate binders) may be necessary, and cimetidine may be helpful in controlling gastric ulceration.

REFERENCES

1. Cotter SM, Kanki PJ, Simon M: Renal disease in five tumor-bearing cats treated with Adriamycin. *JAAHA* 21:405–412, 1985.
2. Ogilvie GK: Chemotherapy induced renal failure, in Wingfield WE (ed): *Veterinary Emergency Medicine Secrets*. Philadelphia, Hanley and Belfus, 2001, pp 261–264.
3. Kirby R: Acute renal failure as a complication of the critically ill animal. *Vet Clin North Am Small Anim Pract* 19:1189–1208, 1989.

Cancer is a documented common cause of sickness and debilitation in cats. More recently, it has become obvious that cancer may induce clinical signs not only directly by altering the body's structure or function but also by indirect means that may actually be more debilitating than the consequences of the primary tumor. These indirect effects are known as *paraneoplastic syndromes* and are of profound importance to practicing veterinarians because of their devastating effects on cats with cancer. The most common paraneoplastic syndromes in feline medicine are thought to be caused by the production of polypeptide hormones, the most common of which have endocrine-like effects. Other paraneoplastic syndromes include hematologic and cutaneous manifestations, hypergammaglobulinemia, cachexia, fever, neurologic syndromes, and hypertrophic osteopathy.

Detection of hormones or hormone-like substances that are directly elaborated or indirectly induced by the tumor can be used as markers for the presence of a tumor. The most obvious examples are the detection of parathormone or insulin-like substances. Clinical evidence of an endocrine-associated paraneoplastic syndrome can also be used as a tumor marker. Complete workups of each condition are essential to unravel the typically vague clinical signs and subtle findings on physical examination. Therapy should primarily be directed at eliminating the underlying malignancy, although modulation of tumor-induced hormones or hormone-like substances is an attractive alternative. In many cases, specific treatment of the paraneoplastic syndrome itself may be essential for the cat's survival.

ENDOCRINE MANIFESTATIONS OF MALIGNANCY

31

Gregory K. Ogilvie and Antony S. Moore

ALTERED CALCIUM HOMEOSTASIS

HYPERCALCEMIA OF MALIGNANCY (also see Chapter 27)

<table>
<tr><td colspan="2" align="center">C L I N I C A L   B R I E F I N G</td></tr>
<tr><td>Diagnosis
History</td><td>Often nonspecific; may include lethargy, anorexia, and vomiting. Increased water consumption and urination are often less obvious than in other companion animals.</td></tr>
<tr><td>Clinical Signs</td><td>Often quite subtle but may include polyuria, polydipsia, vomiting, constipation, bradycardia, skeletal muscle weakness, depression, stupor, coma, and (occasionally) seizures.</td></tr>
<tr><td>Diagnostics</td><td>Laboratory evidence of hypercalcemia and secondary renal damage. The underlying cause of this electrolyte abnormality may be identified via MDB, measurement of ionized calcium levels, bone marrow aspiration, radiographs, ACTH stimulation test, and, if indicated, measurement of PTH or PTH-rP concentrations. Calcium oxalate urolithiasis may be identified.</td></tr>
<tr><td>Treatment</td><td>Treat the underlying cause.
Therapy depends on the severity of clinical and laboratory signs. Consider saline diuresis and furosemide; give prednisone only after a diagnosis has been made.
In refractory cases, consider salmon calcitonin, bisphosphonates, gallium nitrate, and mithramycin.</td></tr>
</table>

Cancer is an underrecognized cause of hypercalcemia in cats.[1-9] In one study of 71 cats with hypercalcemia, the three most common diagnoses were neoplasia (n = 21), renal failure (n = 18), and urolithiasis (n = 11).[4] Primary hyperparathyroidism was diagnosed in 4 cats. Lymphoma and squamous cell carcinoma were the tumors identified most frequently. Calcium oxalate uroliths were diagnosed in 8 of 11 cats with urolithiasis.

Hypercalcemia can be an oncologic emergency and is covered in that context in Chapter 27. The tumors most often associated with the paraneoplastic syndrome of hypercalcemia are squamous cell carcinoma, lymphoma, primary lung tumors, and multiple myeloma, but any neoplastic process has the potential to elevate serum calcium levels. Granulomatous disease, oxalate urolithiasis, and parathyroid tumors are other diagnostic differentials. Parathyroid adenomas have been identified as malignancy-associated causes of hypercalcemia in dogs and cats, but this is not considered a true neoplastic syndrome because parathyroids normally produce parathormone.

Potential causes of hypercalcemia of malignancy include tumor-induced production of[1-6]:

- Osteoclast-activating factors (OAFs), such as interleukins, tumor necrosis factor, lymphotoxin, colony-stimulating factors, and interferon-γ
- 1,25-Dihydroxycholecalciferol (vitamin D)
- Prostaglandins
- Transforming growth factors
- Parathyroid hormone-related peptide (PTH-rP)

The actual cause of hypercalcemia is not as well described in feline patients as in canine or human medicine.

Clinical Presentation

Nonspecific clinical signs predominate.[1,6] Polyuria is not as commonly recognized in cats as in other species. Signs can progress from lethargy, anorexia, nausea, and fatigue to dehydration, azotemia, and coma secondary to hypercalcemia-induced renal failure. Decreased sensitivity of the distal convoluted tubules and collecting ducts to antidiuretic hormone (ADH) causes polyuria and secondary polydipsia. Vasoconstrictive properties of calcium decrease renal blood flow and glomerular filtration rate, resulting in degenerative changes, necrosis, and calcification of the renal

168

epithelium.[1-6] Other clinical signs (e.g., constipation, muscle weakness, central nervous system signs) may arise as a direct effect of the electrolyte abnormality.

Diagnosis (Figure 31-1)

The diagnostic workup should always include a hemogram, biochemical profile, ionized calcium, urinalysis, radiographs, and ultimately bone marrow aspiration and determination of parathormone (PTH) and PTH-rP concentrations. The former is elevated in renal disease and primary hyperparathyroid disease, whereas the latter may be increased in neoplastic disease. PTH-rP appears to be less reliable in cats than in other species, such as dogs. In one study, cats with neoplasia were shown to have a higher serum calcium concentration (13.5 ± 2.5 mg/dl) than cats with renal failure with or without urolithiasis (11.5 ± 0.4 mg/dl).[8] Serum phosphorus concentrations were higher in cats with renal failure than in cats with neoplasia. Despite the fact that the majority of cats with uroliths were azotemic, their serum urea nitrogen (SUN) and creatinine concentrations and urine specific gravity differed from that of cats with renal failure. In essence, cats with renal failure had more advanced signs.

While blood work is important, clinical pathology must be combined with a good history and physical examination to confirm or eliminate the following differentials[1-7]:

- Laboratory error
- Interpretation error
- Hyperproteinemia due to dehydration (controversial)
- Acute renal failure
- Vitamin D and calcium toxicosis
- Granulomatous disorders, such as nocardiosis
- Nonneoplastic bone disorders
- Hypoadrenocorticism

- Calcium oxalate urolithiasis
- True hyperparathyroidism

MDB = minimum database; includes CBC, biochemical profile, urinalysis, FeLV/FIV serology, T_4 testing, and thoracic radiographs (three views).

Calcium values must be interpreted in relation to serum albumin and blood pH. The following correction formula accounts for albumin:

$$\text{Adjusted Calcium (mg/dl)} = (\text{Calcium [mg/dl]} - \text{Albumin [g/dl]}) + 3.5$$

Clinical signs associated with hypercalcemia are intensified when the electrolyte is in the free, ionized fraction, which is increased by acidosis.

Ultimately, it may be difficult to identify malignancy as the cause of hypercalcemia. Laboratory abnormalities that may accompany true hypercalcemia include:

- Elevated SUN
- Normo- or hypophosphatemia
- Hypercalciuria
- Hyperphosphaturia
- Hypernatriuria
- Decreased glomerular filtration rate (determined by exogenous or endogenous creatinine clearance study)

PARANEOPLASTIC SYNDROMES

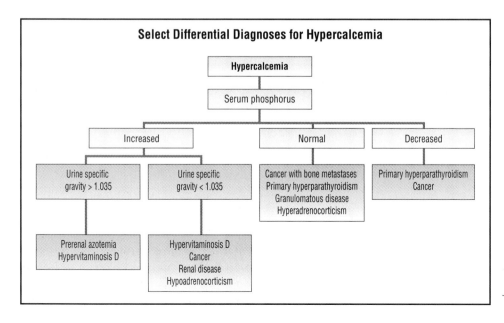

Figure 31-1: *The most common differentials and laboratory findings associated with hypercalcemia in cats.*

Treatment[1-9]

Eliminating the tumor is the first and most important therapy for hypercalcemia of malignancy. Associated clinical signs can range from very mild to a full oncologic emergency. The approach to the treatment of this condition depends on the severity of the clinical signs.

Mild Hypercalcemia, Minimal Clinical Signs

- Restore and maintain hydration and ensure calciuresis, especially during anesthesia and surgery.
- Monitor calcium, phosphorus, and creatinine levels until the underlying cause can be identified and eliminated or until the hypercalcemia and subsequent clinical signs progress to the point that additional therapy is required.
- Avoid nephrotoxic drugs.

Moderate Hypercalcemia, Moderate Clinical Signs

More aggressive management is indicated in these patients:

- Administer IV saline in volumes that exceed daily maintenance needs (>44–66 ml/kg/day) and result in urine output exceeding 2 ml/kg/hour.
- Consider adding potassium chloride to 0.9% NaCl to prevent potassium depletion (20–30 mEq KCl/L of 0.9% NaCl).
- Repeatedly assess all electrolytes, SUN, and serum creatinine concentrations to determine necessary adjustments of fluid rate, type, and potassium content.
- Monitor patients carefully for signs of overhydration and congestive heart failure. IV administration of 0.9% NaCl effectively expands the extracellular fluid volume, increases glomerular filtration rate, decreases renal tubular calcium reabsorption, and enhances calcium and sodium excretion.

MDB = minimum database; includes CBC, biochemical profile, urinalysis, FeLV/FIV serology, T₄ testing, and thoracic radiographs (three views).

In refractory cases, administer:

- Furosemide (2.2–8.8 mg/kg IV or PO bid; often administered concurrently with NaCl to well-hydrated, hypercalcemic patients to prevent calcium reabsorption in the kidneys). This drug is also effective for treating many cases of anuria or oliguria. Furosemide inhibits calcium resorption at the level of the ascending loop of Henle.
- Prednisone (0.5–1.0 mg/kg PO bid) or any other glucocorticoid to inhibit OAF, prostaglandins, vitamin D, and the absorption of calcium across the intestinal tract. Glucocorticoids are cytotoxic to lymphoma and myeloma cells and therefore should not be used until suspect tissue has been submitted for histology and a diagnosis made. Glucocorticoids may also obscure the extent of the tumor and thus delay diagnosis of the neoplasm and prevent accurate staging and definitive therapy.

KEY POINT

Obtain blood and urine samples before any therapy, especially steroids, is instituted to improve the chances of correctly identifying electrolyte abnormalities.

Severe Hypercalcemia, Severe Clinical Signs

This is considered an oncologic emergency; refer to Chapter 27 for specific recommendations. Briefly, treatment is the same as for moderate hypercalcemia. In addition, the use of such agents as calcitonin, mithramycin, prostaglandin-synthetase inhibitors, bisphosphonates, gallium nitrate, and oral phosphate may be considered to control hypercalcemia.[1]

- Calcitonin (4–8 MRC U/kg SQ) can cause a dramatic, rapid reduction in calcium levels; levels may remain low for days.
- Mithramycin (25 µg/kg IV once or twice weekly given through a newly placed IV line); at higher dosages, this agent has anticancer properties.
- Prostaglandin-synthetase inhibitors.
- Bisphosphonates are being explored for use in treating hypercalcemia of malignancy. Etidronate disodium is the most commonly used member of this class in human medicine. Early work in human patients with severe hypercalcemia and severe clinical signs suggests that bisphosphonates are effective in long-term control of chronic hypercalcemia. Unlike phosphates, which bind calcium in the gastrointestinal tract, bisphosphonates bind to hydroxyapatite in bone and inhibit the dissolution of crystals.[1,9]
- Gallium nitrate has recently been approved in human medicine for the treatment of hypercalcemia; it appears to inhibit bone resorption by binding to and reducing the solubility of hydroxyapatite crystals.[1,9]

HYPOCALCEMIA (also see Chapter 24)

C L I N I C A L B R I E F I N G	
Diagnosis	
History	Usually asymptomatic; occasional lethargy and anorexia; may occur after chemical, surgical, or (rarely) radioactive iodine bilateral thyroidectomy.
Clinical Signs	Usually normal; occasional weakness, depression, and seizures.
Diagnostics	MDB, measurement of ionized calcium levels, and (if indicated) PTH concentration.
Treatment	Rarely requires direct treatment; treat the underlying cause.
	In severe cases, administer 10% calcium gluconate IV; oral calcium supplementation, with or without vitamin D, may be effective.

Hypocalcemia secondary to a malignancy or its treatment is much more common in human than feline medicine.

Clinical Presentation

Hypocalcemia is a rare complication of bilateral thyroidectomy and inadvertent parathyroidectomy in cats and an uncommon cause of clinical signs related to cancer. Other causes include magnesium deficiency, which can occur because of prolonged intestinal drainage procedures, parenteral hyperalimentation without magnesium supplementation, and severe liver disease. Hypomagnesemia seems to impair the effect of PTH on its target organs, resulting in hypocalcemia. Tumor lysis syndrome may be associated with hypocalcemia secondary to elevated phosphate levels and can result in partial or generalized seizures; this extremely rare (or underrecognized) condition is an oncologic emergency and is discussed in Chapter 24.

Diagnosis

A diagnosis is made based on an MDB and ionized calcium and (if indicated) PTH levels.

Treatment[1–9]

The underlying cause of hypocalcemia should be identified and treated as soon as possible. Cancer-induced hypocalcemia rarely results in clinical signs or requires therapy. If clinical signs are present, calcium should be administered via slow IV (i.e., 1.0–1.5 ml 10% calcium gluconate/kg given over 10–20 min; maintenance therapy, 2 ml/kg given over 6–8 hr) with electrocardiographic monitoring followed by oral calcium supplements (i.e., calcium lactate, 400–600 mg/kg/day divided into three or four doses). Vitamin D supplementation (1,25-dihydroxycholecalciferol, 0.03 µg/kg/day PO) may be indicated to aid calcium absorption.

ALTERED GLUCOSE HOMEOSTASIS

HYPOGLYCEMIA (also see Chapter 27)

C L I N I C A L B R I E F I N G	
Diagnosis	
History	Uncommon condition; clients may observe subtle clinical signs (e.g., weakness, confusion); seizures are rare.
Clinical Signs	Clinical signs are often paroxysmal and subtle in the early phases of the disease and are followed by seizures, coma, and death.
Diagnostics	MDB, measurement of fasting blood glucose and insulin levels, radiographs, abdominal ultrasonography, exploratory surgery, and biopsy.
Treatment	Treat the underlying cause, typically via surgery.
	Feed frequent meals composed of complex carbohydrates.
	Administer dextrose (infusion), prednisone, somatostatin, and diazoxide ± hydrochlorothiazide.
	Propranolol may be of value in refractory cases.

Hypoglycemia (blood glucose <70 mg/dl), an underrecognized and uncommon paraneoplastic syndrome in cats, can cause a variety of clinical signs ranging from generalized weakness to seizures and death.[9–13] Insulinoma is the most common malignancy associated with hypoglycemia in cats. Nonlymphoid hepatic tumors are a common cause of hypoglycemia in other species, but this tumor type is not as commonly recognized in cats. Insulinomas produce excessive quantities of insulin, which causes very low blood glucose levels. In contrast, hypoglycemia of extrapancreatic tumors is associated with low to low-normal insulin levels.[9–13] Extrapancreatic tumors cause hypoglycemia by secretion of an insulin-like substance, by accelerating the utilization of glucose by the tumor, and by failure of gluconeogenesis and/or glycogenolysis by the liver.[9–13] The most common nonmalignant causes of hypoglycemia include hyperinsulinism, hepatic dysfunction, adrenocortical insufficiency, hypopituitarism, extrapancreatic tumors, starvation, sepsis, and laboratory error. Rarely, hypoadrenocorticism secondary to lymphoma infiltration of the adrenal glands can cause hypoglycemia.[11]

KEY POINT

Subtle neurologic signs, such as weakness and facial twitching, predominate in cats with hypoglycemia because carbohydrate reserve is limited in neural tissue and brain function depends on an adequate quantity of glucose.

Clinical Signs

Hypoglycemia in cats can result in very subtle clinical signs if the condition progresses very gradually. Acute onset results in overt clinical signs that can include such neurologic signs as weakness, disorientation, behavioral changes, facial twitching, seizures, coma, and death.[1,9–13] These signs generally occur in cats when blood glucose falls below 45 mg/dl. Catecholamines, growth hormone, glucocorticoids, and glucagon are released secondary to hypoglycemia and activate compensatory mechanisms to combat hypoglycemia by promoting glycogenolysis.

Diagnosis

It is not currently possible to identify the mechanism responsible for inducing hypoglycemia associated with many extrapancreatic tumors. Insulin-producing tumors (e.g., insulinomas) may be diagnosed by identifying elevated insulin levels in association with low blood glucose concentrations.[1,9–13] Frequent evaluation of glucose and insulin concentrations during a 72 hour fast may be necessary to accurately diagnose insulinoma in some cats. Although

quite controversial and certainly not validated in cats, the amended insulin:glucose ratio has been advocated as a method to help diagnose insulin-producing tumors:

$$\frac{\text{Serum Insulin}\ (\mu U/ml) \times 100}{\text{Serum Glucose}\ (mg/dl) - 30} = \text{Amended Insulin:Glucose Ratio}$$

Values above 30 are suggestive of an insulinoma or other insulin-producing tumor. The reality is that abdominal imaging (radiology and ultrasonography) is indicated for any cat with sustained hypoglycemia and hyperinsulinemia of unknown origin; this should be followed by exploratory abdominal surgery and concurrent supportive care (e.g., IV glucose). Diagnostic imaging helps guide the surgeon and eliminate other causes of hypoglycemia (e.g., hepatic abscess).

Treatment

Surgery is the only way to make a definitive diagnosis and eliminate the underlying cause of malignancy-associated hypoglycemia. Metastases are common in most malignant tumors associated with this condition. Therefore surgery may not be curative but is palliative in many cases. If an insulinoma is suspected, partial pancreatectomy may be indicated. Complications include iatrogenic pancreatitis and diabetes mellitus. To minimize damage to the pancreas and reduce the chance of pancreatitis, careful surgical techniques should be employed; preoperative somatostatin treatment is optimal. Medical management of hypoglycemia is essential before, during, and after surgery because of the serious consequences of hypoglycemia and the high metastatic rate of insulinomas.[1,9–13]

Cats with severe hypoglycemia should be treated with IV administration of 2.5% to 5% dextrose in parenteral fluids, such as 0.9% NaCl or Ringer's solution. Cats that are convulsing should be given 0.5 g dextrose/kg IV slowly over 5 minutes. Prednisone (0.5–2.0 mg/kg PO divided bid) can induce hepatic gluconeogenesis and decrease peripheral utilization of glucose. Diazoxide (10–40 mg/kg PO divided bid), with or without hydrochlorothiazide (2–4 mg/kg PO bid), may be effective in elevating blood glucose levels by inhibiting pancreatic insulin secretion and glucose uptake by tissues, enhancing epinephrine-induced glycogenolysis, and increasing the rate of mobilization of free fatty acids.[11–13] Diazoxide may be difficult to obtain in some countries. Hydrochlorothiazide enhances the hyperglycemic effects of diazoxide. In refractory cases, the β-adrenergic blocking agent propranolol (0.2–1.0 mg/kg PO tid) may be effective in increasing blood glucose levels by blocking insulin release through the blockade of β-adrenergic receptors at the level of the pancreatic beta cell, inhibiting insulin release by membrane stabilization, and altering peripheral insulin receptor affinity.

Combined surgical and medical management of pancreatic tumors has been associated with remission periods of 1 year or more (see Chapter 44). For example, in one study, a functional, insulin-secreting pancreatic (islet cell) carcinoma was diagnosed in a 17-year-old male Siamese.[1,9–13] Diagnosis was made on the basis of clinical signs (i.e., seizures and stupor) that temporarily resolved after hypoglycemia was corrected with oral feeding or IV administration of glucose; the cat had an inappropriately increased serum insulin concentration in the face of hypoglycemia, and prolonged resolution of hypoglycemia occurred after surgical removal of the tumor. A primary islet cell tumor of the pancreas was confirmed by biopsy. The cat died 18 months later, and necropsy revealed metastases to regional lymph nodes and liver. Specimens of the tumor and metastatic lesions both stained positively for insulin. In another report,[12] transient diabetes mellitus developed after an insulinoma was removed in a cat but normalized after 1 week. The cat remained normal until recurrence of ataxia, twitching, and hypoglycemia 7 months postoperatively. The episodes were responsive to administration of exogenous glucose. Treatment consisted of prednisolone, which successfully palliated the hypoglycemic episodes for 2 years, at which time the cat died of unknown causes.

ALTERED SODIUM HOMEOSTASIS (SYNDROME OF INAPPROPRIATE SECRETION OF ANTIDIURETIC HORMONE)

(Also see Chapter 27)

CLINICAL BRIEFING

Diagnosis	
History	Anorexia, depression, lethargy, collapse, confused or unresponsive state, and recent administration of drug that may cause hyponatremia or SIADH.
Clinical Signs	Anorexia, nausea, subtle neurologic symptoms, confusion, and coma.
Diagnostics	MDB (including serum sodium), fractional excretion of sodium, serum osmolality, and adrenal and thyroid function tests.
Treatment	Treat the underlying cause.
	Judicious water restriction.
	Administer demeclocycline and furosemide.
	Lithium carbonate, phenytoin, and hypertonic saline are suggested in refractory cases in other species; efficacy in cats is unknown.

Although the syndrome of inappropriate secretion of antidiuretic hormone (SIADH) is rarely identified in veterinary medicine, it is one of the best characterized and most frequently encountered ectopic hormone syndromes in human medicine.[2] It is likely that SIADH will be identified more frequently in cats as awareness of this syndrome grows.[1,9]

SIADH can be caused by increased expression of ADH from the pituitary gland or can be a true paraneoplastic syndrome secondary to the ectopic production of ADH. In addition, several drugs (including chlorpropamide, vincristine, vinblastine, cyclophosphamide, opiates, histamine, thiazides, barbiturates, and isoproterenol) can indirectly cause SIADH by potentiating the release of ADH.[1,9]

Clinical Signs[2,7,9]

Most cats with SIADH are clinically normal. When serum sodium levels drop to 120 to 125 mEq/L, however, lethargy and mental dullness may be noted. When they drop below 115 mEq/L, more dramatic central nervous system (CNS) problems can develop and may progress to convulsions and coma. When this occurs, the cat must be treated as a medical emergency.

Diagnosis

The diagnosis of SIADH is based on the absence of hypovolemia and dehydration and the following laboratory findings[1,9]:

- Hypoosmolality of plasma despite inappropriately concentrated urine (high sodium)
- Hyponatremia of extracellular fluids
- Urine that is less than maximally dilute
- Absence of volume depletion
- Sustained increased renal fractional excretion of sodium
- Normal renal, pituitary, thyroid, and adrenal function
- Hypophosphatemia may be noted

Drugs that can cause SIADH include chlorpropamide, vincristine, vinblastine, cyclophosphamide, opiates, histamine, thiazides, barbiturates, and isoproterenol.

Spurious or artifactual hyponatremia can occur in cats with marked increases in serum lipids or serum proteins. In addition, in cats with marked hyperglycemia, water can be drawn into the circulatory system, diluting electrolytes and causing hyponatremia.

Treatment

The treatment of choice for patients with SIADH is to eliminate the underlying cause. If clinical signs warrant treatment, additional measures may be helpful.[1,9] Water restriction is effective for mild cases in which the cat can be carefully monitored for over- or underhydration. The objective is to raise the serum sodium level while restricting water intake to approximately 66 ml/kg/day. Demeclocycline antagonizes the actions of ADH on the kidneys and thus causes reversible nephrogenic diabetes insipidus. Possible side effects in humans include nausea, vomiting, skin rashes, and hypersensitivity reactions. Demeclocycline is effective in treating patients with mild to moderate SIADH. Other drugs, such as lithium carbonate and phenytoin, are not as effective. IV hypertonic sodium chloride is generally reserved for patients that have significant clinical signs related to hyponatremia. A more detailed description of its use appears in Chapter 27.

REFERENCES

1. Ogilvie GK: Metabolic emergencies and the cancer patient, in Wingfield WE (ed): *Veterinary Emergency Medicine Secrets.* Philadelphia, Hanley and Belfus, 2001, pp 247–251.
2. Marquez GA, Klausner JS, Osborne CA: Calcium oxalate urolithiasis in a cat with a functional parathyroid adenocarcinoma. *JAVMA* 206:817–819, 1995.
3. Sheafor SE, Gamblin RM, Couto CG: Hypercalcemia in two cats with multiple myeloma. *JAAHA* 32:503–508, 1996.
4. Savary KC, Price GS, Vaden SL: Hypercalcemia in cats: A retrospective study of 71 cases (1991–1997). *J Vet Intern Med* 14:184–189, 2000.
5. Klausner JS, Bell FW, Hayden DW, et al: Hypercalcemia in two cats with squamous cell carcinomas. *JAVMA* 196:103–105, 1990.
6. Mealey KL, Willard MD, Nagode LA, Helman G: Hypercalcemia associated with granulomatous disease in a cat. *JAVMA* 215:959–962, 1999.
7. Anderson TE, Legendre AM, McEntee MM: Probable hypercalcemia of malignancy in a cat with bronchogenic adenocarcinoma. *JAAHA* 36:52–55, 2000.
8. McClain HM, Barsanti JA, Bartges JW: Hypercalcemia and calcium oxalate urolithiasis in cats: A report of five cases. *JAAHA* 35:297–301, 1999.
9. Ogilvie GK: Paraneoplastic syndromes, in Ettinger SJ, Feldman EC (eds): *Textbook of Veterinary Internal Medicine*, ed 5. Philadelphia, WB Saunders, 2000, pp 498–506.
10. Brennan MD: Hypoglycemia in association with non-islet cell tumors, in Service FJ (ed): *Hypoglycemic Disorders: Pathogenesis, Diagnosis, and Treatment.* Boston, GK Hall, 1983, pp 143–151.
11. Chastain CB, Panciera D, Walters C (eds): Hypoadrenocorticism as the primary manifestation of lymphoma in two cats. *Small Anim Clin Endocrinol* 9:19, 1999.
12. Hawks D, Peterson ME, Hawkins KL, Rosebury WS: Insulin-secreting pancreatic (islet cell) carcinoma in a cat. *J Vet Intern Med* 6:193–196, 1992.
13. O'Brien TD, Norton F, Turner T, Johnson KH: Pancreatic endocrine tumor in a cat: Clinical, pathological, and immunohistochemical evaluation. *JAAHA* 26:453–457, 1990.

32

HEMATOLOGIC MANIFESTATIONS OF MALIGNANCY

Gregory K. Ogilvie and Antony S. Moore

ERYTHROCYTOSIS

CLINICAL BRIEFING

Diagnosis

History — Cats are often asymptomatic; lethargy, anorexia, polyuria, and polydipsia may be noted by owners.

Clinical Signs — Most often: lethargy and anorexia; less commonly: polyuria, polydipsia, and red mucous membranes.

Diagnostics — MDB, blood gas analysis, erythropoietin levels, abdominal radiographs, cardiovascular examination, bone marrow aspiration, renal imaging, and, if needed, splenic aspiration or needle core biopsy. Increased number of RBCs on CBC and hyperviscosity of the blood resulting in appearance of "sludging" in retinal vessels may be detected. The key clinical/pathologic features of true paraneoplastic syndrome are increased erythropoietin concentration, normal blood oxygenation, extramedullary hematopoiesis, and hyperplastic erythroid series on bone marrow examination. Nonparaneoplastic syndromes (including primary erythrocytosis) are characterized by: normal blood oxygenation and erythropoietin levels and malignant erythron on bone marrow examination. Secondary erythrocytosis caused by hypoxemia is associated with elevated erythropoietin concentration, enlargement of liver and spleen caused by extramedullary hematopoiesis, and decreased arterial oxygen concentration, whereas secondary erythrocytosis caused by renal disease is accompanied by evidence of renal disease on MDB, normal arterial or venous oxygenation, and enlargement of spleen and liver caused by extramedullary hematopoiesis.

Treatment — Treat the underlying cause and institute supportive care.
Phlebotomy and concurrent crystalloid fluid therapy.
Hydroxyurea in selected cases.

An increase in the number of red blood cells (RBCs; i.e., erythrocytosis) is occasionally seen in feline patients, but only a small fraction of these cases can be classified as true paraneoplastic syndromes and are an indirect result of malignancy.[1-8] Erythrocytosis can also be caused by dehydration and secondary volume contraction, pulmonary and cardiac disorders, venoarterial shunts, and polycythemia vera. Erythrocytosis can produce significant clinical signs and a diagnostic dilemma.

An elevated RBC mass secondary to malignancy occurs either directly by tumor production of erythropoietin or an erythropoietin-like molecule or indirectly because of hypoxia produced by the physical presence of a tumor that induces erythropoietin production. Erythropoietin is normally pro-

duced by the kidney in dogs and cats; thus it is not surprising that kidney tumors are associated with erythrocytosis.[4] When erythrocytosis is secondary to elevated erythropoietin concentrations, four possible mechanisms may be responsible:

- Production of erythropoietin directly by the tumor
- Tumor-induced hypoxia
- Tumor-enhanced induction of erythropoietin
- Tumor-induced change in erythropoietin metabolism[1-6]

Clinical Presentation

Many cats with erythrocytosis are asymptomatic.[1-6] Others exhibit nonspecific signs of lethargy, anorexia, and less commonly, polydipsia and polyuria. If the erythrocytosis is caused by generalized hypoxia, clinical signs referable to decreased oxygenation (e.g., dyspnea, cyanosis) may predominate.

Diagnosis

The diagnosis of erythrocytosis is based on the results of an MDB, blood gas analysis, erythropoietin levels, abdominal radiographs, cardiovascular examination, bone marrow aspiration, renal imaging (radiography, ultrasonography, CT, or MRI), and, if indicated, splenic aspiration or needle core biopsy (Table 32-1).[4] Cats with erythrocytosis of paraneoplastic origin are diagnosed by the presence of a triad of diagnostic results: (1) normal renal structure and function, (2) extramedullary hematopoiesis and a hyperplastic erythroid series in the bone marrow, and (3) normal arterial oxygenation systemically and locally in the kidney.

Cats with secondary polycythemia have decreased arterial oxygen saturation or renal disease.[4,5,7-9] Polycythemia vera is a myeloproliferative disorder that results from clonal proliferation of RBC precursors. The diagnosis generally is made by finding myelodysplastic disease (confirmed by histology and cytology of a bone marrow core biopsy specimen and aspiration), no evidence of local or systemic hypoxia, and lack of elevated erythropoietin concentrations.

Treatment

Most cats with erythrocytosis are asymptomatic and hence require no treatment. Specific therapy for the underlying cause of tissue hypoxia should be instituted in appropriate cases.[1-6] For asymptomatic cats, phlebotomies every 3 to 6 weeks may help reduce the RBC load temporarily. This procedure is performed by withdrawing approximately 20 to 40 ml/kg of blood through a large-bore (e.g., 18 ga) needle while simultaneously replacing the volume being removed with crystalloid fluids. With polycythemia vera, the chemotherapeutic agent hydroxyurea (30 mg/kg/day PO for 7 days then 15 mg/kg/day while watching for myelosuppression) can be used to induce reversible bone marrow suppression and reduce RBC production[1-6] (also see Chapter 37).

TABLE 32-1
Results of Common Diagnostic Tests in Various Classifications of Erythrocytosis

Classification	Erythropoietin Levels	Blood Oxygen	Bone Marrow	Renal Status	Extramedullary Hematopoiesis
(1°) Polycythemia vera	OK to low	OK	Malignant/Dysplatic	OK	No
(2°) Paraneoplastic syndrome	Increased	OK	Hyperplastic	OK	Yes
(2°) Tissue hypoxia	Increased	Low	Hyperplastic	OK	Yes
(2°) Renal disease	Increased	OK	Hyperplastic	Abnormal	Yes

ANEMIA

CLINICAL BRIEFING

Diagnosis

History — Typically nonspecific (e.g., lethargy, weakness, and exercise intolerance may be noted by owners).

Clinical Signs — Pale mucous membranes, lethargy, and weakness.

Diagnostics — MDB, bone marrow aspiration and biopsy, serum iron levels, total iron-binding capacity, slide agglutination test, antinuclear antibody, and Coombs' test (if indicated).

Treatment — Treat the underlying cause.

Consider iron supplementation, erythropoietin, and immune modulation after diagnosis is made.

Transfusion after cross-match.

Anemia occurs frequently in feline cancer patients and may result from increased blood loss, decreased RBC production (e.g., abnormal bone marrow function), or increased RBC destruction (e.g., immune-mediated diseases).[1-6] More specific causes of malignancy-associated anemia can be best understood by categorizing anemia as "regenerative" or "nonregenerative." Causes of regenerative anemia include blood loss (acute: trauma and coagulopathies; chronic: parasitism, GI ulceration or tumors, hematuria, and thrombocytopenia) and hemolysis (*Hemobartonella felis*, immune-mediated hemolytic anemia [uncommon], systemic lupus erythematosus, transfusion reactions, porphyria, disseminated intravascular coagulation, hemangiosarcoma, and such drugs as methylene blue, acetaminophen, benzocaine, and phenazopyridine). Causes of nonregenerative anemia include renal disease, hypoadrenocorticism, chronic disease, poor nutrition, red cell aplasia (FeLV), aplastic anemia (due to chemotherapeutic agents, FeLV, total body irradiation, or such drugs as griseofulvin and chloramphenicol), and myelophthisic disorders.

In chronic disease, an increase in iron stores is seen in the reticuloendothelial cells. Regardless of cause, anemia that is an indirect effect of a tumor is indeed a paraneoplastic syndrome. In most cats, a clear cause of the anemia is not found and a diagnosis of "anemia of chronic disease" is made.

Blood loss anemia is seen in many types of cancer. It can be a direct effect of the cancer or a result of coagulopathies linked with the tumor. Histamine released from mast cell tumors can theoretically activate parietal cells in the stomach, thereby increasing production of hydrochloric acid and inducing gastric or duodenal ulceration and consequent blood loss. This is noted much less commonly in cats than in dogs. If anemia is secondary to blood loss, the cause may be obvious (as with bleeding superficial tumors) or inconspicuous (as with bladder or GI tumors).

Microangiopathic hemolytic anemia often occurs secondary to damage to arteriolar endothelium or fibrin deposition within the artery.[1,4-6] Disseminated intravascular coagulation (DIC) is an important cause of this type of anemia. DIC, also called *consumptive coagulopathy* or *defibrination syndrome*, refers to a complex syndrome in which excessive intravascular coagulation leads to multiple-organ microthrombosis and paradoxic bleeding. In DIC, bleeding is caused by the inactivation or excessive consumption of platelets and clotting factors secondary to enhanced fibrinolysis. DIC is not a specific disorder but rather a common pathway in a variety of clinical situations. Moreover, DIC constitutes a dynamic phenomenon in which marked changes in the patient's status and in the results of coagulation tests occur rapidly and repeatedly during the course of treatment.

In cats, immune-mediated hemolytic anemia is sometimes triggered by tumors. The result is premature destruction of RBCs by immune mechanisms.[1,4-6] Antibodies can be directed against the RBC or a hapten (e.g., virus or drug) that is associated with the RBC.

Chemotherapy-induced nonregenerative anemia is common in cats. It is frequently associated with chronic drug therapy. Although chemotherapeutic agents often decrease the number of white blood cells (WBCs) and platelets, anemia associated with administration of chemotherapeutic agents is generally mild and not associated with clinical signs.

Less common causes of cancer-induced anemia include leukoerythroblastic anemia, hematopoietic dysplasia, hypersplenism, erythrophagocytosis, megaloblastic anemia, and red cell aplasia.[1,4-6]

> **KEY POINT**
>
> *Surgical removal is the treatment of choice for erythropoietin-producing tumors or tumors that induce regional or systemic hypoxia. Phlebotomies and hydroxyurea can be used if needed.*

Clinical Presentation

Many of the mechanisms described work alone or in concert to decrease the population of RBCs.[1,4-6] Although clinical signs relating to the anemia may be overshadowed by aspects of the underlying neoplastic condition, the anemia can nevertheless impair the quality of life in cats with cancer. The majority of patients remain asymptomatic if anemia develops gradually or the number of RBCs decreases only slightly. As the anemia progresses, lethargy and exercise intolerance may arise. Mucous membranes may be pale.

Diagnosis (Figure 32-1)

A CBC, biochemical profile, and bone marrow aspiration are needed to determine the cause of anemia; serum iron levels, total iron-binding capacity, Coombs' or slide agglutination test, and/or antinuclear antibody testing may be needed as well. The anemia must first be classified as regenerative or nonregenerative. If the anemia is regenerative (i.e., corrected aggregate reticulocyte count of 0.04 or greater) and serum proteins are decreased, blood loss may be considered.[4,7,9] If serum proteins are increased, differentials of RBC destruction by immune-mediated diseases (e.g., immune-mediated hemolytic anemia), physical trauma (e.g., DIC, parasites), or toxins (e.g., methylene blue) must be considered. If the anemia is nonregenerative, bone marrow aspiration or biopsy should be performed to evaluate erythroid hypoplasia (such causes as anemia of chronic disease, endocrine deficiencies, renal disease, or lead toxicity), aplastic anemia (such causes as FeLV), myeloproliferative disorders, and iron deficiency.

> *MDB = minimum database; includes CBC, biochemical profile, urinalysis, FeLV/FIV serology, T$_4$ testing, and thoracic radiographs (three views).*

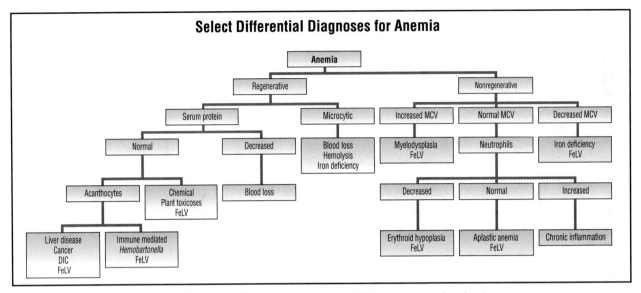

Figure 32-1: *Diagnostic differentials and laboratory findings associated with anemia (MCV = mean corpuscular volume).*

Anemia of chronic disease in cancer patients is associated with a shortened erythrocyte life span, depressed bone marrow response, and disordered iron metabolism and storage.[4,7,9] Clinically, this type of anemia is recognized as normocytic and normochromic, with normal bone marrow cellularity and reticuloendothelial iron sequestration. Blood loss anemia is recognized clinically when the RBCs are microcytic and hypochromic because of decreased hemoglobin synthesis.[4,7,9] Poikilocytosis, microleptocytosis, inadequate reticulocytosis, increased total iron-binding capacity, decreased serum iron concentrations, and elevated platelet counts may also be seen with blood loss. Hemolysis and schistocytosis are the hallmarks of microangiopathic hemolytic anemia. The diagnosis of immune-mediated hemolytic anemia is based on finding antibody or complement on the surface of the patient's RBCs by a Coombs' test or slide agglutination test paired with nonregenerative anemia. Histologically, chemotherapy-induced changes include bone marrow hypoplasia of the erythroid or other cell lines that subsequently cause inadequate reticulocytes and decreased red cell mass with normal erythrocytic indices.[4,7,9]

Treatment

As with all paraneoplastic syndromes, the best treatment is to eliminate the underlying cause.[4,5,7,8] Symptomatic treatment is usually needed only if the anemia produces clinical signs or if the cat is to undergo surgery. If acute correction of the condition is warranted, it is common to administer a blood transfusion after a cross-match has been performed (see Box, above). A more detailed description can be found in Chapter 20.

Human recombinant erythropoietin (75–100 U/kg/day SQ three times a week; decrease to once or twice weekly

General Rule: Amount to Transfuse

$$[(2.2 \times wt_{kg}) \times 30] \times \frac{(PCV_{desired} - PCV_{recipient})}{PCV_{donor}}$$

Note: 2.2 ml of whole blood/kg or 1 ml/kg of packed RBCs raises PCV 1% (transfused whole blood has a PCV of 40%). The rate of transfusion is 40 ml/30 minutes with close patient monitoring.

when the desired hematocrit level is reached) is being used more commonly for a variety of anemias.[5] Because recombinant erythropoietin is somewhat species-specific, patients may develop antibodies that may cross-react with their own erythropoietin. Recombinant erythropoietin is most effective when endogenous erythropoietin levels are low and adequate erythrocyte precursors are present in the bone marrow and other structures. If anemia is attributable to blood loss, the source of bleeding should be identified and eliminated. Medical management of immune-mediated hemolytic anemia can include oral prednisone (2 mg/kg/day); in addition, oral azathioprine (1 mg/kg/day for 2–4 days, then 0.3 mg/kg every other day) may be indicated if resolution of the underlying neoplastic condition is delayed.[4–6] Azathioprine should be used with caution in cats as this species is more sensitive to the adverse effects of this antimetabolite than dogs and humans. Cyclosporine (5 mg/kg bid; dose adjusted by monitoring blood levels) is sometimes effective, but cats should be watched for intussusception, an uncommon side effect associated with oral administration.

THROMBOCYTOPENIA

CLINICAL BRIEFING

Diagnosis

History	Bleeding from any site and into any body cavity without an obvious cause.
Clinical Signs	If onset is gradual, cats are often asymptomatic or may show petechiation, ecchymotic hemorrhages, bleeding from any site without cause, pale mucous membranes, weakness, and shock.
Diagnostics	MDB, bone-marrow aspiration, and coagulation profile, including ACT, OSPT, APTT, fibrinogen, antithrombin III, platelet factor III, and FDPs.

Treatment	Treat the underlying cause.
	Consider immunomodulation or low-dose vincristine, depending on cause and severity of thrombocytopenia.
	Transfusion with fresh whole blood or platelet-rich plasma.

Mechanisms associated with diminished platelet numbers in cats with cancer include reduced platelet production from bone marrow, sequestration of platelets in capillaries, increased platelet consumption (as in DIC), increased platelet destruction, and reduction of hematopoietic growth factors. Consumption of platelets is considered the primary hemostatic abnormality in cats with tumors.[10,11]

The prevalence of feline thrombocytopenia (<200,000 platelets/μl) was determined and reported in one study.[11] Cats were divided into six categories based on clinical diagnoses: 29% had infectious disease, 20% had neoplasia, 7% had cardiac disease, 2% had primary immune-mediated disease, 22% had multiple diseases, and 20% had disorders of unknown etiology. The mean platelet count for all thrombocytopenic cats was 52,000/μl. Bleeding disorders (hemorrhage or thrombosis) were observed in 29% of thrombocytopenic cats and were more likely to be associated with neoplasia, cardiac disease, and platelet counts less than or equal to 30,000/μl. DIC was diagnosed in 12% of the cats. Infections and/or neoplasia affecting the bone marrow were the most common diseases associated with thrombocytopenia. FeLV and myeloproliferative neoplasia accounted for approximately 44% of the specific diagnoses in thrombocytopenic cats.

KEY POINT

Vincristine and platelet transfusions should be administered only when the thrombocytopenia is transient and the cat is stable, as in instances of transient thrombocytopenia following chemotherapy.

Diminished platelet numbers and elevated plasma-fibrinogen concentrations are common in cats with extensive tumors involving the spleen or bone marrow.[10,11] DIC, a common cause of platelet consumption, may occur in cats with tumors involving these structures.[11] Eliminating the neoplastic condition and administering IV fluids and heparin may be of therapeutic value in these patients. Immune-mediated thrombocytopenia also significantly decreases platelet numbers in some cats with cancer.[10,11]

Clinical Presentation

Cats with thrombocytopenia may be clinically normal or may bleed for no reason into any part of the body. For example, affected cats may bleed excessively from a simple venipuncture, and petechial or ecchymotic hemorrhages may be noted on physical examination.

Diagnosis (Figure 32-2)

A thorough history, physical examination, CBC, platelet count, clotting profile, and bone marrow evaluation are essential to diagnose and evaluate the cause of thrombocytopenia.[4,10,11] This information helps to determine whether thrombocytopenia results from decreased production (e.g., tumor-induced myelophthisis, chemotherapy-induced marrow suppression), increased consumption (e.g., DIC secondary to any malignancy), or increased blood loss. If DIC is suspected, prolongation of clotting times (activated clotting time [ACT], one-step prothrombin time [OSPT], activated partial thromboplastin time [APTT]), and elevated fibrinogen levels) may be identified. Thrombocytopenia attributable to an immune mechanism is diagnosed when antibodies against bone marrow megakaryocytes are detected. In addition, thrombocytopenia can be a true paraneoplastic syndrome, which is diagnosed by eliminating all other causes and determining whether the cat responds to removal of an apparently unrelated tumor.

PARANEOPLASTIC SYNDROMES

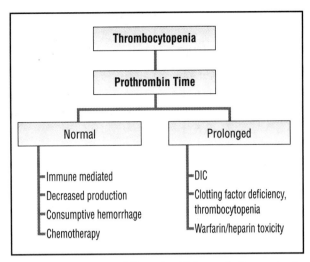

Figure 32-2: *Diagnostic differentials and laboratory findings associated with thrombocytopenia.*

Treatment

Cats with thrombocytopenia should be kept quiet. The primary treatment for the paraneoplastic syndrome is removal of the tumor.[4,10,11] Malignancy-associated, immune-mediated thrombocytopenia has been successfully resolved in cats by administering immunosuppressive drugs, such as prednisone (2 mg/kg daily) or azathioprine (1 mg/kg daily for 4 days followed by 0.3–1 mg/kg every other day).[1,4-6] Azathioprine should be used with caution in cats as they are more sensitive to the adverse effects of this antimetabolite than dogs and humans. Cyclosporine may be helpful in refractory cases, but cats should be watched for intussusception, an uncommon side effect associated with oral administration. When thrombocytopenia is secondary to a malignancy, vincristine (0.5–0.75 mg/m²) can be used to increase the number of platelets temporarily; response is directly proportional to the number of megakaryocytes and the rate of platelet removal from the body. Platelet counts increase 4 days after vincristine is given. Platelet-rich plasma transfusions can be administered to specific patients that are or have a high likelihood of bleeding uncontrollably. As can be expected, special equipment and a large number of donor cats are required to significantly enhance platelet numbers, which is why this procedure is rarely performed. The amount of random donor platelet transfusion is generally about 3 U/m² body surface area or 0.1 U/kg body weight. Each unit should be administered with 30 to 60 ml of plasma.

LEUKOCYTOSIS

CLINICAL BRIEFING

Diagnosis

History	Affected animals are usually asymptomatic but may be lethargic and anorectic.
Clinical Signs	Bone marrow packing can result in shifting leg lameness due to bone pain, lethargy, and rarely splenomegaly if the reticuloendothelial system is actively clearing abnormal cells.
Diagnostics	CBC, bone marrow aspiration and biopsy, and special stains for abnormal cells; thoracic and abdominal radiographs and MDB to identify other causes.

Treatment

Treat the underlying cause.
Treat any underlying infection.

An increased WBC count attributable to either increased production, decreased loss, or decreased destruction is common in feline cancer patients.[4,5,12,13] Any cell line can be involved. When leukocytosis is a remote effect of underlying malignancy, the laboratory finding may be classified as a paraneoplastic syndrome. Paraneoplastic leukocytosis in cats arises from a variety of malignancies. Cases of leukocytosis caused by malignant clonal proliferation of a specific WBC line are not considered paraneoplastic syndromes. The mechanism of malignancy-associated leukocytosis is unknown but may involve the direct or indirect production of hematopoietic growth factors (e.g., granulocyte colony-stimulating factor, granulocyte-macrophage colony-stimulating factor, or interleukin-3) or may occur as a result of tissue necrosis and granulocyte breakdown with positive feedback that increases neutrophil production.[4,5]

Clinical Presentation

Cats with paraneoplastic leukocytosis are often clinically normal. Human patients occasionally describe bone pain due to the high proliferative rate in the bone marrow. Rarely, splenomegaly may be found if the reticuloendothelial system is attempting to actively clear the abnormal cells.

Diagnosis

The diagnosis is based on a CBC and bone marrow examination. Occasionally, special stains may be performed by the clinical pathology laboratory to determine whether the increased number of leukocytes is from a neoplastic clone. Thoracic and abdominal radiographs as well as an MDB should be considered to determine other possible causes for the leukocytosis.

Treatment

The condition generally has no clinical significance and thus requires no therapy. However, clinicians should be aware of and treat any underlying infection that may exist in these cats.

MDB = minimum database; includes CBC, biochemical profile, urinalysis, FeLV/FIV serology, T_4 testing, and thoracic radiographs (three views).

REFERENCES

1. Giger U, Gorman NT: Acute complications of cancer and cancer therapy, in Gorman NT (ed): *Oncology*. New York, Churchill Livingstone, 1986, pp 147–168.
2. Peterson ME, Randolph JF: Diagnosis and treatment of polycythemia vera, in Kirk RW (ed): *Current Veterinary Therapy VIII*. Philadelphia, WB Saunders, 1983, pp 406–408.
3. Hammond D, Winnick S: Paraneoplastic erythrocytosis and ectopic erythropoietin. *Ann N Y Acad Sci* 230:219–226, 1974.
4. Ogilvie GK: Paraneoplastic syndromes, in Ettinger SJ, Feldman EC (eds): *Textbook of Veterinary Internal Medicine*, ed 5. Philadelphia, WB Saunders, 2000, pp 498–506.
5. Ogilvie GK: Anemia, thrombocytopenia, and hypoproteinemia, in Wingfield WE (ed): *Veterinary Emergency Medicine Secrets*. Philadelphia, Hanley and Belfus, 2001, pp 265–268.
6. Griffin TW, Rosenthal PE, Costanza ME: Paraneoplastic and endocrine syndromes, in Cady B (ed): *Cancer Manual*, ed 7. Boston, American Cancer Society, 1986, pp 373–390.
7. Madewell BR, Feldman BF: Characterization of anemias associated with neoplasia in small animals. *JAVMA* 176:419–425, 1980.
8. Hackner SG: Approach to the diagnosis of bleeding disorders. *Compend Contin Educ Pract Vet* 17:331–349, 1995.
9. Rentko VT, Cotter SM: Feline anemia: The classifications, causes, and diagnostic procedures. *Vet Med* 85:584–604, 1990.
10. Ogilvie GK: Anemia, thrombocytopenia, and hypoproteinemia, in Wingfield WE (ed): *Veterinary Emergency Medicine Secrets*. Philadelphia, Hanley and Belfus, 1997, pp 230–234.
11. Jordan HL, Grindem CB, Breitschwerdt EB: Thrombocytopenia in cats: A retrospective study of 41 cases. *J Vet Intern Med* 7:261–265, 1993.
12. Sharkey LC, Rosol TJ, Grone A, et al: Production of granulocyte colony-stimulating factor and granulocyte-macrophage colony-stimulating factor by carcinomas in a dog and a cat with paraneoplastic leukocytosis. *J Vet Intern Med* 10:405–408, 1996.
13. Center SA, Randolph JF, Erb HN, Reiter S: Eosinophilia in the cat: A retrospective study of 312 cases (1985–1986). *JAAHA* 26:349–358, 1990.

PARANEOPLASTIC SYNDROMES

HYPERGAMMAGLOBULINEMIA

Gregory K. Ogilvie and Antony S. Moore

33

CLINICAL BRIEFING

Diagnosis	
History	Anorexia, weight loss, polyuria, polydipsia, and seizures.
Clinical Signs	Bleeding from any site, petechial and ecchymotic hemorrhages, evidence of volume expansion, cardiovascular problems, blindness due to retinal hemorrhages, and bone pain.
Diagnostics	MDB, immunoelectrophoresis demonstrating monoclonal gammopathy in blood and urine, bone marrow aspiration and cytology, retinal examination, coagulation profile (ACT, OSPT, APTT, fibrinogen, antithrombin III, platelet factor III, and FDPs), blood pressure, and abdominal radiographs and/or ultrasonography to help confirm or eliminate neoplastic etiology.
Therapy	Eliminate underlying cause via surgery, chemotherapy (e.g., melphalan and prednisone), and/or radiation therapy.
	Restore tissue perfusion with fluids, stabilize cardiovascular system, and if needed, reduce viscosity with fluids, plasmapheresis, or plasma harvests from patient.

Multiple myeloma is the most common cause of hypergammaglobulinemia, also known as *M-component disorder* or *hyperviscosity syndrome*, in cats.[1-17] This condition results from excessive secretion of immunoglobulin (including IgG, IgA, IgM, and light-chain protein classes) by a monoclonal line of immunoglobulin-producing cells. Light chains, also known as Bence-Jones proteins, may be present in urine. Other tumors that may be associated with the production of large quantities of immunoglobulins include lymphoma, lymphocytic leukemia, a variety of solid tumors, and primary macroglobulinemia.[1,5-16] Paraneoplastic syndromes occur only in tumors that increase globulin concentration as an indirect, distant effect.

Clinical Presentation

Clinical signs seen in cats with M-component disorders arise from increased viscosity associated with elevated globulins and from the tumor's direct effect on surrounding structures. Reported clinical findings include:

- Anorexia
- Weight loss
- Polyuria/polydipsia
- Seizures and other neurologic findings
- Stupor
- Hemorrhage
- Pallor
- Prolonged capillary refill time

- Heart murmur
- Splenomegaly

Hemorrhage results from elevated levels of proteins that interfere with normal platelet function.[1-6,10,11] Hyperviscosity syndrome, or "sludging" of blood within the vessels, causes polydipsia, central nervous system (CNS) signs, retinopathies, visual disturbances, secondary renal problems, and congestive heart failure. Renal decompensation often succeeds renal amyloidosis or Bence-Jones proteinuria; increased serum viscosity decreases renal perfusion, and concentrating ability is impaired. Neurologic signs arise when altered blood flow and diminished delivery of oxygen to neural tissues produce CNS hypoxia. Increased blood volume and viscosity place greater demands on the heart, which in turn can result in cardiomegaly, murmurs, and, in some rare cases, congestive heart failure. Hypergammaglobulinemia can produce decompensation of stable preexisting cardiac conditions or lead to the development of a hypertrophic cardiomyopathy-like state.

Diagnosis

Each case of hypergammaglobulinemia must be assessed to determine the underlying cause by performing the following baseline tests[1-3,5,6,8]:

- CBC, biochemical profile, and urinalysis
- Blood pressure measurement

- Immunoelectrophoresis of serum and urine (± Bence-Jones protein test of urine)
- Bone marrow aspiration and cytology
- Thoracic and abdominal radiographs
- Survey skeletal radiographs (± nuclear scintigraphy of skeletal system)
- Retinal examination
- Coagulation profile (activated partial thromboplastin time [APTT], one-step prothrombin time [OSPT], activated clotting time [ACT], platelet count, fibrin degradation products [FDPs], and antithrombin III)
- *Ehrlichia* titer

Initial screening tests are primarily performed to detect evidence of bone marrow involvement by tumor or *Ehrlichia*, monoclonal gammopathy, renal failure secondary to hyperglobulinemia, coagulopathy distinct from increased globulins, lytic bone lesions suggestive of multiple myeloma, myelophthisis, or hypertension and bleeding. Because it determines not only whether monoclonal gammopathy is present but also which class of immunoglobulins is involved, immunoelectrophoresis is usually preferred to general electrophoresis. Multiple myeloma is diagnosed by the presence of monoclonal gammopathy, Bence-Jones proteinuria or monoclonal proteinuria, "punched-out" bone lesions that may be detected with a nuclear bone scan, and more than 20% to 30% plasma cells in the bone marrow. Resolution of clinical signs occurs when malignancy is controlled. If increased globulin concentrations are in response to *Ehrlichia* infection, titers should disclose the organism.

Treatment

The treatment of choice for multiple myeloma is melphalan (0.1 mg/kg PO daily for 10 days, then 0.05 mg/kg daily) and prednisone (0.5 mg/kg PO daily for 21 days, then every other day thereafter); this combination produces a survival time of 4 to 12 months.[1-6,8] Radiation therapy for areas of bone involvement may be palliative. Plasmapheresis rapidly reduces protein levels and is useful in cases where hyperviscosity requires symptomatic treatment.[1-3] If plasmapheresis is not available, blood from a cat with clinically significant hypergammaglobulinemia can be harvested; the plasma can then be removed and the RBCs resuspended in an equal volume of 0.9% NaCl for immediate reintroduction into the

KEY POINT

Because plasmapheresis requires specialized equipment, blood can be harvested from cats with clinically significant hypergammaglobulinemia; the plasma can then be removed and the RBCs resuspended in an equal volume of 0.9% NaCl for immediate reintroduction into the patient.

patient. Other supportive care involves fluid therapy for dehydration. Because myeloma cells are believed to secrete a substance that suppresses macrophage and lymphocyte function, antibiotics may be indicated (see Chapter 37).

REFERENCES

1. Ogilvie GK: Paraneoplastic syndromes, in Withrow SJ, MacEwen EG (eds): *Clinical Veterinary Oncology.* Philadelphia, JB Lippincott, 1989, pp 29–40.
2. Ogilvie GK: Paraneoplastic syndromes, in Ettinger SJ, Feldman EC (eds): *Textbook of Veterinary Internal Medicine,* ed 5. Philadelphia, WB Saunders, 2000, pp 498–506.
3. Griffin TW, Rosenthal PE, Costanza ME: Paraneoplastic and endocrine syndromes, in Cady B (ed): *Cancer Manual,* ed 7. Boston, American Cancer Society, 1986, pp 373–390.
4. Ogilvie GK: Metabolic emergencies and the cancer patient, in Wingfield WE (ed): *Veterinary Emergency Medicine Secrets.* Philadelphia, Hanley and Belfus, 2001, pp 247–251.
5. MacEwen EG, Hurvitz AI: Diagnosis and management of monoclonal gammopathies. *Vet Clin North Am Small Anim Pract* 7:119–132, 1977.
6. Larsen AE, Carpenter JL: Hepatic plasmacytoma and biclonal gammopathy in a cat. *JAVMA* 205:708–710, 1994.
7. Yamada T, Matsuda M, Samata T, et al: Immunochemistry and physiochemistry on a feline monoclonal IgA and Bence Jones proteins. *Nippon Juigaku Zasshi* 50:63–69, 1988.
8. Hribernik TN, Barta O, Gaunt SD, Boudreaux MK: Serum hyperviscosity syndrome associated with IgG myeloma in a cat. *JAVMA* 181:169–170, 1982.
9. MacEwen EG, Hurvitz AI: Diagnosis and management of monoclonal gammopathies. *Vet Clin North Am Small Anim Pract* 7:119–132, 1977.
10. Lane IF, Roberts SM, Lappin MR: Ocular manifestations of vascular disease: Hypertension, hyperviscosity, and hyperlipidemia. *JAAHA* 29:28–36, 1993.
11. Forrester SD, Greco DS, Relford RL: Serum hyperviscosity syndrome associated with multiple myeloma in two cats. *JAVMA* 200:79–82, 1992.
12. Ford SL, Schaer M: Shock syndrome in cats. *Compend Contin Educ Pract Vet* 15:1517–1526, 1993.
13. Ward DA, McEntee MF, Weddle DL: Orbital plasmacytoma in a cat. *J Small Anim Pract* 38:576–578, 1997.
14. Weber NA, Tebeau CS: An unusual presentation of multiple myeloma in two cats. *JAAHA* 34:477–483, 1998.
15. Eastman CA: Plasma cell tumors in a cat. *Feline Pract* 24:26–31, 1996.
16. Carr AP, Johnson GS: A review of hemostatic abnormalities in dogs and cats. *JAAHA* 30:475–481, 1994.
17. Mandel NS, Esplin DG: A retroperitoneal extramedullary plasmacytoma in a cat with a monoclonal gammopathy. *JAAHA* 30:603–608, 1994.

PARANEOPLASTIC SYNDROMES

CANCER CACHEXIA AS A MANIFESTATION OF MALIGNANCY

34

Gregory K. Ogilvie and Antony S. Moore

CLINICAL BRIEFING

Diagnosis

History — Initial stages vague and often associated with "aging"; owners may note lethargy, anorexia, and later in the disease, weight loss despite adequate nutritional intake.

Clinical Signs — Lack of weight gain; later in the syndrome, weight loss despite adequate energy intake; increased toxicoses in response to radiation therapy, surgery, and chemotherapy; decreased response to therapy.

Diagnostics — Hypoalbuminemia, hyperlactatemia, and hyperinsulinemia are seen later in the syndrome and are associated with alterations in carbohydrate, lipid, and protein metabolism.

Therapy — Eliminate underlying cause with surgery, chemotherapy, and radiation therapy.

Feed diet with minimal amounts of carbohydrates, modest amounts of high quality protein, and moderate amounts of fats (possibly enriched with n-3 eicosanoids).

Encourage oral feeding when possible; use nasogastric, gastrostomy, or jejunostomy tube feeding when necessary.

Parenteral support should be employed if enteral feeding fails.

Cancer cachexia is a complex clinical syndrome of inefficient metabolic processes impacting quality and length of life. The dramatic metabolic alterations associated with cancer cachexia occur before clinical evidence of weight loss and cachexia are detectable.[1-8] In the terminal stages of cancer, this condition produces involuntary weight loss even when caloric intake is adequate.[1-4] As with all other paraneoplastic syndromes, this condition is a remote effect of cancer. This paraneoplastic syndrome is encountered by every practitioner who treats cats with cancer. The actual cause of cancer cachexia is unknown, but its metabolic effects are wide ranging and thus impair quality of life, response to therapy, and overall survival. A detailed description of this paraneoplastic syndrome and its treatment are found in Chapter 19.

Clinical Presentation

Cats with cancer cachexia show no clinical signs of the paraneoplastic syndrome in the early stages. As the syndrome progresses, weight loss is noted despite a good appetite. Later, weight loss, anorexia, lethargy, and depression predominate.

Diagnosis

As discussed, alterations occur early in the course of malignant disease. Cats in the preclinical or silent phase of cancer cachexia may show only exercise intolerance, lethargy, and anorexia. Later in the course of the disease, there is overt wasting and loss of body condition despite adequate nutritional intake. This is followed by death due to failure of one or more organ systems. Hypoalbuminemia, hyperlactatemia, and hyperinsulinemia are often noted in later stages of disease.

KEY POINT

Dramatic alterations in metabolism are documented in cancer patients even before clinical evidence of cachexia is noted; these alterations fail to resolve following remission achieved via surgery or chemotherapy.

Treatment

Detailed therapeutic strategies are found in Chapter 19. Some general principles include:

- Ensuring that the patient consumes an adequate quantity of highly bioavailable nutrients presented in a palatable form.

- A diet composed of limited amounts of carbohydrates, high quality but relatively modest amounts of bioavailable proteins, and a modest amount of fat may be ideal for supporting cancer patients without enhancing tumor growth.
- Cats should be fed enterally whenever possible. If appropriate, methods such as minimizing dehydration, nausea, and discomfort with nursing care and appropriate drugs, warming the food, increasing palatability, and using pharmacologic agents (e.g., megestrol acetate, benzodiazepine derivatives, cyproheptadine) to enhance appetite and stimulate oral feeding should be employed before considering nasogastric, gastrostomy, or jejunostomy tube feeding.
- When enteral feeding is not feasible, parenteral feeding of a diet with minimal simple carbohydrates should be employed.
- Avoid diets with simple carbohydrates as the principle source of calories.
- When possible, avoid lactate- and glucose-containing fluids, as they may cause an elevation in lactate and insulin.. A clear exception is in cases of septic shock or during an insulin overdose, when glucose-containing fluids may be specifically required to treat hypoglycemia.
- Adequate calories should be provided; however, it may not be necessary to provide more nutrients than needed by disease-free cats. The following formula is a gen-

MDB = minimum database; includes CBC, biochemical profile, urinalysis, FeLV/FIV serology, T_4 testing, and thoracic radiographs (three views).

eral approximation of the amount of metabolizable food to feed (Kcal/day):

$$2 \times (30 \times \text{body weight [kg]}) + 70$$

REFERENCES

1. Ogilvie GK, Vail DM: Nutrition and cancer: Recent developments. *Vet Clin North Am Small Anim Pract* 20:1–15, 1990.
2. Ogilvie GK, Marks SL: Cancer, in Hand MS, Thatcher CD, Remillard RL, Roudebush P (eds): *Small Animal Clinical Nutrition*, ed 4. Topeka, KS, Mark Morris Institute, 2000, pp 887–906.
3. Vail DM, Ogilvie GK, Wheeler SL: Metabolic alterations in patients with cancer cachexia. *Compend Contin Educ Pract Vet* 12:381–387, 1990.
4. Ogilvie GK: Alterations in metabolism and nutritional support for veterinary cancer patients: Recent advances. *Compend Contin Educ Pract Vet* 15:925–937, 1993.
5. Ogilvie GK: Paraneoplastic syndromes, in Withrow SJ, MacEwen EG (eds): *Clinical Veterinary Oncology*. Philadelphia, JB Lippincott, 1989, pp 29–40.
6. Ogilvie GK: Paraneoplastic syndromes, in Ettinger SJ, Feldman EC (eds): *Textbook of Veterinary Internal Medicine*, ed 5. Philadelphia, WB Saunders, 2000, pp 498–506.
7. Selting KA, Ogilvie GK, Lana SE, et al: Serum alpha 1 acid glycoprotein concentrations in healthy and tumor bearing cats. *J Vet Intern Med* 14:503–506, 2000.
8. Chlebowski RT, Heber D: Metabolic abnormalities in cancer patients: Carbohydrate metabolism. *Surg Clin North Am* 66:957, 1986.

PARANEOPLASTIC SYNDROMES

MISCELLANEOUS CONDITIONS— FEVER, NEUROLOGIC SYNDROMES, AND HYPERTROPHIC OSTEOPATHY

35

Gregory K. Ogilvie and Antony S. Moore

FEVER

<table>
<tr><td colspan="2" align="center">C L I N I C A L   B R I E F I N G</td></tr>
<tr><td>Diagnosis</td><td></td></tr>
<tr><td>History</td><td>Lethargy and anorexia.</td></tr>
<tr><td>Clinical Signs</td><td>Lethargy, anorexia, increased body temperature, and weight loss (if condition is prolonged).</td></tr>
<tr><td>Diagnostics</td><td>Confirm that elevated body temperature persists when patient is relaxed and at rest. Rule out infections and inflammatory or immune-mediated causes with MDB, echocardiogram, antinuclear antibody test, and cultures of blood, urine, and if indicated, lung. Confirm/eliminate meningitis and disease of the hypothalamus with history, physical examination, brain-imaging studies, and a CSF tap (if indicated).</td></tr>
<tr><td>Treatment</td><td>Eliminate the underlying cause.</td></tr>
<tr><td></td><td>Therapy depends on the severity of clinical and laboratory parameters; consider fluids and steroidal and nonsteroidal antiinflammatory agents</td></tr>
</table>

Fever is a common complication of cancer and other infectious and noninfectious conditions.[1-3] In many cases, pyrexia is caused by infection, although other noninfectious causes, such as drug toxicity and adrenal insufficiency, have been associated with fever. Elevated body temperature can also be a sign of neoplastic disease.[2] Tumor-associated fever is usually defined as unexplained elevated body temperature that coincides with the presence of a tumor. Tumor-induced fevers may result from release of pyrogens from tumor cells as well as from normal leukocytes or other normal cells. Tumor-elaborated pyrogens may act on the hypothalamus to reset temperature regulation of the body. Although the incidence of cancer-associated fever is unknown in cats, up to 40% of fevers of unknown origin in humans have been found to be caused by cancer.[3]

Clinical Signs

Clinical signs are directly related to the underlying malignant disease, elevated body temperature, and associated increase in energy expenditure. Depression, anorexia, lethargy, and weight loss may result.

Diagnosis

The diagnosis of this paraneoplastic syndrome is made by excluding all other causes and identifying a neoplastic disease. The condition is confirmed when the pyrexia resolves after the tumor is eliminated. All non-tumor-related causes of increased body temperature are eliminated via CBC, biochemical profile, urinalysis, blood and urine cultures, thoracic radiographs, echocardiography (looking for bacterial endocarditis), and (if indicated) an antinuclear antibody test, brain imaging study (computed tomography [CT], magnetic resonance imaging [MRI]), myelogram, and cerebrospinal fluid (CSF) tap to evaluate for hypothalamic dysfunction (the hypothalamus governs thermoregulation).

Treatment

This paraneoplastic syndrome can be used as a tumor marker to document response to therapy.[1-3] Excessive body temperature that induces clinical signs and is directly related to malignant disease can be treated symptomatically with fluid therapy, antipyretics, or nonsteroidal antiinflammatory agents. Resolution of the underlying malignant condition usually eliminates the fever.

NEUROLOGIC SYNDROMES

C L I N I C A L B R I E F I N G	
Diagnosis	
History	Abnormalities referable to the brain, spinal cord, peripheral nerves, and muscle and neuromuscular junctions.
Clinical Signs	Clinical signs are often subtle in the early phases but can include behavioral abnormalities, CNS upper motor neuron dysfunction, and central and peripheral nervous system lower motor neuron dysfunction.
Diagnostics	MDB and evaluation of thyroid and adrenal function; specific nervous system diseases are diagnosed by imaging techniques (e.g., CT, MRI, myelogram), CSF tap (if indicated), electrodiagnostics, biopsy of nervous tissue, and response tests (e.g., with edrophonium chloride).
Treatment	Treat the underlying cause. Immunosuppressive therapy may be indicated.

In both human and veterinary patients, the remote effects of cancer on the nervous system induce a wide variety of clinical signs[1-6] of unknown causes. This paraneoplastic syndrome is quite common in humans but rarely noted in feline medicine. Cats exhibit neurologic signs secondary to endocrine, fluid, and electrolyte disturbances attributable to neoplasia. Examples of these include hypercalcemia, hyperviscosity syndrome, and hepatoencephalopathy. The neurologic syndrome of myasthenia gravis secondary to thymoma (e.g., megaesophagus and acetyl cholinesterase-responsive neuropathy), although rare in cats, is well described in the literature.[1-6]

Clinical Signs

Manifestations of neurologic paraneoplastic syndromes comprise virtually any change in normal nervous system function. Abnormalities include behavioral changes; peripheral and spinal cord neuropathies; and alterations in the function of the cerebrum, cerebellum, medulla, and neuromuscular junction in both humans and cats (Table 35-1).

Diagnosis

The diagnosis of this paraneoplastic syndrome includes eliminating nonneoplastic causes using a CBC, biochemical profile, urinalysis, tests of the thyroid and adrenal axes, brain or spinal cord imaging (CT, MRI, and contrast radiography), biopsy of the affected nerves, CSF tap, and (if indicated) electrodiagnostics.

Treatment

Elimination of the neoplastic condition may resolve neurologic syndromes. Immune-mediated conditions of the central or peripheral nervous system may require the use of immunosuppressive therapy, including glucocorticoids.

TABLE 35-1
Paraneoplastic Syndromes of the Nervous System and Resulting Neurologic Syndromes[1-6]

Site Involved	Syndrome
Brain	Cerebellar degeneration
	Optic neuritis
	Progressive multifocal leukoencephalopathy
Spinal cord	Subacute necrotic myelopathy
	Subacute motor neuropathy
Peripheral nerves	Sensory neuropathy
	Peripheral neuropathy
	Autonomic gastrointestinal neuropathy
Muscle and neuromuscular junction	Dermatomyositis and polymyositis
	Myasthenic syndrome (Eaton-Lambert syndrome)
	Myasthenia gravis

HYPERTROPHIC OSTEOPATHY

CLINICAL BRIEFING

Diagnosis	
History	Shifting leg lameness.
Clinical Signs	Swollen, warm extremities; may also involve ribs and pelvis.
Diagnostics	Radiographs of affected bones to demonstrate unique periosteal reaction. Search for underlying malignancy with MDB, followed by abdominal radiography or ultrasonography.
Treatment	Treat the underlying cause.
	Administer antiinflammatory agents.

Hypertrophic osteopathy is an uncommon, but also underrecognized, disease that primarily occurs in the extremities. The disease primarily affects dogs and is rare in cats. This paraneoplastic syndrome is often associated with primary and metastatic lung tumors.[2] Other neoplastic and nonneoplastic conditions that have been associated with this disorder include esophageal sarcoma, rhabdomyosarcoma of the urinary bladder, pneumonia, heartworm disease, congenital and acquired heart disease, and focal lung atelectasis.[2] Other factors include hyperestrogenism, deficient oxygenation, and increased blood flow.[2]

Clinical Signs

The disease produces an increase in peripheral blood flow and a periosteal proliferation along the shafts of long bones, often beginning with the digits and extending as far proximally as the femur and humerus. Soft tissue proliferation occurs initially and is succeeded by osteophytes, which tend to radiate from the cortices at a 90 degree angle. The cause of this unique syndrome is unknown, although many theories exist.

Diagnosis (Figure 35-1)

Radiographs of the affected limb and the contralateral ex-

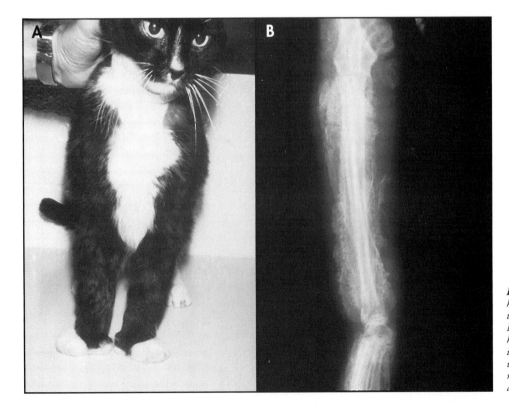

Figure 35-1: *This cat with hypertrophic osteopathy has thickening of the front limbs (**A**). Radiograph of a limb affected with hypertrophic osteopathy showing an increased soft tissue density and a unique osteophyte reaction that radiates outward at a 90-degree angle from the cortex of the bone (**B**).*

tremity often show an increased soft tissue density and a unique osteophyte reaction that radiates outward at a 90-degree angle from the cortex of the bone. When hypertrophic osteopathy is identified, the thorax (and abdomen, when indicated) should be radiographed to identify the underlying cause. Although a biopsy is definitive, the classic history, physical examination findings, and radiographic changes are often sufficient to permit a definitive diagnosis of hypertrophic osteopathy.

Treatment

Prednisone offers temporary improvement in clinical signs and may reduce swelling.[1,2] Removal of the tumor can effect almost immediate resolution of clinical signs; regression of bony and soft tissue changes may take months or years. Other suggested treatments include the use of analgesics, unilateral vagotomy on the side of the lung lesion, incision through the parietal pleura, subperiosteal rib resection, or bilateral cervical vagotomy.

REFERENCES

1. Ogilvie GK: Paraneoplastic syndromes, in Withrow SJ, MacEwen EG (eds): *Clinical Veterinary Oncology*. Philadelphia, JB Lippincott, 1989 pp 29–40.

2. Ogilvie GK: Paraneoplastic syndromes, in Ettinger SJ, Feldman EC (eds): *Textbook of Veterinary Internal Medicine*, ed 5. Philadelphia, WB Saunders, 2000, pp 498–506.

3. Griffin TW, Rosenthal PE, Costanza ME: Paraneoplastic and endocrine syndromes, in Cady B (ed): *Cancer Manual*, ed 7. Boston, American Cancer Society, 1986, pp 373–390.

4. Duncan ID: Peripheral neuropathy in the dog and cat. *Prog Vet Neurol* 2:111–121, 1990.

5. Manana KR, Luttgen PJ: Endocrine-associated neuropathies in dogs and cats. *Compend Contin Educ Pract Vet* 16:24–37, 1994.

6. Braund KG: Remote effects of cancer on the nervous system. *Semin Vet Med Surg Small Anim* 5:262–273, 1990.

PARANEOPLASTIC SYNDROMES

LYMPHOMA

Antony S. Moore and Gregory K. Ogilvie

36

CLINICAL BRIEFING

Common Presentation	Clinical signs vary because the disease affects multiple organs and systems.
Alimentary Lymphoma	Most common type; usually affects older, FeLV-negative cats.
Mediastinal Lymphoma	Usually affects young, FeLV-positive cats, often of Siamese/Oriental breed.
Spinal Lymphoma	Usually affects FeLV-positive cats. Demographics may be changing as FeLV infection is becoming less common.
Staging and Diagnosis	MDB (FeLV and FIV serology particularly important), abdominal ultrasonography, and bone marrow aspiration; CT scan or MRI needed to detect CNS lymphoma.
Treatment	
Initial	Chemotherapy combinations that include doxorubicin are most successful. Cats that are FeLV negative and physically well have the best prognosis.
Adjunctive	Radiation, always in conjunction with chemotherapy, may have a role in apparently localized lymphoma.
Supportive	Nutritional support is mandatory for inappetent cats. Administer appetite stimulants as needed and antiemetics therapeutically and prophylactically.

Incidence, Signalment, and Etiology

Lymphoma has long been considered the most common neoplasm in cats, largely because of its association with FeLV infection. Prior to the 1950s, reports of lymphoma were scarce.[1] However, this disease accounted for 20% to 40% of all feline neoplasms diagnosed in surveys published prior to the mid 1980s, with the highest prevalence in the northeastern United States.[2-4] Recent data suggest that lymphoma is less common now than it was a decade ago, which coincides with the decrease in FeLV infection rates.[5] Feline lymphoma is a heterogenous disease entity and difficult to classify anatomically or to "stage" in the manner used for dogs.

Cats of any age may be affected; lymphoma has been diagnosed in cats ranging in age from 4 months[6,7] to 19 years. There appears to be an early age peak as well as one at 7 to 8 years of age.[3,7] Lymphoma affecting the mediastinum appears to be more common in younger cats.[2,7-11] Although early reports found that most affected cats were DSHs or DLHs,[12]

MDB = minimum database; includes CBC, biochemical profile, urinalysis, FeLV/FIV serology, T₄ testing, and thoracic radiographs (three views).

other studies have found that Siamese/Oriental purebreds are at high risk for developing lymphoma.[3,13,14] This may relate to a higher risk of FeLV infection in catteries. Siamese cats also appeared more likely to have mediastinal lymphoma.[13] Male cats have predominated in large studies[3,7,15,16] and were statistically more likely to have lymphoma in an Australian study.[14] This may relate to males being more likely to roam and hence become infected with FeLV or FIV.

Virus particles were first identified in cats with lymphoma in the 1960s. Household clusters of lymphoma in cats led to speculation that horizontal transmission might occur.[18,19] Subsequently, a "C-type virus" was isolated and shown to be able to induce lymphoma after transmission.[20] From that time through the mid 1980s, the majority of reported lymphoma cases in cats occurred in association with FeLV infection. Cats with lymphoma often tested positive for FeLV antigen on ELISA serology. Lymphoma cells in cats with FeLV have been shown to contain provirus in addition to cytoplasmic and surface FeLV structural antigens. In addition, they have feline oncornavirus associated cell membrane antigen (FOCMA), which is probably a modified viral envelope glycoprotein and is considered to be a tumor-specific antigen.[21-23]

Approximately 25% of cats that test FeLV positive will develop lymphoma during their lifetime.[24,25] The time from first evidence of persistent viremia to tumor induction ranges from 1 to 41 months, with most cats affected between 5 to 17 months.[26,27] Tumorigenesis may be faster in younger cats. (Interestingly, FeLV vaccination did not appear to reduce the risk of FeLV infection in one group of cats with lymphoma.[15])

KEY POINT

Young FeLV-positive cats and young Siamese cats appear predisposed to developing mediastinal lymphoma.

Classically, FeLV integrates into the *myc* oncogene or transduces the *myc* oncogene to cause tumors.[28] An excellent review on this subject has been published by Rezanka and colleagues.[27] Other studies have identified portions of the FeLV viral genome and mechanisms that are specific for lymphomagenesis.[29–31] As with other tumors, mutations in the tumor suppressor gene, *p53*, are associated with some feline lymphomas[32]; however, the relationship of such mutations to viral infection is unclear.

Although lymphomas are seen in cats that do not have a positive serum antigen test for FeLV, the virus may still be implicated in tumorigenesis in many of these cats. Recombinant proviruses can be found in approximately 75% of lymphomas occurring in FeLV-positive cats,[33] but 5% of lymphomas in FeLV-negative cats also contained provirus.[34] More recently, the use of immunohistochemistry to stain for viral proteins and polymerase chain reaction (PCR) to amplify viral sequences has enabled researchers to detect FeLV in many cats that are seronegative for FeLV antigen.[35–37] PCR is the most sensitive technique to detect FeLV and therefore is more accurate than serology for predicting whether a tumor is virally induced.[35–38] The incidence of FeLV seropositivity in one U.S. study was only 25%, but PCR was not used and the true rate may be higher.[15] An Australian study showed that while seropositivity was only 2%, FeLV provirus could be amplified by PCR from 26% of the same cats.[37] This low rate of FeLV in Australia compared with the United States may reflect a difference in populations of cats between the two countries.

FIV has also been implicated in the development of feline lymphoma. The true independent contribution of this virus to tumorigenicity has been difficult to determine since FIV often occurs in conjunction with FeLV.[39] Of 353 cats with FeLV infection, 51 (14%) also had FIV infection. The risk of FeLV-positive cats developing lymphoma is approximately 60 times higher than that of FeLV/FIV-negative cats. The risk for FIV-positive cats is five times higher, and cats that are positive for both FeLV and FIV are nearly 80 times more likely to develop lymphoma than cats that are not infected with either virus.[39]

FIV is capable of inducing lymphoma by itself and may be responsible for some of the cases of FeLV-negative lymphoma dating back as far as 1968.[39] Although the prevalence of lymphoma in FeLV-positive cats is low in Australia, approximately 45% of cats with lymphoma test FIV positive on Western blot, implying a greater role for FIV in this disease.[a]

Many of the FIV-associated lymphomas appear to be multicentric, involving multiple extranodal sites based on case reports. This is true in the United States,[40] Europe (including the United Kingdom),[41,42] and Australia.[43] Many of these lymphomas appear to be of B lymphocyte origin.[41,42]

The anatomic distribution of lymphoma appears to be somewhat determined by the cat's viral status (Tables 36-1 and 36-2).

Lymphoma may also develop spontaneously, as evidenced by its presence in specific-pathogen free (SPF) cats.[44] Chromosomal abnormalities have been detected in lymphoma cells from virus-negative cats.[45]

Classically, feline lymphoma has been believed to be of T lymphocyte derivation, based largely on identification of T cells by rosette formation with guinea pig erythrocytes.[46] With the finding that feline monocytes also form rosettes,[47]

KEY POINT

Polymerase chain reaction to amplify viral sequences is the most sensitive method for detecting FeLV.

[a]R. Malik, personal communication.

TABLE 36-1
Anatomic Distribution of Feline Lymphoma Related to FeLV Status and Average Age in Cats Diagnosed in the 1970s[9]

Type of Lymphoma	No. of Cats	FeLV Positive (%)	FeLV Negative (%)	Mean Age (yr)
Multicentric	198	80.3	19.7	4
Mediastinal	174	77.0	23.0	2.5
Alimentary	69	23.2	76.8	8
Extranodal	13	38.5	61.5	8.6

TABLE 36-2
Anatomic Distribution of Lymphoma in Cats Diagnosed from 1968 to 1988[39]

Type of Lymphoma	Status			
	FeLV+/FIV−	FeLV−/FIV+	FeLV+/FIV+	FeLV−/FIV−
Multicentric	41	3	15	5
Thymic	33	0	1	10
Alimentary	1	1	2	9
Other	1	0	1	4
Unclassified	20	2	6	6
TOTAL	**96**	**6**	**25**	**34**

it is now believed that many of the tumors previously thought to be of T cell origin may be null cell, immature thymocyte, or monocyte in origin.[27,31,48]

Application of immunohistochemical staining for monoclonal antibodies to lymphocyte antigens has allowed researchers to more specifically characterize feline lymphomas.[49–51] In one study investigating 70 cases of lymphoma, 67% were of T cell derivation, 27% were B cell, and 6% were null cell[38]; FeLV infection was equally common in T and B cell lymphomas and in all age groups. Intestinal lymphomas were more likely to be of B cell origin, while skin lymphomas were all of T cell derivation.

Of 130 cats from three U.S. institutions, only 33 (25%) had lymphoma of T cell derivation.[15] Of 118 Australian cats, lymphomas were of T cell derivation in 28 (26%), B cell in 74 (70%), and null cell in 5 (4%).[52] The percentage of FeLV-positive cats in both studies was low, as appears to be true in since the 1980s when the practices of FeLV testing and vaccination and separating infected cats became generally accepted.[15,37,53]

The decline in the number of cats with FeLV has been noted in the United States[5] and Australia[37] and is presumably due to the practice of vaccination, either because vaccines protect against disease or because the practice of serologic testing before vaccination has enabled detection and separation of seropositive cats. The change in FeLV prevalence has also mirrored a change in feline lymphoma. The classic mediastinal or multicentric diseases of T lymphocytes in young cats—the forms of lymphoma most commonly associated with FeLV—have declined in prevalence in the last decade. Instead, alimentary lymphoma in older, FeLV-negative cats has become more common. These changes in the incidence, signalment, and etiology of lymphoma have also meant changes in treatment outcomes and supportive strategies.

Clinical Presentation and History

Lymphoma is a heterogenous disease in cats, and classification techniques that have attempted to describe groupings usually contain a "miscellaneous" or "other" category for those cats that do not fit the overall scheme. This heterogeneity means that there are few, if any, common clinical signs in all cats with lymphoma. Thus this book discusses the various forms of lymphoma in terms of the anatomic sites affected: Nasal, laryngeal, and tracheal lymphoma is covered in Chapter 47, cardiac lymphoma in Chapter 48, and cutaneous lymphoma in Chapter 50. Lymphoma of rare locations is included in the appropriate chapters, while more common types are discussed here.

Staging and Diagnosis

Most studies have divided cats with lymphoma into one of four groups. The *thoracic* or *mediastinal* group includes solitary tumors in the anterior mediastinum, *alimentary* includes gastrointestinal (GI) tumors with associated lymph node involvement, *multicentric* includes tumors with lymphadenopathy or spleen or liver involvement, and *unclassified* includes lymphoma affecting the eye, skin, nasal cavity, central nervous system (CNS), and other extranodal sites. Confusion with this system arises because some authors include renal lymphoma in the alimentary group,[7] some classify it in the multicentric group,[9] some group all abdominal tumors together,[8] and others consider renal lymphoma as a separate entity.[54] A recent study attempted to reclassify lymphoma as abdominal (as above), mediastinal, nodal (lymph nodes only), and atypical (unclassified extranodal locations); these authors also included a mixed category to define combinations from all other groups (Table 36-3).[14] The variation in these classification systems emphasizes the confusing nature of this disease, and attempts to subclassify lymphoma have not been shown to be prognostically important.

Another group of researchers attempted to "stage" cats by extent of disease regardless of anatomic site.[55] Application of this staging system appeared to be prognostic in their studies,[54,56] but other investigations have failed to validate this system.[15] Any cat with lymphoma should be thoroughly examined and the extent of disease determined by a MDB (FeLV and FIV serology particularly important), abdominal ultrasonography, and bone marrow aspiration. Many cats with apparently localized lymphoma will be found to have other sites of involvement. Feline lymphoma should always be considered to be multisystemic.

Thoracic radiography is indicated to detect a mediastinal mass, pleural effusion, or pulmonary involvement. In cats, lymphoma of the lungs may take the form of a nodule or mass[14] rather than the diffuse pattern seen in dogs.

Abdominal ultrasonography is an excellent method to identify GI lymphoma, enlarged abdominal lymph nodes, and renal abnormalities.[57] It is also ideal for guiding fine-needle aspiration or needle core biopsy of abdominal organs.[58] Ultrasonography without biopsy was not very helpful in the diagnosis of hepatic lymphoma in one study. Only two of five cats subsequently shown to have lymphoma in the liver had an abnormal liver on ultrasonography.[59]

Hematologic and serum biochemical profiles are of limited value in diagnosing lymphoma in cats. One survey found that approximately half of the cats with lymphoma were anemic and two thirds had a neutrophilic leucocytosis.[60] Serum biochemical changes were related to the primary site of involvement: Hypoalbuminemia was common in cats with alimentary lymphoma and azotemia occurred most commonly in cats with renal lymphoma. Signalment and histologic criteria had no influence on these findings.[60]

Bone marrow aspiration is warranted even in cats with a normal hemogram, particularly in cats that test FeLV positive[61] or that have signs of spinal disease. Approximately 70% of cats with spinal lymphoma have concurrent bone marrow involvement.[62] In these cats, it is less invasive to collect bone marrow to make a diagnosis of lymphoma than it is to do surgical exploration, decompression, and biopsy of an extradural mass.

Histologically, feline lymphoma most closely resembles non-Hodgkin's lymphoma in humans. The specific histologic appearance associated with Hodgkin's disease in humans is rarely described in cats.[64–66] Eight older (4.5 to 18 years) DSHs with a solitary enlarged mandibular or cervical lymph node were found to have a B cell lymphoma similar to Hodgkin's disease; there was no evidence of FeLV or FIV in these cats.[67] Histologically, the majority of lymphomas in cats are high or intermediate grade; low-grade tumors account for only 10% of cases.[68]

Well-differentiated (low-grade) lymphomas appear to be diagnosed mainly in the GI tract,[68] where they may represent progression from "lymphocytic-plasmacytic gastroenteritis" or inflammatory bowel disease. It might be difficult histologically to differentiate early low-grade lymphoma

TABLE 36-3
Anatomic Distribution of Feline Lymphoma (1950–2000)

Country	Years of Study	No. (%) of Cats with Specified Tumor Type				
		Mediastinal	Alimentary	Multicentric	Extranodal	Total
Scotland[10]	1954–1964	5 (10)	24 (50)	14 (30)	5 (10)	48
Northeastern United States[7]	1958–1970	38 (25)	70[a] (47)	28 (19)	14 (9)	150
Japan[2]	1964–1972	20 (71)	8 (29)			28
California[8]	1970–1978	402 (23)	694[a] (40)	637 (37)		1733
New York[9]	Before 1981	174 (38)	69 (15)	198[a] (44)	13 (3)	454
Yugoslavia[63]	Before 1990	4 (14)	5 (18)	19[a] (68)		28
Canada[38]	Before 1996	10 (14)	13 (19)	42 (60)	5 (7)	70
United States (multicenter)[15]	1988–1996	17 (13)	50 (38)	45[a] (34)	19 (15)	131
Australia[13]	1984–1994	14 (23)	12 (20)	18 (30)	16 (27)	60
Australia[14]	1997–1998	9 (8)	Nodal 20 (17)	Abdominal 43 (36) Mixed 39 (33)	7 (6)	118
TOTAL		**693 (24)**	⊢——— 2048 (73) ———⊣		**79 (3)**	**2820**

[a]Includes renal lymphoma.

from severe inflammatory bowel disease.[3] The finding of well-differentiated GI lymphoma may improve the chance for long-term survival compared with cats that have high-grade lymphoma because well-differentiated GI tumors may be more responsive to chemotherapy.[10,69]

Despite prognostic utility in dogs, histologic methods for measuring cell proliferation (proliferating cell nuclear antigen [PCNA]) or nuclear activity (silver-staining nucleolar organizer region [AgNOR] staining) have not been shown to classify feline lymphoma into any prognostic groupings.[15,70]

Paraneoplastic syndromes are uncommon in cats with lymphoma. Hypercalcemia has been reported in three cats with lymphoma, all of which were FeLV positive[71–73]; their serum calcium levels were 12.2 to 16.2 mg/dl, and serum albumin levels were normal to low. A decrease in serum calcium was noted concurrently with tumor regression in one cat.[72] The distribution of lymphoma was varied: Two had mediastinal lymphoma,[72,73] and one had liver and alimentary involvement.[71] In dogs, hypercalcemia is often associated with a T cell phenotype. This information was unavailable in these cats, although one had monoclonal IgG gammopathy and hyperviscosity, implying a B cell derivation.[71] One hypercalcemic cat had dystrophic mineralization of the pulmonary alveoli and bronchi.[73] Three other cats had mineralization and bone formulation within their mediastinal lymphoma,[74,75] but serum calcium was not measured. In a larger series of cats, only 4 of 84 had elevated serum calcium levels, and there was no correlation with T cell phenotype.[60] Parathyroid hormone-related peptide (PTH-rP) levels may also be elevated and can be measured in cats using a commonly available human assay. Normal levels are below 0.2 pmol/L.[76]

Although uncommon, hyperviscosity associated with monoclonal gammopathy is a possible paraneoplastic syndrome. Two cats in addition to the one cited above[71] had an IgG monoclonal gammopathy and multicentric lymphoma.[77]

Associated glomerulonephritis has been described in FeLV-positive cats with various forms of lymphoma.[78–80] Because serum protein electrophoresis was not available for these cats, it is difficult to say whether glomerular IgG deposition was a result of a paraneoplastic gammopathy.

> **KEY POINT**
>
> *In addition to the MDB (with FeLV and FIV serology), the diagnostic workup of any cat with lymphoma should include abdominal ultrasonography and bone marrow aspiration.*

Unusual paraneoplastic syndromes have also been described in cats with lymphoma. An FeLV-negative cat with hepatic and alimentary B cell lymphoma developed ischemic cutaneous necrosis of the hind feet.[81] Another cat developed myoclonic tremors or seizures that affected all skeletal muscles; despite multicentric involvement with lymphoma, there was no neoplastic muscle infiltrate to explain this paraneoplastic condition.[82] Adrenal gland involvement in two cats with multicentric lymphoma led to an acute hypoadrenal (Addisonian) crisis.[83] Both cats were weak, lethargic, and anorexic and had hyperkalemia and hyponatremia in addition to azotemia. Involvement of the adrenal gland appears to be rare in cats with lymphoma.[84]

Immunosuppression due to lymphoma or FeLV infection may lead to secondary infections in cats. Cats with concurrent FeLV and lymphoma have been diagnosed with *Cryptococcal* rhinitis,[85] generalized *Sarcocystis,*[86] and multiple osteolytic lesions due to *Histoplasma capsulatum.*[87] All three of these cats were less than 3 years of age. Two cats with lymphoma but no evidence of FeLV (13 and 15 years old) were diagnosed with *Cryptosporidium* enteritis[88] and *Salmonella typhimurium* septicemia,[89] respectively. Both cats had intestinal lymphoma. A 5-year-old cat had *Toxoplasmosis* in addition to lymphoma and leukemia.[90]

LYMPHOMA OF THE GI TRACT AND MESENTERIC LYMPH NODES

Incidence, Signalment, and Etiology

In many surveys, lymphoma involving the mesenteric nodes and intestinal tract is called *alimentary lymphoma.* Many studies have identified this as the most common form of lymphoma, particularly in recent years when 40% to 50% of feline lymphoma cases have involved the alimentary system.[14,15] Although cats as young as 5 months may have intestinal lymphoma,[14] the median age is 10 to 12 years,[14,15,70,91–93] which is significantly older than the general population of cats with lymphoma.[15]

The majority of affected cats (141 of 178 cats [79%]) have been DSHs.[14,70,91,93–97] Siamese was the next most commonly affected breed (13 cats [7%]), followed by other purebred shorthairs (10 cats), including Abyssinian, Burmese, and Russian Blue.[14,70,93] There were only 5 (3%) DLHS[91,93,95,97] and 9 purebred longhaired cats (including Maine Coon, Himalayan, and Persian)[14,70,95,97,98] in this group (99 males and 79 females).

Cats with alimentary lymphoma are significantly less likely than other cats with lymphoma to test positive for

FeLV antigen.[15] Of 127 cats for which FeLV status was known, 9 were antigen positive (7%).[15,70,91,93] One cat that was serologically negative subsequently proved positive on bone marrow immunohistochemistry. In cats with alimentary lymphoma, FeLV is much more likely to be detected by PCR than by serology.[35] Of 50 cats tested for FIV, 3 were antibody positive.[70,91] An Australian study showed that FIV may be more prevalent than FeLV in B cell tumors of the abdominal cavity, including the intestinal tract; approximately 45% of cats were FIV positive[a] but only 26% were FeLV positive in that study.

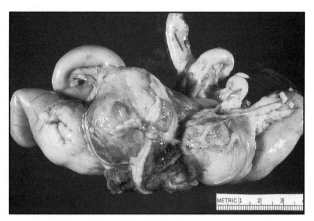

Figure 36-1: *Intestinal adhesions and associated lymphadenopathy created a large irregular abdominal mass in a 4-year-old cat with intestinal lymphoma. This tumor had perforated the intestine to cause localized peritonitis.*

KEY POINT

Alimentary tract lymphoma occurs most commonly in older cats that are serologically FeLV negative.

Clinical Presentation and History

Clinical signs in most cats are chronic and have been present for 1 to 3 months before presentation.[91] The most common clinical signs are anorexia and weight loss, and these may be the only signs referable to the GI tract.[93] Vomiting appears to be less common, occurring in less than 50% of cats presented.[93,94] The histologic type of lymphoma may influence the distribution of lymphoma within the GI layers and therefore the clinical signs. Well-differentiated lymphoma is more likely to affect the superficial mucosal layers. In one study of 39 cats with well-differentiated intestinal lymphoma, all but 4 had vomiting or diarrhea.[69] Other signs that are less specific to alimentary lymphomas are lethargy, depression, weakness, polydipsia/polyuria (often with concurrent renal involvement),[92] pica, and abdominal swelling.

An abdominal mass is often palpable[93,96,98,99] and may perforate, causing septic peritonitis (Figure 36-1).[91] Cats with lymphoblastic GI lymphoma are more likely to have a palpable abdominal mass than cats with well-differentiated lymphoma,[69] whereas cats with well-differentiated lymphoma are more likely to have thickened bowel loops.[69]

There is some debate about whether inflammatory bowel disease (IBD) may transform into lymphoma or is merely found in conjunction with lymphoma (i.e., a reaction to the tumor).[93] Of 49 cats with alimentary lymphoma, 6 had been previously treated for IBD with prednisone (treatment range, 3 months to 2 years; median, 9 months).[91,93] In at least one of these studies, cats that had received corticosteroids prior to diagnosis fared neither better nor worse than other cats with alimentary lymphoma. Persistent signs that do not respond to traditional therapy for IBD should be investigated for underlying lymphoma. This may require exploratory laparotomy and full-thickness intestinal biopsies.

Staging and Diagnosis

Most commonly, alimentary lymphoma involves the small intestine, either as a diffuse segmental thickening or generalized thickening throughout the small intestinal tract.[92] Involvement of the cecum or colon is less common.[92,100,101] Although lymphoma is the most common gastric tumor in cats, the stomach is still an uncommon site compared with the small intestine. Lymphoma is usually localized to one segment of the intestinal tract (Figure 36-2).[92,93]

Most cats have involvement of mesenteric lymph nodes in addition to an intestinal mass or have multiple adhesions to the intestine that make it unresectable. In four studies comprising a total of 140 cats, only 31 cats were considered to have resectable lesions.[14,70,91,93] Concurrent infiltration of the spleen or liver with lymphoma may be less common than involvement of the kidneys.[14,92] Other sites of involvement reported include bone marrow,[70,91,93] larynx,[96] lung,[91,93] pleura,[91,93] eye,[14,93] skin,[14,93] or pancreas.[14,93] This emphasizes

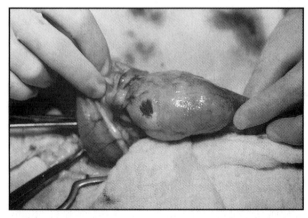

Figure 36-2: *Occasionally, an intestinal lymphoma will be localized, as shown here, but usually extends over a much larger segment. When lymphoma is localized, surgical excision may relieve obstruction but needs to be combined with chemotherapy to provide long-term control. (Courtesy of J. Berg)*

the importance of assessing the entire body and determining the location of all disease by complete staging.

Abdominal radiography can discern an abdominal mass, but such masses are usually already evident on abdominal palpation. A barium meal may show decreased transit time,[96,102] but the length of time to perform this procedure (1 to 3 hours) and the difficulties associated with oropharyngeal intubation for barium administration make this option less attractive.[91]

Ultrasonography requires less time and patient manipulation and can be used to evaluate other abdominal organs. Ultrasonographic findings in a cat with lymphoma include thickening of the gastric or intestinal wall; this thickening is usually symmetric for intestinal lesions but may be asymmetric for gastric lesions (Figure 36-3). In addition, there is loss of the normal layered appearance and often a hypoechoic mass within the GI tract. Abdominal lymphadenopathy is common (in contrast to intestinal carcinoma, which is generally a solitary lesion without lymph node involvement and best treated with surgery—illustrating the importance of obtaining a biopsy).[57,95] Ultrasonography can be used to safely guide fine-needle aspiration or needle core biopsy of an intestinal lymphoma[57,58,91,95] and is the imaging modality of choice.

Endoscopy has a limited ability to diagnose intestinal lymphoma. In one study, the diagnostic efficiency of gastroscopy was 32% and that of duodenoscopy was 36%. This is probably due to the small size of samples that can be obtained with endoscopy. It is possible to collect biopsy samples of superficial mucosa that show IBD but "miss" the underlying lymphoma (Figure 36-4). Less commonly, an inflammatory lesion may be misdiagnosed as lymphoma.[104] Endoscopy is also unable to evaluate the jejunum, ileum, and cecal regions where most intestinal lymphomas occur.

There is some discrepancy as to the derivation of intestinal lymphoma. In two studies totaling 107 cats, only 20 cats had T cell GI lymphoma.[15,52] This concurs with early studies that showed most alimentary lymphomas to be of B cell derivation. In contrast, a small California study showed 10 of 13 cats to have T cell lymphoma.[91] Whether lymphoma is of T or B cell origin does not seem to influence prognosis.[15]

Most cats with intestinal lymphoma also have involvement of mesenteric nodes and intraabdominal adhesions that make the lymphoma surgically unresectable.

Well-differentiated lymphoma accounted for only 6 of 57 cats with alimentary lymphoma in one study[52] and 3 of 28 cats in another study.[93] In contrast, a California group found that 50 of 67 cats with intestinal lymphoma had a well-differentiated type of tumor. By their definition, any biopsy with "packets" of five or more lymphocytes in direct apposition and located between epithelial cells was lymphoma. Well-differentiated lymphoma arises in the superficial mucosa and invades underlying layers, rarely creating clinically obvious masses. In that study, most cats (92%) were diagnosed via endoscopic biopsy.[69] In contrast to lymphoblastic lymphoma, which often involves only the stomach, well-differentiated lymphoma is primarily an intestinal disease involving the stomach only by extension.

Cats that had areas of both well-differentiated and lymphoblastic lymphoma were identified but were not included in the analysis.[69] In another report, a cat with well-differentiated intestinal lymphoma had lymphoblastic lymphoma in its mesenteric node.[105]

The use of AgNOR counts was not found to predict survival or response in cats with intestinal lymphomas,[15,70] and measures of proliferative activity were likewise unhelpful in

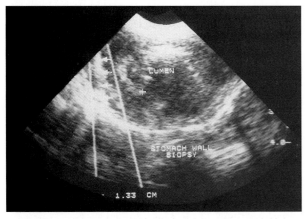

Figure 36-3: *Lymphoma may cause massive thickening of the gastric wall. Ultrasonography allows "staging" of other organs and guides needle biopsy, as seen in this image. (Courtesy of D. Penninck)*

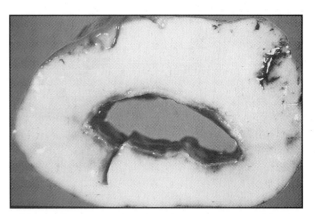

Figure 36-4: *Complete transmural, circumferential lymphoma as seen in this 13-year-old cat may not be diagnosed by endoscopic biopsy due to an intact mucosa. Surgical- or ultrasonographic-guided biopsy is preferred. (Courtesy of G.H. Theilen)*

predicting outcome.[15] In a large histopathology study, biopsy samples from cats with alimentary lymphoma had significantly fewer mitoses than samples from cats with lymphoma at other sites.[68]

Treatment

It is uncommon for lymphoma to be localized to the intestinal tract without lymph node or other organ involvement, and thus surgical resection alone should not be relied on for treatment. Even though there are individual reports of wide intestinal resection causing long-term (2 to 3 years) remissions in cats with lymphoma,[96,100] recurrence is usually rapid.[96,99] Of five cats treated surgically to relieve intestinal obstruction, one achieved complete remission (CR) for more than 13 months but the others died of lymphoma within 3.5 months.[69] Chemotherapy is necessary to treat other sites of disease. In two studies, resection of an intestinal mass prior to chemotherapy did not seem to improve survival compared with chemotherapy alone.[93,100]

Supportive care is mandatory for cats with lymphoma involving the GI tract. The disease is often chronic, and these patients are frequently thin and anorectic and/or vomiting. In addition, many of the chemotherapeutics employed have the potential to make these symptoms worse. For some cats, placement of an esophagostomy or gastrostomy feeding tube is essential to allow adequate nutrition, especially during the induction of remission. In addition, a tube enhances the caregiver's ability to administer oral medication (Figure 36-5). However, if the cat is vomiting or has gastric involvement, a jejunal feeding tube may be needed (see Chapter 19). In cats for which enteral feeding is impossible, parenteral (IV) feeding of a complete diet is warranted. Cats will often start to eat once a tumor responds to treatment, but nutritional support is vital in the meantime. In addition to assisted feeding techniques, the use of oral appetite stimulants as well as good general nursing care is essential to improve nutritional status.

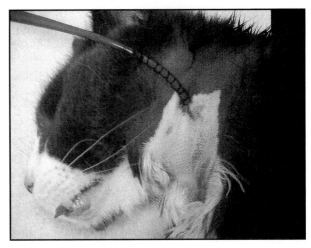

Figure 36-5: *An esophagostomy tube allows anorectic cats to be fed during the early stages of treatment.*

Cats may lose a large percentage of their body weight in a period as short as a week; any weight loss should be considered unacceptable and prompt one or more of the interventions described previously.[93]

Chemotherapy is the principal modality used to treat lymphoma. Multiple-agent chemotherapy using vincristine, cyclophosphamide, and prednisone (COP) was the basis for treating 38 cats.[93,99,102,105,106] Additional drugs such as L-asparaginase[105] or cytosine arabinoside[99] did not seem to alter the outcome. In case reports, two cats had long (more than 12 months) survivals. In a large study, only 9 (32%) of 28 cats attained CR following therapy.[93] The overall median survival for these 28 cats was 50 days (range, 2 to 2,120 days). In comparison, the cats that achieved CR had a median survival of 213 days (7 months), and 4 lived longer than a year. This is in contrast to two studies with a total of 16 cats that were treated in the late 1970s in which 11 cats had a CR and 1 had a partial remission (PR)[97,106]; median remission was approximately 6 months. It is possible that these cats were selected for treatment on the basis of good health.[106] Clinical signs of illness are strongly correlated with poor response to treatment.[15,93]

A more aggressive protocol utilizing COP plus doxorubicin and L-asparaginase was used to treat 70 cats.[69,70,97,100] Eleven cats with colonic lymphoma had a median survival of 3 months, which was not significantly different from 8 cats that did not receive chemotherapy. Some cats had surgical excision of the tumor, and thus response to chemotherapy could not be assessed.[100] The remaining 59 cats received chemotherapy alone.[69,70,91] Thirty-two cats (54%) achieved a CR (median duration, 4[70] to 10[91] months). Seventeen cats had a PR, although survival times were shorter than in cats that achieved a CR.[70,91] These remission rates (CR plus PR) were better than those achieved with COP alone, although survival times for cats achieving a CR were similar.[93] This implies that CR to chemotherapy determines survival; this was the only prognostic factor found in these studies.[70,91,93] It is possible that the addition of doxorubicin improved outcome by increasing the CR rate.[15,107]

It should be noted that some cats have short-term responses that last less than 3 weeks. Rapid tumor recurrence in these cats does not seem to respond to further chemotherapy, and median survival times are usually less than 1 month.[70,93] Similarly, cats that fail to respond to initial chemotherapy rarely respond to other chemotherapy drugs, including doxorubicin, idarubicin, L-asparaginase, and chlorambucil.[93]

In contrast, when a cat relapses after having had a durable (longer than 6 months) remission induced by chemotherapy, the chances of a second remission are good, particularly if relapse occurs after chemotherapy has been discontinued. Three cats relapsed when COP chemotherapy was discontinued, and all achieved a second remission.[102] Six cats that had a CR to chemotherapy had a second remission when treated with the same protocol[91] and maintained that remission for a median of 3 months. Another cat responded to doxorubicin and mitoxantrone on relapse and maintained a second remission for 10 months.[91]

A separate syndrome of well-differentiated lymphoma has been reported in cats with intestinal involvement. In one study, response to COP chemotherapy was no better than in cats with high-grade intestinal lymphoma.[93] In contrast, a series of 29 cats with well-differentiated lymphoma were treated with prednisone and chlorambucil alone; 20 cats (69%) achieved a CR for up to 49 months (median, 16 months).[69] The median survival for all 29 cats regardless of response was 17 months, while those achieving CR lived a median of 23 months. In contrast, 11 cats with lymphoblastic lymphoma in the same study received multiple-agent chemotherapy but only 2 (11%) had a CR.[69] Most cats were diagnosed by endoscopic biopsy. Recent reports of the unreliability of endoscopic biopsy in diagnosing lymphoma[103,104] creates some skepticism regarding the diagnosis described in that report.[69] As discussed, GI lymphoma is best diagnosed by ultrasound-guided needle core biopsy or by surgery.[57]

> **KEY POINT**
>
> *Nutritional support is mandatory for a successful outcome in cats treated for alimentary lymphoma.*

LYMPHOMA OF LARGE GRANULAR LYMPHOCYTES

Incidence, Signalment, and Etiology

Since 1986,[108,109] there have been increasing numbers of reports of cats with round cell tumors that are clinically indistinguishable from lymphoma; this has been termed *large granular lymphoma* or *neoplasm of globule leukocytes*. The principal histologic differentiation between the two entities appeared to be that cytoplasmic granules within globule leukocyte cells stained with phosphotungstic acid–hematoxylin whereas large granular lymphoma did not. Recent studies have utilized lymphoid markers to show that all these tumors are probably derived from lymphocyte subpopulations (cytotoxic T lymphocytes or natural killer [NK] cells)[110–113] and that all are the same disease, which we have termed *lymphoma of large granular lymphocytes* (LLGL).

This tumor type is considered uncommon, possibly as a result of the staining characteristics of the intracytoplasmic granules. These granules are best seen with Wright-Giemsa-based stains rather than the hematoxylin-eosin stains used for biopsy specimens. This means that the tumor type is often not diagnosed unless cytology of a fine-needle aspirate or fluid analysis is performed. A recent study suggested that nearly 10% of feline lymphomas may be of this subtype.[113] It is probably best considered a subtype of alimentary lymphoma based on the distribution of lesions.

This tumor type had been reported in 42 cats (22 females and 20 males; most were neutered).[90,108,111–122] LLGL has not been described in purebreds, and only 7 affected cats were DLHs.[116,118,119] Although it has been reported in cats as young as 2.5 years of age,[120] LLGL mainly affects older cats (median age, approximately 9 years).

Clinical Presentation and History

Most LLGLs affect the alimentary tract, with the true extent of disease being much wider. The most common presenting sign was decreased appetite or anorexia (27 cats), which was exacerbated by chronic or intermittent vomiting in 16 cats. Most cats had lost weight. Other less common signs included lethargy (8 cats), diarrhea (5 cats), icterus (6 cats), and hematuria (2 cats).

On physical examination, the most common finding was a palpable abdominal mass from $5 \times 2 \times 2$ cm to $8 \times 6 \times 4$ cm in size.[108,117] These masses are composed of mesenteric lymph nodes and/or intestinal masses, as is commonly seen in cats with alimentary lymphoma. Four cats presented with a perforation of the intestine associated with tumor infiltration.[112,114]

Staging and Diagnosis

Complete staging, including MDB, abdominal ultrasonography, bone marrow aspiration, and a biopsy, should be performed prior to initiating treatment.

Lymphoma of large granular lymphocytes is considered a subtype of alimentary lymphoma.

CBC results may demonstrate a neutrophilic leukocytosis, often with a left shift.[109,111,113,118,122] Total neutrophil counts can be very high (ranging up to 50,000), leading one investigator to suggest that the neoplastic cells may produce cytokines that stimulate granulopoiesis.[111] LLGL cells have been shown to produce interleukin-2 (IL-2) and interleukin-3 (IL-3). Most cats have a normal circulating lymphocyte count, but some cats have a leukemic differential with total counts as high as 250,000.[112,113,118] One cat had more than 5,000 normoblasts/μl. The percentage of circulating large granular lymphocytes (LGLs) has varied in studies, ranging from 2.5%[108] to more than 40%.[113,118] It should be noted, however, that normal cats may circulate these cells and have between 3% and 13% circulating LGLs.[118] This means that the presence of circulating LGLs in the absence of disease may not indicate lymphoma.

In one study, 10 of 11 cats were hypoalbuminemic, presumably due to intestinal loss and decreased liver production of albumin; 8 of these cats also were hyperbilirubinemic.[118]

Thoracic radiographs may demonstrate a mediastinal mass and/or pleural effusion. Ascites is uncommon,[111,116,117,122] and pericardial effusion is rare.[122] Cytology of pleural or ascitic fluid is usually positive for LGLs, and the granules are easily seen using Wright-Giemsa stain.

Bone marrow cytology has demonstrated LGL infiltration in a small number of cats,[108,117,120] usually in association with circulating cells. Most tested cats have been FeLV negative, although one was positive[111] and one had latent FeLV cultured from bone marrow.[116] Of the very few cats tested for FIV, only one was positive.[118]

A possible differential for an abdominal mass and granulated round cells on cytology would be a mast cell tumor; but histopathologic evidence of histamine reactivity should be absent in LLGL.[112] Other more specific testing to diagnose LLGL can be performed using a T cell marker to CD3 or an NK cell marker.[113] In addition, perforin, a potent mediator of cytotoxicity found in granules of cytotoxic T cells and NK cells, may be demonstrated using a monoclonal antibody.[110,112]

Although LLGL usually affects the small intestinal tract and/or mesenteric nodes, extension to involve the large intestine[109,111–113,120,122] or stomach[113,122] may occur. The most commonly affected organs are the liver (15 cats), spleen (10 cats), kidney (6 cats), and pancreas (4 cats). A mediastinal mass was seen in 6 cats and pleural effusion in 4. It should be noted, however, that just as with lymphoma of any type in cats, other organs such as the heart, lung, adrenal gland, brain, bladder, or skin may also be involved. Peripheral lymph nodes are rarely affected.[115,119]

Treatment

Chemotherapy is the treatment of choice for LLGL, and as is the case with other types and locations of feline lymphoma, responses are mixed. The pattern of response is very similar to that seen in cats with GI lymphoma.

Of 13 cats treated with chemotherapy, CR of 6 to 21 months (median, 20 months) was seen in 4 cats. Chemotherapy for these animals included prednisone, vincristine, cyclophosphamide, and L-asparaginase in two cats, L-asparaginase and vincristine in one cat, and prednisone, vincristine, and cyclophosphamide in the fourth.[119,120] Another cat had a 50% response to L-asparaginase but relapsed quickly.[117] Intraperitoneal administration of L-asparaginase caused a CR for 6 months in a cat with LLGL of the liver even though it was resistant to other chemotherapy.[b] A solitary small intestinal mass was resected in one cat, and there was no evidence of disease until recurrence in the mesenteric lymph nodes 13.5 months later.[121]

[b]Moore AS: Personal observation.

MEDIASTINAL LYMPHOMA

Incidence, Signalment, and Etiology

Mediastinal lymphoma is most often presented as being the characteristic form of the disease in cats. Studies before 1980 found this to be a common type of lymphoma, accounting for 20% to 40% of cases in the United States,[7,9,124] 10% to 50% of cases in the United Kingdom,[10,125] and 70% of cases in Japan.[2] Recent surveys have found much lower prevalence rates for mediastinal lymphoma (i.e., less than 15% of cases in the United States[15,107,126] and approximately 25% of cases in Australia[13,14]).

Although the prevalence may have changed, the signalment and etiology of this disease have not. While there is a wide range in ages of affected cats, the median age has been less than 5 years in all studies.[14,15,125,127,128] This is significantly younger than the median age of all cats with lymphoma.[14,15]

The Siamese/Oriental purebreds seem to be at higher risk for developing mediastinal lymphoma and account for 30%[14,128] to 90%[13,125] of cats with this form of the disease. Young Siamese cats appear to be at particularly high risk.[14]

FeLV appears to play a prominent etiologic role in mediastinal lymphoma in cats. The majority of reported cats were FeLV positive,[128-132] and in one large survey, 75% of cats with mediastinal lymphoma were FeLV positive.[15] Therefore despite a decrease in the prevalence of mediastinal lymphoma, it remains a disease of mainly young, FeLV-positive cats, often of the Siamese/Oriental breeds.

Clinical Presentation and History

Dyspnea due to the presence of a large mediastinal mass and/or pleural effusion is a common presenting sign, although it may not be obvious to the owner. Dyspnea was the major cause of owner concern in only 13 of 30 cats with mediastinal lymphoma in one study,[125] but an additional 9 cats were found to be dyspneic by the veterinarian. Regurgitation or dysphagia in addition to dyspnea was a cause for owner concern in 23 of 60 cats.[125,128] Other less specific causes for presentation to a veterinarian were anorexia, weight loss, enlarged lymph nodes, cough, and ptyalism. Regurgitation due to esophageal compression may be mistaken for vomiting by owners.[133] The clinical signs are usually acute, being present for less than 4 weeks in nearly all cats.[128]

KEY POINT

Dyspnea due to a large mediastinal mass, pleural effusion, and/or regurgitation due to esophageal compression are the most common signs of mediastinal lymphoma.

On physical examination, dull rostral lung fields on auscultation are common. The anterior thorax may be incompressible (75% of cats in one study[125]), or there may be a palpable mass at the thoracic inlet.

Lymphadenopathy, particularly affecting lymph nodes of the head, neck, and axilla, is common. In two studies with a total of 59 cats, 22 (37%) had peripheral lymphadenopathy due to lymphoma in addition to the mediastinal mass, and this was the most common secondary site for lymphoma in these animals.[14,128]

Invasion of intrathoracic structures may lead to effusion, which exacerbates the dyspnea. In extreme cases, invasion of a vital structure can occur, leading to a life-threatening condition. A cat with cranial vena cava syndrome (occlusion of venous return to the heart) had a mediastinal lymphoma that invaded the vena cava and lungs.[132] The tumor may grow very quickly—one study reported a cat with mediastinal lymphoma that weighed 250 g and had not been detectable 3 weeks earlier (Figure 36-6).

Staging and Diagnosis

An MDB (especially FeLV/FIV serology) should be obtained. Thoracic radiographs may demonstrate an anterior

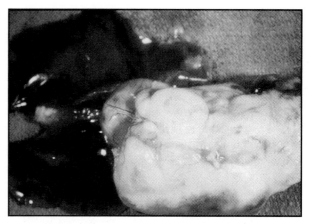

Figure 36-6: *Mediastinal lymphoma may be massive and occupy most of the thoracic cavity. Dyspnea may be exacerbated by pleural effusion. (Courtesy of S.M. Cotter)*

mediastinal mass causing dorsal tracheal elevation and, less commonly, caudal displacement of the carina.[125]

A mediastinal mass may be obscured by pleural effusion. Drainage of this fluid can be therapeutic and palliative in addition to helping obtain a diagnosis. Cytologic examination is nearly always diagnostic for lymphoma.[125,129] Approximately 15% of cats have a chylous-appearing effusion[125] that often also contains lymphoblasts (Figure 36-7).[129,135]

Because imaging is enhanced in the presence of fluid, thoracic ultrasonography is an excellent alternative but should not be performed until the cat is stabilized clinically via thoracocentesis (Figures 36-8 and 36-9). Ultrasonography may guide collection of needle aspiration or Tru-cut biopsy specimen, which is necessary to differentiate lymphoma from thymoma in older cats.

Complete staging is important to determine extent of disease and as a guide for therapy. In three groups totaling 89 cats with mediastinal lymphoma, 43 had evidence of

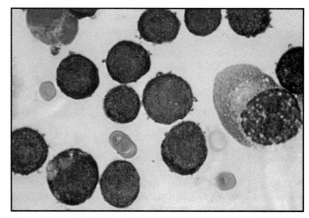

Figure 36-7: *Cytology of pleural effusion is usually diagnostic due to the presence of a large number of lymphoblasts. This sample is from a 3-year-old cat. (Courtesy of S.M. Cotter)*

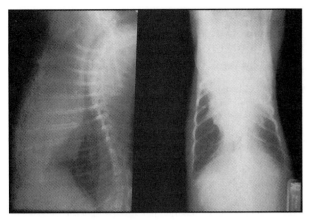

Figure 36-8: Thoracic radiographs showing an anterior mediastinal mass in a 3-year-old cat with lymphoma. (Courtesy of S.M. Cotter)

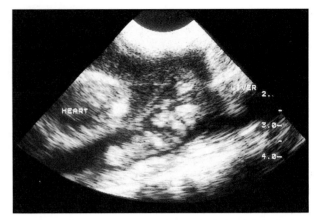

Figure 36-9: Pleural effusion may obscure radiographic detail in a cat with mediastinal lymphoma. Ultrasonography allows detailed examination of the mass and helps guide biopsy specimen collection. (Courtesy of D. Penninck)

lymphoma at sites other than the mediastinum.[14,125,128] The most commonly affected secondary sites were peripheral lymph nodes (particularly head, superficial cervical, and axillary[14]) and intrathoracic and abdominal lymph nodes (including sublumbar nodes).[128] Less common secondary sites were the liver, spleen, and kidney. Blood or bone marrow involvement is uncommon, which serves to emphasize the importance of complete staging. Abdominal ultrasonography and bone marrow aspiration should be performed in addition to the tests outlined above.

KEY POINT

Biopsy is required to differentiate lymphoma from thymoma in older cats.

Mediastinal lymphoma was thought to be a disease of T cells, even early in the description of this disease.[136] Recent use of monoclonal antibodies has confirmed that 50%[52] to 85%[15] of mediastinal lymphomas are T cell derived and that they are significantly more likely to be of this phenotype than the general population of lymphomas.[15,52] Most young cats have T cell lymphoma, but older cats often have B cell mediastinal lymphoma. The finding of T cell phenotype did not appear to influence prognosis in one study.[15]

Treatment

Surgery does not have a role in the treatment of mediastinal lymphoma.[133] Radiation therapy, although anecdotally believed to improve response rates in cats with mediastinal lymphoma, has not been critically evaluated as an adjunct to chemotherapy. The potential for pulmonary damage is high if large doses of radiation are used.

Mediastinal lymphoma is considered to be one of the more chemotherapy-responsive anatomic forms of lymphoma.[137] In early studies, response rates ranged from over 90%[106,127] to less than 50%.[97] Cats receiving combination chemotherapy seemed to have a better response if prednisone[97] and maintenance treatment were used.[134] Prednisone alone, however, is probably ineffective.[131]

With the exception of a few anecdotal reports of long-term survival,[137] the best median remission (6 months) in the 1980s was obtained with COP. Other studies found median remission times of 8 to 10 weeks.[15,97,127] In two studies, cats that had mediastinal lymphoma and no other site involvement had better remission duration and survival.[56,127] The prognosis for young, FeLV-negative cats appears to be excellent.[a] In general, FeLV-negative cats with lymphoma that achieve a CR to therapy are likely to have long remissions, particularly if doxorubicin is added to the treatment protocol.[15,107]

CNS LYMPHOMA

BRAIN

Incidence, Signalment, and Etiology

The true incidence of intracranial lymphoma is currently unknown. The results of published studies appear to conflict, and thus assessing clinical signs and being aware of the possibility of brain involvement is important. In two studies, only 4 of 54 cats with CNS lymphoma had brain involvement.[138,139] In contrast, a recent study found that 15 of 18 cats with CNS lymphoma had signs of intracranial disease due to lymphoma.[140] Perhaps this recent study reflects a decrease in the number of cats with spinal lymphoma rather than an increased incidence of lymphoma of the brain.

Most reported cats have been DSHs[138,140,141]; the only purebreds reported were a Siamese[142] and two Persians.[143,144] Age ranges seem to be similar as for cats with other forms of lymphoma, and there is no gender predilection. Most cats with lymphoma of the brain have been FeLV negative,[140,142,143] whereas cats with spinal lymphoma are usually FeLV positive.

Clinical Presentation and History

Of 15 affected cats, seizures were seen in 10 and 4 had prolapsed nictitans with cranial nerve and CNS signs on examination.[140] Less frequent findings were ataxia (3 cats), circling and blindness (2 cats), and anorexia and lethargy with neurologic deficits noted on physical examination (2 cats).

Other cats have shown disorientation and circling for up to 2 months[141,142] as well as blindness,[141] seizures, aggression, hyperesthesia, and intention tremors.[143] Two cats had signs referable to cranial nerve involvement in addition to an intracranial mass.[138,144]

Staging and Diagnosis

A complete neurologic examination is warranted in any cat with CNS signs. Although meningioma is a more common brain tumor, lymphoma is an important differential diagnosis in cats with neurologic deficits.

Cerebrospinal fluid (CSF) analysis may provide a cytologic diagnosis of lymphoma. However, only 5 of 11 cerebellomedullary cisternal CSF taps were diagnostic in one study.[140] Therefore a negative result should in no way rule out a diagnosis of lymphoma.

Computed tomography (CT) is an excellent way to diagnose a mass lesion due to lymphoma. Five of six cats with brain lymphoma had a solitary ring-enhancing mass effect on CT.[140] Magnetic resonance imaging (MRI) may be even better able to visualize small lesions. However, if the lymphoma is infiltrative without a discrete mass, or localized to the vasculature as in one reported cat,[142] MRI may detect only a nonspecific increase in cortical density.

The majority of CNS lymphomas appear to be of B cell derivation.[15,52] Only two cases of T cell brain lymphomas have been confirmed and occurred in purebred cats; both had an unusual vascular distribution.[142,143]

Sixteen of 20 cats autopsied had evidence of lymphoma at other sites,[14,138,140,142] most commonly the kidneys (9 cats), liver (5 cats), spleen (4 cats), and mesenteric lymph nodes (4 cats). Three cats also had pulmonary involvement in the form of a single pulmonary nodule.[14] It is unclear from the literature how many cats with brain lymphoma had bone marrow involvement. These findings emphasize the importance of complete staging, including an MDB (with FIV/FeLV serology), abdominal ultrasonography, and bone marrow aspiration in addition to CT or MRI in cats with suspected CNS lymphoma.

Treatment

Corticosteroids alone had little effect on survival in seven cats.[140,142] Average survival was fewer than 5 weeks,[140] and any clinical improvement was transient.[142]

Three cats were already being treated with chemotherapy when they developed CNS brain signs. Cytosine arabinoside (a chemotherapeutic drug that crosses the blood-brain barrier) was added to the treatment protocol of two of these cats but did not cause any clinical improvement.[140]

MDB = minimum database; includes CBC, biochemical profile, urinalysis, FeLV/FIV serology, T$_4$ testing, and thoracic radiographs (three views).

Radiation therapy is probably the treatment of choice for CNS lymphoma of the brain, particularly if the rest of the spinal tract is not affected. Concurrent chemotherapy is warranted, however, because of the high rate of involvement of other anatomic sites. In one cat, radiation alone (total dose, 36 Gy) induced remission for 6 months.[141] Palliative radiation (24 Gy) and chemotherapy resulted in a 7 month remission in another cat.[140] A cat with systemic lymphoma that developed brain signs was treated with radiation and cytosine arabinoside but lived only an additional 40 days.[140] At present, the best therapeutic option for brain lymphoma is unknown; however, radiation used as primary therapy early in the course of the disease may be the most appropriate option if combined with chemotherapy.

SPINAL CORD

Incidence, Signalment, and Etiology

Based on the literature, CNS lymphoma is much more likely to affect the spinal cord than the brain.[139] The age range of cats with spinal lymphoma was 6 months[138,139] to 17 years,[62,145] and more than 60% were 3 years or younger.[62,139,145–156] Of 46 cats for which breed information was recorded, there were 30 DSHs, 7 DLHs, 7 Siamese, 1 Burmese, and 1 Russian Blue. There were 40 males and 28 females reported. Unlike cats with lymphoma of the brain, cats with spinal lymphoma often have associated FeLV infection; 41 of 45 tested cats (90%) were FeLV positive.[62,139,148–153,155] As the incidence of FeLV decreases, a concurrent decrease in spinal lymphoma might be expected. A recent study appeared to confirm this, with a higher proportion of CNS lymphoma seen in the brain rather than the spinal cord.[140]

Of six cats tested for FIV in one study, none tested positive.[139] A cat with FIV but not FeLV has been reported with spinal lymphoma and mast cell disease.[155]

Clinical Presentation and History

The most common presenting sign is posterior paresis or paralysis, usually bilateral at onset (Figure 36-10). Of 44 cats for which the information was available, 35 had hindlimb signs and 20 of those presented with bilateral hindlimb paresis.[62,149] Hindlimb paresis progressed to paralysis in 2 cats; this progression took 5 days in 1 cat and 2 weeks in the other.[145] The remaining cats were paralyzed when presented.

In one study, nociception was intact in 8 of 10 paralyzed cats.[62] None of the cats with hindlimb signs progressed to tetraparesis, which is most consistent with a solitary spinal lesion. Most cats had shown signs for 2 weeks or less.

Nine of 44 cats had signs of forelimb paresis or paralysis. The condition was unilateral in 5 cats—presenting as lameness or weakness and sometimes accompanied by a "dropped" shoulder or elbow—but progressed to quadriplegia or tetraparesis over a period of 1 month in 1 cat and 2 months in a second cat.[149,154] Another 4 cats were tetraplegic on presentation.[62,146,151]

KEY POINT

Spinal lymphoma is the most common cause of bilateral posterior paresis or paralysis in cats.

Other neurologic signs included focal hyperesthesia in 27 of 44 cats[162,139] (which manifested in one cat only when its back was rubbed[147]), urinary retention, tail paralysis, and dyschezia.[146,149,152] In one study, 10 of 21 cats had bladder paralysis, the origin of which was upper motor neuron in 8 cats and lower motor neuron in 2.[62] Most cats were constitutionally well; only 8 of 44 cats showed weight loss, and listlessness or anorexia was rare.[62,139] One cat with concurrent mediastinal lymphoma was dyspneic.[146] Lymph-

adenopathy or skin lesions due to other sites of lymphoma were uncommon.[62,139,149]

Staging and Diagnosis

Primary lymphoma of the spinal cord is rare in cats.[153] Signs are usually caused by compression of the cord from the extradural space that leads to demyelination and necrosis. Rarely, an extradural lymphoma may invade the cord itself.[138] The lymphoma lesion usually extends over two or three vertebral spaces[139] but may reach a length of 4 cm (Figure 36-11).[138] The lesion is solitary in most cats; in five reports totaling 65 cats, only 10 cats had multiple levels of spinal cord involvement.[62,138,139,146,156]

Plain radiography rarely shows evidence of a lesion. Spinal lymphoma will only occasionally invade the adjacent vertebra to result in radiographically detectable lesions.[62,138,146] Myelography is very useful in precisely locating the spinal lesion. Evidence of an extradural mass was detected in 11 (asymmetric in 9, symmetric in 2) of 16 cats that received a myelogram in one study. Three cats had evidence of an intramedullary mass; all of these cats had lymphoma that infiltrated from the spinal nerve roots in the brachial plexus and across the subarachnoid space, thereby causing hemorrhage in the cord.[139] Myelograms appeared normal despite the presence of lymphoma in 2 of these 16 cats. With wider availability, MRI may become the imaging modality of choice, although results have not yet been reported for spinal lymphoma in cats.

CSF analysis often shows only nonspecific indications of an inflammatory process. CSF analysis demonstrated lymphoblasts in 7 of 27 cats with spinal lymphoma.[139,149] Three cats that had extension of lymphoma intradurally[139] had increased numbers of segmented neutrophils but no lymphoblasts on CSF cytology. CSF collection for diagnosis is probably unwarranted unless all other extraspinal sites prove negative for lymphoma (see below).

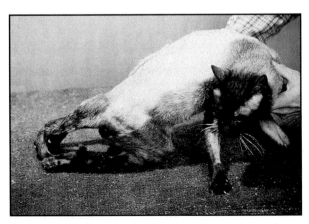

Figure 36-10: Posterior paralysis in cats is most commonly due to lymphoma. (Courtesy of J. Berg)

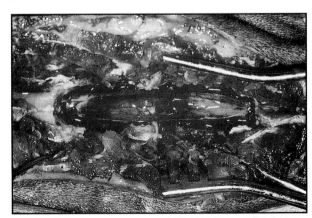

Figure 36-11: Surgical exposure of an extradural lymphoma in a cat. Diagnosis may be made in most cats by bone marrow aspiration, thereby avoiding unnecessary surgery and allowing timely use of chemotherapy. (Courtesy of J. Berg).

Fluoroscopic guided fine-needle aspiration of the mass was performed in two cats.[62] The diagnosis was confirmed cytologically in both animals, and the procedure did not exacerbate neurologic signs.

More than half of the cats with spinal lymphoma have involvement of other sites. In one study, lymphoma was detected via bone marrow aspiration in 11 of 16 cats[62]; in another study, some cats had circulating lymphoblasts.[51] Careful scrutiny of a blood smear and bone marrow aspirate is warranted in cats showing signs of spinal neurologic disease, particularly in FeLV-positive animals. When bone marrow aspiration is performed early in the diagnostic process, more invasive procedures such as surgical biopsy or fine-needle aspiration of the spinal lesion or CSF collection may be unnecessary.

The kidney is another very common secondary site of involvement, seen in 22 of 42 cats with spinal lymphoma.[62,139,145] Mesenteric lymph node and liver involvement are also common.[62,145–147,150,153,154,156] The spleen, mediastinum, eyes, heart, and lungs are less commonly involved. Rarely, lymphoma can be seen in peripheral lymph nodes, the adrenal gland, pancreas, and bladder. In one study,[62] a secondary site of lymphoma was identified during a full autopsy in 11 of 13 cats, emphasizing the need for complete staging, including an MDB (with FIV/FeLV serology), abdominal ultrasonography, and bone marrow aspiration as outlined at the beginning of this chapter.

Treatment

Little has been written specifically about treatment for spinal lymphoma in cats. Because most cats have extradural lymphoma, the blood-brain barrier should not interfere with the efficacy of chemotherapy.

Corticosteroids alone have been used in a number of cats; most studies report the use of prednisone,[62] although drugs such as flumethasone have also been used.[148] Most responses to corticosteroids alone have been classified as transient or slight.[146,149,150] Some cats appeared to return to normal but relapsed when corticosteroids were discontinued. Responses to second treatments were often less dramatic or of shorter duration.[148,153] More recent studies have documented either no or short-term (4 to 10 weeks) response[62,140] when corticosteroids were used alone.

> **KEY POINT**
>
> *Most cats with spinal lymphoma have other sites of involvement. The bone marrow is commonly infiltrated, and thus bone marrow aspiration may be a less invasive method of obtaining a diagnosis compared with spinal surgery.*

The use of combination chemotherapy (COP) has been reported in 11 cats. Six cats had a complete return to normal function for 5 to 62 weeks (median, 32 weeks).[62,106,151] One of the longest responders had undergone surgical decompression prior to receiving chemotherapy.[62]

Combination chemotherapy with L-asparaginase, vincristine, and prednisone was reported for four cats with spinal lymphoma.[139] Three of these cats also received radiation therapy to the lesion. One cat survived 60 weeks, but the others had systemic lymphoma that caused their death within the first 20 weeks.[139]

Based on responses of lymphoma at other sites, the best treatment for spinal lymphoma is probably combination chemotherapy that includes doxorubicin. Adjunctive radiation therapy may result in more rapid tumor shrinkage, which is important to reduce the risk of pressure-induced myelonecrosis. Surgery has little role in the treatment of this disease.

RENAL LYMPHOMA

Incidence, Signalment, and Etiology

Most studies of feline lymphoma assign cats with renal involvement to either the alimentary[7,8] or multicentric[9,63] category, which confuses the distinction between these two groups. Other investigators have separated cats with renal involvement on the basis of potentially different biologic behavior[54] or included them as having abdominal tumors, which were then subclassified as solitary or mixed according to a new staging scheme.[14]

Of 69 cats with renal involvement,[14,54,157–159] most (55) were DSHs or DLHs, 8 were Siamese (7 of 36 in an Australian study[14]), 2 were Burmese, 2 were Abyssinian, and 2 were other shorthaired purebreds; there were 45 males and 24 females. The median age of affected cats was 7.5 years,[14,15,54] although affected cats as young as 16 months have been reported.[14] In earlier studies, more than half the cats with renal lymphoma were infected with FeLV, whereas only 25% of cats with renal lymphoma were FeLV infected in a more recent survey.[15]

Clinical Presentation and History

The most common clinical signs seen in cats with renal lymphoma are related to acute renal insufficiency due to cortical infiltration by lymphoma cells. Affected cats are depressed and anorectic, have lost weight, and are usually polydipsic and polyuric despite clinical dehydration. The time between owner recognition of initial signs and presentation to the veterinarian is usually only 4 to 6 weeks.[158,159]

Renomegaly with irregular cortical protrusions is usually bilateral and easily detected on abdominal palpation (Figure 36-12). Occasionally, renal involvement will be subclinical in a cat with other areas of lymphoma involvement.

KEY POINT

Renal lymphoma is always bilateral.

Staging and Diagnosis

Renal involvement is always bilateral.[14] It is uncommon to have renal lymphoma without other organ or system involvement. Of 68 cats for which the information was known, only 18 had lymphoma confined to the kidneys.[14,54,157] Of the remaining 50 cats, other sites of lymphoma were limited to the abdominal cavity in 20 cats (mesenteric nodes alone or with involvement of liver, spleen, or GI tract; Figure 36-13).[14,54,159] The rest of the cats had involvement of multiple sites, including peripheral or sternal lymph nodes, adrenal gland, lungs, heart, bone marrow, eyes, skin, or CNS.[54,157,158]

One group of researchers felt that the risk of relapse in patients with CNS lymphoma was higher when renal lymphoma was also present.[54] No other study has confirmed that association, and it may represent the heterogeneity of feline lymphoma rather than an absolute association. In a group of 23 cats presented for primary CNS lymphoma, 10 had evidence of renal involvement.[139] In another study, renal lymphoma was seen in combination with nasal lymphoma (1 cat), pulmonary lymphoma (2 cats), and ocular lymphoma (3 cats) but not CNS lymphoma.[14]

For staging, an MDB (including FeLV/FIV serology) should be obtained. Most cats are anemic, primarily due to lymphoma but also due to renal failure if signs have been chronic. A serum chemistry profile and urinalysis will allow critical evaluation of renal function. One study showed that the level of azotemia did not provide strong prognostic information,[54] probably because lymphoma is infiltrative and will allow functional recovery of the renal cortex if treated promptly. Cats that are azotemic, however, should be treated with crystalloid diuresis to limit the damage caused by lymphoma while waiting for chemotherapy to take effect.

Staging should include thoracic radiography to look for involvement of intrathoracic structures. Abdominal ultrasonography allows examination of kidneys for degree of cortical involvement and can also detect other abdominal organ involvement. Occasionally, renal lymphoma may coexist with another congenital malformation, such as polycystic kidneys,[158] emphasizing the need for biopsy as well as ultrasonographic examination. Ultrasound-guided percutaneous fine-needle aspiration or Tru-cut renal biopsy should confirm the diagnosis; biopsy is preferred.

Renal lymphoma appears to be mainly B cell in origin. Of 44 cats with renal lymphoma, 38 had B cell, 5 had T cell, and 1 had null cell lymphoma.[15,52] These findings could not be correlated with prognosis.

Treatment

A combination chemotherapy protocol using vincristine, L-asparaginase, prednisone, cyclophosphamide, and methotrexate was used to treat 28 cats with renal lymphoma.[54] Ten of the 28 also received cytosine arabinoside (600 mg/m² SQ divided into two daily doses every 4 weeks). This drug was added to the protocol because 10 of the 18 previously treated cats had relapsed with CNS lymphoma and cytosine arabinoside is known to cross the blood-brain barrier in humans and dogs. Overall, tumor size was reduced

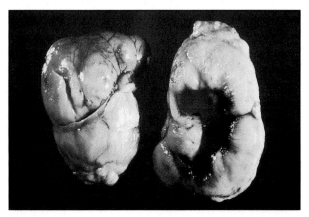

Figure 36-12: *Renal lymphoma is always bilateral, causing enlargement and irregular contours of the kidneys, which may be easily palpated, as seen in this necropsy specimen from an 8-year-old cat. (Courtesy of G.H. Theilen).*

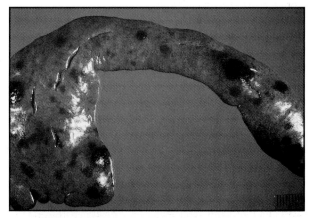

Figure 36-13: *Lymphoma is rarely confined to one site. All organs, including the spleen, should be evaluated for concurrent disease. Splenic lymphoma in addition to renal lymphoma was seen in a 15-year-old cat.*

by more than 75% in 17 of the 28 cats, and this remission lasted a median of 127 days (range, 20 days to more than 6 years). Of those cats with renal involvement alone, average survival time was shorter in cats with FeLV infection.[54]

Two of three cats with renal lymphoma treated with COP had CRs, lasting 2 months in one animal and 36 months in the other.[106] Only one of six cats treated with a similar protocol achieved a remission, but it was still alive 2.5 years later.[97] The median survival for all six cats in the latter group was 5 months.[97] Three other cats treated with COP plus cytosine arabinoside had partial responses and lived between 1 and 7 weeks.[157-158]

In a large group of 145 cats treated with a variety of chemotherapeutic agents, 10 had renal lymphoma (median remission duration, 13 weeks).[15] This duration was not significantly worse than for cats with lymphoma of any other site.

LYMPHADENOPATHY

Benign lymphadenopathy is more common than lymphoma-induced lymphadenopathy in cats, and generalized peripheral lymphadenopathy of any cause is an uncommon finding. In a study of 132 cats, generalized lymphadenopathy was most commonly a result of idiopathic causes, with bacterial, allergic, inflammatory, or neoplastic (nonlymphoma) causes identified in only 50 cats.[160]

Fourteen cats with peripheral lymphadenopathy were all young (age range, 5 months to 2 years) DSHs.[160] Eight of these cats were not systemically ill, but the others showed signs of fever, lethargy, or anorexia. Many of the cats were FeLV positive, and one developed lymphoma 2 years later. Lymphadenopathy resolved in eight cats after treatment with antibiotics and/or corticosteroids, but resolution took 4 to 7 months in some cats. One cat with recurrent lymphadenopathy was treated successfully with COP chemotherapy over a period of 5 years. It is possible that the paracortical hyperplasia seen histologically was due to viral (FeLV) infection.

Lymph nodes were examined in 17 cats (age range, 4 to 13 years) with natural FIV infection.[161] Six of these cats had lymphadenopathy consisting of follicular hyperplasia, and all cats showed evidence of erythrophagocytosis with mixed lymphoblastic, histiocytic, and plasmacytoid cells.[161]

In younger cats with generalized lymphadenopathy, a biopsy, an MDB (with FeLV/FIV serology), thoracic radiographs, and abdominal ultrasound should be performed. It may be prudent to perform PCR, which is considered to be a more sensitive technique for detecting FeLV, prior to starting immunosuppressive treatments such as chemotherapy. Clinicians should not rely on fine-needle aspiration to diagnose lymphoma in cats with peripheral lymphadenopathy. Older cats should also be tested for viral causes, and Western blot analysis for FIV may be warranted.

MDB = minimum database; includes CBC, biochemical profile, urinalysis, FeLV/FIV serology, T_4 testing, and thoracic radiographs (three views).

Solitary or localized lymphadenopathy in cats is also rare. Nine domestic cats (with an overrepresentation of DLHs) were diagnosed with unilateral cervical or inguinal node (seven cats) or bilateral inguinal node (two cats) enlargement (1.5 to 5 cm in diameter). On biopsy, the follicular structure was unchanged but the interfollicular pulp was replaced with vascular channels. This was not considered to be a neoplastic lesion.[162] Of six cats monitored after lymph node excision, none had recurrence of lymphadenopathy or other disease 3 to 36 months later (average, 15 months).

NODAL LYMPHOMA

The best investigation of nodal lymphoma was included in a study of 118 cats with lymphoma.[14] Forty-seven (40%) had involvement of one or more of the peripheral lymph nodes. Most commonly, a solitary lymph node was involved (18 cats), with regional involvement (i.e., two or more adjacent nodes) seen in 13 cats and generalized lymph node involvement in 16. The nodes of the head and neck were most commonly involved in all groups. More than half the cats (11 of 18, 6 of 13, and 10 of 16) had other organ or system involvement.[14]

When the immunophenotype of these lymphomas was studied, 27 were of B cell origin, 14 were of T cell origin, and 2 were of null cell origin.[52]

In another study, six cats had generalized lymphadenopathy with nodes that were 2 to 3 cm in diameter.[163] These cats were 1 to 4 years of age, and three were Maine Coons. Histologically, none were considered to have high-grade lymphoma. The lymphadenopathy resolved without treatment in all cats within 5 to 120 days, and all cats were alive 1 to 7 years later.[163] Low-grade lymphoma may have a long clinical course even without treatment.

Lymphadenopathy in cats is more likely to result from idiopathic, nonneoplastic causes than from lymphoma.

Recently, nine cats were diagnosed with mandibular or cervical lymphadenopathy that was solitary in seven cats and involved only two nodes in the other cats.[164,165] Nodes measured 2 to 5 cm in diameter. All cats were DSHs between the ages of 4.5 and 18 years (median, 11 years). All were negative for FeLV and FIV by PCR. Histologically, there was obliteration of follicular architecture by a mixture of lymphocytes, lymphoblasts, and histiocytic lymphocytes as well as giant multinucleate cells with bizarre mitoses that

were immunologically B cells. Three cats had no recurrence 6 months or more after surgical excision of the affected node, while another cat had two recurrences at 6 month intervals before responding to COP chemotherapy. Interestingly, all cases were diagnosed between 1995 and 1998, and no similar lesion was found in archives dating back to 1900.

The heterogenous population of lymphoid cells makes it impossible to distinguish between lymphoma and a reactive lymph node on fine-needle aspiration cytology. Biopsy is therefore mandatory for diagnosis, and excisional biopsy may prove therapeutic in select cats. The extent of disease should be determined by examining an MDB (including FeLV/FIV serology), abdominal ultrasound, and bone marrow aspiration; in addition, if chemotherapy is considered and serology is negative, cats with lymphadenopathy should be tested for FeLV and FIV by PCR and Western blot.

LYMPHOMA OF THE EYE

Ocular manifestation of lymphoma is an uncommon clinical entity, although microscopic and subclinical ocular disease in cats with systemic lymphoma is rarely investigated by veterinarians. Unilateral or bilateral ocular lymphoma may precede systemic disease in some cats[166–168] but more commonly occurs concurrently with multicentric lymphoma. In one study, 5 of 13 cats with ocular involvement at necropsy had bilateral eye involvement.[167] Of 17 cats with ocular lymphoma that were tested for FeLV, 7 were positive; serologic testing for FIV was positive in 1 of 2 cats tested.

Ocular lymphoma is usually part of systemic lymphoma in cats.

In a large study of 50 feline eyes affected with ocular lymphoma, the uvea was affected most commonly. The iris was involved diffusely by lymphoma in 10 eyes, and a nodule formed in 35 eyes. Only the choroid was affected in 5 eyes.[168] The cornea was infiltrated with lymphoma in 13 cats, but secondary corneal changes were common in other eyes. Secondary inflammatory changes were seen in 25 of the 50 eyes. In 19 cats this manifested as anterior chamber cellular debris that was mixed with lymphoma cells (Figure 36-14). Similarly, the vitreous was infiltrated with lymphoma in 7 cats and with a mixture of lymphoma and inflammatory cells in another 7 cats. Retinal infiltration with lymphoma was seen in only 5 cats, but 15 had a secondary retinal detachment. Glaucoma secondary to tumor infiltration or anterior synechiae was seen in 10 cats.

Diagnosis of lymphoma in these cats was made on biop-

sy, but it may be possible to use a fine-gauge needle to aspirate the cellular infiltrate of the anterior chamber. The mixture of tumor and inflammatory cells may make cytologic diagnosis difficult. Ocular involvement may rarely extend to the retrobulbar space, causing exophthalmos.[169]

Enucleation was used as a single therapy in 10 cats. None of these animals received multidrug chemotherapy after enucleation, although some received corticosteroids.[168] Despite an average survival of 14 months and one long-term survival of 31 months, there was marked

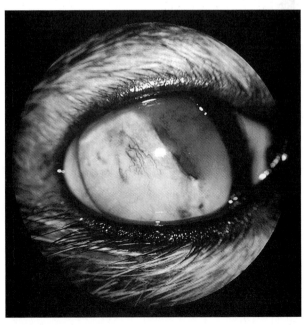

Figure 36-14: *Ocular involvement with lymphoma may be a tumor mass or a mixture of neoplastic and inflammatory cells, as in this 14-year-old cat.*

variation in survival times. Most of the cats treated with enucleation alone or enucleation and steroids were free of systemic signs at diagnosis.[166,168] However, multicentric disease is seen in many cats with ocular involvement.[168] Clinicians should always assume that lymphoma is a systemic disease[170,171] and thus can rarely be successfully treated with local therapies. Complete staging, including an MDB, abdominal ultrasound, and bone marrow aspiration, should be performed, and chemotherapy should be offered as the standard of care.

OTHER EXTRANODAL LYMPHOMAS

BONE

Involvement of the skeletal system with lymphoma is rare in cats. An FeLV-negative cat with bilateral lytic tarsal lesions was found to have lymphoma when biopsy samples were collected from associated soft tissue (Figure 36-15).[172] Four related male DSHs (2–4 years old) with lymphoma of the distal radius and ulna showed rapidly progressive disease and died with multicentric lymphoma within 5 months.[173] Lymphoma of the extradural spinal canal will sometimes invade bone of the surrounding vertebrae.[138,145,146,158]

Treatment was not attempted in any of the cats described above, but multiple-agent chemotherapy, which is recommended for cats with lymphoma of other sites, is probably the treatment of choice. Radiation therapy may provide palliation of individual bone lesions but should always be considered an adjunct to chemotherapy. Information regarding the effectiveness of radiation for bone lymphoma has not been published.

ORAL CAVITY

There are few reports of cats with lymphoma involving the oral cavity. As with other lymphomas, each patient should be appropriately staged prior to starting treatment. Chemotherapy should be used in addition to radiation therapy for the treatment of extranodal lymphoma.

One cat with gingival lymphoma had a partial, albeit short, response to COP chemotherapy.[106] Two cats with oral lymphoma located in the maxilla or mandible were treated with radiation therapy. One had a CR for nearly 6 months before developing lymphoma in lymph nodes distant from the original site. The other cat had only a short-term response before developing lymphoma outside the treatment area.[174]

LUNG

There is little information on lymphoma of the lung in cats, although it may take the form of solitary pulmonary nodules rather than the diffuse pattern typically seen in dogs.[14] As with other lymphomas, each patient should be appropriately staged prior to starting treatment. Systemic chemotherapy is most likely to be effective in these cats.

NASAL AND DERMAL LYMPHOMA

Nasal and dermal lymphoma are covered in Chapters 47 and 50, respectively.

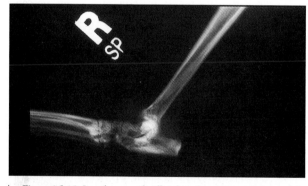

Figure 36-15: Lymphoma rarely affects bone but may cause lysis around a joint due to extension from surrounding tissue.

PROGNOSTIC FACTORS

Stage of disease, as defined by Mooney,[55] was significantly related to response in one study[56] in which cats with stage I lymphoma had higher response rates (93%) than those with stage IV or V disease (40% to 60%); in addition, cats with stage I and II lymphoma had longer survival times (7.6 months versus 3 months). This five-stage system is more complex than the one used for dogs, and the difficulties in applying it may explain why it has not shown prognostic value in other studies.

Response to treatment has been shown to be one of the few prognostic factors for cats with lymphoma.[15,97,126] In one large study of 145 cats, cats achieving CR had a median response duration of 7 months and median survival of 8.5 months compared with 3 weeks and 7 weeks, respectively, if they achieved PR.

Similarly, a cat with FeLV antigenemia is less likely to have a long survival, possibly due to development of other diseases as well as the lymphoma.[15,56,126] Both CR duration (4 weeks versus 5 months) and survival (5 weeks versus 6 months) were shorter for cats with FeLV. In contradiction to these findings, FeLV test status was not an independent predictor of survival in another study.[126]

In one study, cats were classified as having substage "b" lymphoma if they were "constitutionally unwell" (sick) and substage "a" lymphoma if they were otherwise well. Cats with substage "b" had a median survival of 3.5 months compared with a 9.5 month median survival for cats with substage "a" lymphoma.[15] This same effect of illness has been seen in other studies[93,126] and underscores the importance of supportive care for these cats while chemotherapy is being administered.

In the same study, additional prognostic factors identified that were not independent of those listed above included the following: Cats with nasal lymphoma had longer remissions and survival times; cats with Mooney stages I to III disease had longer remission and survival times than cats with stages IV and V disease; cats that received doxorubicin as part of their treatment had longer remissions; and cats with a high proliferative fraction of their tumor cells had longer survival times.[15]

TREATMENT

Information regarding treatment of lymphoma at specific sites was provided in the previous sections. The following is a more general overview of treatment for feline lymphoma.

Regardless of the primary site of lymphoma, survival times in untreated cats tend to be very short. In one study, the majority of cats that were not treated died within 2 weeks,[175] although FeLV-negative cats appeared to live a little longer.[9] In another group of 39 untreated cats, only 2 cats lived longer than 4 months.[10] Cats with lymphoma treated with supportive care had an average survival of only 5 days.[176]

CHEMOTHERAPY

Single Agent Chemotherapy

Cyclophosphamide, vincristine, and prednisone form the basis for most chemotherapy protocols. The individual drugs had been shown, albeit anecdotally, to have significant activity in the treatment of feline lymphoma, sometimes resulting in long-term control.[177–180] In these early reports, vinblastine was also found to be useful[178] while L-asparaginase had some limited activity[178] and chlorambucil had questionable efficacy.[177]

Idarubicin is an anthracycline derivative that is more active in vitro and less cardiotoxic than its parent compound, daunorubicin. In addition, the drug is active by both parenteral and oral routes of administration. Idarubicin treatment (2 mg/day PO for 3 consecutive days, repeated every 21 days) resulted in CR in 2 cats with lymphoma. In another investigation of the utility of idarubicin for treatment of feline lymphoma, 18 cats that achieved remission following COP therapy were treated from week 4 with idarubicin as a single agent. The median remission duration for these cats was 183 days (range, 30 to 825 days), with 1 cat still alive and off treatment at 351 days and another at 825 days. One cat died of unknown causes after 220 days of remission.[107] The dose-limiting toxicities were leukopenia and anorexia, as has been reported with other anthracycline derivatives such as doxorubicin. The ease and noninvasive nature of oral administration make idarubicin an attractive option for clients, although the drug is available only in Europe.

Mitoxantrone (6.5 mg/m^2 IV every 3 weeks) did not seem to effectively treat feline lymphoma; only 1 of 11 cats had an objective response to treatment.[181]

COP Protocol (Cyclophosphamide, Vincristine, and Prednisone)

The COP protocol used most often involves a 4 week induction period (Table 36-4) followed by maintenance therapy every 3 weeks for a total of 1 year, at which time all treatment is ceased.[106] Cats that were treated with the 4 week induction period alone had a median remission of less than 2 months[164] compared with median remissions of 4.5 to 28 months for cats that received the complete protocol,[106] which implies that maintenance therapy is important.

Vincristine, even at a dose of 0.5 mg/m^2, can be myelosuppressive, and careful hematologic monitoring 1 week after each treatment is warranted until a safe dose has been established for each patient.[182]

Thirty-eight cats were treated with COP and maintenance therapy for various anatomic forms of lymphoma.[106] The CR rate varied from 100% for multicentric lymphoma to 50% for extranodal lymphoma. Similarly, the median duration of remission ranged from 4.5 months for alimentary lymphoma to 28 months for cats with peripheral nodal lymphoma. All groups contained individuals that lived longer than a year. The overall CR rate was 30 of 38 cats (74%), with 6 cats having a partial response and 2 having no response. The duration of CR ranged from 2 to 42 months.[106]

More recent reports of the use of COP protocol have not found the same efficacy.[107] A group of 38 cats treated in the 1990s differed from the earlier cats in that this later group was less likely to be FeLV positive or have mediastinal lym-

TABLE 36-4
COP Protocol for Treatment of Lymphoma[106]

Agent	Week						
	1	2	3	4	7	10	13[a]
Vincristine (0.75 mg/m² IV)	•	•	•	•	•	•	• →
Cyclophosphamide (300 mg/m² PO [to nearest 25 mg])	•			•	•	•	• →
Prednisone (10 mg PO daily throughout the protocol)	•						→

[a]After week 13, administer protocol every 3 weeks for a total treatment period of 1 year, then stop therapy.

phoma. Eighteen of the 38 cats (47%) had a CR. The median response duration was less than 3 months, and no cat had a remission lasting longer than 6 months. All cats with mediastinal, nasal, or peripheral nerve lymphoma responded (*n* = 5), and 6 of 11 cats with multicentric lymphoma, 5 of 12 with alimentary lymphoma, and 2 of 9 with renal lymphoma responded.[107] The changing demographics for feline lymphoma as described previously may be responsible for the altered response to chemotherapy.

COP Plus L-Asparaginase and Methotrexate

A similar protocol to COP in which some cats received L-asparaginase and all 62 cats received methotrexate did not seem to induce more remissions than those achieved with COP. Overall, the median survival for all 62 cats was only 7 weeks. The highest response rate (70%) was seen in cats with multicentric lymphoma.[97]

KEY POINT

Multiple-drug chemotherapy, as used in dogs, is the most likely to result in CR.

The overall CR rate to this protocol was 52%, (median duration, 5 months). All groups had individual long-term survivors; nine cats were alive for a median of 2 years after diagnosis.[97] Six of these cats had multicentric lymphoma, two had alimentary lymphoma, and one had renal lymphoma. [97]

Another group of 103 cats received COP plus methotrexate and L-asparaginase.[56] Responses were classified as a CR if there was a 75% or greater reduction in tumor volume. Sixty-four cats (62%) had a CR (median survival, 7 months); 30% of the cats showing a CR were alive 1 year after starting treatment. Cats with stage I or II lymphoma had longer remission and survival times; cats that tested FeLV positive lived for a shorter time but were equally likely to respond to chemotherapy.

Doxorubicin

The utility of doxorubicin in combination chemotherapy for feline lymphoma was first suggested in 1980.[176] Four cats with lymphoma (sites unspecified) were treated with vincristine, prednisone, L-asparaginase, and doxorubicin. One cat had a CR and two cats had PR (median remission, 7.5 months). The response rate and duration were better than those seen in six cats treated with cyclophosphamide in place of doxorubicin.[176] These findings were supported by a multi-institutional study that found that cats receiving doxorubicin as part of their chemotherapy protocol were likely to have a longer remission duration than those receiving protocols that did not include doxorubicin (9 months versus 3 months, respectively).[15]

Further evidence of the utility for doxorubicin as a component of multiple-agent chemotherapy came from a study in which cats that had achieved a CR to COP were randomized to either continue COP maintenance or to receive doxorubicin alone. Median remission was 3 months in cats receiving COP only and 9.5 months in those receiving doxorubicin.[107] The long-term survivors in the study received both doxorubicin and COP. This protocol spanned only 6 months, which is a much shorter maintenance phase than most other protocols, which continue for 1 or more years. This implies that shorter protocols may be adequate to treat feline lymphoma when effective multiple-drug combinations are used

Two studies that investigated the efficacy of doxorubicin as an induction agent found that fewer than 30% of cats had a CR.[183,184] This contrasts with the situation in dogs, in which doxorubicin is a very effective single agent in the treatment of lymphoma. It thus appears that doxorubicin is best used in combination with other chemotherapeutic agents.

COP Plus Doxorubicin, L-Asparaginase, and Methotrexate

One of the most widely used protocols for the treatment of feline lymphoma is described in *Current Veterinary Ther-*

TABLE 36-5
CVT X Protocol for Treatment of Lymphoma[185]

Agent	Week 1	2	3	4	5	6	8	10	12	14[a] →
Vincristine (0.025 mg/kg IV)	•			•			•		•	
L-Asparaginase (400 IU/kg IV)	•									
Cyclophosphamide (10 mg/kg IV)		•			•			•		
Doxorubicin (20 mg/m² IV)			•			•				
Methotrexate (0.8 mg/kg IV)										•
Prednisone (5 mg PO bid daily throughout protocol)	•————————————————————————————————→									

[a]After week 14, continue protocol as described for weeks 8 to 14 for 12 months; the same drugs are then administered at 3 week intervals for 6 months, followed by monthly intervals for another 6 months.

apy X (Table 36-5).[185] Reports of the efficacy of this protocol in the treatment of alimentary lymphoma[70,97,100] were discussed in the sections on GI lymphoma and mesenteric lymph nodes earlier in this chapter. A similar protocol was used to treat 132 cats with lymphoma of all stages and anatomic sites (11 cats were FeLV positive and 4 cats were FIV positive).[126] Most cats (100 cats [76%]) were clinically ill, and most had GI lymphoma. CR was seen in 88 cats (67%). Remission times for all cats ranged from 0 days to over 5 years (median, 5 months). Response to therapy and whether the cat was sick appeared to be the only factors to influence survival.

MDB = minimum database; includes CBC, biochemical profile, urinalysis, FeLV/FIV serology, T₄ testing, and thoracic radiographs (three views).

A similar protocol was used to treat Australian cats with lymphoma, and the median survival was only about 6 months in this group of FeLV-negative, but often FIV-positive, cats.[a]

Methotrexate may cause diarrhea and inappetence due to enterotoxic effects. One study found that a complex diet with intact protein may help prevent this toxicity, whereas purified diets with an amino acid base may exacerbate enterotoxicosis.[186] This is important to consider when an enteral feeding tube is used.

Investigational Chemotherapy Drugs

Ifosfamide is an alkylating agent related to cyclophosphamide. It must be given IV and causes hemorrhagic cystitis in dogs and humans unless mesna is given concurrently. Ifosfamide anecdotally causes remission in cats with lymphoma. The current investigational dosage is 900 mg/m² given as described in Chapter 11.[c]

CCNU is an alkylating agent that is highly absorbed orally and crosses the blood-brain barrier. Recent work indicates that the dosage of this drug in cats is 50 to 60 mg/m² PO every 6 weeks (myelosuppression, particularly neutropenia, can be prolonged for 5 or more weeks).[187] CCNU has efficacy in treatment of canine lymphoma and has shown efficacy in treating feline lymphoma.

The MOPP protocol (mechlorethamine HCl, vincristine, prednisone, and procarbazine) combines two alkylating agents with vincristine and prednisone. A 28 day cycling MOPP protocol was reported to be effective when other chemotherapy failed to induce remission (Table 36-6).[188]

Twenty-three cats, most of which had GI lymphoma, were treated with MOPP when a combination chemotherapy protocol failed. Ten cats had a CR and four cats had a PR (median remission duration, 166 days). Mild anorexia was seen in two cats, and five cats showed significant leukopenia or anemia. Overall, the protocol was well tolerated. Anorexia with MOPP protocol is most likely to resolve when procarbazine is reduced to alternate day administration or given concurrently with metoclopramide.

RADIATION THERAPY

Radiation has limited application in the treatment of feline lymphoma. Indications for radiation would be in the treatment of an apparently localized (usually extranodal) lymphoma or to cause rapid reduction in tumor bulk for comfort (e.g., a large mediastinal lymphoma causing dyspnea). Radiation therapy alone can occasionally cause long

[c]Rassnick KM: Personal communication.

TABLE 36-6
MOPP Protocol for Treatment of Lymphoma[188]

Agent	Week											
	1	2	3	4	5	6	7	8	9	10	11	12[a] →
Vincristine (0.75 mg/m^2 on days 1 and 8)	•	•			•	•			•	•		
Mechlorethamine HCl (3.0 mg/m^2 IV on days 1 and 8)	•	•			•	•			•	•		
Procarbazine (10 mg PO daily for 14 days)	• →				• →				• →			
Prednisone (5 mg/cat PO q12h for 14 days)	• →				• →				• →			

[a]Cycle repeats every 4 weeks.

remissions but should be used in conjunction with chemotherapy as lymphoma should always be considered to be a systemic disease.

Radiation doses for treatment of lymphoma can be quite low as cell division is not needed for cell death (unlike carcinomas and sarcomas). This means that side effects may often be considerably reduced in lymphoma patients.

Radiation therapy was noted to cause short-term responses in feline lymphoma as early as the 1960s[178] but has been critically evaluated in only one series of 10 cats.[174] Three of three cats with nasal lymphoma, two of three cats with retrobulbar lymphoma, and one cat each with oral, subcutaneous, and mediastinal lymphoma all had a CR to therapy. The other two cats had short-term (6 to 9 weeks) partial responses.[174] With the exception of the subcutaneous tumor, which recurred outside the treated area within a month, the other CRs lasted 6.5 months to more than 5 years (median, 2 years). Lymphoma recurred in lymph nodes in two cats within a year, and three cats in this study received some chemotherapy in addition to radiation. As stated, however, radiation should always be used with concurrent chemotherapy.

Radiation was found to be effective in the treatment of other cats with nasal lymphoma[189]; results of that study are in Chapter 47.

Care should be taken when using radiation therapy. The massive and rapid death of lymphoma cells after even a single dose of radiation can lead to life-threatening metabolic changes known as *tumor lysis syndrome*. This syndrome was reported in one cat following radiation for mediastinal lymphoma and leukemic blood count.[190] Aggressive fluid therapy and correction of acid-base and electrolyte disturbances (acidosis, hyperkalemia, hyperphosphatemia, hyperuricemia) are necessary to avoid patient death.

IMMUNOTHERAPY

Immunotherapy is an interesting area of research for feline lymphoma; at present, however, there are no practical modalities for use in clinical practice. Future research and commercial development of this area may lead to some clinically useful treatments.

An intriguing study looked at 39 cats treated for lymphoma using various blood products and components.[191,192] All but one cat were FeLV positive. The site of the lymphoma was not reported in all cases, although most were mediastinal or multicentric. In this study, any tumor reduction of 20% or more was considered to be a PR.

There were nine treatment groups in this study. Serum from normal cats without FeLV or lymphoma (normal cat serum [NCS]) was diluted 1:1 with normal saline and given IV (total dose, 200 ml) over 1.5 hours three times a week for 2 weeks. A second group of cats was treated with NCS that had been heated to 56°C for 1 hour (heat-inactivated NCS) and then stored at −80°C. A third group of cats received heat-inactivated serum that had not been stored. The fourth group received NCS that was "inactivated" using cobra venom (which inactivates "late" complement components). The fifth and sixth groups received fresh normal cat plasma (NCP) at a dose of 10 to 15 ml/cat (low dose) or 50 ml/cat (high dose), respectively. A seventh group received frozen stored NCP, and an eighth group received whole cat blood (WCB) at a dose of 50 to 100 ml. The ninth group received serum obtained from cats with FeLV and lymphoma. Results are tabulated in Table 36-7.

Although marked regressions were seen in cats treated with NCS and WCB, there was a risk of transfusion reaction or DIC occurring due to continued use of blood products.[192] In addition, all but one cat died of lymphoma

TABLE 36-7
Responses of Cats with Lymphoma to Various Blood Components[191,192]

Treatment	No. of Cats	CR	PR	NR
NCS	9	5	3	1
Stored HI NCS	6	4	2	0
Nonstored HI NCS	3	0	0	3
CV-inactivated NCS	4	0	3	1
Low-dose NCP	4	0	0	4
High-dose NCP	6	2	1	3
Stored NCP	?			All
WCB	7	As for NCS[a]	As for NCS[a]	
LCS	3	0	0	3

[a]Actual numbers are unavailable; same response rates as seen with NCS.
CR = complete remission; CV = cobra venom; HI = heat inactivated; LCS = leukemic cat serum; NCP = normal cat plasma; NCS = normal cat serum; NR = no response; PR = partial response; WCB = whole cat blood.

within 3 months. The exception was the cat that tested FeLV negative, which was alive and in CR 2 years after treatment.[192]

Another reported immunotherapeutic approach perfused the patient's serum over a column of *Staphylococcus aureus* Cowan I strain. A cell wall protein (Protein A) from the bacteria is thought to bind with the F_C component of certain immunoglobulins, thereby clearing IgG and IgG immune complexes from the blood.[193,194] Removal of immunosuppressive complexes presumably allows increased antibody synthesis against the viral membrane antigens and possibly the tumor. In addition to activation of antibody synthesis, induction of gamma interferon,[195] potentiation of natural killer cell activity, and blast transformation of B and T cell lymphocytes has been ascribed to protein A. In early studies, about 50% of cats with FeLV would become FeLV negative after this treatment, possibly due to enhanced antibody response to FeLV *gp70*.[197]

Sixteen FeLV-positive cats with lymphoma were treated using extracorporeal infusion of their serum over a *S. aureus* column twice weekly for 10 to 20 weeks. Eleven of the 16 had a CR, and 9 of these 11 also became FeLV negative. Two cats had extended remissions, one for 7 months and the other for 35 months.[195,197,198]

Protein A administered directly to cats with lymphoma by intravenous[196] or intraperitoneal[195] routes caused partial responses that lasted as long as treatment was continued.[196] Other strains of *S. aureus* have been shown to have similar effects, and some investigators believe that bacterial products other than protein A may also be responsible for the responses.[199]

Fibronectin (heparin precipitate from plasma) is an enhancer of macrophage-mediated tumoricidal activity and indirectly increases T cell blastogenesis. Eighteen cats with lymphoma were treated with fibronectin; two cats had a CR and seven had a PR.[194] Duration of remission was not reported.

Other nonspecific immunotherapies such as acemannan[200] and immunoreglin[201] have caused anecdotal improvement in FeLV-positive cats but have not been evaluated for treatment of lymphoma. Immunotherapy for feline lymphoma remains an intriguing but unexplored possibility, particularly in combination with chemotherapy or radiation therapy.

SUPPORTIVE CARE

If treatment for lymphoma is contemplated in a cat that is already sick ("substage b"), nutritional support should be provided. An esophagostomy tube may be used if esophageal motility is not a problem and nausea is well controlled; similarly, a gastrostomy tube may provide long-term access for feeding. A jejunostomy tube should be considered if the stomach is involved, but it must be placed surgically (other tubes can be placed endoscopically). The use of appetite stimulants is often helpful when chemotherapy is being administered, particularly in cats that are already inappetent or anorectic from lymphoma; see Chapter 19 for details.

Hair coat changes with chemotherapy are common in longhaired breeds (Figures 36-16 and 36-17) and are often seen in shorthaired cats as well. These changes resolve within months of discontinuing chemotherapy.

CURRENT RECOMMENDATIONS

Cats with lymphoma are best treated with a combination protocol that includes doxorubicin, such as that published in *CVT X* (Table 36-5),[185] as cats that receive doxorubicin are likely to have better outcomes. Dosages as published in this book are higher than those in the *CVT-X* protocol and may be substituted safely. In addition, the use of MOPP

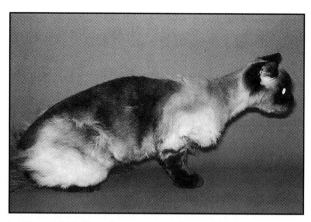

Figure 36-16: *Chemotherapy may cause hair coat changes and whisker loss, as in this 1-year-old FeLV-negative Himalayan treated with COP for mediastinal lymphoma.*

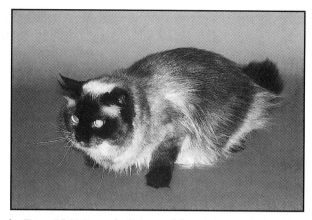

Figure 36-17: *Regrowth of hair coat of the cat in Figure 36-16 occurred within 6 months of finishing chemotherapy, and the cat was still alive and in remission 11 years later.*

chemotherapy for induction of remission in cats with lymphoma in addition to combination protocols should be assessed. Radiation therapy is valuable in the treatment of extranodal lymphomas and should be combined with chemotherapy. Supportive care is mandatory, as many cats with lymphoma are very ill.

NONDOMESTIC FELIDAE

FeLV appears to be a rare infection in nondomestic Felidae. Transient positive ELISA or IFA tests have been associated with lymphadenopathy in a clouded leopard *(Neofelis nebulosa)* and nonspecific illness in a cheetah *(Acinonyx jubatus).* Other cats with a positive test have been clinically normal, including cheetahs and a leopard cat *(Felis bengalensis).* FeLV-positive cats that were followed with serial testing became antigen "negative" within 2 to 9 weeks and at least one developed neutralizing antibodies and FOCMA. Tissues from a margay, ocelot, leopard cat, cheetah, jaguar, Chinese leopard, African lion, and Bengal tiger failed to show evidence of FeLV. However, cells from the ocelot, tiger, and lion can be infected in vitro with FeLV, making the risk to these species from affected domestic cats difficult to dismiss. A recent survey of *Felis silvestris* (Scottish wildcat) found a 10% prevalence of FeLV in a wild population but no evidence of FIV. A similar survey of *Felis silverstris* in Europe found two of eight captured cats were positive for FeLV, and both cats were thin and in poor condition. No cat had evidence of FIV. Serosurveys of wild *Felis bengalensis* in Taiwan and Vietnam showed no evidence of FeLV or FIV in this population or in the domestic cat population.

Lymphoma is very rare in nondomestic Felidae; it has been reported in a female cheetah *(Acinonyx jubatus obergi),* a jaguar *(Panthera onca),* and two lions. One of these lions, an aged male, tested negative for FeLV, and the lymphoma was apparently restricted to the spleen and associated lymph nodes. A young male cougar *(Felis concolor)* with FeLV and an uncharacterized leukemia noted on bone marrow aspirate died prior to treatment being initiated.

REFERENCES

1. Nielsen SW, Holzworth J: Visceral lymphosarcoma of the cat. *JAVMA* 122:189–197, 1953.
2. Takahashi R, Goto N, Ishii H, et al: Pathological observations of natural cases of feline lymphosarcomatosis. *Jap J Vet Sci* 36:163–173, 1974.
3. Carpenter JL, Andrews LK, Holzworth J: Tumors and tumor-like lesions, in Holzworth J (ed): *Diseases of the Cat Medicine and Surgery.* Philadelphia, WB Saunders, 1987, pp 407–596.
4. Nielsen SW: Spontaneous hematopoietic neoplasms of the domestic cat [monograph]. *Natl Cancer Inst* 32:73–94, 1969.
5. Cotter SM: Feline viral neoplasia, in Greene CE (ed): *Infectious Diseases of the Dog and Cat,* ed 3. Philadelphia, WB Saunders, 1998, pp 71–83.
6. Anderson WI, Miller DM, Davis JM: Multicentric lymphosarcoma in a kitten. *Modern Vet Pract* 66:206, 1985.
7. Meincke JE, Hobbie Jr WV, Hardy Jr WD: Lymphoreticular malignancies in the cat: Clinical findings. *JAVMA* 160:1093–1099, 1972.
8. Slayter MV, Farver TB, Schneider R: Feline malignant lymphoma: Log linear multiway frequency analysis of a population involving the factors of sex and age of animal and tumor cell type and location. *Am J Vet Res* 45:2178–2181, 1984.
9. Hardy Jr WD: Hematopoietic tumors of cats. *JAAHA* 17:921–940, 1981.
10. Crighton GW: Clinical aspects of lymphosarcoma in the cat. *Vet Rec* 83:122–126, 1968.
11. Sabine M, Wright RG, Love DN: Studies on feline lymphosarcoma in the Sydney area. *Aust J Exp Biol Med Sci* 52:331–340, 1974.
12. Holzworth J: Leukemia and related neoplasms in the cat: I. Lymphoid malignancies *JAVMA* 136:47–69, 1960.
13. Court EA, Watson ADJ, Peaston AE: Retrospective study of 60 cases of feline lymphosarcoma. *Aust Vet J* 75:424–427, 1997.
14. Gabor LJ, Malik R, Canfield PJ: Clinical and anatomical features of lymphosarcoma in 118 cats. *Aust Vet J* 76:725–732, 1998.
15. Vail DM, Moore AS, Ogilvie GK, Volk LM: Feline lymphoma (145 cases): Proliferation indices, cluster of differentiation 3 immunoreactivity, and their

association with prognosis in 90 cats. *J Vet Intern Med* 12:349–354, 1998.

16. Dorn CR, Taylor DON, Schneider R, et al: Survey of animal neoplasms in Alameda and Contra Costa Counties, California: II Cancer morbidity in dogs and cats from Alameda County. *J Natl Cancer Inst* 40:307–318, 1968.

17. Jarrett WFH, Crawford EM, Martin WB, Davie F: Leukemia in the cat. *Nature* 202:566–568, 1964.

18. Schneider R, Frye FL, Taylor DON, Dorn CR: A household cluster of feline malignant lymphoma. *Cancer Res* 27:1316–1322, 1967.

19. Schneider R: Feline malignant lymphoma: Environmental factors and the occurrence of this viral cancer in cats. *Int J Cancer* 10:345–350, 1972.

20. Theilen GH, Dungworth DL, Kawakami TG, et al: Experimental induction of lymphosarcoma in the cat with "C"-type virus. *Cancer Res* 30:401–408, 1970.

21. Cotter SM, Hardy Jr WD, Essex M: Association of feline leukemia virus with lymphosarcoma and other disorders in the cat. *JAVMA* 166:449–454, 1975.

22. Hardy Jr WD, Zuckerman EE, MacEwen EG, et al: A feline leukemia and sarcoma virus-induced tumor-specific antigen. *Nature (Lond)* 270:249–251, 1977.

23. Snyder Jr HW, Singhal MC, Zuckerman EE, et al: The feline oncornavirus-associated cell membrane antigen (FOCMA) is related to, but distinguishable from, FeLV-C gp70. *Virology* 131:315–327, 1983.

24. Reinacher M, Theilen GH: Frequency and significance of feline leukemia virus infection in necropsied cats. *Am J Vet Res* 48:939–945, 1987.

25. Reinacher M: Diseases associated with spontaneous feline leukemia virus (FeLV) infection in cats. *Vet Immunol Immunopathol* 21:85–95, 1989.

26. Francis DP, Cotter SM, Hardy Jr WD, Essex M: Comparison of virus positive and virus negative cases of feline leukemia and lymphoma. *Cancer Res* 39:3866–3870, 1979.

27. Rezanka LJ, Rojko JL, Neil JC: Feline leukemia virus: Pathogenesis of neoplastic disease. *Cancer Invest* 10:371–389, 1992.

28. Miura T, Tsujimoto H, Fukasawa M, et al: Structural abnormality and over-expression of the *myc* gene in feline leukemias. *Int J Cancer* 40:564–569, 1987.

29. Pantginis J, Beaty RM, Levy LS, Lenz J: The feline leukemia virus long terminal repeat contains a potent genetic determinant of T-cell lymphomagenicity. *J Virology* 71:9786–9791, 1997.

30. Pandey R, Bechtel MK, Su Y, et al: Feline leukemia virus variants in experimentally induced thymic lymphosarcomas. *Virology* 214:584–592, 1995.

31. Athas GB, Choi B, Prabhu S, et al: Genetic determinants of feline leukemia virus-induced multicentric lymphomas. *Virology* 214:431–438, 1995.

32. Okuda M, Umeda A, Sakai T, et al: Cloning of the feline p53 tumor-suppressor gene and its aberration in hematopoietic tumors. *Int J Cancer* 58:602–607, 1994.

33. Casey JW, Roach A, Mullins JE, et al: The U3 portion of feline leukemia virus DNA identifies horizontally acquired proviruses in leukemia cats. *Proc Natl Acad Sci USA* 78:7778–7782, 1981.

34. Sheets RL, Pandey R, Jen W-C, Roy-Burman P: Recombinant feline leukemia virus genes detected in naturally occurring feline lymphosarcomas. *J Virology* 67:3118–3125, 1993.

35. Jackson ML, Haines DM, Meric SM, Misra V: Feline leukemia virus detection by immunohistochemistry and polymerase chain reaction in formalin-fixed, paraffin-embedded tumor tissue from cats with lymphosarcoma. *Can J Vet Res* 57:269–276, 1993.

36. Gregory CR, Madewell BR, Griffey S, Torten M: Feline leukemia virus-associated lymphosarcoma following renal transplantation in a cat. *Transplantation* 1097–1099, 1991.

37. Gabor LJ, Jackson ML, Trask B, et al: Feline leukemia virus status of Australian cats with lymphosarcoma. Submitted for publication, 2000.

38. Jackson ML, Wood SL, Misra V, Haines DM: Immunohistochemical identification of B and T lymphocytes in formalin-fixed, paraffin-embedded feline lymphosarcomas: Relation to feline leukemia virus status, tumor site, and patient age. *Can J Vet Res* 60:199–204, 1996.

39. Shelton GH, Grant CK, Cotter SM, et al: Feline immunodeficiency virus and feline leukemia virus infections and their relationships to lymphoid malignancies in cats: A retrospective study (1968–1988). *J Acquir Immune Defic Syndr* 3:623–630, 1990.

40. Hutson CA, Rideout BA, Pedersen NC: Neoplasia associated with feline immunodeficiency virus infection in cats of Southern California. *JAVMA* 199:1357–1362, 1991.

41. Callanan JJ, Jones BA, Irvine J, et al: Histologic classification and immunophenotype of lymphosarcomas in cats with naturally and experimentally acquired feline immunodeficiency virus infections. *Vet Pathol* 33:264–272, 1996.

42. Poli A, Abramo F, Baldinotti F, et al: Malignant lymphoma associated with experimentally induced feline immunodeficiency virus infection. *J Comp Pathol* 110:319–328, 1994.

43. Alexander R, Robinson WF, Mills JN, et al: Isolation of feline immunodeficiency virus from three cats with lymphoma. *Aust Vet Practit* 19:93–97, 1989.

44. Jarrett O, Edney ATB, Toth S, Hay D: Feline leukaemia virus-free lymphosarcoma in a specific pathogen free cat. *Vet Rec* 115:249–250, 1984.

45. Gulino SE: Chromosome abnormalities and oncogenesis in cat leukemias. *Cancer Genet Cytogenet* 64:149–157, 1992.

46. Holmberg CA, Manning JS, Osburn BI: Feline malignant lymphomas: Comparison of morphologic and immunologic characteristics. *Am J Vet Res* 37:1455–1460, 1976.

47. Wellman ML, Kociba GJ, Rojko JL: Guinea pig erythrocyte rosette formation as a non-specific cell surface receptor assay in the cat. *Am J Vet Res* 47:433–437, 1986.

48. Rojko JL, Kociba GJ, Abkowitz JL, et al: Feline lymphomas: Immunological and cytochemical characterization. *Cancer Res* 49:345–351, 1989.

49. Darbès J, Majzoub M, Hermanns W: Evaluation of the cross-reactivity between human and feline or canine leucocyte antigens using commercially available antibodies. *J Vet Diagn Invest* 9:94–97, 1997.

50. Monteith CE, Chelack BJ, Davis WC, Haines DM: Identification of monoclonal antibodies for immunohistochemical staining of feline B lymphocytes in frozen and fomalin-fixed paraffin-embedded tissues. *Can J Vet Res* 60:193–198, 1996.

51. Shimojima M, Pecoraro MR, Maeda K, et al: Characterization of anti-feline CD8 monoclonal antibodies. *Vet Immunol Immunopathol* 61:17–23, 1998.

52. Gabor LJ, Canfield PJ, Malik R: Immunophenotypic and histological characterization of 109 cases of feline lymphosarcoma. *Aust Vet J* 77:436–441, 1999.

53. Moore AS: Treatment of feline lymphoma. *Feline Pract* 24:17–20, 1996.

54. Mooney SC, Hayes AA, Matus R, MacEwen EG: Renal lymphoma in cats: 28 cases (1977–1984). *JAVMA* 191:1473–1477, 1987.

55. Mooney SC, Hayes AA: Lymphoma in the cat: An approach to diagnosis and management. *Semin Vet Med Surg Small Anim* 1:51–57, 1986.

56. Mooney SC, Hayes AA, MacEwen EG, et al: Treatment and prognostic factors in lymphoma in cats: 103 cases (1977–1981). *JAVMA* 194:696–699, 1989.

57. Pennick DG, Moore AS, Tidwell AS, et al: Ultrasonography of alimentary lymphosarcoma in the cat. *Vet Radiol* 35:299–304, 1994.

58. Penninck DG, Crystal MA, Matz ME, Pearson SH: The technique of percutaneous ultrasound guided fine-needle aspiration biopsy and automated microcore biopsy in small animal gastrointestinal diseases. *Vet Radiol Ultrasound* 34:433–436, 1993.

59. Lamb CR, Hartzband LE, Tidwell AS, Pearson SH: Ultrasonographic findings in hepatic and splenic lymphosarcoma in dogs and cats. *Vet Radiol* 32:117–120, 1991.

60. Gabor LJ, Canfield PJ, Malik R: Haematological and biomedical findings in cats in Australia with lymphosarcoma. *Aust Vet J* 78:456–461, 2000.

61. Fritz D, Saignes C-F, Hopfner C: Usefulness of bone marrow biopsy for the diagnosis of deep-seated lymphomas in cat: One case. *Revue Méd Vét* 147:681–686, 1996.

62. Spodnick GJ, Berg J, Moore FMCSM: Spinal lymphoma in cats: 21 cases (1976—1989). *JAVMA* 200:373–376, 1992.

63. Todorovic D, Gafner F, Knezevic M, Kovacevic S: Lymphosarcoma in cats. *Acta Veterinarian (Beograd)* 40:341–344, 1990.

64. Nakayama H, Nakanaga K, Ogihara S, et al: Three cases of feline lymphosarcoma with formation of multinucleated giant cells. *Jpn J Vet Sci* 46:225–228, 1984.

65. Roperto F, Damiano S, Galati P: Hodgkin's disease in a cat. *Zbl Vet Med A* 30:182–188, 1983.

66. Walton RM, Hendrick MJ: Feline Hodgkin's-like lymphosarcoma: 20 cases (1992–1998) [abstract 64]. *Vet Pathol* 36:496, 1999.

67. Day MJ, Kyaw-Tanner M, Silkstone MA, et al: T-cell-rich B-cell lymphoma in the cat. *J Comp Pathol* 120:155–167, 1999.

68. Valli VE, Jacobs RM, Norris A, et al: The histological classification of 602 cases of feline lymphoproliferative disease using the national cancer institute working formulation. *J Vet Diagn Invest* 12:295–306, 2000.

69. Fondacaro JV, Richter KP, Carpenter JL, et al: Feline gastrointestinal well differentiated lymphocytic lymphoma: 39 cases [abstract 123]. *J Vet Intern Med* 13:257, 1999.

70. Rassnick KM, Mauldin GN, Moroff SD, et al: Prognostic value of argyrophilic nucleolar organizer region (AgNOR) staining in feline intestinal lymphoma. *J Vet Intern Med* 13:187–190, 1999.

71. Dust A, Norris AM, Valli VEO: Cutaneous lymphosarcoma with IgG monoclonal gammopathy, serum hyperviscosity and hypercalcemia in a cat. *Can Vet J* 23:235–239, 1982.

72. Engelman RW, Tyler RD, Kay NK: Hypercalcemia in cats with feline-

leukemia-virus-associated leukemia-lymphoma. *Cancer* 56:777–781, 1985.

73. Chew DJ, Schaer M, Liu SK, Owens J: Pseudohyperparathyroidism in a cat. *JAAHA* 11:46–52, 1975.

74. Qureshi SR, Olander HJ: Feline lymphosarcoma with heterotopic bone. *JAAHA* 13:616–618, 1977.

75. Thilsted JP, Bolton RG: Thymic lymphosarcoma with bony metaplasia in a cat. *Vet Pathol* 22:424–425, 1985.

76. Provencher-Bollinger A, Graham PA, Refsal KR, et al: Detection of parathyroid hormone related peptide (PTHrP) in serum of cats with hypercalcemia of malignancy [abstract 12]. *Proc Am Soc Vet Clin Pathol Vet Pathol* 36:483, 1999.

77. Kehoe JM, Hurvitsz AI, Capra JD: Characterization of three feline paraproteins. *J Immunol* 109:511–516, 1972.

78. Glick AD, Horn RG, Holscher M: Characterization of feline glomerulonephritis associated with viral-induced hematopoietic neoplasms. *Am J Pathol* 92:321–327, 1978.

79. Jeraj KP, Hardy R, O'Leary TP, et al: Immune complex glomerulonephritis in a cat with renal lymphosarcoma. *Vet Pathol* 22:287–290, 1985.

80. Anderson LJ, Jarrett WFH: Membranous glomerulonephritis associated with leukaemia in cats. *Res Vet Sci* 12:179–180, 1971.

81. Ashley PF, Bowman LA: Symmetric cutaneous necrosis of the hind feet and multicentric follicular lymphoma in a cat. *JAVMA* 214:211–214, 1999.

82. Daniels-McQueen SM, Directo AC, Palomo HA: Chorea in a cat with malignant lymphoma. *Vet Med Small Anim Clin*: 413–415, 1974.

83. Parnell NK, Powell LL, Hohenhaus AE, et al: Hypoadrenocortism as the primary manifestation of lymphoma in two cats. *JAVMA* 8:1208–1211, 1999.

84. Farrelly J, Hohenhaus AE, Peterson ME, et al: Evaluation of pituitary-adrenal function in cats with lymphoma. *Proc 19th Annu Conf Vet Cancer Soc*:33, 1999.

85. Madewell BR, Holmberg CA, Ackerman N: Lymphosarcoma and cryptococcosis in a cat. *JAVMA* 175:65–68, 1979.

86. Edwards JF, Ficken MD, Luttgen PJ, Frey MS: Disseminated sarcocystosis in a cat with lymphosarcoma. *JAVMA* 193:831–832, 1988.

87. Aronson E, Bendickson JC, Miles KG, et al: Disseminated histoplasmosis with osseous lesions in a cat with feline lymphosarcoma. *Vet Radiol* 27:50–53, 1986.

88. Lent SF, Burkhardt JE, Bolka D: Coincident enteric crytosporidiosis and lymphosarcoma in a cat with diarrhea. *JAAHA* 29:492–496, 1993.

89. Hohenhaus AE, Rosenberg MP, Moroff SD: Concurrent lymphoma and salmonellosis in a cat. *Can Vet J* 31:38–40, 1990.

90. Järplid B, Feldman BF: Large granular lymphoma with toxoplasmosis in a cat. *Comp Haematol Int* 3:241–243, 1993.

91. Zwahlen CH, Lucroy MD, Kraegel SA, Madewell BR: Results of chemotherapy for cats with alimentary malignant lymphoma: 21 cases (1993–1997). *JAVMA* 213:1144–1149, 1998.

92. Head KW, Else RW: Neoplasia and allied conditions of the canine and feline intestine. *Small Anim Intest Neoplasia* 190–208, 1981.

93. Mahony O, Moore AS, Cotter SM: Alimentary lymphoma in cats: 28 cases (1988–1993). *JAVMA* 207:1593–1598, 1995.

94. Brodey RS: Alimentary tract neoplasms in the cat: A clinicopathologic survey of 46 cases. *Am J Vet Res* 27:74–80, 1966.

95. Groothers AM, Biller DS, Ward H, et al: Ultrasonographic appearance of feline alimentary lymphoma. *Vet Radiol Ultrasound* 35:468–472, 1994.

96. Patterson DF, Meier H: Surgical intervention in intestinal lymphosarcoma in two cats. *JAVMA* 127:495–498, 1955.

97. Jeglum KA, Whereat A, Young K: Chemotherapy of lymphoma in 75 cats. *JAVMA* 190:174–178, 1987.

98. Wieser JR: What is your diagnosis? *JAVMA* 205:685–686, 1994.

99. Weller RE, Hornof WJ: Gastric malignant lymphoma in two cats. *Modern Vet Pract* 60:701–704, 1979.

100. Slawienski MJ, Mauldin GE, Mauldin GN, Patnaik AK: Malignant colonic neoplasia in cats: 46 cases (1990–1996). *JAVMA* 211:878–881, 1997.

101. Loupal G, Pfeil C: Tumoren im darmtrakt der katze unter besonderer Berücksightigung der nicht-hämatopoetischen Geschwülste. *Berl Münch Teirärztl Wschr* 97:208–213, 1984.

102. Strand RD: Treatment of recurrent feline intestinal lymphoma. *Mod Vet Pract* 67:823–824, 1986.

103. Münster M: Effizienz der endoskopie bei magen-darm-erkrankungen von hund und katze. *Der Praktische Tierarzt* 4:309–312, 1993.

104. Wasmer ML, Willard MD, Helman RG, Edwards JF: Food intolerance mimicking alimentary lymphosarcoma. *JAAHA* 31:463–466, 1995.

105. Gores BR, Berg J, Carpenter JL, Ullman SL: Chylous ascites in cats: Nine cas-

es (1978–1993). *JAVMA* 205:1161–1164, 1994.

106. Cotter SM: Treatment of lymphoma and leukemia with cyclophosphamide, vincristine, and prednisone: II. Treatment of cats. *JAAHA* 19:166–172, 1983.

107. Moore AS, Cotter SM, Frimberger AE, et al: A comparison of doxorubicin and COP for maintenance of remission in cats with lymphoma. *J Vet Intern Med* 10:372–375, 1996.

108. Franks PT, Harvey JW, Calderwood Mays M, et al: Feline large granular lymphoma. *Vet Pathol* 23:200–202, 1986.

109. Honor DJ, DeNicola DB, Turek JJ, et al: A neoplasm of globule leukocytes in a cat. *Vet Pathol* 23:287–292, 1986.

110. Konno A, Hashimoto Y, Kon Y, Sugimura M: Perforin-like immunoreactivity in feline globule leukocytes and their distribution. *J Vet Med Sci* 56:1101–1105, 1994.

111. Goitsuka R, Tsuji M, Matsumoto Y, et al: A case of feline large granular lymphoma. *Jpn J Vet Sci* 50:593–595, 1988.

112. Kariya K, Konno A, Ishida T, et al: Globule leukocyte neoplasm in a cat. *Jpn J Vet Sci* 52:403–405, 1990.

113. Darbés J, Majzoub M, Breuer W, Hermanns W: Large granular lymphocyte leukemia/lymphoma in six cats. *Vet Pathol* 35:370–379, 1988.

114. Finn JP, Schwartz LW: A neoplasm of globule leucocytes in the intestine of a cat. *J Comp Pathol* 82:323–326, 1972.

115. Moore FM, Kaufman J: What is your diagnosis? *Vet Clin Pathol* 18:37–38, 2000.

116. Cheney CM, Rojko JL, Kociba GJ, et al: A feline large granular lymphoma and its derived cell line. *In Vitro Cell Dev Biol* 26:455–463, 1990.

117. Buracco P, Guglielmino R, Abate O, et al: Large granular lymphoma in an FIV-positive and FeLV-negative cat. *J Small Anim Pract* 33:279–284, 1992.

118. Wellman ML, Hammer AS, DiBartola SP, et al: Lymphoma involving large granular lymphocytes in cats: 11 cases (1982–1991). *JAVMA* 201:1265–1269, 1992.

119. McEntee MF, Horton S, Blue J, Meuten DJ: Granulated round cell tumor of cats. *Vet Pathol* 30:195–203, 1993.

120. Drobatz KJ, Fred R, Waddle J: Globule leukocyte tumor in six cats. *JAAHA* 29:391–396, 1993.

121. McPherron MA, Chavkin MJ, Powers BE, Seim III HB: Globule leukocyte tumor involving the small intestine in a cat. *JAVMA* 204:241–245, 1994.

122. von Beust BR, Guscetti F, Kohn B: Neoplasien ausgehend von großen granulierten lymphzyten bei hund und katze. *Tierarztl Prax* 23:70–74, 1995.

123. Goitsuka R, Ohno K, Matsumoto Y, et al: Establishment and characterization of a feline large granular lymphoma cell line expressing interleukin 2 receptor α–chain. *J Vet Med Sci* 55:863–865, 1993.

124. Tobey JC, Houston DM, Breur GJ, et al: Cutaneous T-cell lymphoma in a cat. *JAVMA* 204:606–609, 1994.

125. Gruffydd-Jones TJ, Gaskell CJ, Gibbs C: Clinical and radiological features of anterior mediastinal lymphosarcoma in the cat: A review of 30 cases. *Vet Rec* 104:304–307, 1979.

126. Mauldin GE, Mooney SC, Meleo KA, et al: Chemotherapy in 132 cats with lymphoma (1988–1994). *Proc 15th Vet Cancer Soc*:35–36, 1995.

127. Shimoda T: Clinicopathological findings in 12 cases of feline thymic lymphoma. *J Jpn Vet Med Assoc* 46:227–230, 1993.

128. Day MJ: Review of thymic pathology in 30 cats and 36 dogs. *J Small Anim Pract* 38:393–403, 1997.

129. Forrester SD, Fossum TW, Rogers KS: Diagnosis and treatment of chylothorax associated with lymphoblastic lymphosarcoma in four cats. *JAVMA* 198:291–294, 1991.

130. Fossum TW, Forrester SD, Swenson CL, et al: Chylothorax in cats: 37 cases (1969–1989). *JAVMA* 198:672–678, 1991.

131. Murphy MG: Thymic lymphosarcoma in a cat. *Irish Vet J* 41:332–334, 1987.

132. Sottiaux J, Franck M: Cranial vena caval thrombosis secondary to invasive mediastinal lymphosarcoma in a cat. *J Small Anim Pract* 39:352–355, 1998.

133. Hinko PJ, Rickards DA, Morse Jr EM: Malignant lymphoma of thymus gland. *Feline Pract* 2:17–18, 1972.

134. Cotter SM, Essex M, McLane MF, et al: Chemotherapy and passive immunotherapy in naturally occurring feline mediastinal lymphoma, in Hardy Jr WD, Essex M, McClelland AJ (eds): *Feline Leukemia Virus.* New York, Elsevier North Holland, Inc, 1980, pp 219–225.

135. Gruffydd-Jones TJ, Flecknell PA: The prognosis and treatment related to the gross appearance and laboratory characteristics of pathological thoracic fluids in the cat. *J Small Anim Pract* 19:315–328, 1978.

136. Mackey L, Jarrett W, Jarrett O, Wilson L: B and T cells in a cat with thymic lymphosarcoma. *J Natl Cancer Inst* 54:1483–1485, 1975.

137. Freitag WA, Norsworthy GD: Lymphosarcoma treatment. *Feline Pract* 6:11–14, 1976.

138. Zaki FA, Hurvitz AI: Spontaneous neoplasms of the central nervous system of the cat. *J Small Anim Pract* 17:773–782, 1976.

139. Lane SB, Kornegay JN, Duncan JR, Oliver Jr JE: Feline spinal lymphosarcoma: A retrospective evaluation of 23 cats. *J Vet Intern Med* 8:99– 104, 1994.

140. Noonan M, Kline KL, Meleo K: Lymphoma of the central nervous system: A retrospective study of 18 cats. *Compend Contin Educ Pract Vet* 19:497–504, 1997.

141. LeCouteur RA, Fike JR, Cann CE, et al: X-ray computed tomography of brain tumors in cats. *JAVMA* 183:301–305, 1983.

142. Lapointe J-M, Higgins RJ, Kortz GD, et al: Intravascular malignant T-cell lymphoma (malignant angioendotheliomatosis) in a cat. *Vet Pathol* 34:247–250, 1997.

143. Fondevila D, Vilafranca M, Pumarola M: Primary central nervous system T-cell lymphoma in a cat. *Vet Pathol* 35:550–553, 1998.

144. Allen JG, Amis T: Lymphosarcoma involving cranial nerves in a cat. *Aust Vet J* 51:155–158, 1975.

145. Northington JW, Juliana MM: Extradural lymphosarcoma in six cats. *J Small Anim Pract* 19:409–416, 1978.

146. Schappert HR, Geib LW: Reticuloendothelial neoplasms involving the spinal canal in cats. *JAVMA* 150:753–757, 1967.

147. Fox JG, Gutnick MJ: Horner's syndrome and brachial paralysis due to lymphosarcoma in a cat. *JAVMA* 160:977–980, 1972.

148. Rowe WS, Bradford TS, Martin P: Posterior paralysis due to lymphosarcoma. *Feline Pract* 7:34–36, 1977.

149. Heavner JE: Neural lymphomatosis in cats. *Mod Vet Pract* 59:122–124, 1978.

150. Mitchell M: Feline spinal lymphosarcoma—A case report. *Southwest Vet* 33:72–75, 1980.

151. Ogilvie GK: Extradural lymphoma in a cat. *Vet Med Report* 1:57–61, 1988.

152. Suess Jr RP, Martin RA, Shell LG, et al: Vertebral lymphosarcoma in a cat. *JAVMA* 197:101–103, 1990.

153. Parker AJ, Park RD: Myelographic diagnosis of a spinal cord tumor in a cat. *Feline Pract* 4:28–33, 1974.

154. Chrisman CL: Electromyography in the localization of spinal cord and nerve root neoplasia in dogs and cats. *JAVMA* 166:1074–1079, 1975.

155. Barr MC, Butt MT, Anderson KL, et al: Spinal lymphosarcoma and disseminated mastocytoma associated with feline immunodeficiency virus infection in a cat. *JAVMA* 202:1978–1980, 1993.

156. Swaim SF, Shields RP: Paraplegia in the cat. *Vet Med Small Anim Clin* 66:787–798, 1971.

157. Weller RE, Stann SE: Renal lymphosarcoma in the cat. *JAAHA* 19:363–367, 1983.

158. Podell M, DiBartola SP, Rosol TJ: Polycystic kidney disease and renal lymphoma in a cat. *JAVMA* 201:906–909, 1992.

159. Osborne CA, Johnson KH, Kurtz HJ, Hanlon GF: Renal lymphoma in the dog and cat. *JAVMA* 158:2058–2070, 1971.

160. Moore FM, Emerson WE, Cotter SM, Delellis RA: Distinctive peripheral lymph node hyperplasia of young cats. *Vet Pathol* 23:386–391, 1986.

161. Brown PJ, Hopper CD, Harbour DA: Pathological features of lymphoid tissues in cats with natural feline immunodeficiency virus infection. *J Comp Pathol* 104:345–355, 1991.

162. Lucke VM, Davies JD, Wood CA, Whitbread TJ: Plexiform vascularization of lymph nodes: An unusual but distinctive lymphadenopathy in cat. *J Comp Pathol* 97:109–119, 1987.

163. Mooney SC, Patnaik AK, Hayes AA, MacEwen EG: Generalized lymphadenopathy resembling lymphoma in cats: Six cases (1972–1976). *JAVMA* 190:897–900, 1987.

164. Steele KE, Saunders GK, Coleman GD: T cell-rich B-cell lymphoma in a cat. *Vet Pathol* 34:47–49, 1997.

165. Day MJ, Kyaw-Tanner M, Silkstone MA, et al: T-cell rich B-cell lymphoma in the cat. *J Comp Pathol* 120:155–167, 1999.

166. Carlton WW: Intraocular lymphosarcoma: Two cases in Siamese cats. *JAAHA* 12:83–87, 1976.

167. Peiffer Jr RL, Wilcock BP: Histopathologic study of uveitis in cats: 139 cases (1978–1988). *JAVMA* 198:135–138, 1991.

168. Corcoran KA, Peiffer Jr RL, Koch SA: Histopathologic features of feline ocular lymphosarcoma: 49 cases (1978–1992). *Vet Comp Ophthalmol* 5:35–41, 1995.

169. Hittmair K, Walzer C: Generalisierte lymphidezellige infiltration des fettgewebes und exophthalmus bei einer leukosekranken katze. *Wien Tierärztl Mschr* 79:81–86, 1992.

170. Meincke JE: Reticuloendothelial malignancies, with intraocular involvement in the cat. *JAVMA* 148:157–161, 1966.

171. Saunders LZ, Barron CN: Intraocular tumors in animals. *Br Vet J* 120:25–35, 1964.

172. Barclay SM: Lymphosarcoma in tarsi of a cat. *JAVMA* 175:582–583, 1979.

173. Wilson JW: Reticulum cell sarcoma of long bone terminating as respiratory distress. *Vet Med Small Anim Clin* 68:1393–1401, 1973.

174. Elmslie RE, Ogilvie GK, Gillette EL, McChesney-Gillette S: Radiotherapy with and without chemotherapy for localized lymphoma in 10 cats. *Vet Radiol* 32:277–280, 1991.

175. Squire RA: Feline lymphoma: A comparison with the Burkitt tumor of children. *Cancer* 19:447–453, 1966.

176. Ladiges WC, Zeidner NS: An overview of feline cancer therapy. *Feline Pract* 10:38–43, 1980.

177. Brick JO, Roenigk WJ, Wilson GP: Chemotherapy of malignant lymphoma in dogs and cats. *JAVMA* 153:47–52, 1968.

178. Carpenter JL, Holzworth J: Treatment of leukemia in the cat. *JAVMA* 158:1130–1131, 1971.

179. Squires RA, Bush M: The therapy of canine and feline lymphosarcoma, in: *Unifying Concepts of Leukemia*. Basel, Switzerland, Bibl Haemat Karger, 1973, pp 189–197.

180. McClelland RB: Chemotherapy in reticulum-cell sarcoma in five dogs and a cat and in mast cell leukemia in a cat. *Cornell Vet* 61:477–481, 1971.

181. Ogilvie GK, Moore AS, Obradovich JE, et al: Toxicoses and efficacy associated with the administration of mitoxantrone to cats with malignant tumors. *JAVMA* 202:1839–1844, 1993.

182. Hahn KA, Fletcher CM, Legendre AM: Marked neutropenia in five tumor-bearing cats one week following single agent vincristine sulfate chemotherapy. *Vet Clin Pathol* 25:121–123, 1996.

183. Peaston AE, Maddison JE: Efficacy of doxorubicin as an induction agent for cats with lymphosarcoma. *Aust Vet J* 77:442–444, 1999.

184. Kristal O, Lana SE, Moore AS, et al: Single agent chemotherapy with doxorubicin for feline lymphoma. *Proc 18th Vet Cancer Soc*:25, 1998.

185. Matus RE: Chemotherapy of lymphoma and leukemia, in Kirk RW (ed): *Current Veterinary Therapy X. Small Animal Practice*. Philadelphia, WB Saunders, 1989, pp 482–488.

186. Marks SL, Cook AK, Griffey S, et al: Dietary modulation of methotrexate-induced enteritis in cats. *Am J Vet Res* 58:989–996, 1997.

187. Rassnick KM, Geiger TL, Williams LE, et al: Phase I evaluation of CCNU (lomustine) in tumor-bearing cats. *J Vet Internal Med* 15:196–199, 2001.

188. Mauldin GE, Mooney SC, Mauldin GN: MOPP chemotherapy for cats with refractory lymphoma. *Proc 17th Vet Cancer Soc*:98, 1997.

189. Klein MK, Powers BE, Johnson CS, et al: Feline nasal lymphoma: A retrospective analysis. Submitted for publication, 1999.

190. Calia CM, Hohenhaus AE, Fox PR, Meleo KA: Acute tumor lysis syndrome in a cat with lymphoma. *J Vet Intern Med* 10:409–411, 1996.

191. Hardy Jr WD, Hess PW, MacEwan EG, et al:: Treatment of feline lymphosarcoma with feline blood constituents, in: *Comparative Leukemia Research. Bibliotheca Haematologica*. Basel, Switzerland, Karger, 43:518–521, 1976.

192. Kassel RL, Old LJ, Day NK, et al: Plasma mediated leukemic cell destruction: Current status. *Blood Cells* 3:605–621, 1977.

193. Snyder Jr HW, Jones FR, Day NK, Hardy Jr WD: Isolation and characterization of circulating feline leukemia virus-immune complexes from plasma of persistently infected pet cats removed by ex vivo immunosorption. *J Immunol* 128:2726–2730, 1982.

194. MacEwan EG: Current concepts in cancer therapy: Biologic therapy and chemotherapy. *Semin Vet Med Surg (Small Anim)* 1:5–16, 1986.

195. Engelman RW, Good RA, Day NK: Clearance of retroviremia and regression of malignancy in cats with leukemia-lymphoma during treatment with staphylococcal protein A. *Cancer Detect Prevent* 10:435–444, 1987.

196. Harper HD, Sjöquist J, Hardy Jr WD, Jones FR: Antitumor activity of protein A administered intravenously to pet cats with leukemia or lymphosarcoma. *Cancer* 55:1863–1867, 1985.

197. Snyder Jr HW, Singhal MC, Hardy Jr WD, Jones FR: Clearance of feline leukemia virus from persistently infected pet cats treated by extracorporeal immunoadsorption is correlated with an enhanced antibody response to FeLV gp 70. *J Immunol* 132:1538–1543, 1984.

198. Jones FR, Grant CK, Snyder Jr HW: Lymphosarcoma and persistent feline leukemia virus infection of pet cats: A system to study responses during extracorporeal treatments. *J Biol Resp Modif* 3:286–292, 1984.

199. Gordon BR, Matus RE, Hurvitz AI, et al: Perfusion of plasma over *Staphylococcus aureus:* Release of bacterial product is related to regression of tumor. *J Biol Resp Modif* 3:266–270, 1984.

200. Sheets MA, Unger BA, Giggleman Jr GF, Tizard IR: Studies of the effect of acemannan on retrovirus infections: Clinical stabilization of feline leukemia virus-infected cats. *Mol Biother* 3:41–45, 1991.

201. Ray Jr WJ, Gilliland CD, McMichael JC, et al: *Informational Brochure: Immunoregulin Biologic Response Modifier.* Immunovet, Inc., 1982, pp 1–10.

202. Citino SB: Transient FeLV viremia in a clouded leopard. *J Zoo Anim Med* 17:5–7, 1986.

203. Briggs MB, Ott RL: Feline leukemia virus infection in a captive cheetah and the clinical and antibody response of six captive cheetahs to vaccination with a subunit feline leukemia virus vaccine. *JAVMA* 189:1197–1199, 1986.

204. Rasheed S, Gardner MB: Isolation of feline leukemia virus from a leopard cat cell line and search for retrovirus in wild felidae. *J Natl Cancer Inst* 67:929–933, 1981.

205. Daniels MJ, Golder MC, Jarret O, MacDonald DW: Feline viruses in wild-cats from Scotland. *J Wildl Dis* 35:121–124, 1999.

206. Artois M, Remond M: Viral diseases as a threat to free-living wild cats *(Felis silvestris)* in Continental Europe. *Vet Rec* 134:651–652, 1994.

207. Ikeda Y, Miyazawa T, Nakamura K, et al: Serosurvey for selected virus infections of wild carnivores in Taiwan and Vietnam. *J Wildl Dis* 35:578–581, 1999.

208. Miyazawa T, Ideda Y, Maeda K, et al: Seroepidemiological survey of feline retrovirus infections in domestic and leopard cats in northern Vietnam in 1997. *J Vet Med Sci* 60:1273–1275, 1998.

209. Effron M, Griner L, Benirschke K: Nature and rate of neoplasia found in captive wild mammals, birds and reptiles at necropsy. *J Natl Cancer Inst* 59:185–198, 1977.

210. Butler R, Wrigley RH, Horsey R, Reuter R: Chondrosarcoma in a Sumatran tiger *(Panthera tigris sumatrae). J Zoo Anim Med* 12:80–84, 1981.

211. Douglass EM: Lymphosarcoma and blockage of the biliary duct in an African lion *(Panthera leo). Vet Med Small Anim Clin* 74(11):1637–1641, 1979.

212. Meric SM: Suspected feline leukemia virus infection and pancytopenia in a western cougar. *JAVMA* 185:1390–1391, 1984.

BONE MARROW DISORDERS

Antony S. Moore and Gregory K. Ogilvie

37

It is more realistic to think of neoplastic disorders of bone marrow as a disease continuum rather than a number of discrete pathophysiologic entities. The earliest stages in myeloproliferative disease reflect decreased or inappropriate bone marrow production; signs may indicate functional problems without overt evidence of neoplasia. When cytopenias and morphologic abnormalities are detected, the condition is termed *myelodysplasia* (MDS) or *preleukemia*. MDS may progress to a true neoplastic process or leukemia; the term *aleukemic leukemia* is used when only the bone marrow, and not peripheral blood, is involved. Leukemia may affect any of the cell lines in the marrow, and the nomenclature reflects the type of cell from which the leukemia is derived. Clinically, it is important to distinguish chronic leukemias and myeloproliferative diseases from acute leukemias and to differentiate between acute lymphoid leukemia (ALL) and acute nonlymphoid leukemia (ANLL; Figure 37-1).

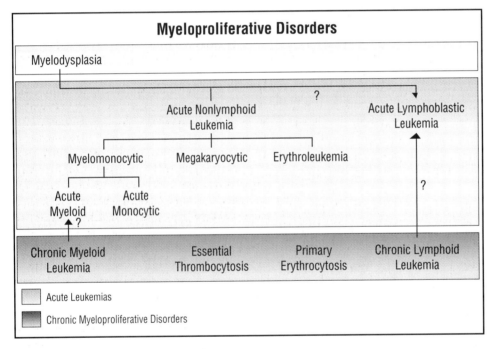

Figure 37-1: Myelodysplasia may progress to ANLL or ALL. Chronic myeloproliferative disorders, such as chronic lymphoid leukemia and chronic myeloid leukemia are rare in cats and seldom progress to an acute leukemia. (The question marks indicate uncertainty about whether the pathway exists in cats.)

MYELODYSPLASIA (PRELEUKEMIA)

CLINICAL BRIEFING

Common Presentation	No age, gender, or breed predilection; usually progresses to acute leukemia in cats (most affected cats are FeLV antigenemic). Clinical signs reflect cytopenias (e.g., fever and neutropenia or petechiation and thrombocytopenia).
Staging and Diagnosis	Differentiated from leukemia by less than 30% blast cells in a dysplastic bone marrow. Perform MDB (particularly FeLV serology).
Treatment Supportive Differentiating Agents	Antibiotics and transfusions of blood and blood products. Cytosine arabinoside and retinoids (investigational); corticosteroids and erythropoietin (investigational).

Incidence, Signalment, and Etiology

MDS is considerably more common in cats than in dogs, largely because of the role of FeLV. Experimental infection of cats with FeLV leads to the development of myeloid and erythroid leukemias, and it is possible that certain strains of the virus determine the pathologic outcome. Subgroup C FeLV has been associated with pure red cell aplasia, whereas defective FeLV may cause MDS.[1]

KEY POINT

Most cats with myelodysplasia are FeLV antigenemic.

MDS is distinguished from the acute leukemias by the presence of less than 30% abnormal blast cells in the bone marrow aspirate. The distinction may be clinically irrelevant, however, as affected cats are frequently very ill and survival beyond 1 week after diagnosis is rare.[2] Cats with MDS are usually FeLV positive[3-5] and are often young, although affected cats without detectable FeLV[3,6] have been described. In one study, 15 of 21 cats with MDS were FeLV antigenemic.[2] Ages ranged from 6 months to 15 years (median, 3 years). Most cats were DSHs or DLHs, and 75% were male. In one cat, MDS progressed to ANLL 90 days after peripheral blood changes (macrocytic red blood cells and large platelets) were seen.[7]

Clinical Presentation and History

Cats with MDS are usually anorectic and lethargic.[3,6,8] Weight loss and fever are occasionally noted. Despite pancytopenia, some cats are initially asymptomatic but usually progress to show signs similar to those just listed.[3] Clinical examination may reveal pallor, weight loss, and often hepatosplenomegaly. Retinal hemorrhages have been described in cats with MDS.[2] Clinical signs are rarely present more than 3 weeks prior to presentation and may be of shorter duration.[2]

KEY POINT

Myelodysplasia is characterized by a bone marrow that contains abnormalities in cellular maturation but less than 30% blast cells.

Staging and Diagnosis

Bone marrow aspiration is warranted in any cat with non-regenerative anemia or other unexplained cytopenias. Although clinical signs usually relate to anemia, pancytopenia is the most common finding on the hemogram.[3,4,6] In one study, all but 1 of 21 cats with MDS were anemic. Large platelets are often seen in circulation. Bone marrow cytology usually reveals hypercellular marrow that often shows a preponderance of early granulocyte precursors with morphologic abnormalities (Figure 37-2). In one study of 16 cats with MDS, 9 (56%) had evidence of myelofibrosis.[9] Progression to acute leukemia (ALL or ANLL) may be rapid or may occur after many months of persistent cytopenias.[3,4,7]

MDB = minimum database; includes CBC, biochemical profile, urinalysis, FeLV/FIV serology, T_4 testing, and thoracic radiographs (three views).

Treatment

Supportive therapy, such as transfusions, antibiotics (for cats that are febrile or severely neutropenic), corticosteroids, and anabolic steroids, have been used in cats with MDS. Some authors recommend monitoring asymptomatic cats with serial blood counts and providing supportive care only to animals that develop life-threatening cytopenias. The use of differentiating agents, such as low-dose cytosine arabinoside, has not been reported for cats. In one study of 21 cats, 1 cat lived for 6 weeks (after two blood transfusions), 1 for 5 months, and 1 for 9 months; the 2 cats with longer survival times had no cytopenias at diagnosis.[2] One cat treated with supportive therapy developed ANLL within 15 weeks of treatment. Another untreated cat developed ANLL after 11 months of persistent neutropenia. Chemotherapy is not warranted for MDS, and the prognosis is very poor. Anecdotal evidence supports the use of corticosteroids at immunosuppressive doses in combination with erythropoietin (100 U/kg three times a week until improvement is noted, then once or twice a week for maintenance).

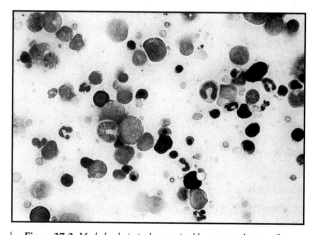

Figure 37-2: *Myelodysplasia is characterized by a preponderance of precursors, often with morphologic abnormalities. This feline marrow shows megaloblastic changes with giant band neutrophils. Fewer than 30% blast forms are present, so the diagnosis is myelodysplasia rather than leukemia. (Courtesy of S.M. Cotter)*

ACUTE LEUKEMIAS

ACUTE NONLYMPHOID LEUKEMIA (ANLL; ACUTE MYELOID LEUKEMIA)

CLINICAL BRIEFING

Common Presentation	Young cats (median age, 4 years); possible male predilection; FeLV antigenemia present in 90% or more of affected cats; disease is rapidly progressive; organ infiltration is common. Rapid onset of inappetence and lethargy; clinical signs reflect cytopenias; hepatosplenomegaly.
Staging and Diagnosis	MDB (particularly FeLV serology) and bone marrow aspiration. Because of the poor prognosis, it is not clinically relevant to distinguish between subtypes of ANLL.
Treatment Supportive Chemotherapy	Antibiotics and transfusions of blood and blood products. Rarely efficacious; may try cytosine arabinoside.

Incidence, Signalment, and Etiology

Both ANLL and ALL are more common in cats than in dogs. Most cats present with ANLL, but progression from MDS to ANLL has been described.[7] In one study, ANLL was more common than MDS and occurred in 39 of 60 cats with nonlymphoid hematopoietic neoplasms.[2]

The age range of cats with ANLL is 7 months to 16 years (median, 4 years).[2,10] No obvious gender predilection was found in one study of 39 cats,[2] although a review of 110 cases[10] found that 78 cats were male and 32 were female. Most affected cats are DSHs or DLHs.[2]

FeLV is associated with ANLL, and FeLV antigen has been detected in 88% to 97% of cats with ANLL.[1,2,11–13] In one study, the only cats not infected with FeLV may have

KEY POINT

FeLV infection is frequently associated with both ANLL and ALL in cats.

had hypereosinophilic disease and not ANLL.[11] As the number of cats infected with FeLV has declined,[14] the number of cats presenting with ANLL has also decreased. It is uncommon to see reports of this disease after 1985.

Clinical Presentation and History

Cats with ANLL have a rapid onset of clinical signs that are often initially noted by owners 2 to 11 days before presentation.[10] Many affected cats have shown signs for less than 1 week.[17]

Clinical signs are nonspecific and are related to cytopenias as well as circulating leukemic cells. Inappetence, lethargy, weakness, and weight loss are most common. One third of cats with ANLL have an enlarged spleen (Figure 37-3) and/or liver, and some cats may have peripheral lymphadenopathy.[2,10,15–17] Fever (presumably due to concurrent neutropenia and sepsis) may be present, and some cats are dyspneic, possibly due to profound anemia[2,10] or secondary pneumonia.[17] Retinal hemorrhages may occur in cats with ANLL.[2]

Staging and Diagnosis

Absolute classification of the cell of origin for any feline acute leukemia is difficult on the basis of morphologic criteria alone. As with dogs, it is clinically important to distinguish ANLL from ALL using cytochemical stains or immunohistochemistry.[13]

Anemia is common in cats with ANLL and occurs in nearly all affected cats.[2,10,13,16] Median packed cell volume (PCV) is 14%.[10] An inappropriate number of nucleated RBCs were seen in 62 of 110 cats with ANLL, and the av-

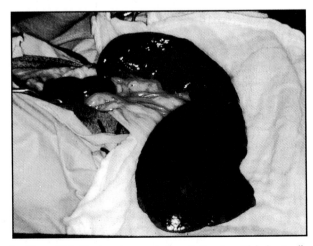

Figure 37-3: *Massive splenomegaly due to infiltration with leukemic cells in a cat with ANLL. (Courtesy of S.M. Cotter)*

erage count in these cats was 83/100 leukocytes.[10] Normoblastemia was common in another group of cats with ANLL (Figure 37-4).[17] It should be remembered that the finding of normoblastemia alone does not provide a diagnosis of MDS or leukemia and may be secondary to a number of nonneoplastic causes.[18] Other cytopenias, such as neutropenia, may be seen.[10] Cytopenias may simply be due to overcrowding and growth inhibition of the marrow by malignant cells. One study, however, found that more than 60% of cats with ANLL had myelofibrosis.[9] FeLV may play a role in bone marrow suppression.[11] Hypercalcemia along with soft tissue mineralization may occur in cats with ANLL.[19,20] Glomerulonephritis may occur secondary to immune complex deposition.[21]

Not all cats have circulating blast cells, which causes white cell counts to vary widely (1,300–369,000/µl).[2] Bone marrow aspiration may be necessary to confirm a diagnosis. A bone marrow aspirate containing more than 30% abnormal blast cells is diagnostic for either ALL or ANLL; a finding of less than 30% blast cells with abnormal maturation is consistent with MDS. Megaloblastic changes in the red cell series in the bone marrow often accompany ANLL. These changes are not due to folate/vitamin B_{12} deficiency and do not respond to supplementation.[17,22] Cats with either ANLL or ALL are likely to have malignant cellular infiltrates in sites other than bone marrow. In one study, such infiltrates were found in the spleen, liver, kidney, and lymph nodes, whereas cats with MDS had no other organ infiltration.[2]

Cells derived from the erythroid series may give rise to erythremic myelosis, erythroleukemia, or reticuloendotheliosis; all these terms are used to describe ANLL of this derivation.[23–30] Granulocytic leukemias are rare[31–38] and monocytic leukemias even more so.[39,40] Involvement of the megakaryocytic series is rare,[13,41–43] as are myelomonocytic leukemias.[44–46] The differentiation makes little difference to the clinical picture, however, and the prognosis does not appear to alter for various subtypes. Some cats may have a primitive stem cell leukemia that causes variable peripheral types of leukemic cells.[47]

KEY POINT

Chemotherapy for ANLL in cats has not met with any success. The prognosis for these animals is very poor.

Treatment

Most cats with ANLL are euthanized at diagnosis,[2] but supportive treatment, including transfusions, is occasionally used. Four cats were treated this way; one lived 14 days, one 19 days, one 44 days, and one 72 days.[2,44] In another study, three cats treated with transfusions lived for a median of 14 days[10]; two of these cats were also treated with plasmapheresis or cytosine arabinoside and L-asparaginase. Chemotherapy is rarely used. Cyclophosphamide,[24] vinblastine, cytosine arabinoside, L-asparaginase, and 6-thioguanine appear to do little to alter the course of the disease,[48] although occasional short-term partial remissions are reported.[35,39] 6-MP (6-mercaptopurine) caused rapid resolution of ANLL in one cat, but the dose (2.5 mg/kg/day) caused lethal myelosuppression.[49] When a daunorubicin derivative, idarubicin, was used to treat five cats with ANLL, none responded to treatment.[50]

Immunotherapy with Staph A caused a reduction in serum calcium (which had been elevated) and clinical improvement in a cat with ANLL for about a month before it died.[19]

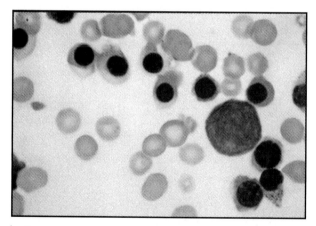

Figure 37-4: *Massive normoblastemia and circulating blast cells characterized by large prominent nucleoli in a cat with ANLL. Normoblastemia alone is not diagnostic of leukemia. (Courtesy of S.M. Cotter)*

ACUTE LYMPHOID (LYMPHOBLASTIC) LEUKEMIA (ALL)

CLINICAL BRIEFING

Common Presentation	Young cats (median age, 5 years); no breed or gender predilection; most cats are FeLV antigenemic. Rapid onset of anorexia and weight loss. Lymphadenopathy is common, which may make differentiating ALL from lymphoma difficult.

(continued)

MANAGEMENT OF SPECIFIC DISEASES

Staging and Diagnosis	MDB (particularly FeLV serology) and bone marrow aspiration; abdominal ultrasonography to rule out lymphoma.
Treatment Supportive	Antibiotics and transfusions of blood and blood products.
Chemotherapy	COP protocol may give 65% remission rate for median remission of 7 months.

Incidence, Signalment, and Etiology

ALL is less common than lymphoma in cats, accounting for 15 of 53 cats (28%) in one study of lymphoid malignancies.[51] Cats with ALL have a similar signalment to cats with ANLL. The average age of affected cats is younger than 5 years; in a review of 57 cases, ages ranged from 6 months to 14 years.[10] There is no obvious gender or breed predilection. FeLV infection is frequently associated with ALL, although this association is less common than that between FeLV and ANLL.[2,11,12]

Clinical Presentation and History

As with ANLL, clinical signs of ALL are nonspecific; anorexia, lethargy, weight loss, and fever are most commonly reported. Lymphadenopathy is common in cats with ALL,[10] making it difficult to distinguish from advanced lymphoma.

Staging and Diagnosis

The staging scheme for cats with ALL is as described for feline lymphoma. Because blast cells found in the circulation or in bone marrow aspirates are difficult to identify definitively on morphologic criteria alone, cytochemical staining is warranted for all cases of acute leukemia. In addition, immunohistochemical staining for lymphoid cell types will differentiate ALL from ANLL. Most cats with ALL are anemic; the average PCV is 16%.[10] Leukopenia may be present.[10] Blast cells may account for up to 83% of circulating cells (average, 18%; Figure 37-5). Some cats with ALL have cytopenia without circulating blasts, and thus bone marrow

aspiration is warranted in any cat with nonregenerative anemia or other unexplained cytopenias.

Treatment

In a report of 15 cats treated with COP protocol (vincristine, 0.75 mg/m^2 IV; cyclophosphamide, 300 mg/m^2 PO every 3 weeks; and prednisone, 40 mg/m^2 PO sid; see Chapter 36), 4 cats achieved complete remission (CR) and 6 cats achieved partial remission (PR).[51] Remission lasted 1 to 24 months (median, 7 months). The prognosis for cats with ALL is considerably better than for cats with ANLL.

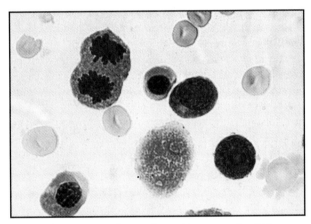

Figure 37-5: *A mitotic figure and normoblasts are seen in addition to lymphoblasts in this blood sample from a 3-year-old tricolor cat with ALL; lymphoblasts accounted for 24% of the white cell count. (Courtesy of S.M. Cotter)*

CHRONIC LEUKEMIA

CHRONIC LYMPHOID (LYMPHOBLASTIC) LEUKEMIA (CLL)

CLINICAL BRIEFING

Common Presentation	Nonspecific; often asymptomatic and slow to progress.
Staging and Diagnosis	Mature lymphocytosis; differentiate from reactive lymphocytosis and well-differentiated lymphoma as described for ALL.
Treatment Observation	Repeated monitoring of blood counts may be all that is required for asymptomatic animals.
Chemotherapy	Prednisone and chlorambucil provide long-term remissions in symptomatic cats.

Incidence, Signalment, and Etiology

Chronic lymphocytic leukemia (CLL) is an uncommon myeloproliferative disease characterized by an increased number of circulating lymphocytes with normal morphology; the bone marrow is often infiltrated with similar cells. This disease is very rare in cats. Three cases were reported in old castrated male cats[52] and one case in an 11-year-old female cat.[53] We are aware of three other cases (12-year-old castrated male, 5-year-old castrated male, and 12-year-old spayed female).[a] White cell counts were above 55,000/μl in five cats, and it was 13,500/μl in one. Three cats were FeLV and FIV negative on serology.

Clinical Presentation and History

Cats may be asymptomatic, in which case the diagnosis may be made only when a hemogram is evaluated for some other reason. Anemia may be a feature of this disease in cats, although hematocrit levels were normal in three of six cats. Appetite may be normal, but weight loss, mild diarrhea, and lethargy may occur.

Staging and Diagnosis

Unlike the situation in animals with acute leukemias, definitive diagnosis of chronic leukemias is rarely problematic. Hematologic evaluation reveals a lymphocytosis composed of well-differentiated cells. "Reactive" forms are occasionally noted. Circulating mature lymphocytosis in

---

[a]Moore AS: personal observations.

cats should prompt clinicians to have a bone marrow aspirate evaluated cytologically to confirm the diagnosis; bone marrow cytology in cats with chronic leukemia discloses infiltration by small lymphocytes. This infiltration explains other hematologic abnormalities, such as nonregenerative anemia and thrombocytopenia, which are usually mild. Severe cytopenias are rare because marrow is seldom replaced. Infiltration of the bone marrow with more than 15% mature lymphocytes confirms the diagnosis of CLL in cats. Unlike dogs, normal cats may have lymphocytes accounting for as much as 5% of their bone marrow.

Treatment

Observation of asymptomatic cats with CLL may be justified. One cat with splenomegaly, thrombocytopenia, and presumed hypersplenism secondary to CLL remained neutropenic and anemic after chlorambucil administration; the animal was then treated with splenectomy, and all medications were discontinued. The cat was still asymptomatic with a stable lymphocytosis 5 years later. Two cats treated with prednisone achieved remissions of several months[52,53]; another cat failed to respond to vincristine and prednisone.[53] Chlorambucil and prednisone resulted in a long remission in one cat.[52] Two cats remained in remission (one for 1 year and the other for 3 years) when a combination of chlorambucil (2 mg/cat qod) and prednisone (40 mg/m² qod) was administered.[a] The prognosis for cats with CLL seems to be similar to that for dogs with CLL, and the combination of chlorambucil and prednisone is the treatment of choice for symptomatic cats.

HYPEREOSINOPHILIC DISEASE

CLINICAL BRIEFING

Common Presentation	Adult cats (median age, 8 years); females may be predisposed; cats may have widespread organ infiltration; affected cats often have a chronic history of GI signs.
Staging and Diagnosis	Allergic diseases and eosinophilic granuloma complex must be ruled out in patients with mature eosinophilia. Perform MDB, abdominal ultrasonography, and bone marrow aspiration.
Treatment	Prednisone and hydroxyurea may be palliative (under investigation).

Incidence, Signalment, and Etiology

Hypereosinophilic disease is a rare condition that is diagnosed by exclusion rather than by other defined criteria. Causes of mature eosinophilia in cats include flea-allergy dermatitis and eosinophilic granuloma complex,[54] although the eosinophil count in these conditions does not usually reach the levels seen with hypereosinophilic disease. In a review of 13 cases, all but 1 occurred in adult cats (median

age, 8 years[55]; range, 10 months to 10 years), and 9 cats were female.

The term *eosinophilic leukemia* is used when eosinophilia is not ordered and immature blast forms are seen in increased numbers, either in the circulation or in the bone marrow.[56,57] Hypereosinophilia is usually an ordered progression, similar to chronic myelogenous leukemia, although metamyelocyte forms may be seen in the circulation.

Clinical Presentation and History

Hypereosinophilia in cats is usually associated with gastrointestinal (GI) signs, presumably arising from GI infiltration by eosinophils. Affected cats often have diarrhea, weight loss, vomiting, and anorexia.[56] On physical examination, bowel loops may be thickened, lymphadenopathy is palpable, and splenomegaly and hepatomegaly may be detected. Fever and pruritus (from cutaneous involvement) are less commonly noted.[56] Clinical signs have often been present for a long time.[56]

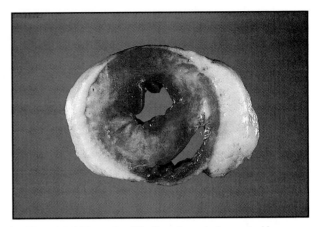

Figure 37-6: *Hypereosinophilic disease in cats is characterized by widespread infiltration of sites such as the intestine, spleen, liver, and lymph nodes. Note the massive infiltration of the cardiac ventricular walls and pericardium in this sample from a 15-year-old male cat.*

KEY POINT

Hypereosinophilia is usually associated with GI signs due to eosinophilic infiltration of bowel and lymph nodes.

Staging and Diagnosis

Diagnosis is usually made on the basis of mature hypereosinophilia without other causes. Eosinophil counts ranged from 3,200 to 130,000 cells/µl (mean, 42,000 cells/µl) in one study.[56] No other cell lines were affected. Cats may be mildly anemic. Bone marrow may be heavily infiltrated with eosinophil precursors. Numerous other organs, most commonly the small intestine, spleen, mesenteric lymph nodes, and liver, may be involved (Figure 37-6).[55]

Cats with eosinophilia should be carefully evaluated for causative diseases; when these have been excluded, bone marrow aspiration should be performed. The finding of an increased number of eosinophil precursors without a preponderance of blast forms is diagnostic for hypereosinophilic disease.

Treatment

Treatment for this disease is not very efficacious. Prednisone was used to treat six cats; the drug decreased eosinophil counts in some cats and improved the attitude in others, but five cats died of their disease within 4 months. Hypereosinophilia resolved following prednisone (2 mg/kg PO bid) administration in one cat, which became normal for 8 months.[58] After the animal relapsed, increasing prednisone doses and adding hydroxyurea (15 mg/kg/day) had no effect on the disease. Hydroxyurea was likewise ineffective in treating another cat.[59] Treatment using hydroxyurea in combination with prednisone may be warranted but is still considered investigational. Care should be exercised when using hydroxyurea (outlined below).

PRIMARY ERYTHROCYTOSIS (POLYCYTHEMIA VERA)

CLINICAL BRIEFING

Common Presentation	Median age, 6 years; male predominance; hyperviscosity causes signs of neurologic disturbances (e.g., seizures and ataxia) and dark mucous membranes.
Staging and Diagnosis	Rule out relative and secondary polycythemia in patients with mature erythrocytosis; MDB, abdominal ultrasonography for renal tumor, arterial blood gas analysis, and determination of serum erythropoietin levels.
Treatment Supportive Chemotherapy	Periodic removal of blood (phlebotomy) is palliative. Hydroxyurea gives long-term control.

Polycythemia is characterized by an increase in the PCV, hemoglobin concentration, and RBC count. This increase may follow changes in plasma volume, such as occur with dehydration, and is termed *relative polycythemia*. Absolute polycythemia may be primary (polycythemia vera, primary erythrocytosis) or secondary to an increase in serum erythropoietin. Conditions that cause secondary polycythemia include systemic hypoxia arising from cardiopulmonary disease, hemoglobinopathies, or high altitude. Erythropoietin may also be secreted by tumors, particularly renal tumors, leading to secondary polycythemia. In cats, some renal tumors are reported to increase serum erythropoietin levels (see Chapter 43).

Polycythemia vera results from a clonal proliferation of the erythroid series and does not require erythropoietin for continued stimulus. In humans, this disorder usually includes thrombocytosis and hepatosplenomegaly and progresses to myelofibrosis or acute leukemia. These manifestations are not reported in cats, and thus *primary erythrocytosis* may be a more appropriate term.

KEY POINT

Phlebotomy to remove 20 ml of blood/kg body weight will reduce PCV by approximately 15%.

Incidence, Signalment, and Etiology

Polycythemia vera is defined as an increase in the red cell mass accompanied by thrombocytosis and organomegaly. The condition does not progress to myelofibrosis or leukemia, which again makes *primary erythrocytosis* a better term for the disease in cats, which are rarely affected. It is characterized by an increase in the number of erythrocytes in the presence of normal or low serum erythropoietin levels.

In a review of 11 reported cases of primary erythrocytosis,[60] affected cats ranged in age from 3 to 15 years (median, 6 years). Male cats were predominantly affected (8 of 10 cats). There was no obvious breed predisposition.

KEY POINT

Care should be taken when administering large, single doses of hydroxyurea to cats as methemoglobinemia may occur.

Clinical Presentation and History

Neurologic disturbances, such as seizures, are common in cats with erythrocytosis and occurred in 7 of 11 reported cases.[60] Blindness, ataxia, or abnormal behavior may be present. Less common signs include depression, lethargy, anorexia, polyuria, and polydipsia. Dark mucous membranes may be noted. Splenomegaly is rare, and hepatomegaly has not been recorded.

Staging and Diagnosis

To confirm a diagnosis of primary erythrocytosis in a normally hydrated cat, secondary erythrocytosis should be ruled out. Causes of secondary erythrocytosis include cardiopulmonary diseases, other causes of hypoxia, and abnormal production of erythropoietin due to renal neoplasia. Thoracic radiographs should be obtained to evaluate cardiopulmonary structures; if cardiac disease is suspected, echocardiography should be performed. Hypoxemia can be ruled out by performing blood gas analysis. Renal structure may be assessed by ultrasonography, and biopsy samples should be collected from any suspicious lesions. Serum erythropoietin levels can confirm the diagnosis, although this test is still in the process of being validated for use in cats. In 11 reported cases of primary erythrocytosis, initial PCV was 63% to 82%.[60] Increases in white cell counts were seen in 3 cats, and the platelet count was increased in 1 cat. Serum erythropoietin level was low or normal in the 8 cats from which a sample was obtained.[60]

MDB = minimum database; includes CBC, biochemical profile, urinalysis, FeLV/FIV serology, T_4 testing, and thoracic radiographs (three views).

Treatment

Two cats did not receive treatment; one survived for 6 weeks[61] and the other for more than 20 weeks.[62] Phlebotomy alone every 2 to 3 months was used to manage one cat for longer than 20 months.[63]

Hydroxyurea, alone or in combination with phlebotomy, was used to treat eight cats; all survived more than 1 year, and two survived more than 6 years.[60] The dose of hydroxyurea to induce and maintain remission is variable. Doses of less than 500 mg require capsules to be split, which introduces inaccuracy and risk of drug exposure to the handler. A cat treated with a single hydroxyurea dose of 500 mg developed severe methemoglobinemia and hemolytic anemia with Heinz bodies[a]; therefore, although some cats tolerate 500 mg orally every 5 to 7 days, it may be prudent to start treatment at 125 mg/cat every 2 days for 2 weeks, followed by 250 mg/cat twice weekly for 2 weeks and then as often as needed to maintain a normal hematocrit. Cats treated with hydroxyurea should be hospitalized for 24 hours following treatment to check for methemoglobinemia each time the dose is increased; it may be prudent to store blood collected prior to treatment for autotransfusion if necessary. Signs of methemoglobinemia include dyspnea and dark-brown mucous membranes.

MULTIPLE MYELOMA

Multiple myeloma is diagnosed when malignant plasma cells in the bone marrow are found in conjunction with a monoclonal gammopathy, lytic bone lesions, or light-chain (Bence-Jones) proteinuria. The presence of two of these four criteria is sufficient to make the diagnosis of multiple myeloma. Although extramedullary plasma cell tumors in the retrobulbar space, GI tract, and skin of cats have been associated with a monoclonal gammopathy, they are discussed separately in Chapters 40, 41, and 50, respectively. Cats with lymphoma may also show a monoclonal gammopathy, and these cats are described in Chapter 36.

C L I N I C A L B R I E F I N G	
Common Presentation	Nonspecific signs of lethargy, anorexia, and weight loss usually predominate; epistaxis and melena as a result of monoclonal gammopathy; light-chain proteinuria; plasma cells in bone marrow; lytic lesions in bones. Mostly in older cats. Neurologic signs occasionally predominate.
Staging and Diagnosis	MDB and survey radiographs of the spine, skull, and pelvis; bone marrow aspiration, serum protein electrophoresis and immunoelectrophoresis; Bence-Jones urine protein test or urinary protein electrophoresis; serum viscosity; fundic examination.
Treatment Initial	Chemotherapy with prednisone and melphalan is most successful. Plasmapheresis if serum viscosity is high.
Adjunctive	Cyclophosphamide or doxorubicin may induce remission when cats fail to respond to initial treatment.
Supportive	Plasmapheresis if serum viscosity is high. Antibiotics for bacterial infections secondary to immunosuppression.

Incidence, Signalment, and Etiology

Thirty-three cats with multiple myeloma have been reported in the literature; most were DSHs, although there were also three DLHs,[64–66] a Persian,[67] a Manx,[68] an Abyssinian,[69] and a Burmese.[70] Affected cats ranged in age from 19 months to 17 years (median, 12 years). Only two cats were younger than 6 years,[71] including a 19-month-old that may have had lymphoma.[72] Eighteen of the cats were castrated males, and FeLV was detected in one cat with multiple myeloma.[72]

Clinical Presentation and History

When abnormal plasma cells produce excessive amounts of abnormal globulin, there may be a concurrent decrease in the production of normal immunoglobulins and hence the patient may become immunosuppressed. Bone marrow infiltration by neoplastic plasma cells may result in cytopenias, thereby exacerbating susceptibility to infection. Most affected cats are anemic.

Nonspecific clinical signs such as listlessness, lethargy, inappetence, and weight loss are common in cats with multiple myeloma[15,64,67–70,72–80] and may have been present for months to years.[67,73,74] Vomiting was usually intermittent.

Tumor cell infiltration of bone and associated lysis may cause pain in the limbs or spine.[65,75,76] A pathologic fracture may occur if lysis is severe.[65] Extradural accumulation of neoplastic cells may compress the spinal cord; one cat with a cervical epidural mass presented with ataxia.[15]

Bleeding tendencies may be seen as a result of interference with platelet function by the abnormal protein, and extremely high protein levels lead to hyperviscosity. Hyperviscosity is most common when the tumor produces IgM (due to its large size), IgA (due to polymerization of the molecule), or very high levels of IgG.[78] Abnormal globulin levels also interfere with clotting factors and platelet function. Clinical signs associated with these abnormalities in cats include epistaxis,[69,76] melena,[69] retinal hemorrhages causing blindness,[72,77] and acute neurologic disturbances such as circling,[77] behavior changes,[15] and seizures.[68,77,78]

Renal damage may occur secondary to deposition of immunoglobulin light chains in the tubules. Polyuria associated with azotemia was reported as a presenting sign in some cats[72–74,78]; two of these animals were also hyperviscous.[72,78]

Staging and Diagnosis

Appropriate staging of the myeloma patient should begin with the MDB. Radiography may be also helpful to identify organomegaly or lytic bone lesions.

Multiple myeloma is diagnosed when malignant plasma cells

in the bone marrow are found in conjunction with a monoclonal gammopathy, lytic bone lesions, or light-chain (Bence-Jones) proteinuria. The presence of two of these four criteria is sufficient to make the diagnosis of multiple myeloma.

Serum chemistry profile may reveal the most common reason for suspecting multiple myeloma in cats—an elevated serum protein, or more specifically, a high serum globulin level. Total serum protein in affected cats ranged from 8.1[71] to 16.5[81] mg/dl (median, 12 mg/dl). One cat had a normal serum protein level.[80] Serum globulin in affected cats ranged from 4.2[70] to 14.8[76] mg/dl (median, 6.7 mg/dl). Serum protein electrophoresis should be performed for any cat with high serum globulin levels. Production of a single immunoglobulin by neoplastic plasma cells is measured on protein electrophoresis as a monoclonal "spike" or monoclonal gammopathy. Serum protein electrophoresis demonstrated a monoclonal gammopathy in most reported cats, although cats without a monoclonal spike have been reported[65,80] and one cat had polyclonal gammopathy.[75] These three cats were diagnosed as having multiple myeloma by fulfilling two of the remaining three criteria listed above. Hypercalcemia has been seen in association with multiple myeloma in other species but has not been reported in cats.

Further characterization of the monoclonal gammopathy requires serum protein immunoelectrophoresis. The most common immunoglobulin class for multiple myeloma in cats is IgG; IgA is less common. Some authors identify patients with IgM monoclonal gammopathy as having macroglobulinemia. Fourteen cats have been shown to have IgG gammopathy,[68,70,71,77,78,82] while only two have had IgA gammopathy[64,70] and three have had IgM monoclonal gammopathy (or macroglobulinemia).[71–73]

A CBC should be evaluated in addition to a serum chemistry profile. Anemia is the most common finding; of 33 reported cats, 10 had a hematocrit between 8% and 29%.[70,73,74,76,77,83] Two of these anemic cats were also thrombocytopenic,[73,76] one was neutropenic,[77] and one was pancytopenic.[73] Although rare, it may be possible to detect circulating abnormal plasma cells in cats with multiple myeloma.

Bone marrow aspiration should be performed in all cats with suspected or confirmed myeloma. The extent of bone marrow infiltration by normal or pleomorphic-appearing plasma cells varies from complete obliteration[73,76,77] to relatively few plasma cells.[64] In at least four cats, plasma cells were found to have obliterated the normal bone marrow elements.[73,76,77] In these cats, bone marrow aspiration is important not only in staging but also in directing supportive care during chemotherapy. These cats may have a higher risk for infection when myelosuppressive chemotherapy is started and should be monitored closely.

Lytic bone lesions are uncommon in cats with multiple myeloma but may affect the axial or the appendicular skeleton.[65,66,71,75,76] Therefore the skull, spine, pelvis, and long bones should be radiographed in addition to the thorax (Figure 37-7). This is particularly important if pain is part of the clinical history. Immunoglobulin was classified in only one of five reported cats with bone lesions, and it was IgG.[71] If a spinal lesion is suspected but no radiographic bone lesions are detected, an extradural mass may be present[15,66,68] and myelography or MRI may delineate the mass. If bone lesions are suspected but not present on survey radiographs, a bone scan using technetium may be used; however, the rarity of bone lesions makes this procedure unnecessary in most cats.

In addition to a routine urinalysis and culture, urine should be submitted for either Bence-Jones protein quantification or urine protein electrophoresis. Remember that urine "dipsticks" cannot detect light chains and measure only albumin. Elevated urine protein may signal glomerular damage or a secondary bacterial cystitis rather than Bence-Jones proteinuria. The Bence-Jones heat precipitation test was positive in 11 of 23 cats with myeloma.[70,71,75,78–80] Immunoglobulin light chains were detected on urine immunoelectrophoresis as well as by heat precipitation in 2 of these 11 cats,[78,80] and another 3 cats had a positive urine immunoelectrophoresis.[73,77,78] One cat with a negative Bence-Jones assay had light chains detected by the more sensitive urine immunoelectrophoresis,[73] suggesting that this may be a better test to use. The presence of light chains in the urine may increase the risk of nephrotoxicity due to formation of intratubular protein aggregates. It is important to monitor renal function before and during treatment, particularly in cats with Bence-Jones proteinuria.[66,74,78,79]

Hyperviscosity occurs when the concentration of serum globulin rises sufficiently to affect hemodynamics. Interference with coagulation, retinal hemorrhage, and central nervous system signs may occur. Serum viscosity can be measured if hyperviscosity is suspected. Normal values for serum viscosity in cats are based on a small number of ani-

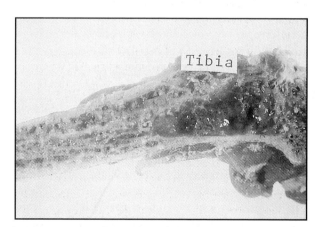

Figure 37-7: Lytic bone lesions are uncommon in cats with multiple myeloma but can occur in either the axial skeleton or the appendicular skeleton, as shown here.

mals; however, a value of less than 2.5 is usually used.[64,77–79] Serum viscosity was not measured in all reported cats; of 12 cats so tested, 6 had hyperviscosity (range, 3.5 to 6.7; median, 6.2).[64,71,72,77–79] These cats had IgM,[72] IgG,[77,78] or IgA monoclonal gammopathy.[64] Ventricular hypertrophy, possibly as a compensatory mechanism for serum hyperviscosity, has been noted in a few cats.[66,68,78] Hyperviscosity was confirmed in only 2 of these cats.[78] Retinal hemorrhages were seen in 2 hyperviscous cats,[72,78] and a coagulation profile was normal in a cat with mild hyperviscosity (3.5).[64] A fundic examination should be performed in affected cats to detect retinal hemorrhage or detachment.

Bone marrow infiltration together with interference with normal immune function due to decreased levels of normal immunoglobulin may leave cats susceptible to infection. Sepsis was a cause of death in some cats,[75,78] while others had localized infections: *Staphylococcus*, *Proteus*, *Sporothrix schenckii*, and *Microsporum canis* in the skin,[70] *Nocardia* and *Salmonella* pleuritis,[64,70] spiral bacteria in the gastric mucosa,[69] and *Histoplasma capsulatum*.[65] Careful monitoring and prompt appropriate antimicrobial treatment is mandatory for cats undergoing treatment for multiple myeloma.

Other organs have been found to be infiltrated by plasma cells in affected cats. Liver and spleen are commonly involved,[15,64–67,72,73,75–78,80,82] with the kidneys,[65,72] skin,[65,73] or intestinal tract[64] less commonly affected. Abdominal ultrasonography should be performed in affected cats to obtain a pretreatment baseline evaluation and to obtain samples for cytology or histopathology. Some cats with primary GI plasma cell neoplasia may also develop multiple myeloma (see Chapter 41). As mentioned, extramedullary sites of plasma cell tumors or a diagnosis of lymphoma should be pursued in cats with a monoclonal gammopathy that do not have multiple myeloma.

MDB = minimum database; includes CBC, biochemical profile, urinalysis, FeLV/FIV serology, T₄ testing, and thoracic radiographs (three views).

Treatment

Treatment involves supportive care (which may be needed before definitive chemotherapy is initiated) and chemotherapy. Transfusion of whole blood may be necessary in severely anemic cats. Azotemia should prompt crystalloid fluid therapy until definitive treatment can be started. Broad-spectrum antibiotics are necessary and should be given prophylactically, particularly in neutropenic cats. Sepsis is potentially fatal in these cats because of the com-

promised state of their immune system.[78]

The ideal treatment for multiple myeloma in cats is currently unknown; however, melphalan, prednisone, and possibly doxorubicin should be used as first line chemotherapy. Prednisone (30 mg/m² to a maximum of 4 mg/kg daily) in combination with melphalan (1.5 mg/m² PO daily for 10 days and then every other day) is the standard chemotherapy for multiple myeloma in cats. The use of this combination has been reported for 12 cats. There was no response to treatment in 7 of these cats,[65,70,71,78] although tumor progression appeared to slow in 1 of the 7.[65] Clinical and serum biochemical improvements were seen in the other 5 cats, although 4 experienced relapses (1 cat each at 2.5,[78] 6, 7, and 9 months[70]); the fifth was lost to follow up 1 month after starting treatment.

The addition of vincristine did not seem to improve response, and this agent had to be discontinued within 3 weeks due to GI toxicity in two cats.[78] The combination of vincristine, cyclophosphamide, and prednisone (COP) was ineffective in another cat.[65]

Cyclophosphamide was not helpful in a cat that had failed to respond to melphalan and prednisone.[78] Another cat responded to cyclophosphamide and prednisone until treatment was discontinued after 3 weeks, at which time the disease progressed and the cat was euthanized.[80] Chlorambucil and prednisone did not seem to induce remission in another cat.[76] Doxorubicin showed short-term efficacy in a cat that had failed to respond to melphalan and prednisone.[a]

Treatment with corticosteroids alone is unlikely to be anything but palliative. Two cats treated with either prednisone[69] or dexamethasone[64] died within 2 days due to progression of multiple myeloma. Another cat had remission from seizures for 3 months prior to tumor progression,[68] and a fourth had a 4 month remission; both of these animals were treated with prednisone alone.[74]

Plasmapheresis may be used to rapidly reduce immunoglobulin levels and is particularly helpful if hyperviscosity is present. There are technical difficulties in using machines specifically for plasmapheresis due to the very small blood volume of cats. Despite these limitations, plasmapheresis did result in clinical improvement when performed every 2 weeks in a cat that was not responding to chemotherapy.[78] Radiation therapy is presently unexplored for treatment of myeloma in the cat.

Supportive care is as important as chemotherapy in the treatment of cats with multiple myeloma. Fluid therapy, attention to possible sepsis with judicious prophylactic use of antibiotics, antiemetic treatment, and nutritional support are essential. Because of the presence of immunosuppression and the risk of sepsis, extreme care must be taken if assisted feeding techniques, such as esophagostomy/gastrostomy tubes, are used.

NONDOMESTIC FELIDAE

A 21-year-old male jaguar *(Panthera onca)* died after experiencing rear limb lameness, anorexia, and ataxia for 2 weeks. Total serum protein was 11.1 mg /dl, and the globulin level was 9.0 mg/dl. The cat was hypercalcemic, azotemic, and anemic. Serum protein electrophoresis showed a monoclonal gammopathy, and the bone marrow was obliterated by plasma cells.[84] Radiographs of the pelvis showed lytic lesions, although none were present on other survey radiographs. This cat also had an adrenocortical adenocarcinoma and a metastatic pheochromocytoma.

REFERENCES

1. Tzavaras T, Stewart M, McDougall A, et al: Molecular cloning and characterization of a defective recombinant feline leukaemia virus associated with myeloid leukaemia. *J Gen Virol* 71:343–354, 1990.

2. Blue JT, French TW, Kranz JS: Non-lymphoid hematopoietic neoplasia in cats: A retrospective study of 60 cases. *Cornell Vet* 78:21–42, 1988.

3. Madewell BR, Jain NC, Weller RE: Hematologic abnormalities preceding myeloid leukemia in three cats. *Vet Pathol* 16:510–519, 1979.

4. Maggio LHR, Cotter SM, Dainak N, et al: Feline preleukemia: An animal model of human disease. *Yale J Biol Med* 51:469–476, 1978.

5. Evans RJ, Gorman NT: Myeloproliferative disease in the dog and cat: Definition, aetiology and classification. *Vet Rec* 121:437–443, 1987.

6. Harvey JW, Shields RP, Gaskin JM: Feline myeloproliferative disease: Changing manifestations in the peripheral blood. *Vet Pathol* 15:437–448, 1978.

7. Raskin RE, Krehbiel JD: Myelodysplastic changes in a cat with myelomonocytic leukemia. *JAVMA* 187:171–174, 1985.

8. Gorman NT, Evans RJ: Myeloproliferative disease in the dog and cat: Clinical presentations, diagnosis and treatment. *Vet Rec* 121:490–496, 1987.

9. Blue JT: Myelofibrosis in cats with myelodysplastaic syndrome and acute myelogenous leukemia. *Vet Pathol* 25:154–160, 1988.

10. Grindem CB, Perman V, Stevens JB: Morphological classification and clinical and pathological characteristics of spontaneous leukemia in 10 cats. *JAAHA* 21:227–236, 1985.

11. Hardy Jr WD: Hematopoietic tumors of cats. *JAAHA* 17:921–940, 1981.

12. Cotter SM, Hardy Jr WD, Essex M: Association of feline leukemia virus with lymphosarcoma and other disorders in the cat. *JAVMA* 166:449–454, 1975.

13. Colbatzky F, Hermanns W: Acute megakaryoblastic leukemia in one cat and two dogs. *Vet Pathol* 30:186–194, 1993.

14. Cotter SM: Feline viral neoplasia, in Greene CE (ed): *Infectious Diseases of the Dog and Cat*, ed 3. Philadelphia, WB Saunders, 1998, pp 71–83.

15. Carpenter JL, Andrews LK, Holzworth J: Tumors and tumor-like lesions, in Holzworth J (ed): *Diseases of the Cat. Medicine and Surgery*, Philadelphia, WB Saunders, 1987, pp 407–596.

16. Holzworth J: Leukemia and related neoplasms in the cat. II. Malignancies other than lymphoid. *JAVMA* 136:107–121, 1960.

17. Ward JM, Sodikoff CH, Schalm OW: Myeloproliferative disease and abnormal erythrogenesis in the cat. *JAVMA* 155:879–888, 1969.

18. Hammer AS, Wellmann M: Leukoerythroblastosis and normoblastemia in the cat. *JAAHA* 35:471–473, 1999.

19. Engelman RW, Tyler RD, Kay NK: Hypercalcemia in cats with feline-leukemia-virus-associated leukemia-lymphoma. *Cancer* 56:777–781, 1985.

20. Zenoble RD, Rowland GN: Hypercalcemia and proliferative, myelosclerotic bone reaction associated with feline leukovirus infection in a cat. *JAVMA* 175:591–595, 1979.

21. Glick AD, Horn RG, Holscher M: Characterization of feline glomerulonephritis associated with viral-induced hematopoietic neoplasms. *Am J Pathol* 92:321–327, 1978.

22. Hirsch VM, Dunn J: Megaloblastic anemia in the cat. *JAAHA* 19:873–880, 1983.

23. Falconer GJ, Irving AC, Watson PR, Ludwig J: A case of erythremic myelosis in a cat. *NZ Vet J* 28:83–84, 1980.

24. Giles RC, Buhles WC, Montgomery CA: Myeloproliferative disorder in a cat. *JAVMA* 165:456–457, 1974.

25. Gilmore CE, Gilmore VH, Jones TC: Reticuloendotheliosis, a myeloproliferative disorder of cats: Comparison with lymphocytic leukemia. *Pathol Vet* 1:161–183, 1964.

26. Maede Y, Murata H: Erythroleukemia in a cat with special reference to the fine structure of primitive cells in its peripheral blood. *Jpn J Vet Sci* 42:531–541, 1980.

27. Groulade P, Guilhon JC: Syndrome érythrémique chez le chat. *Bull Acad Vet France* 39:127–131, 1966.

28. Watson ADJ, Huxtable CRR, Hoskins LP: Erythremic myelosis in two cats. *Aust Vet J* 50:29–33, 1974.

29. Zawidzka ZZ, Janzen E, Grice HC: Erythremic myelosis in a cat. A case resembling Di Guglielmo's syndrome in man. *Pathol Vet* 1:530–541, 1964.

30. Saar C: Erythrämie und erythroleukämie bei der katze bericht über je einen fall. *Berl Münch Teirärztl Wschr* 21:423–426, 1968.

31. Cotter SM, Holzworth J: Disorders of the hematopoietic system, in Holzworth J (ed): *Diseases of the cat. Medicine and Surgery*. Philadelphia, WB Saunders, 1987, pp 755–807.

32. Case MT: A case of myelogenous leukemia in a cat. *Zentralbl Veterinärmed A* 17:273–277, 1970.

33. Eyestone WH: Myelogenous leukemia in the cat. *J Natl Cancer Inst* 12:599–613, 1951.

34. Gilbride AP: Myelogenous leukemia in a cat complicated by otitis media. *Can J Comp Med* 28:207–211, 1964.

35. Henness AM, Crow SE: Treatment of feline myelogenous leukemia. Four case reports. *JAVMA* 171:263–266, 1977.

36. Meier H, Patterson DF: Myelogenous leukemia in a cat. *JAVMA* 128:211–214, 1956.

37. Reid JA, Marcus LC: Granulocytic leukemia in a cat. *J Small Anim Pract* 7:421–425, 1966.

38. Fraser CJ, Joiner GN, Jardine JH, Gleiser CA: Acute granulocytic leukemia in cats. *JAVMA* 165:355–359, 1974.

39. Henness AM, Crow SE, Anderson BC: Monocytic leukemia in three cats. *JAVMA* 170:1325–1328, 1977.

40. Saar C, Reichel C: Einige besondere leukoseformen bei der katze. *Praktische Tierarzt* 5:443–450, 1983.

41. Holscher MA, Collins RD, Cousar JB, et al: Megakaryocytic leukemia in a cat. *Feline Pract* 13:8–12, 1983.

42. Michel RL, O'Handley P, Dade AW: Megakaryocytic myelosis in a cat. *JAVMA* 168:1021–1025, 1976.

43. Sutton RH, McKellow AM, Bottrill MB: Myeloproliferative disease in the cat: A granulocytic and megakaryocytic disorder. *NZ Vet J* 26:273–279, 1978.

44. Miyamoto T, Takeda T, Kuwamura M, et al: An unusual feline case of suspected myelomonocytic leukemia with severe leukopenia. *Feline Pract* 27:15–17, 1999.

45. Loeb WF, Rininger B: Myelomonocytic leukemia in a cat. *Vet Pathol* 12:464–467, 1975.

46. Stann SE: Myelomonocytic leukemia in a cat. *JAVMA* 174:722–725, 1979.

47. Engleman RW, Tyler RD, Mosier DA: Changing manifestations of a chronic feline haematopoietic proliferative disease during immunotherapy with staphylococcal protein A. *J Comp Pathol* 96:177–188, 1986.

48. Crow SE, Madewell BR, Henness AM: Feline reticuloendotheliosis: A report of four cases. *JAVMA* 170:1329–1332, 1977.

49. Carpenter JL, Holzworth J: Treatment of leukemia in the cat. *JAVMA* 158:1130–1131, 1971.

50. Moore AS, Ruslander D, Cotter SM, et al: Efficacy of, and toxicoses associated with, oral idarubicin administration in cats with neoplasia. *JAVMA* 206:1550–1554, 1995.

51. Cotter SM: Treatment of lymphoma and leukemia with cyclophosphamide, vincristine, and prednisone: II. Treatment of cats. *JAAHA* 19:166–172, 1983.

52. Cotter SM, Holzworth J: Disorders of the hematopoetic system, in Holzworth J (ed): *Diseases of the Cat. Medicine and Surgery*. Philadelphia, WB Saunders, 1987, pp 755–807.

53. Thrall MA: Lymphoproliferative disorders: Lymphocytic leukemia and plasma cell myeloma. *Vet Clin North Am Small Anim Clin* 11:321–347, 1981.

54. Center SA, Randolph JF, Erb HN, Reiter S: Eosinophilia in the cat: A retrospective study of 312 cases (1975 to 1986). *JAAHA* 26:349–358, 1990.

55. Neer TM: Hypereosinophilic syndrome in cats. *Compend Contin Educ Pract Vet* 13:549–555, 1991.

56. Simon N, Holzworth J: Eosinophilic leukemia in a cat. *Cornell Vet* 7:579–597, 1967.

57. Silverman J: Eosinophilic leukemia in a cat. *JAVMA* 158:199, 1971.

58. Harvey RG: Feline hypereosinophilia with cutaneous lesions. *J Small Anim Pract* 31:453–456, 1990.

59. Scott DW, Randolph JF, Walsh KM: Hypereosinophilic syndrome in a cat. *Feline Pract* 15:22–30, 1985.

60. Watson ADJ, Moore AS, Helfand SC: Primary erythrocytosis in the cat: Treatment with hydroxyurea. *J Small Anim Pract* 35:320–325, 1994.

61. Reed C, Ling GV, Gould D, Kaneko JJ: Polycythemia vera in a cat. *JAVMA* 157:85–91, 1970.

62. Duff BC, Allan GS, Howlett CR: A presumptive case of polycythemia vera in a cat. *Aust Vet Pract* 3:78–79, 1973.

63. Foster ES, Lothrop Jr CD: Polycythemia vera in a cat with cardiac hypertrophy. *JAVMA* 192:1736–1738, 1988.

64. Hawkins EC, Feldman BF, Blanchard PC: Immunoglobulin A myeloma in a cat with pleural effusion and serum hyperviscosity. *JAVMA* 188:876–878, 1986.

65. Eastman CA: Plasma cell tumors in a cat. *Feline Pract* 24:26–31, 1996.

66. Jacobs T: Multiple myeloma in a cat with paraparesis. *Feline Pract* 22:28–32, 1994.

67. Holzworth J, Meier H: Reticulum cell myeloma in a cat. *Cornell Vet* 47:302–316, 1957.

68. Mills JN, Eger CE, Robinson WF, et al: A case of multiple myeloma in a cat. *JAAHA* 18:79–82, 1982.

69. Ward DA, McEntee MF, Weddle DL: Orbital plasmacytoma in a cat. *J Small Anim Pract* 38:576–578, 1997.

70. Drazner FH: Multiple myeloma in the cat. *Compend Contin Educ Pract Vet* 4:206–216, 1982.

71. MacEwen EG, Huruitz AI: Diagnosis and management of monoclonal gammopathies. *Vet Clin North Am Small Anim Clin* 7:119–132, 1977.

72. Williams DA, Goldschmidt MH: Hyperviscosity syndrome with IgM monoclonal gammopathy and hepatic plasmacytoid lymphosarcoma in a cat. *J Small Anim Pract* 23:311–323, 1982.

73. Saar C, Saar U, Opitz M, et al: Paraproteinämische retikulosen bei der katze. *Berl Münch Teirärztl Wschr* 86:11–15, 1973.

74. Mandel NS, Esplin DG: A retroperitoneal extramedullary plasmacytoma in a cat with a monoclonal gammopathy. *JAAHA* 30:603–608, 1994.

75. Weber NA, Tebeau CS: An unusual presentation of multiple myeloma in two cats. *JAAHA* 34:477–483, 1998.

76. Hay LE: Multiple myeloma in a cat. *Aust Vet Pract* 8:45–48, 1978.

77. Hribernik TN, Barta O, Gaunt SD, Boudreaux MK: Serum hyperviscosity syndrome associated with IgG myeloma in a cat. *JAVMA* 181:169–170, 1982.

78. Forrester SD, Greco DS, Relford RL: Serum hyperviscosity syndrome associated with multiple myeloma in two cats. *JAVMA* 200:79–82, 1992.

79. Forrester SD, Fossum TW, Rogers KS: Diagnosis and treatment of chylothorax associated with lymphoblastic lymphosarcoma in four cats. *JAVMA* 198:291–294, 1991.

80. Farrow BRH, Penny R: Multiple myeloma in a cat. *JAVMA* 158:606–611, 1971.

81. Bertoy RW, Brightman AH, Regan K: Intraocular melanoma with multiple metastases in a cat. *JAVMA* 192:87–89, 1988.

82. Kehoe JM, Hurvitsz AI, Capra JD: Characterization of three feline paraproteins. *J Immunol* 109:511–516, 1972.

83. Rowland PH, Linke RP: Immunohistochemical characterization of lambda light-chain-derived amyloid in one feline and five canine plasma cell tumors. *Vet Pathol* 31:390–393, 1994.

84. Port CD, Maschgan ER, Pond J, Scarpelli DG: Multiple neoplasia in a jaguar (*Panthera onca*). *J Comp Pathol* 91:115–122, 1981.

TUMORS OF THE SKELETAL SYSTEM 38

Antony S. Moore and Gregory K. Ogilvie

OSTEOSARCOMA

CLINICAL BRIEFING

Common Presentation	Appendicular and axial skeleton equally affected. Hindlimb and skull are the most common sites. Extraosseous osteosarcoma may be injection (vaccine) associated sarcomas.
Staging and Diagnosis	MDB, lymph node palpation, CT scan for axial tumors. Metastasis (typically to lungs) is uncommon regardless of primary site.
Treatment	
Initial	
Appendicular	Amputation.
Axial	Excision if possible.
Parosteal	Surgical excision.
Adjunctive	
Appendicular	Chemotherapy (e.g., carboplatin or doxorubicin) may be indicated.
Axial	Palliative or curative-intent radiation for incomplete excision; chemotherapy (e.g., carboplatin or doxorubicin) may be indicated.
Supportive	Pre- and postoperative anesthesia; esophagostomy/gastrostomy tube if surgery involves the head; fluid therapy/appetite stimulants as needed.

Osteosarcoma is the most common primary bone tumor in cats but accounts for only 1.5% to 6.0% of all tumors diagnosed in this species.[1–6] Osteosarcoma in cats has been described under three general categories: appendicular, axial, and parosteal. A literature search found reports of 126 osteosarcomas of the appendicular skeleton, 92 of the axial skeleton, and 14 parosteal tumors. Appendicular osteosarcomas are less likely to metastasize in cats than in dogs.

APPENDICULAR OSTEOSARCOMA

Incidence, Signalment, and Etiology

Appendicular osteosarcoma occurs most frequently in DSHs. Of 101 reported cases in which breed was noted, there were 5 DLHs with appendicular tumors.[7–9] One Persian cat had a tibial osteosarcoma,[10] and one had an ischial lesion.[9] Reported cats tend to be older; in two studies that distinguished cats with appendicular or axial osteosarcoma, the average age for those with appendicular tumors was 8 to 9 years (range, <1 year to 17 years).[11,12] These figures seem to agree with other large studies.[4,7] There does not seem to be a gender predilection for appendicular os-

teosarcoma.[11,12]

The cause of osteosarcoma in cats is obscure, although the near equal numbers of tumors occurring in the axial and appendicular skeleton implies that size and weight-bearing are not as significant factors as in dogs.

Exposure to radiation was reported to induce appendicular osteosarcoma in one cat.[13] As in dogs and humans, fractures or repair thereof has been associated with tumor formation, albeit rarely. There have been six reports of osteosarcoma occurring in cats at the site of a previous fracture repaired using an intramedullary pin. The period from fixation to tumor diagnosis varied from 6[13] to 12[14] months in two early reports. In two larger studies, tumors were associated with a diaphyseal femoral fracture repaired 10 months previously,[11] an epiphyseal femoral fracture repaired 1 year previously,[11] an epiphyseal femoral fracture repaired 5 years previously,[11] a tibial fracture repaired 5 years previously,[11] and one other fracture site for which the time sequence was not reported.[12]

Clinical Presentation and History

Appendicular osteosarcoma is much more likely to occur

in the hindlimbs than in the forelimbs. The distribution of lesions described in the literature is summarized in Figure 38-1. The three most commonly reported sites are the proximal tibia, distal femur, and proximal humerus (Figures 38-2 to 38-5).

KEY POINT

Pathologic fracture at the site of an appendicular osteosarcoma is common in cats.

Chronic lameness is the most common reason for presentation[11]; the mean duration of lameness is approximately 3 months,[2,4] although some cats have been lame up to a year prior to presentation.[15] Lameness may suddenly get worse if a pathologic fracture occurs. In one study,[13] 5 of 39 cats had a pathologic fracture at the site of an appendicular tumor; pathologic fractures have also been seen in 9 of 39 other cats with appendicular osteosarcoma.[7,9,10] The high rate of pathologic fractures may be a consequence of the primary osteolytic nature of these tumors, as seen on radiographs (Figure 38-4). One study noted that appendicular osteosarcoma was more likely to appear as lysis than as an axial osteosarcoma on radiographs[11] (Table 38-1). A possible explanation for this osteolytic appearance, which is noted radiographically and histologically, is the high proportion of nonosteogenic cells (fibrosarcomatous and giant cells) in many of these tumors.[4]

Staging and Diagnosis

While feline osteosarcoma appears less likely to metastasize than its canine counterpart, accurate diagnosis with appropriate attention to staging is necessary to offer prognostic information and treatment options to caregivers. Although needle core biopsies are helpful in determining an initial, tentative diagnosis, results should be treated as preliminary only and the entire tumor should be submitted for histopathologic evaluation once amputation is performed. The predominance of giant cell components in these tumors may have led to the series of manuscripts describing giant cell sarcomas of bone.[16–19] It is possible that these tumors were osteosarcomas.

KEY POINT

Needle core biopsies should not be relied on for definitive diagnosis; the entire tumor should be submitted after amputation.

Cats with a suspected osteosarcoma should be staged prior to definitive surgery. In addition to a MDB, regional lymph nodes should be palpated and, if enlarged, samples obtained for biopsy. Abdominal ultrasound should be performed if clinically indicated.

Metastasis at the time of diagnosis appears to be rare. Of 41 cats that were autopsied,[2,4,15,20–22] only 9 had metastasis, even though one of the tumors had been present for a year.[15] Of these 9 cats, 8 had pulmonary metastases, and 7 of those had lymph node metastases (3 renal, 2 pleural, 1 cerebral,

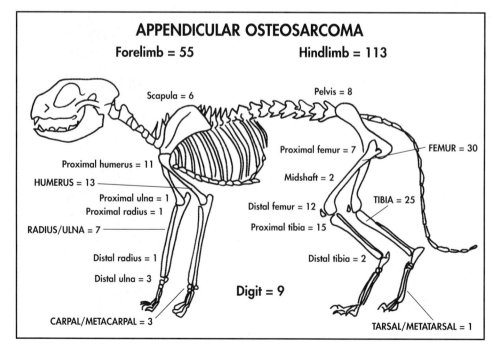

APPENDICULAR OSTEOSARCOMA

Forelimb = 55   Hindlimb = 113

Scapula = 6   Pelvis = 8
                                       Proximal femur = 7   FEMUR = 30
Proximal humerus = 11   Midshaft = 2
HUMERUS = 13
Proximal ulna = 1   Distal femur = 12   TIBIA = 25
Proximal radius = 1   Proximal tibia = 15
RADIUS/ULNA = 7
Distal radius = 1   Distal tibia = 2
Distal ulna = 3   Digit = 9
CARPAL/METACARPAL = 3   TARSAL/METATARSAL = 1

Figure 38-1: Distribution of osteosarcoma affecting the appendicular skeletal system of cats (compiled from literature). Numbers do not add up because of inconsistent data.

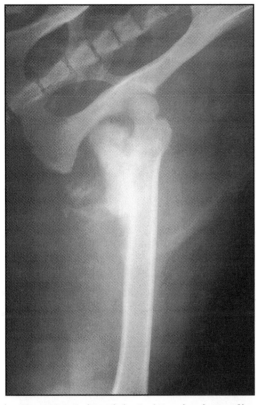

Figure 38-2: Radiograph showing lysis and production of bone in a proximal femoral osteosarcoma in an 8-year-old male Maine Coon.

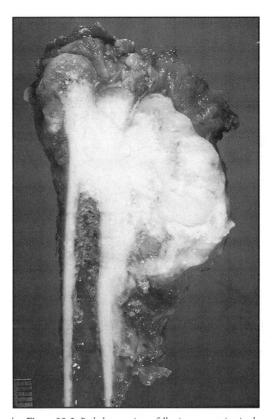

Figure 38-3: Pathology specimen following amputation in the cat in Figure 38-2.

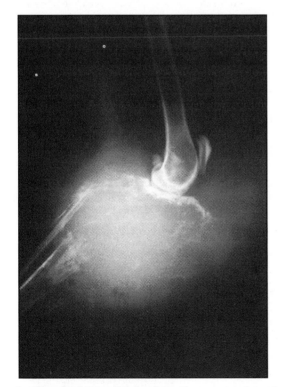

Figure 38-4: Primarily lytic radiographic appearance of a proximal tibial osteosarcoma. (Courtesy of K.M. Rassnick)

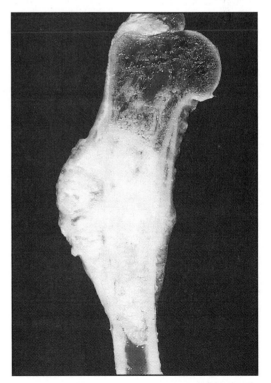

Figure 38-5: Sclerotic osteosarcoma in the right humerus of a 14-year-old DSH.

TABLE 38-1
Radiographic Appearance of Lesions in 33 Cats with Osteosarcoma[11]

Appearance		No. of Cats	
		Appendicular	Axial
Lytic	1	9	—
	2	4	1
	3	6	4
	4	3	2
Sclerotic	5	—	4

and 1 iliac). The ninth cat had liver metastases only.[2,4,11] A cat with a giant cell tumor (possibly osteosarcoma) had pulmonary and renal metastases.[17] In addition, 3 of 16 cats with skeletal tumors had metastases—1 to the lung, 1 to the lung and regional lymph node, and 1 to the spleen—although it is unclear whether all these cats had osteosarcoma.[1] Thoracic radiographs taken at the time of diagnosis disclosed pulmonary metastases in only 2 of 59 cats.[7,11,23] Elevations in alkaline phosphatase (ALP) have been correlated with a poor prognosis in dogs and humans with osteosarcoma. Serum ALP levels were normal in 17 cats with appendicular osteosarcoma.[7] While hypertrophic osteopathy (HO) has not yet been described in cats with osteosarcoma, a cat with a tibial osteosarcoma had metatarsal lesions that appeared to be HO in the published radiographs.[24]

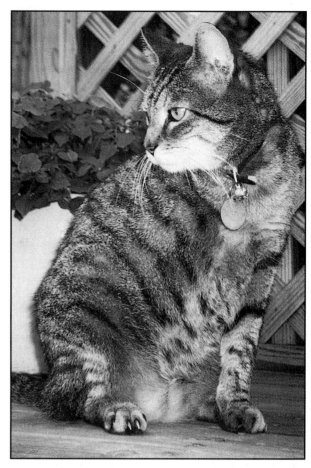

Figure 38-6: *Cats tolerate amputation well and remain very active after surgery. (Courtesy of D. Ruslander)*

KEY POINT

Metastases are uncommon in cats with osteosarcoma and tend to be pulmonary when they do occur.

Treatment

Amputation of the affected limb provides pain relief with little impact on the mobility of cats. In addition, amputation alone may be curative in many cats with osteosarcoma. Thus amputation appears to be the treatment of choice for appendicular osteosarcoma (Figure 38-6). The median survival for cats treated with amputation alone was 20 months in one study.[11] Of 26 cats in three studies that had amputation performed, 16 were alive with no evidence of disease 5 to 64 months following surgery.[7,10,11] Of the 8 cats that died, 1 developed metastases (5 months after amputation),[10] 1 developed a local recurrence,[7] and the other 6 cats died of unrelated causes.[7,11] In another study, 15 of 24 cats treated surgically with curative intent were alive an average of 17 months after surgery.[12]

Adjuvant chemotherapy has not been widely recom-

mended due to the low metastatic potential for these tumors. Given the efficacy of carboplatin and doxorubicin for canine osteosarcoma, there may be a place for these drugs in the adjuvant therapy of feline osteosarcoma. True efficacy would be difficult to demonstrate, however, owing to the excellent prognosis for cats with this tumor.

KEY POINT

Long survival times following amputation alone are possible in cats with appendicular osteosarcoma.

A response to liposome-encapsulated doxorubicin therapy in one cat may indicate a role for this drug in some cats with osteosarcoma,[25] but its function as an adjunct to surgery is far from clear based on existing reports.[8,26] One cat with an osteosarcoma of the ilium received cyclophosphamide, vincristine, and methotrexate every 2 weeks for 4 months, and the tumor decreased in size by 80% for 13 months. At recurrence, there was no response to the same treatment.[7]

AXIAL OSTEOSARCOMA

Incidence, Signalment, and Etiology

Osteosarcoma of the axial skeleton occurs most commonly in DSHs. A Persian with a sacral tumor[10] and a Siamese with a nasal tumor[27] have been described.

As is true for appendicular tumors, axial osteosarcoma occurs mainly in older cats (average age, 10.5 years; range, <1 to 18 years,[11,12] which was significantly older than cats with appendicular tumors in one study[12]). The three youngest cats reported had nasal[11] or mandibular[7] osteosarcoma. Seventeen male cats and 22 female cats had osteosarcoma of the axial skeleton.[11]

Clinical Presentation and History

Axial osteosarcoma is considerably more common in the skull than in the rest of the axial skeleton (Figure 38-7). Signs associated with these tumors vary depending on tumor site and size. Cats are often presented for a large mass or swelling,[5,7,27] and deformity of the skull may lead to nasal stertor, nasal discharge, or sneezing,[11,27] exophthalmos,[4,11,23] behavior changes,[4,7] loose teeth,[11] otitis,[11] or dyspnea[7] (Figures 38-8 to 38-15).

Tumors of the spine may cause paresis or ataxia[23,28]; the latter was noted to be present for as long as 7 months in one cat.[29] Other signs are lameness,[7] constipation,[7] and urinary incontinence.[28] These tumors seem to have a more sclerotic appearance than their appendicular counterparts[11] (Table 38-1), and they appear to consist primarily of proliferative periosteal bone.[7]

Staging and Diagnosis

Appropriate staging should include an MDB and evaluation of the regional lymph nodes. Diagnosis is best made by needle core biopsies from the tumor prior to planning a definitive procedure. Advanced imaging techniques, such as a CT scan or MRI, are very helpful if surgery or radiation therapy is planned. These imaging modalities can identify tumor margins for the surgeon or radiation therapist.

It is unclear in some reports whether metastases that occurred were from axial or appendicular osteosarcomas.[2,4,11] These cats were discussed in the section on appendicular tumors. Of the 18 cats with known axial osteosarcoma, none had metastases at the time of diagnosis.[7,23,27,29,30] Elevations in ALP have been reported to be correlated with a poor prognosis in dogs and humans with osteosarcoma. Serum ALP levels were normal in 5 cats with axial osteosarcoma.[7]

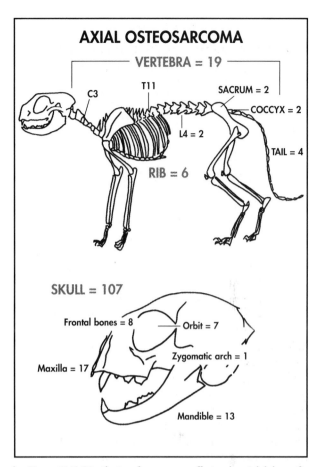

Figure 38-7: Distribution of osteosarcoma affecting the axial skeleton of cats (compiled from literature). Numbers do not add up because of inconsistent data. C=cerebral; L=lumbar; T=thoracic.

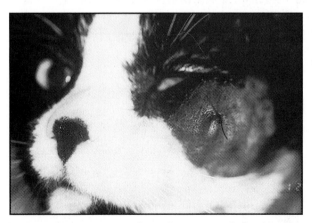

Figure 38-8: Osteosarcoma affecting the zygomatic arch of a 14-year-old cat (photograph taken after needle biopsy). (Courtesy of K.M. Rassnick)

Treatment

Cats rarely live a long time without treatment for axial osteosarcoma. Of eight cats with osteosarcoma of the skull that were not treated, survival times ranged from 2 weeks to 15 months (median, 4 weeks).[11]

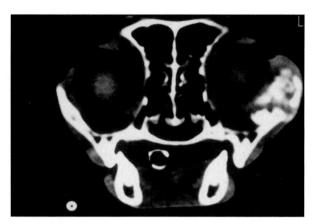

Figure 38-9: Prior to surgery on the cat in Figure 38-8, a CT scan was obtained to delineate margins and assess whether postoperative radiation therapy would be necessary. (Courtesy of K.M. Rassnick)

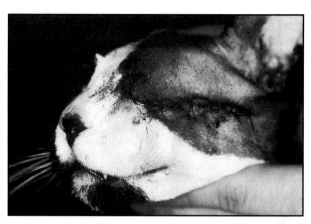

Figure 38-10: Cat in Figure 38-8 after surgical excision of osteosarcoma. Note that an orbitectomy was necessary to obtain adequate surgical margins. (Courtesy of K.M. Rassnick)

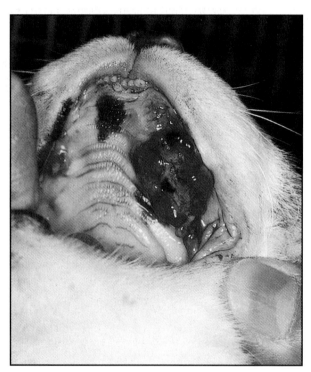

Figure 38-11: Osteosarcoma of the maxilla. Surgery was not an option, so radiation therapy was planned after CT scan.

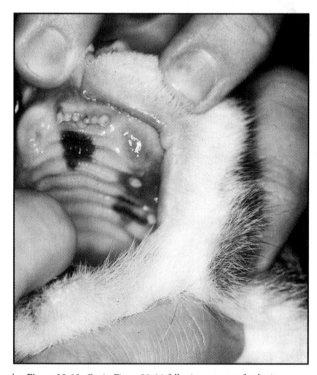

Figure 38-12: Cat in Figure 38-11 following a course of radiation therapy; note the marked reduction in tumor size.

MDB = minimum database; includes CBC, biochemical profile, urinalysis, FeLV/FIV serology, T_4 testing, and thoracic radiographs (three views).

Local tumor recurrence is the reason for euthanasia in most cats with axial osteosarcoma that undergo treatment.

Given the location of the majority of these tumors, it is not surprising that surgical excision is rarely complete. However, even with incomplete resection, survival times for cats with axial osteosarcoma may be longer than 1 year.[11] In one study, tumors recurred within 3 months of surgery in three cats that had incomplete resection of skull osteosarcoma.[7] In contrast, another study reported that seven cats with incomplete excision of axial osteosarcoma survived a median of 13 months (range, 3 weeks to 2 years).[11] Another cat with a small oral osteosarcoma had a complete curative excision.[11]

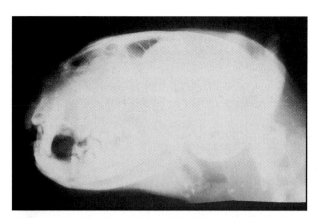

Figure 38-13: *Nasal osteosarcoma (as shown in a 7-year-old cat) is uncommon but best treated with radiation therapy. (Courtesy of S.M. Cotter)*

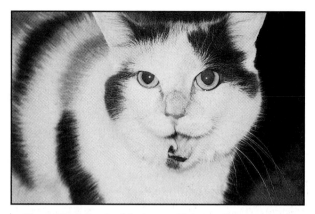

Figure 38-15: *Function following mandibulectomy for osteosarcoma is usually excellent; however, a postoperative gastrostomy tube is mandatory until the cat is eating.*

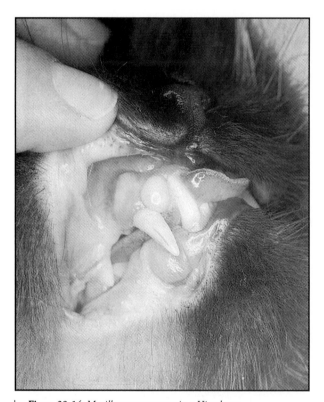

Figure 38-14: *Maxillary osteosarcoma in a Himalayan.*

Complete excision is similarly difficult in cats with vertebral osteosarcoma. One cat with a lesion at T11 improved neurologically following surgery but was euthanized soon afterward.[29] In another cat, incomplete excision was followed by chemotherapy; the tumor recurred after 5 years, and a second incomplete surgery led to a second remission of 1,705 days. The cat was euthanized at the second recurrence.[30] Two cats with osteosarcoma of the tail had complete surgical excision of the tumors and were alive an average of 16 months after surgery.[12]

KEY POINT

Even with incomplete resection, survival times for cats with axial osteosarcoma may be greater than 1 year.

The long survival times seen in some cats with known incomplete surgery makes it difficult to assess the efficacy of adjuvant therapies, however, with the apparently low rate of metastasis, radiation therapy would appear to be a logical adjunct to treatment. Two cats treated with adjuvant radiation were among the longest survivors in one case series.[12] In other single case reports, one cat with osteosarcoma of the skull received radiation therapy following incomplete excision and the tumor recurred 16 months later.[7] In another cat with nasal osteosarcoma, 42 Gy administered in seven equal weekly fractions caused a complete remission of the tumor and the tumor had not recurred 24 months later.[27]

Four cats with mandibular osteosarcoma that had hemimandibulectomies and received one to five doses of doxorubicin (25 mg/m² every 3 weeks) survived more than 5 years without recurrence.[a]

Supportive Care

Pre- and postoperative analgesia is essential. Nutritional support is important in all patients and helps minimize the effects of treatment and improve healing.

PAROSTEAL OSTEOSARCOMA

Incidence, Signalment, and Etiology

Other terms for this disease in the veterinary literature include *juxtacortical osteosarcoma, juxtacortical osteogenic sarcoma, parosteal osteogenic sarcoma, ossifying parosteal sar-*

---

[a]Moore AS, Ogilvie GK: Personal observations.

coma, and *parosteal osteoma.*[31] It is best described as osteosarcoma that does not disrupt the cortex of the underlying bone.[11] The presentation and progression of parosteal osteosarcoma appear remarkably similar to those of osteosarcoma with cortical destruction. In a group of 90 cats with osteosarcoma, only 1 had a parosteal osteosarcoma.[12]

Of the 14 feline cases reported in the literature, 7 occurred in DSHs.[7,9–11,23,31,32] Most cats described are older than 10 years of age.[9,31,32] There does not seem to be a gender predilection.[9,10]

Clinical Presentation and History

In 10 of the 14 reported cats, parosteal osteosarcoma occurred in the appendicular skeleton. The other 4 cats (all from the same study) had tumors that occurred in the skull[10] (Figure 38-16). In a group of 50 cats with appendicular osteosarcoma, only one cat had a parosteal osteosarcoma (site not recorded).[12]

The clinical presentation is related to location of the lesion. In cats with appendicular parosteal tumors, the reason for presentation is lameness, which had been present for more than a year in one cat.[32] In five cats, a mass of 3 to 5 cm was noted by the owners[10,31]; growth of this mass was rapid (it doubled in 4 months) in one cat.[31] One cat with a mandibular lesion was presented for dyspnea due to pharyngeal obstruction.[10]

Staging and Diagnosis

No evidence of metastases was present at the time of diagnosis in eight cats,[9,10,23,32] but one cat had a humeral lesion and pulmonary metastases that did not contain osteoid.[31] Details regarding metastasis could not be determined in five other cats with juxtacortical tumors of the appendicular skeleton.[7,11] Despite the lack of documented cases of metastases, thoracic radiographs (as part of the MDB) are suggested. A CT scan or MRI may be helpful in planning surgery for a parosteal osteosarcoma of the axial skeleton, particularly if it is unclear from radiographs whether the cortex is disrupted. These imaging techniques are mandatory prior to surgery if adjunctive radiation therapy is considered.

Treatment

The behavior of juxtacortical osteosarcoma appears remarkably similar to that of osteosarcoma with cortical destruction. A biopsy prior to the definitive procedure is essential to guide subsequent therapy. Skull lesions were excised in two cats; one was tumor free 4 months after surgery and the other was still tumor free 15 months after surgery[10] (Figures 38-17 to 38-19). In another cat, radiation therapy was started but not completed as the cat's condition deteriorated and it was euthanized.[32] Surgery, either alone or with adjuvant radiation therapy for incompletely excised tumors, is probably the initial treatment of choice.

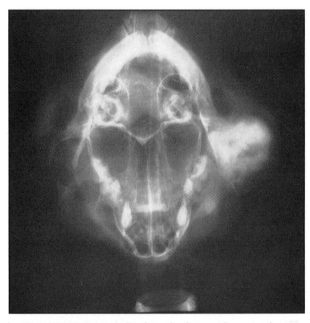

Figure 38-17: *Open-mouth radiographs of a cat with a parosteal osteosarcoma arising from the ramus of the mandible.*

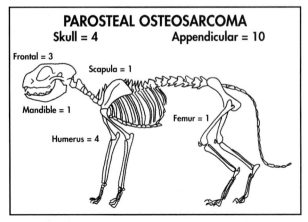

Figure 38-16: *Distribution of parosteal osteosarcomas in cats (compiled from literature). Numbers do not add up because of inconsistent data.*

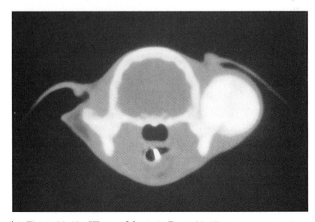

Figure 38-18: *CT scan of the cat in Figure 38-17.*

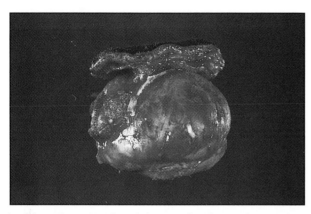

Figure 38-19: Surgically excised specimen from the cat in Figure 38-17. Surgical excision should be curative because metastasis is rare.

EXTRAOSSEOUS OSTEOSARCOMA

Although injection-related sarcomas are most commonly fibrosarcomas, osteosarcoma is the second most common histologic type. An extraosseous osteosarcoma occurring at a nonparosteal location should be treated as a soft tissue sarcoma, particularly if it occurs at the site of previous vaccination (see Chapter 51).

In a case series of 48 cats with extraskeletal osteosarcoma, 44 tumors were found in the subcutaneous tissue and 30 of these 44 were found at common vaccination sites.[12] Other sites recorded were the intestine or omentum (3 cats) and mammary tissue (1 cat).[12] These cats appeared to fare worse after treatment than cats with appendicular tumors.

GIANT CELL TUMORS OF BONE

CLINICAL BRIEFING

Common Presentation	Rare; probable variant of osteosarcoma or synovial sarcoma; appendicular more common than axial.
Staging and Diagnosis	MDB, lymph node palpation; CT scan for axial tumors. Metastasis is uncommon.
Treatment	
Initial	
Appendicular	Amputation.
Axial	Excision if possible.
Adjunctive	
Appendicular	Chemotherapy probably not warranted; treat as for osteosarcoma.
Axial	Radiation for incomplete excision.
Supportive	Pre- and postoperative analgesics. Esophagostomy/gastrostomy tube if surgery involves the head. Fluid therapy/appetite stimulants as needed.

Incidence, Signalment, and Etiology

This is a tumor of uncertain histogenesis. The "giant cells" are thought to be osteoclasts, but this has not been proven. With the high proportion of giant cells seen in feline osteosarcomas,[4] it is possible that the tumors in some early reports may have been osteosarcomas. One author found osteoid spicules in two feline giant cell tumors, suggesting that these were osteosarcomas.[33] To further confuse the issue, some giant cell tumors appear to be of tendon sheath origin and may be synovial sarcomas[5,34] or extraskeletal soft tissue sarcomas.[35]

Of the seven reported giant cell tumors that involved bone, two were described in studies of bone tumors and details were not available.[1,36] One giant cell tumor occurred in a 6-year-old castrated male DSH; the tumor was a 9 cm mass that involved the thoracic wall from the third to the seventh

rib and caused lysis of two of these ribs.[19] The other four cats had lytic appendicular tumors in the tibia,[18] distal femur,[9,17] or ulna[16]; these tumors did not cross the adjacent joint. The tibial lesion was in an 8-year-old Persian, while the others were in two 1-year-old and one 8-year-old DSHs.[9]

Clinical Presentation and History

Cats with giant cell tumors are often presented to the veterinarian for lameness or swelling. The duration of clinical signs can be prolonged. For example, one cat had been lame for more than a year and had a 6 cm diameter mass.[18]

Staging and Diagnosis

No metastases were noted in four of the cats[9,16,18,19]; one cat had metastases to the lung and kidney at the time of presentation.[17] In one young cat, C-type viral particles were observed in the giant cell tumor, although a causal relationship was not established.[16] Despite the lack of documented cases of metastases, thoracic radiographs are suggested as part of the MDB. Just as for cats with osteosarcoma, CT scan or MRI may be helpful in planning surgery for a giant cell sarcoma of the axial skeleton. These imaging techniques are mandatory prior to surgery if adjunctive radiation therapy is considered.

Treatment

This tumor is best treated as a variant of osteosarcoma.

Amputation is the treatment of choice. If amputation is not a logical option, radiation may be palliative. Chemotherapy is unproven for this tumor type. Amputation of the affected hindlimb was performed in one cat,[9] and this animal was free of metastases or tumor recurrence a year later.

Supportive Care

Analgesia and nutritional support should be considered for all patients.

OSTEOMA

CLINICAL BRIEFING

Common Presentation	Axial skeleton affected more commonly than the appendicular skeleton. Tumor may grow rapidly and cause a mass effect.
Staging and Diagnosis	Care should be taken in interpreting needle biopsies as the tumor may be osteosarcoma. MDB; lymph node palpation; CT scan for axial tumors. Metastasis not reported.
Treatment	
Initial	Surgical excision.
Adjunctive	Radiation for incomplete excision. Chemotherapy not warranted.
Supportive	Pre- and postoperative analgesia. Esophagostomy/gastrostomy tube if surgery involves the head. Fluid therapy/appetite stimulants as needed.

Incidence, Signalment, and Etiology

Some pathologists have considered osteoma to be an end product of inflammatory processes, such as fibrous dysplasia, with ossifying fibroma occurring as an intermediate stage.[4,33] Another report distinguished between osteoma and osteoid osteoma,[10] with the latter having a sclerotic mantle of bone. All such tumors are included in this section.

Of the 10 cats with one of the above diagnoses, signalment was available for 7.[4,9,10,23,37,38] Six were domestic cats (one DLH), and one was Siamese.[37] Ages ranged from 4 to 17 years (median, 10 years); five cats were female, and one was a castrated male.

Clinical Presentation and History

This tumor can occur throughout the skeletal system, and its presence can cause discomfort. Despite the benign nature of the tumor, it can grow to a large size. For example, the largest tumor recorded ($2 \times 2 \times 3$ cm) was on the mandible.[9] The other tumors were all 1 to 1.5 cm in diameter.

Of the 10 reported osteomas, the tumor occurred in the appendicular skeleton in four cats. A pathologic fracture of the humerus caused acute lameness in one cat,[23] one tumor occurred on the toe of a forepaw,[4] and another tumor oc-

cured in the "hip."[5] An osteoma causing lameness was adjacent to, but did not disrupt the cortex of, the olecranon.[38]

KEY POINT

Osteomas occur in similar sites to osteosarcoma and may respond to radiation therapy.

The skull was affected in four cats, but clinical details were available for only three. The sella turcica was involved in one cat[10]; in another, a mass that had been present for 12 months grew rapidly over 1 month but caused no clinical problems.[37] A large mandibular ossifying fibroma caused dysphagia and drooling in one cat.[19]

Of the remaining two cats, one had a chest wall osteoma[5]; the other had an osteoma of vertebra T10, which caused paresis and inability to groom.[10]

Staging and Diagnosis

It may be difficult to diagnose an osteoma using incisional biopsy techniques, and the entire resected specimen should be submitted for pathology to confirm an initial diagnosis. Similarly, it is probably prudent to stage cats with these tumors as if they had an osteosarcoma, and thus thoracic radiographs are indicated. Regional radiographs or a CT examination is often quite helpful in determining the extent of the tumor and can assist in directing therapy.

As would be predicted by the benign nature of this tumor, no metastases were seen in any of the reported cats, even those with a long clinical history.[9,37]

Treatment

Surgery appears to be the treatment of choice for lesions in which the margins can be assured, but radiation therapy may have a role in the treatment of nonresectable osteomas. Surgical removal was performed in one cat with a toe lesion,[4] one with a zygomatic arch lesion,[37] and one with an olecranon lesion.[38] There was no recurrence noted at an un-

known period, 6 months, and 14 weeks later, respectively.

A cat with a mandibular lesion was treated with 40 Gy of radiation therapy administered in 10 fractions over 22 days. The tumor did not progress, and clinical signs resolved until regrowth was noted 26 months after radiation.[9]

MDB = minimum database; includes CBC, biochemical profile, urinalysis, FeLV/FIV serology, T_4 testing, and thoracic radiographs (three views).

Supportive Care

Pre- and postoperative analgesia can be helpful in some patients. Nutritional support is also necessary.

CHONDROSARCOMA

CLINICAL BRIEFING

Common Presentation	Second most common primary bone tumor. May arise from a chondroma. Appears to be slow growing. Axial lesions more common than appendicular lesions.
Staging and Diagnosis	Care should be taken in interpreting needle biopsies as the tumor may be an osteosarcoma. MDB and lymph node palpation, CT; scan for axial tumors. Metastasis is rare.
Treatment Initial	Surgical excision.
Adjunctive	Radiation for incomplete excision. Chemotherapy probably not warranted.
Supportive	Pre- and postoperative analgesia. Esophagostomy/gastrostomy tube if surgery involves the head. Fluid therapy/appetite stimulants as needed.

Incidence, Signalment, and Etiology

Chondrosarcoma appears to be the second most common primary bone tumor in cats. Although fibrosarcomas may invade bone, they are rarely primary bone tumors. The locations of chondrosarcomas are indicated in Figure 38-20. While more than 30 chondrosarcomas of bone have been reported in the literature, data is incomplete for many of the affected cats. Of those for which gender was recorded, there were 16 females (15 spayed) and 10 males (6 castrated).[1,6] Of the 15 cats for which breed information was provided, 9 were DSHs,[5,9,10,39–41] 4 were Siamese,[2,9,10,42] and 1 was a Persian.[41] Most cats were older (age range, 4 to 15 years; median, 8 years). Both of the 4-year-old cats were Siamese. One cat with multilobular chondroma of the skull was found to have areas of chondrosarcoma within the benign matrix.[43]

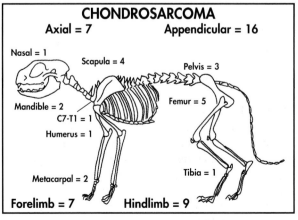

Figure 38-20: *Distribution of chondrosarcoma affecting the skeleton in cats (compiled from literature). Numbers do not add up because of inconsistent data.*

Clinical Presentation and History

Some cats with chondrosarcoma have long histories of clinical signs. Symptoms are primarily related to the location of the lesion. One cat with a nasal tumor had a 2 year history of sneezing.[4] Lameness was the presenting sign in five cats with appendicular tumors.[9,10,40] Five other cats were presented for a noticeable mass.[9,10,41–43] One of these cats had a mass for 6 years,[10] and another had a carpal mass for 13 months.[41] One cat with a mandibular lesion had subluxation of the temporomandibular joint,[10] and a cat with a C7 to T1 vertebral lesion had hemiparesis for 6 months before becoming paralyzed.[39] There have been no reports of chondrosarcomas of the rib in cats, whereas most chondrosarcomas in dogs are found in this location.

Staging and Diagnosis

There was no evidence of metastasis at the time of diagnosis in any of the 15 cats for which this information was available. In 1 cat, metastasis occurred 7 weeks after amputation of a scapular lesion, but this is the only reported occurrence of metastasis.[41] Care should be taken in interpreting needle biopsies from bone tumors in cats since cartilaginous areas may predominate in osteosarcoma. While the metastatic rate for osteosarcoma is low, it appears to be higher than that for chondrosarcoma. Despite the lack of documented cases of metastasis, thoracic radiographs (as part of the MDB) are suggested. Just as for cats with osteosarcoma, CT scan or MRI may be helpful in planning surgery for a chondrosarcoma of the axial skeleton. These imaging techniques are mandatory prior to surgery if adjunctive radiation therapy is considered.

Treatment

Amputation is the treatment of choice for appendicular chondrosarcoma in cats and can result in long-term survival. In cats that had an appendicular tumor removed by amputation, survival times were as follows: 2 years without recurrence after hemipelvectomy in a cat with a pelvic tumor,[44] 18 months following scapulectomy in another cat,[9] 23 months in a cat with a carpal/metacarpal tumor,[9] and 7 months in a fourth cat.[10] A cat with carpal/digital chondrosarcoma had two local excisions; the tumor recurred in 3 months each time. A third local excision coupled with immunotherapy provided only another 4 weeks of palliation, and the leg was then amputated. Recurrence was seen 7 months later.[41] A cat with a scapular chondrosarcoma developed pulmonary metastases 7 weeks after amputation and only 10 weeks after initial signs were noted.[41] Signs were palliated for 6 months following excision of a nasal chondrosarcoma in one cat before the tumor recurred.[4]

KEY POINT

Treatment of chondrosarcoma is similar to that for osteosarcoma.

In tumors that are incompletely excised, radiation may offer good tumor control, as it does in dogs. However, the one cat treated with radiation for a pelvic tumor died during therapy, and efficacy for this modality remains unproven.[9] Chemotherapy is also unproven for the adjuvant treatment of chondrosarcoma and is probably not warranted as the metastatic rate is very low.

Supportive Care

Analgesia should be employed before and after surgery. Nutritional support is also indicated.

NONDOMESTIC FELIDAE

Lameness in a 4-year-old Sumatran tiger *(Panthera tigris sumatrae)* led to diagnosis of chondrosarcoma of the left humeral head. No treatment was attempted, and no metastases were found on autopsy.[45]

OSTEOCHONDROMATOSIS

CLINICAL BRIEFING

Common Presentation	Solitary lesions are found in older, FeLV-negative cats; multiple lesions are found in younger, FeLV-positive cats. Both solitary and multiple tumors may affect both the appendicular and axial skeleton. Siamese cats may be predisposed to both.
Staging and Diagnosis	MDB (FeLV serology important); survey radiographs of skeletal system; thorough physical examination to check for multiple lesions.
Treatment *Initial* Solitary	Surgical excision.

Multiple	Surgery not an option except for palliation; other treatments directed at support and palliation only.
Adjunctive	
Solitary	Radiation for incomplete excision.
Multiple	Radiation may be palliative for individual lesions.
Supportive	Radiation may reduce pain associated with individual lesions. Esophagostomy/gastrostomy tube if radiation involves the head or the patient has difficulty eating. Analgesia and appetite stimulants as needed.

Incidence, Signalment, and Etiology

The occurrence of rapidly growing osteochondromas in mature animals appears to be a uniquely feline phenomenon. Similar lesions in dogs and humans occur prior to epiphyseal closure, and the tumors usually cease to grow when the patient reaches maturity. In cats, progression of the lesion(s) is often rapid and can occur in patients older than 1 year. Two distinct groups appear in the literature. Cats with solitary osteochondroma are usually older. The average age of 13 cats in one survey was 6.3 years (range, 1 to 11 years)[4]; in other studies, one cat was 12 years old[9] and one was 4 years old.[6] In contrast, cats with multiple tumors are younger (average age, 3.2 years; range, 1.5 to 6 years).[4,9,46–49]

KEY POINT

Multiple osteochondromas may be associated with FeLV infection in young cats.

Breed information was available for 13 of 14 cats with multiple tumors. Four were Siamese,[4,46,47,50] and the rest were either DSHs (*n* = 8) or DLH (*n* = 1).[49] Three of the 15 cats with solitary tumors were Siamese, although breed was not reported for all cats.[4,9] Both genders are equally represented in reported cases of solitary or multiple osteochondromas.

FeLV has been implicated in the etiology of multiple osteochondrosarcoma in cats. Two cats were observed to have budding C-type viral particles in the tumor but not in other tissues,[49,50] and five of six cats tested were positive for FeLV antigen.[4,9] Two cats had lymphoma histologically intermingled with their multiple osteochondromas. Of these cats, one (6 years of age) was FeLV positive[4] but testing was not available for the second cat (3 years of age). In the latter cat,[48] osteochondroma of the temporal bone underwent malignant transformation to osteosarcoma.

Clinical Presentation and History

Clinical signs depend on the number, size, and location

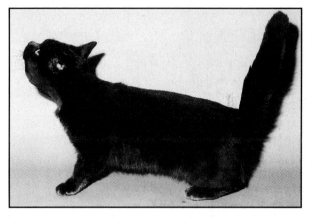

Figure 38-21: *Unusual posture in a cat with a solitary spinal osteochondroma. Surgery and radiation therapy are the therapeutic options after a CT scan is obtained.*

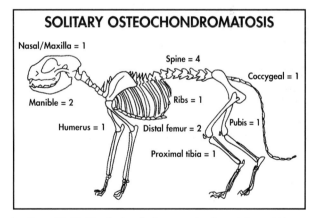

Figure 38-22: *Distribution of solitary osteochondroma lesions, which most commonly occur in older, FeLV-negative cats.*

of tumors (Figure 38-21). Reported sites for these tumors are illustrated in Figures 38-22 and 38-23.

Osteochondromas appear smooth and firm and may reach an enormous size. One scapular lesion measured 14 × 7 cm.[4] The tumors often grow rapidly,[46] both initially and after surgical excision. The duration of signs prior to presentation in seven of eight cats with multiple lesions was 2 weeks to 3 months.[9,46–49]

Signs due to appendicular and rib lesions are lameness

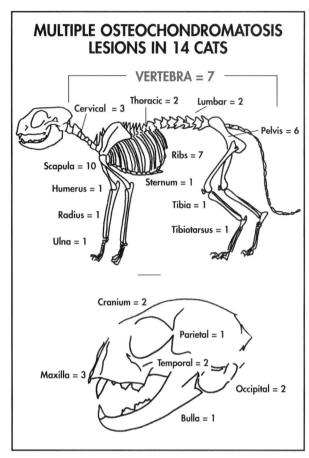

MULTIPLE OSTEOCHONDROMATOSIS LESIONS IN 14 CATS

VERTEBRA = 7

Cervical = 3 | Thoracic = 2 | Lumbar = 2
Pelvis = 6
Scapula = 10
Ribs = 7
Humerus = 1
Sternum = 1
Radius = 1
Tibia = 1
Ulna = 1
Tibiotarsus = 1

Cranium = 2
Parietal = 1
Temporal = 2
Maxilla = 3
Occipital = 2
Bulla = 1

Figure 38-23: Distribution of multiple osteochondromatosis lesions. These tumors are usually seen in young, FeLV-positive cats.

and discomfort, while cats with skull lesions may be presented for dyspnea, sneezing, or dysphagia.[9] One cat with a solitary pelvic lesion was presented for constipation.[9] In other cats, owners noticed a mass with no obvious associated clinical signs. A cat with two tumors in the dura was presented with stupor and blindness[4].

Staging and Diagnosis

Staging can be completed by obtaining a histologic biop-sy, regional radiographs, and an MDB. Survey radiographs and an FeLV test should be performed in cats with suspected osteochondroma. Radiographically, these tumors appear as pedunculated or sessile bony growths that seem to blend with the supporting skeletal structure and occur primarily in the axial skeleton. Both scapulae are often involved, and this is the most commonly affected site in the appendicular skeleton. FeLV testing should be performed in cats that have a solitary tumor, particularly in young cats, and a search for other, potentially clinically "silent" tumors should be made via both radiography and a thorough physical examination. For example, a young, FeLV-positive cat with multiple lesions had nasal tumors up to 0.4 cm in diameter that were not causing clinical signs and that were discovered on necropsy.[4]

KEY POINT

Complete staging is required to rule out the existence of multiple osteochondroma lesions.

Treatment

Surgical resection of an osteochondroma in a cat with multiple lesions rarely provides palliation. Surgery was attempted in three cats; regrowth occurred in 2 months in one cat, 3 months in the second cat, and 8 months in the third, and new lesions also appeared.[9,46,47] Two surgical attempts were made 3 years apart to remove a solitary lesion of the pubis in one cat; the animal had a long period of palliation.[9]

The difficulty of complete surgical removal and the low likelihood of metastasis would seem to make radiation therapy a palliative option for solitary lesions. However, no reports regarding the efficacy of this treatment modality exist. Similarly, there are no reports of chemotherapy for this tumor type.

Supportive Care

Analgesia and supportive nutritional therapy should be employed.

HEMANGIOSARCOMA

CLINICAL BRIEFING

Common Presentation	Very rare primary bone tumor. Appendicular location reported, rarely nasal.
Staging and Diagnosis	MDB and lymph node palpation. Metastasis appears to be common.
Treatment Initial	None reported; surgical excision may be palliative.

| Adjunctive | None reported; radiation therapy may be palliative for a localized lesion. Chemotherapy with doxorubicin or carboplatin may be effective for metastatic disease (unproven). |
| Supportive | Pre- and postoperative analgesia. Esophagostomy/gastrostomy tube if surgery involves head. Fluid therapy/appetite stimulants as needed. |

Like fibrosarcoma, this tumor most frequently invades bone,[10] but four cats appear to have had primary lesions; signalment was not complete for all cats. Three cats were older (12, 17, and 18 years of age), two were male, and one was a DSH.[23,51] Two cats had proximal humeral lesions, and one of these animals had extensive pulmonary metastases.[23] The third cat had a pathologic fracture of the proximal tibia, and the fourth was a 2-year-old female that had been experimentally exposed to radiation. This animal had pulmonary metastases from a femoral hemangiosarcoma and a separate femoral osteosarcoma.[13]

There are no reports of treatment for hemangiosarcoma of the bone in cats, mainly due to the presence of metastases at diagnosis. If metastases are present, amputation could only be considered to be palliative. Chemotherapy may be an option, but owners should be made aware of the grave prognosis if macroscopic metastatic disease is present. Adjuvant chemotherapy should be offered for cats in which the tumor has not visibly spread. Readers are referred to the section on hemangiosarcoma in Chapter 42 for information regarding chemotherapy options.

OTHER BONE TUMORS

CLINICAL BRIEFING

More details for each tumor type may be found in the relevant chapters.

FIBROSARCOMA

Incidence, Signalment, and Etiology

There have been reports of 24 fibrosarcomas included in reviews of feline bone tumors, but most appear to involve bone by extension and invasion rather than as a primary tumor. The majority of these tumors affected the maxilla, mandible, or other areas of the oral cavity.[10,23] Less commonly, the digits,[10] carpus,[5,10,52] or the ribs, humerus, sacrum, or scapula[10,23,26] were affected.

MDB = minimum database; includes CBC, biochemical profile, urinalysis, FeLV/FIV serology, T_4 testing, and thoracic radiographs (three views).

There appear to be reports of only four cats with primary fibrosarcoma of bone: a 13-year-old spayed female DSH with a proximal femoral lesion,[4] an 11-year-old male with a humeral lesion,[23] a 9.5-year-old castrated male DLH with a distal ulnar tumor,[53] and a cat in which fibrosarcoma occurred at the site of a Jonas intramedullary splint 6 months after fixation and 1 month after removal of the device from the femur.[54]

Clinical Presentation and History

Clinical signs are related to the location of the primary tumor and the presence of metastatic disease. All four cats described above were lame, and the cat with the humeral lesion had a pathologic fracture and had been lame for 18 months.[23] One cat had metastases to the iliac lymph nodes and lungs at the time of diagnosis,[4] but no metastases were described for the other three cats.

Staging and Diagnosis

A histologic diagnosis should be obtained by biopsy; however, care should be taken in interpreting needle biopsies from bone tumors in cats since fibrosarcomatous areas may predominate in osteosarcoma. Staging should determine the extent of the primary and metastatic disease if present and ascertain the condition of the patient. Based on the limited data available, the regional lymph nodes should be carefully assessed in addition to collecting an MDB.

Treatment

Surgery is the treatment of choice. Adjunctive therapy such as radiation or chemotherapy depends on the tumor location and confirmation of the diagnosis. A combination of surgery, radiation therapy, and chemotherapy appears to result in the best outcomes for cats with soft-tissue sarcomas (see Chapter 51). Two of the cats reported in

MANAGEMENT OF SPECIFIC DISEASES

the literature were treated by amputation. One had no recurrence or evidence of metastasis 18 months after surgery,[53] and the other died of unknown causes 6 months after surgery.[54]

SQUAMOUS CELL CARCINOMA

Squamous cell carcinoma (SCC) frequently invades the bones of the skull from an oral mucosal tumor, and it may mimic a primary bone tumor by causing a massive cortical bony reaction.[55] SCC is also reported to invade the digits.[10,23] Further discussion is provided in the chapters on gastrointestinal tumors and skin tumors (Chapters 41 and 50, respectively).

KEY POINT

A bony swelling of the mandible is more likely to be SCC than osteosarcoma.

SYNOVIAL TUMORS

CLINICAL BRIEFING

Common Presentation	Rare tumor in cats; invasive.
Staging and Diagnosis	MDB and regional radiographs of the affected area. Lymph node palpation with fine-needle aspiration and biopsy if enlarged.
Treatment	
Initial	Amputation.
Adjunctive	Radiation therapy as for soft tissue sarcomas if excision is incomplete or surgery is not possible. Chemotherapy unproven, but doxorubicin or carboplatin could be considered.
Supportive	Pre- and postoperative analgesia. Esophagostomy/gastrostomy tube if surgery involves the head. Fluid therapy/appetite stimulants as needed.

Incidence, Signalment, and Etiology

There have been only seven reported cases of mesenchymal tumors arising from the synovium. In reading the descriptions, it is hard to clinically distinguish between many of these tumors and soft tissue sarcomas. Bony invasion was reported in three cats—one with a tumor in the tibiotarsal joint,[2] one with a tumor in the carpus,[56] and one with a tumor in the elbow.[57] Ages of reported cats ranged from 6 to 16 years (median, 18 years); four were male (three of which were castrated), and one was a spayed female.[58] For the four cats in which breed was recorded, three were DSHs and one was a British shorthair.[57–59]

Clinical Presentation and History

The presenting complaint in four cats was swelling or a mass that affected the foot,[18] the extensor aspect proximal to the front paw,[59] or the foreleg from elbow to carpus.[34] A swelling of the toe in the right hind foot was ulcerated in one cat.[58] Lameness was the presenting complaint in the three cats with bony involvement. The duration of signs was 2 months in one cat,[57] 12 months in another cat,[56] and 15 months in the third cat.[2]

Staging and Diagnosis

Because of the lack of specific information about the biologic behavior of this tumor, regional radiographs, an MDB, and a histologic biopsy should be obtained prior to the definitive surgery to assist in directing therapy. In select circumstances, an excisional biopsy may be recommended if the results will not alter therapy or the client's willingness to treat the animal.

No metastases were noted in any of the reported cats, including one with a 15 month history[2] and one that was treated for 18 months.[59] A cat with a synovial sarcoma developed metastases after amputation[b] (Figure 38-24).

Treatment

Local excision is unlikely to be successful in cats with synovial tumors as they appear to commonly invade surrounding tissue, similar to other soft tissue sarcomas. Amputation is the preferred treatment; if this is not an option, excisional surgery followed by radiation therapy (as described in Chapter 51) may improve local tumor control. Chemotherapy is unproven, but doxorubicin or carboplatin may be beneficial.

[b]Moore AS: Personal observation.

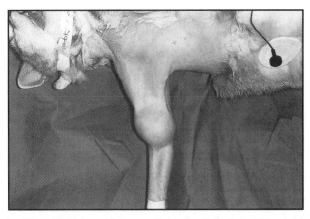

Figure 38-24: *Synovial sarcoma affecting the elbow of a cat. This tumor metastasized to the regional lymph node and lungs.*

Surgery was the only treatment in four reported cats. Amputation was performed in one cat with an elbow lesion, and there was no evidence of tumor 8 months later.[57] Toe amputation in one cat was unsuccessful; the tumor recurred locally 3 months after surgery, at which time the animal was euthanized.[58] In the third cat, local excision of a carpal tumor was performed twice in 18 months, with recurrences at 7 months after the first surgery and 4 months after the second.[59] Another cat had no evidence of tumor recurrence 7 months after local excision.[60]

Supportive Care

Analgesia and nutritional support should be employed.

REFERENCES

1. Cotchin E: Further examples of spontaneous neoplasms in the domestic cat. *Br Vet J* 112:263–272, 1956.
2. Engle GC, Brodey RS: A retrospective study of 395 feline neoplasms. *JAAHA* 5:21–31, 1969.
3. Patnaik AK, Liu S-K, Hurvitz AI, McClelland AJ: Nonhematopoietic neoplasms in cats. *J Natl Cancer Inst* 54:855–860, 1975.
4. Carpenter JL, Andrews LK, Holzworth J: Tumors and tumor-like lesions, in Holzworth J (ed): *Diseases of the Cat. Medicine and Surgery.* Philadelphia, WB Saunders, 1987, pp 407–596.
5. Nielsen SW: Neoplastic diseases, in Catcott EJ (ed): *Feline Medicine and Surgery.* Santa Barbara, CA, American Veterinary Publications, 1964, pp 156–176.
6. Schmidt RE, Langham RF: A survey of feline neoplasms. *JAVMA* 151:1325–1328, 1967.
7. Bitetto WV, Patnaik AK, Schrader SC, Mooney SC: Osteosarcoma in cats: 22 cases (1974–1984). *JAVMA* 190:91–93, 1987.
8. Madewell BR, Leighton RL, Theilen GH: Amputation and doxorubicin for treatment of canine and feline osteogenic sarcoma. *Europ J Cancer* 14:287–293, 1978.
9. Turrel JM, Pool RR: Primary bone tumors in the cat: A retrospective study of 15 cats and literature review. *Vet Radiol* 23:152–166, 1982.
10. Liu S-K, Dorfman HD, Patnaik AK: Primary and secondary bone tumours in the cat. *J Small Anim Pract* 15:141–156, 1974.
11. Kessler M, Tassani-Prell M, von Bomhard D, Matis U: Das osteosarkom der katze: epidemiologische, klinische und röntgenologische befunde bei 78 tieren (1990–1995). *Tierärztl Prax* 25:275–283, 1997.
12. Heldman E, Anderson MA, Wagner-Mann C: Feline osteosarcoma: 145 cases (1990–1995). *JAAHA* 36:518–521, 2000.
13. Berman E, Wright JF: What is your diagnosis? *JAVMA* 162:1065–1066, 1973.
14. Fry PD, Jukes HF: Fracture associated sarcoma in the cat. *J Small Anim Pract* 36:124–126, 1995.
15. Stubbs EL: Osteogenic chondrosarcoma in a cat. *JAVMA* 79:644–646, 1931.
16. Popp JA, Simpson CF: Feline malignant giant cell tumor of bone associated with C-type virus particles. *Cornell Vet* 66:528–535, 1976.
17. Howard EB, Kenyon AJ: Malignant osteoclastoma (giant cell tumor) in the cat with associated mast-cell response. *Cornell Vet* 57:398–409, 1967.
18. McClelland RB: A giant-cell tumor of the tibia in a cat. *Cornell Vet* 31:86–87, 1941.
19. Thornburg LP: Giant cell tumor of bone in a cat. *Vet Pathol* 16:255–257, 1979.
20. Bennett D, Campbell JR, Brown P: Osteosarcoma associated with healed fractures. *J Small Anim Pract* 20:13–18, 1979.
21. Thrasher JP, Riser WH: What is your diagnosis? *JAVMA* 141:1501–1502, 1962.
22. Goncalves M, Baptista R: Sarcoma osteogenico em felino. *Rep Trab* 14:63–66, 1982.
23. Quigley PJ, Leedale AH: Tumors involving bone in the domestic cat: A review of fifty-eight cases. *Vet Pathol* 20:670–686, 1983.
24. Purdy JG: Osteogeneic sarcoma in a cat. *Can Vet J* 2:156, 1961.
25. Thamm DH, MacEwen EG, Chun R, et al: Phase I clinical trial of Doxil, a stealth liposome encapsulated doxorubicin, in cats with malignant tumors. *Proc 17th Annu Conf Vet Cancer Soc:38,* 1997.
26. Trout NJ, Pavletic MM, Kraus KH: Partial scapulectomy for management of sarcomas in three dogs and two cats. *JAVMA* 207:585–587, 1995.
27. Lord PF, Kapp DS, Schwartz A, Morrow DT: Osteogenic sarcoma of the nasal cavity in a cat: Postoperative control with high dose-per-fraction radiation therapy and metronidazole. *Vet Radiol* 23:23–26, 1982.
28. Wolvekamp WThC, Boor-vd Putten IME, Gruys E: Wat is uw diagnose? *Tijdschr Diergeneesk* 101:1393–1397, 1976.
29. O'Brien D, Parker AJ, Tarvin G: Osteosarcoma of the vertebra causing compression of the thoracic spinal cord in a cat. *JAAHA* 16:497–499, 1980.
30. Levy MS, Mauldin G, Kapatkin AS, Patnaik AK: Nonlymphoid vertebral canal tumors in cats: 11 cases (1987–1995). *JAVMA* 5:663–664, 1997.
31. Griffith JW, Dubielzig RR, Riser WH, Jezyk P: Parosteal osteosarcoma with pulmonary metastases in a cat. *Vet Pathol* 21:123–125, 1984.
32. Banks WC: Parosteal osteosarcoma in a dog and a cat. *JAVMA* 158:1412–1415, 1971.
33. Pool RR: Tumors of bone and cartilage, in Moulton JE (ed): *Tumors in Domestic Animals.* Berkeley, University of California, 1990, pp 157–230.
34. Nielsen SW: Extraskeletal giant cell tumor in a cat. *Cornell Vet* 42:304–311, 1952.
35. Alexander JW, Riis RC, Dueland R: Extraskeletal giant cell tumor in a cat. *Vet Med Small Anim Clin* 70:1161–1166, 1975.
36. Whitehead JE: Neoplasia in the cat. *Vet Med Small Anim Clin* 357–358, 1967.
37. Knecht CD, Greene JA: Osteoma of the zygomatic arch in a cat. *JAVMA* 171:1077–1078, 1977.
38. Jabara AG, Paton JS: Extraskeletal osteoma in a cat. *Aust Vet J* 61:405–407, 1984.
39. Shell L, Sponenberg P: Chondrosarcoma in a cat presenting with forelimb monoparalysis. *Comp Small Anim* 9:391–398, 1987.
40. Hinko PJ, Burt JK, Fetter AW: Chondrosarcoma in the femur of a cat. *JAAHA* 15:737–739, 1979.
41. Brown NO, Patnaik AK, Mooney SC, et al: Soft tissue sarcomas in the cat. *JAVMA* 173:744–779, 1978.
42. Alden CL, Helzer LL: Humeral chondrosarcoma in a cat. *Modern Vet Pract* 214–216, 1981.
43. Morton D: Chondrosarcoma arising in a multilobular chondroma in a cat. *JAVMA* 186:804–806, 1985.
44. Herron ML: The musculoskeletal system, in Catcott EJ (ed): *Feline Medicine and Surgery,* ed 2. Santa Barbara, CA, American Veterinary Publications, 1975, pp 355–361.
45. Butler R, Wrigley RH, Horsey R, Reuter R: Chondrosarcoma in a Sumatran tiger *(Panthera tigris sumatrae).* *J Zoo Anim Med* 12:80–84, 1981.
46. Brown RJ, Trevethan WP, Henry VL: Multiple osteochondroma in a Siamese cat. *JAVMA* 160:433–435, 1972.
47. Riddle WE, Leighton RL: Osteochondromatosis in a cat. *JAVMA* 156:1428–1430, 1970.
48. Doige CE: Multiple osteochondromas with evidence of malignant transformation in a cat. *Vet Pathol* 24:457–459, 1987.
49. Pool RR, Harris JM: Feline osteochondromatosis. *Feline Pract* 5:24–30, 1975.
50. Pool RR, Carrig CB: Multiple cartilaginous exostoses in a cat. *Vet Pathol* 9:350–359, 1972.
51. Witt C: What is your diagnosis? *JAVMA* 185:451–452, 1984.

52. Cook JL, Turk JR, Tomlinson JL, et al: Fibrosarcoma in the distal radius and carpus of a four-year-old Persian. *JAAHA* 34:31–33, 1998.

53. Tischler SA, Owens JM: Ulnar fibrosarcoma in a cat. *Modern Vet Pract* 67:39, 1986.

54. Sinibaldi KR, Pugh J, Rosen H, Liu S-K: Osteomyelitis and neoplasia associated with use of the Jonas intramedullary splint in small animals. *JAVMA* 181:885–890, 1982.

55. Madewell BR, Ackerman N, Sesline DH: Invasive carcinoma radiographically mimicking primary bone cancer in the mandibles of two cats. *Cancer* 17:213–215, 1976.

56. Bornstein N, Fayolle P, Moissonnier P: What is your diagnosis? *J Small Anim Pract* 40:205–207, 1999.

57. Silva-Krott IU, Tucker RL, Meeks JC: Synovial sarcoma in a cat. *JAVMA* 203:1430–1431, 1993.

58. Davies JD, Little NRF: Synovioma in a cat. *J Small Anim Pract* 13:127–133, 1972.

59. Hulse EV: A benign giant-cell synovioma in a cat. *J Pathol Bact* 91:269–271, 1966.

60. Thoday KL, Evans JG: Letters to the editor. *J Small Anim Pract* 13:399–402, 1972.

NERVOUS SYSTEM TUMORS

Antony S. Moore and Gregory K. Ogilvie

39

The wide range of cell types found within the central nervous system (CNS) can give rise to an equally wide range of tumors. In feline medicine, obtaining a histologic diagnosis prior to necropsy was once rare and the determination of tumor type was often made solely for academic interest. This trend appears to be changing. With advances in imaging, surgical, and radiation techniques, many CNS tumors are being diagnosed and managed, which has significantly improved survival times. Because of its location and accessibility for biopsy and surgical management, feline meningioma is one such disease.

Tumors of the nervous system are rare in cats, although brain tumors are more common than spinal tumors. Nervous system tumors rarely metastasize; their effects occur as a result of expansion and displacement or destruction of surrounding nervous tissue. Signs may therefore be mild and overlooked by owners until the advent of more serious neurologic disturbances, such as seizures or paresis.

Several good general reviews on CNS tumors and imaging techniques to detect them can be found in the veterinary literature.[1-4] Discussions of computed tomography (CT) and magnetic resonance imaging (MRI) are covered in excellent detail by Kornegay.[5] Details regarding the use of planar brain scintigraphy are found elsewhere.[6] While cerebrospinal fluid (CSF) cytology is rarely diagnostic, a sedimentation technique appeared to increase the diagnostic yield in one study.[7]

BRAIN TUMORS

Brain tumors that have been described in cats include meningioma, gliomas (oligodendroglioma), ependymoma, medulloblastoma, choroid plexus papilloma, and astrocytoma. In this book, pituitary gland tumors are included in Chapter 44.

It should be remembered that cats with nasal tumors may occasionally present with neurologic signs due to erosion of the cribriform plate.[8,9] This form of tumor progression was seen in two cats with esthesioneuroblastoma of the olfactory epithelium.[10] See Chapter 47 for more information about nasal tumors.

KEY POINT

Invasive nasal tumors may cause neurologic signs even in the absence of nasal symptoms.

Brain tumors can have both primary and secondary effects that lead to neurologic signs (see Box on next page). These signs are frequently sufficient to localize the suspected tumor to the spinal cord or a region of the brain, but diagnostic imaging is required to determine the precise anatomic location.

MENINGIOMA

CLINICAL BRIEFING

Common Presentation	Usually solitary; multiple in 20% of cats. Most common in older male cats. Usually affects the cerebral meninges; falcine and basilar locations are rare. Slow growing, but signs may appear acutely. Behavior changes are most common, although weakness, circling, and visual deficits may also occur. Seizures are rare.
Staging and Diagnosis	MDB; skull radiographs only if CT or MRI is not available. Metastases are extremely rare.
Treatment	
Initial	Surgical excision for superficial lesions provides long-term (>2 years) survival. Second surgery possible for recurrence.
Adjunctive	Radiation therapy may reduce recurrence rate and may be used for falcine or basilar tumors. Chemotherapy not warranted, although CCNU is potentially useful (unproven) if other options are unavailable.
Supportive	Postoperative antiinflammatories and analgesics. Appetite stimulants and nutritional support as necessary.

Effects of Brain Tumors[11]

Primary Effects
- Infiltration of nervous tissue
- Compression of adjacent structures

Secondary Effects
- Hydrocephalus
- Disruption of cerebral circulation
- Disturbance of CSF flow
- Elevated intracranial pressure
- Cerebral edema and/or inflammation
- Brain herniation

Incidence, Signalment, and Etiology

Meningiomas are the most common brain tumor in cats and may arise from the meninges anywhere in the brain. They are usually solitary, although multiple tumors are seen in approximately 20% of cats. They are rarely reported in cats younger than 6 years of age,[10,12-15] and the median age in larger studies is 12 years.[12,13,16] On occasion, very old cats (>20 years) are diagnosed with meningioma,[13,16] and it is likely that many older cats have meningiomas that are not causing clinical signs. In three studies, 141 cats with meningiomas were identified at necropsy although only 68 of these cats had clinical signs referable to the nervous system.[10,13,15] These tumors were often tiny ("meningeal whorls") and occurred in the same areas as larger, more clinically relevant tumors.[10,14]

MDB = minimum database; includes CBC, biochemical profile, urinalysis, FeLV/FIV serology, T_4 testing, and thoracic radiographs (three views).

A notable exception to the average age incidence for meningiomas in cats is the occurrence of multiple meningiomas in four of seven cats between 2 and 3 years of age with mucopolysaccharidosis-I deficiency.[15] The tumors were small and did not cause clinical signs. They possibly arose in areas of meningeal fibroplasia caused by the storage disease.

Although not consistent in all studies, males appear to be predisposed to develop meningiomas.[10,12,13,16-18] Of 191 cats reported with meningioma, 123 were male and 68 were female.[8,10,12,13,15-21] DSHs are most commonly affected, with DLHs much less frequently reported. Except for Persians,[12,13] purebred cats are rarely reported; Siamese,[12,13,17] Maine Coon,[12,16] Manx,[20] Russian Blue,[14] and Abyssinian[22] cats appear only occasionally in reports.

Clinical Presentation and History

Most meningiomas are located in the cerebral meninges above the temporal, frontal, parietal, or occipital regions of the brain. Tumors affecting the falcine area are less common, and basilar tumors are even more rare. Occasionally, a meningioma will be located in the third or lateral ventricle or adjacent to the cerebellum. Spinal meningiomas are rare (see Spinal Cord Tumors section).

> **KEY POINT**
>
> *Approximately 20% of cats with meningioma have more than one tumor.*

Cats with meningiomas can have any number of clinical signs as a result of pressure on the CNS beneath the tumor. Meningiomas are slow-growing, and clinical signs, while occasionally acute,[12,22] have usually been present for weeks, months, or even years.[12,13,17] In one study of 42 cats, the median duration of signs was 5 weeks.[12] Behavioral abnormalities are reported most commonly. Owners may describe nonspecific signs such as lethargy, depression, dullness, inactivity, or inappetence. More specific signs, including increased aggression (or rarely, increased affection), disorientation, hiding, staring at the wall, increased vocalization, crouched posture, inappropriate elimination habits, increased sleeping, decreased grooming, and decreased jumping, have also been reported.

The most common signs reported by owners are changes in vision. While some cats may become blind,[22,23] visual deficits are often less severe. In two studies, 48 of 52 cats had visual deficits[12,17] and the majority of cats had bilateral deficits. Circling was another common clinical sign in studies, occurring in approximately 50% of affected cats.[12,13,17] Circling was accompanied by nystagmus in many of these cats, but head tilt was rare. Seizures are less commonly reported, occurring in approximately 20% of cats with meningioma.[12,13,16,17] Although seizures are rare, even small tumors may cause epileptogenic foci due to compression of cerebral tissue.[21]

> **KEY POINT**
>
> *Paresis of one or more limbs is a common clinical sign in cats with meningioma.*

Paresis, usually tetraparesis, occurs in 60% to 80% of cats[12,13]; other gait abnormalities such as ataxia are less common. In one study of 42 cats, tetraparesis was most common (15 cats); monoparesis (10), hemiparesis (6), and paraparesis (4) were less commonly seen.[12] Cranial nerve deficits, commonly affecting cranial nerves V and VII, are noted in 20% or more of cats. Nasal and thoracic wall hyperesthesia were equally common, occurring in approximately 45% of cats.[12]

Acute collapse is rarely seen, but cats will occasionally present decerebrate or in opisthotonus.[12] Meningioma should be considered a likely diagnosis in older cats with weakness, visual deficits, and gait abnormalities, particularly if accompanied by behavioral changes.

Staging and Diagnosis

It is very important to determine the location of a meningioma to plan treatment options for the cat. While neurologic examination may help to localize the lesion within the brain, additional diagnostics are necessary to differentiate neoplasia from other causes of CNS disease. Following a complete neurologic evaluation and examination of the ocular fundus, it is important to pursue imaging techniques for further localization and diagnosis. While most cats have a solitary tumor, multiple meningiomas have been reported in 53 of 266 cats (20%).[8,10,12–18,24]

Radiographs of the skull often appear normal, although hyperostotic, sclerotic lesions may be seen in some cats. The occurrence of these radiographic findings ranges from 40%[16] to 90%[17] of cats. Occasionally, bony lysis of the calvarium will be seen on radiographs.[10,13,17] In one cat the tumor grew out of the calvarium to produce a visible mass.[24] No other brain tumor in cats is expected to cause these radiographic changes.

CSF analysis may be performed but is never diagnostic for meningioma. A mild increase in protein[20] is a nonspecific finding and only suggests an inflammatory process. Electroencephalography (EEG) was successful in localizing the lesion in 5 of 10 affected cats.[17,20]

Planar brain scintigraphy using technetium glucoheptonate has rarely been used. Focal accumulation of the technetium is commonly seen in meningiomas.[6] The widespread availability and superior image quality of CT makes scintigraphy a less appealing option.

Advanced imaging techniques are required for diagnosis and follow-up management of the meningioma patient. Both CT and MRI are helpful, with MRI being the preferred technique and most complete method of visualization, particularly for cerebellar or brainstem lesions in cats. In the cerebrum, CT scanning will often demonstrate the tumor without the need to use contrast agents and allows clinicians to plan appropriate therapy (Figure 39-1). Potentially complicating factors such as hydrocephalus, thickening of the calvarium, or bony lysis are easily identified.[5,8,12,16,19,20] A meningioma most often appears as a superficial space-occupying cerebral lesion in broad-based contact with the calvarium. Such a tumor, rather than one occupying a deep basilar location, is amenable to surgery (Figure 39-2).

> ### KEY POINT
> *CT and MRI scanning are the imaging modalities of choice for meningioma.*

MRI (as explained in detail by Kornegay[5]), is superior to CT scanning for lesions associated with the cerebellum and brainstem.[11] It is difficult to obtain good quality CT images of these locations in cats. Fortunately, MRI is becoming more widely available for veterinary use.[5,22,25] On MRI images, a tumor may be provisionally diagnosed as a meningioma by its location and associated calvarium changes and also if a "dural-tail sign" (i.e., the appearance of a linear enhancement of the dura mater adjacent to a gadolinium [Gd-DTPA] enhancing mass) is present. This tail likely represents tumor extension or a reactive thickened dura mater.[25]

Although metastases appear to be rare, this does not preclude the need for a complete staging procedure, including the MDB. Metastasis has been described in only one 10-

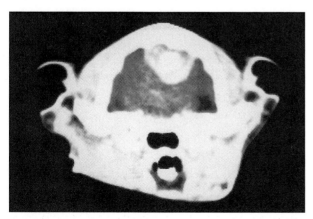

Figure 39-1: *CT allows localization of a brain tumor prior to surgery. A broad-based peripheral mass is most likely a meningioma, as seen in this CT scan. (Courtesy of A. Tidwell)*

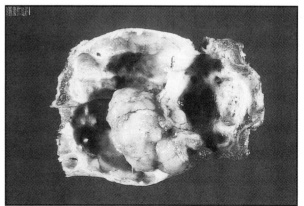

Figure 39-2: *This large, ventrally located meningioma was not able to be resected. Radiation therapy may be an appropriate treatment option for tumors in similar locations that are difficult to access surgically.*

year-old cat, which was reported to have developed miliary lung metastases with pleural effusion along with renal and uterine metastases.[26] Due to the geriatric nature of most patients with suspected meningioma, complete staging is more important to rule in/out concurrent disease. Thoracic radiographs should be obtained to identify metastases as well as to look for any concurrent disease. In addition, radiographs will help to rule in/out metastatic disease from another primary tumor as a differential for CNS lesions.

Treatment

If the location of the tumor allows surgical access, surgery is the treatment of choice for meningioma in cats. Corticosteroids rarely provide palliation of signs, perhaps because the tumor grows slowly, and inflammatory changes are minimal. Seizures may temporarily resolve in cats treated with prednisone,[16] but most cats do not appreciably improve, particularly those that are blind.[19,20,22] Phenobarbital may be necessary to control seizures prior to surgery in some cats.[16]

Meningiomas may be quite large (up to 15 cm³ in one study[12]), and a hemicraniectomy may be required.[17] This type of defect may be strengthened postoperatively by the use of an artificial mesh. The use of a bone burr will facilitate removal of the meningioma and attached dura (Figures 39-3 and 39-4); CT localization will assist in planning an appropriate approach.

Postoperative complications include brain herniation due to an unsuspected second meningioma[16] or more commonly to excessive bleeding and cerebral edema. Herniation is recognized clinically as a rapidly deteriorating neurologic status within 24 hours of surgery and is uniformly fatal.[12,16,17] The incidence of herniation in studies is 10% to 20%.[12,16,17]

Despite the minimal neurologic improvement in cats treated with corticosteroids, preoperative dexamethasone or prednisolone sodium succinate (25–50 mg/kg IV) appears to reduce postoperative inflammation. In addition, hyperventilation (16–18 breaths/min) during anesthesia decreases carbon dioxide concentration, thereby reducing cerebral blood flow, which in turn can help to reduce "brain swelling" and resultant postoperative complications.[16,19]

Intraoperative bleeding may be severe enough to cause anemia. In one study, 13 of 42 cats became anemic due to bleeding and 4 of the 13 required a blood transfusion.[12] A technique of autologous transfusion has been described in which the cat donates 60 ml of blood 1 to 2 weeks before surgery. Cats that receive their own blood during surgery have a decreased risk of transfusion reaction.[27]

Overall, complications resulted in the postoperative death of 12 of 69 cats (17%) in three studies.[12,16,17] Thus careful hemostasis during surgery as well as perioperative management and postoperative care are mandatory for cats undergoing surgery for treatment of a meningioma.

KEY POINT

With careful hemostasis and postoperative care, long-term survival is likely for cats treated surgically for a meningioma.

Neurologic improvement is generally quite rapid following surgery, and most cats can be released to their owners within 5 days (Figure 39-5). Most reported behavioral changes resolve within a week.[16,17,19,20] Visual deficits will also usually resolve rapidly,[17] although some degree of residual impairment was seen in 11 of 31 cats in one study.[12] Visual deficits actually worsened in some cats after surgery, with complete unilateral loss of vision reported in two cats that had partial vision before surgery[17] and in one cat with contralateral blindness.[16] Nystagmus took 6 months to resolve in one cat.[16] Seizures usually resolve rapidly and did so in all six cats in one study.[12] Seizures persisted in another cat after surgery, and phenobarbital treatment was required.[17]

Survival times appear to be very long for cats that survive to be discharged to their owners. Survival beyond 1 year is

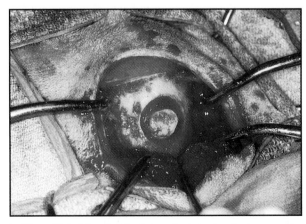

Figure 39-3: A bone burr has been used to incise the calvarium around a small dorsally located meningioma. (Courtesy of K. Kraus)

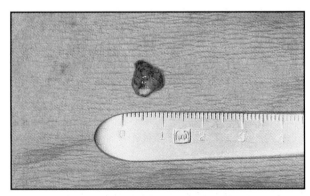

Figure 39-4: The meningioma from the cat in Figure 39-3 has been completely removed. Even small tumors like this can cause neurologic signs. (Courtesy of K. Kraus)

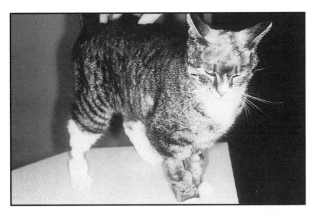

Figure 39-5: A cat 3 days after surgery for meningioma. This surgery is usually associated with an excellent outcome. (Courtesy of J. Berg)

common.[8,16,17,19,20,28] The median survival for cats that were released from the hospital was 22 months, with 66% of the cats alive 1 year and 50% 2 years after surgery.[12]

In two large studies, long-term follow-up information was available for 47 cats.[12,16] Tumor recurrence was confirmed (or suspected due to recurrence of neurologic signs) in 13 cats 1.3 to 69 months after surgery. Interestingly, 2 cats had a new meningioma rather than recurrence[12] and 1 cat had recurrence and an additional pituitary carcinoma.[16] Factors such as tumor location, number of tumors, and age of the cat were not predictive of length of survival in one study.[12]

Cats should be monitored every 3 months for the first year after surgery and every 6 months thereafter. Recurrence of neurologic signs should be investigated as probable tumor recurrence, and a CT or MRI scan should be performed.

A second surgery was performed at the time of tumor recurrence in two cats. One died during surgery,[16] but the other had a second remission of 12 months (first remission lasted 34 months).[12] This would imply that second surgeries may be indicated in select cats that appear to be good anesthetic candidates with no other concurrent disease.

Radiation therapy should be considered in cats that have an incompletely resected meningioma or a surgically inaccessible tumor. Radiation therapy has been reported to successfully treat meningiomas,[11] but detailed reports are not available.

Chemotherapy has not been investigated for this tumor and is not recommended as follow-up or adjunctive therapy due to the low chance of metastasis. If other treatment options such as surgery or radiation therapy are unavailable, CCNU may provide palliation. This drug has anecdotal efficacy for treatment of brain tumors in dogs, but there is currently no information about its use in cats.

NONDOMESTIC FELIDAE

A meningioma was reported in a cheetah (*Acinonyx jubatus jubatus*).[29]

▶ OTHER BRAIN TUMORS

CLINICAL BRIEFING

Common Presentation	Ependymoma, oligodendroglioma, and astrocytoma are the other common tumor types seen in cats. Vestibular signs, weakness, and ataxia are common; seizures are less common.
Staging and Diagnosis	MDB; CT scan helps differentiate from meningioma on basis of tumor location. MRI may be useful for brainstem or cerebellar lesions. Metastases not reported.
Treatment Initial	Because of tumor location, surgery alone is rarely successful. Radiation therapy, alone or following surgery, is the treatment of choice. Long-term survival is possible with ependymoma; survival times for cats with other tumor types are not reported.
Adjunctive	CCNU chemotherapy may be palliative but is unproven in cats.
Supportive	Antiinflammatories or antiseizure medication postoperatively or adjunctively with radiation. Appetite stimulants and supportive care should be administered as needed.

EPENDYMOMA

Incidence, Signalment, and Etiology

The majority of reports of ependymoma in cats are pathology surveys. This tumor has been reported in cats ranging in age from 18 months to 12 years.[10,24,30–33] Most affected cats have been DSHs; one Burmese[30] and two Siamese[10,32] have been reported. One cat was FeLV positive.[32]

Ependymomas arise from the wall of the ventricles. Of 14 cats in which the tumor location was known, six tumors involved the lateral ventricles, five involved the third ventricle, and three involved the fourth ventricle.[10,24,30,34,35]

Clinical Presentation and History

Ependymomas can be quite large and may grow rapidly, as suggested by central necrosis seen on histopathology in some tumors[33] and the short duration of clinical signs (<2 weeks) in most cats.[32–34]

Interference with CSF distribution can lead to hydrocephalus, blindness, disorientation, and incoordination or tetraparesis with normal spinal reflexes.[30,34,35] Vestibular signs may predominate.[31–33] More severe signs of stupor and semicoma may progress to death if herniation occurs.[10,30,35]

Staging and Diagnosis

MRI or CT scan will demonstrate enlargement of ventricles; with contrast enhancement, a mass lesion is usually well demarcated.[30,31] Metastases are not reported, although clusters of malignant cells were found in the CSF of one cat, implying that metastasis by this route may be possible.[32] Therefore an MDB and brain imaging should be pursued to investigate the potential for underlying diseases and to evaluate the extent of the tumor.

KEY POINT

Surgery followed by radiation therapy may allow long survival times in cats with ependymoma.

Treatment

Treatment of ependymoma involves surgery (when indicated), radiation, and supportive or palliative care. Surgery has been described as treatment for two cats with ependymoma. Surgical excision of a tumor that was beneath the cerebellum resulted in worsening clinical signs for 2 weeks before complete recovery occurred.[31] The cat was still normal 2 years later. Similarly, a small (5 × 8 mm) ependymoma was removed from the third ventricle of a cat using a unilateral rostral tentorial craniotomy and suction aspiration. Although postoperative anticonvulsant therapy was required, the cat remained normal for 7 months after surgery.[34]

Surgical excision of an ependymoma followed by radiation therapy resulted in a survival time exceeding 8 months in another cat.[28] Radiation therapy alone (total dose, 36–48 Gy) was used to treat two other cats with papillary ependymoma.[30] One of these cats was still alive 14 months later, while the other initially improved neurologically before regressing 3 weeks after treatment. Prednisone after radiation therapy failed to provide long-term control in this second cat, and the animal was euthanized. Corticosteroids did not improve clinical signs in a cat with an ependymoma[32] but caused dramatic short-term improvement prior to surgical excision in another cat.[34]

GLIOMA (OLIGODENDROGLIOMA)

Incidence, Signalment, and Etiology

Gliomas are rare in cats, although 4 of 10 brain tumors in cats were glial in origin in one study (the other 6 were meningiomas).[36] This high incidence rate does not seem to have been repeated in other studies.[10] Signalment was reported in two cats; both were middle-aged castrated males (one Persian and one DLH).[8,37]

Clinical Presentation and History

Neurologic signs are similar to those seen in cats with other brain tumors. Although one cat had no neurologic signs,[38] other cats have been reported to show hemiparesis, head tilt, circling, and ataxia.[37,39] Another cat had a 1 year history of aggressive behavior and seizures.[8] Two cats with brainstem lesions had cerebellar signs.[40]

Staging and Diagnosis

Predictably, radiographs of the skull are not useful in diagnosing this tumor,[37] and CT or MRI is the preferred imaging technique.[8] Circulating malignant cells could be seen on cytologic examination of CSF in two cats with oligodendroglioma of the brainstem.[40] CSF analysis may be performed (in addition to the MDB), although this procedure has been less helpful in diagnosing other tumor types.

Treatment

As for other types of brain tumors in cats, corticosteroids alone[37] or in combination with phenobarbital[8] resulted in poor, short-term (<2 months) control of signs before euthanasia. Radiation therapy is probably the treatment of choice, although there are no published reports of its efficacy in cats.

ASTROCYTOMA

Incidence, Signalment, and Etiology

Astrocytomas are uncommonly diagnosed tumors that have been shown to affect the frontal and parietal lobes of the cerebrum, the ventricular wall,[41] and the thalamus (Figure 39-6). The age of affected cats ranged from 2[10] to 12[5] years. One reported cat was a Persian.[5]

Clinical Presentation and History

As has been the case in cats with other types of brain tumors, one cat had no neurologic signs[38] while another showed abnormal behavior and hemiparesis for 2 weeks pri-

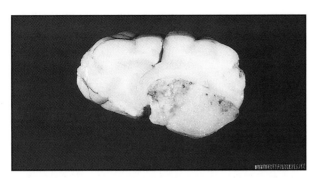

Figure 39-6: An astrocytoma causing necrosis and destruction of the cerebral cortex in a cat. Radiation therapy is the treatment of choice for this tumor.

or to presentation.[5] More chronic symptoms of blindness and behavior changes had been present for 2 months in another cat.[41]

Staging and Diagnosis

As for other brain tumors, CT and MRI are the imaging modalities of choice.

Treatment

No treatment has been described for these tumors in cats. Radiation therapy may be the best option.

MISCELLANEOUS BRAIN TUMORS

An intracranial teratoma caused progressive gait abnormality, visual impairment, depression, and finally tetraparesis in a 4-month-old DSH.[42] Seizures had been present for 1 month. There was obvious facial deformity due to a severe hydrocephalus caused by two large masses. A cerebellar medulloblastoma was diagnosed on necropsy in a 3-month-old kitten.[10]

SPINAL CORD TUMORS

Lymphoma is the most common tumor affecting the spinal cord and is described in Chapter 36. Osteosarcoma of the spine and other extradural tumors may invade or compress the spinal cord, and those tumors are discussed in Chapter 38. Primary spinal cord tumors are rare.

CLINICAL BRIEFING	
Common Presentation	Lymphoma is most common; other tumors are rare. Meningioma, ependymoma, astrocytoma, and sarcomas have been reported.
Staging and Diagnosis	MDB, spinal radiographs, myelogram. MRI if available. (Refer to Chapter 36 for lymphoma staging.) Metastasis is not reported, although lymphoma is often systemic.
Treatment Initial	Surgical excision of extradural or intradural extramedullary meningioma may be possible. Radiation is the primary therapy for intramedullary tumors.
Adjunctive	Radiation therapy may be useful following surgery for meningioma.
Supportive	Postoperative antiinflammatories and analgesics.

MENINGIOMA

Incidence, Signalment, and Etiology

Meningiomas more commonly affect the brain but have been described with variable amounts of clinical detail in the spine of 10 cats.[10,43–47] Three cats were DSHs, and one was a Persian; ages ranged from 6 to 17 years. Six lesions affected thoracic spinal cord sections (T2 in 1 cat and T12 in 2 cats; unspecified in others), and three meningiomas affected the cervical spinal cord. A lumbar lesion was noted in 1 cat.[46] In two studies with a total of 48 symptomatic cats, 3 had a spinal tumor and the other 45 had meningioma of the brain.[10,45]

Clinical Presentation and History

History and clinical signs are consistent with chronic or acute changes in spinal cord function. Hindlimb ataxia of 3 to 5 months' duration progressed to paraplegia in two cats (one with a T2 lesion and the other with a T12 lesion)[43,44] (Figure 39-7). A cat with a meningioma at the C6-C7 region had stable hindlimb paresis over 5 months despite receiving no treatment.[47]

KEY POINT

Lymphoma is the most common spinal cord tumor.

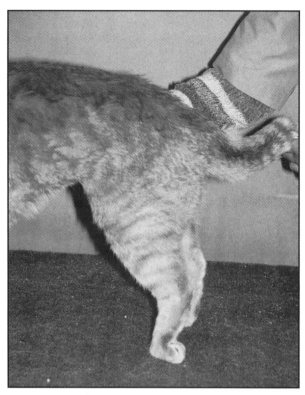

Figure 39-7: *Posterior paresis seen in a cat with a lumbar spinal tumor. The most common cause is extradural spinal lymphoma.*

Staging and Diagnosis

Plain radiographs are unlikely to show any lesion. Bony reaction, such as that occasionally associated with meningiomas in the brain, has not been reported for spinal meningioma.[43,44] Contrast myelogram may demonstrate a partial or complete disruption of the dye column and assist in localization, enabling surgeons to plan an appropriate surgical approach. MRI is superior to myelography or CT in its ability to visualize the tumor and provide information about its size and exact location. Reported spinal meningiomas range in size from 7 to 10 mm.[43,44]

Treatment

Surgery alone or in combination with radiation therapy (as for meningioma of the brain) is probably the treatment of choice. Tumors were completely (three cats) or incompletely (two cats) excised in five cats with histologically benign spinal meningioma of either the intradural-extramedullary space (four cats) or extradural space (one cat). Two of the five cats were euthanized within 2 months of surgery, but the other three lived 9 months to 4 years.[46] Recovery of neurologic function may be rapid: One cat was neurologically normal 5 days after surgery for a cervical meningioma.[47] Palliative therapy with corticosteroids is unlikely to result in significant clinical improvement.[44]

MDB = minimum database; includes CBC, biochemical profile, urinalysis, FeLV/FIV serology, T_4 testing, and thoracic radiographs (three views).

OTHER SPINAL CORD TUMORS

Ependymoma has been described in two cats. The first was 11 years old[48] and had a tumor that affected the cervical spine and caused tetraparesis.[48] The other was 4 years old[10] and had a tumor in the low lumbar spine that caused flaccid paraparesis.[10] No treatment was attempted in one cat, and the other responded briefly to corticosteroids.[10]

Astrocytoma was described in four cats ranging from 1 to 10 years of age, although three cats were 4 years of age or younger.[10,49] Clinical details were available for a 1-year-old Persian with neck pain and monoparesis progressing to hemiparesis. Necropsy revealed a cervical "astroblastoma."[49]

Mesenchymal tumors classified as neurolemmoma,[24] neurofibrosarcoma,[50] and primary sarcoma of the cord[51] have been reported, affecting the thoracic (T4), lumbar (L6), and cervical (C5-T1) cord sections, respectively. These tumors occurred in three DSHs (5 to 19 years of age). Two tumors[24,50] were very invasive, and there was radiographic evidence of lysis of the vertebra in one cat.[50] Signs of lameness and ataxia were acute in two cats.[50,51] Treatment was not described for any of these tumors.

TUMORS OF PERIPHERAL NERVES

Lymphoma is the most common tumor affecting the peripheral nerves in cats (refer to Chapter 36). The peripheral nerves were affected in 4 of 14 cats with CNS tumors.[36] These tumors appeared to derive from the nerve sheath and were classified as neurofibroma, Schwannoma, neuroma, and ganglioneuroma. No other details were available. A 10-year-old DSH had neurofibromatosis of the brachial plexus and caudal thoracic nerves.[10] No other details were available.

Treatment has not been reported for these tumors. Readers should refer to Chapter 51 for more information about nerve sheath tumors of other locations that may also apply here. A combination of surgery and radiation therapy is most likely to be effective.

NONDOMESTIC FELIDAE

A Schwannoma of the larynx in a lion *(Panthera leo)* is described in Chapter 47.[52]

REFERENCES

1. Moore MP, Bagley RS, Harrington ML, Gavin PR: Intracranial tumors. *Vet Clin North Am Small Anim Pract* 26:759–777, 1996.

2. Kraus KH, McDonnell J: Identification and management of brain tumors. *Semin Vet Med Surg (Small Anim)* 11:218–224, 1996.

3. Gavin PR, Fike JR, Hoopes PJ: Central nervous system tumors. *Semin Vet Med Surg (Small Anim)* 10:180–189, 1995

4. Kornegay JN: Central nervous system neoplasia, in Kornegay JN (ed): *Neurologic Disorders. Contemporary Issues in Small Animal Practice.* New York, Churchill Livingston, 1986, pp 79–108.

5. Kornegay JN: Imaging brain neoplasms. Computed tomography and magnetic resonance imaging. *Vet Med Report* 2:372–390, 1990.

6. Dykes NL, Warnick LD, Summers BA, et al: Retrospective analysis of brain scintigraphy in 116 dogs and cats. *Vet Radiol Ultrasound* 35:59–65, 1994.

7. Gevel V, Machus B: Diagnosing brain tumors with a CSF sedimentation technique. *Vet Med Report* 2:403–408, 1990.

8. LeCouteur RA, Fike JR, Cann CE, et al: X-ray computed tomography of brain tumors in cats. *JAVMA* 183:301–305, 1983.

9. Smith MO, Turrell JM, Bailey CS, Cain GR: Neurological abnormalities as the predominant signs of neoplasia of the nasal cavity in dogs and cats: Seven cases (1973–1986). *JAVMA* 195:242–245, 1989.

10. Carpenter JL, Andrews LK, Holzworth J: Tumors and tumor-like lesions, in Holzworth J (ed): *Diseases of the Cat. Medicine and Surgery.* Philadelphia, WB Saunders, 1987, pp 407–596.

11. LeCouter RA: Brain tumors of dogs and cats: Diagnosis and management. *Vet Med Report* 2:332–342, 1990.

12. Gordon LE, Thacher C, Matthiesen DT, Joseph RJ: Results of craniotomy for the treatment of cerebral meningioma in 42 cats. *Vet Surg* 23:94–100, 1994.

13. Nafe LA: Meningiomas in cats: A retrospective study of 36 cases. *JAVMA* 174:1224–1227, 1979.

14. Luginbuhl H: Studies on meningiomas in cats. *Am J Vet Res* 22:1030–1040, 1961.

15. Haskins ME, McGrath JT: Meningiomas in young cats with mucopolysaccharidosis. *J Neuropathol Exp Neurol* 42:664–670, 1983.

16. Gallagher JG, Berg J, Knowles KE, et al: Prognosis after surgical excision of cerebral meningiomas in cats: 17 cases (1986–1992). *JAVMA* 203:1437–1440, 1993.

17. Lawson DC, Burk RL, Prata RG: Cerebral meningioma in the cat: Diagnosis and surgical treatment of ten cases. *JAAHA* 20:333–342, 1984.

18. Smit JD: The lesions found at autopsy in dogs and cats which manifest clinical signs referable to the central nervous system. *J S Afr Vet Med Assoc* 32:47–55, 1961.

19. Fingeroth JM, Hansen B, Myer CW: Diagnosis and successful removal of a brain tumor in a cat. *Comp Anim Pract* 2:6–15, 1988.

20. Shell L, Colter SB, Blass CE, Ingram JT: Surgical removal of a meningioma in a cat after detection by computerized axial tomography. *JAAHA* 21:439–442, 1985.

21. Gonzalez OG, Purpura DP: Epileptogenic effects of an auditory cortex meningioma in a cat. *Cornell Vet* 49:374–379, 1959.

22. Grahn BH, Stewart WA, Towner RA, Noseworthy MD: Magnetic resonance imaging of the canine and feline eye, orbit, and optic nerves and its clinical application. *Can Vet J* 34:418–424, 1993.

23. Ertürk E, Urman HK, Imren HY: Kedide meningioma olayi. *Yazi Dergi Yazi Kuruluna* 27:387–392, 1971.

24. Zaki FA, Hurvitz AI: Spontaneous neoplasms of the central nervous system of the cat. *J Small Anim Pract* 17:773–782, 1976.

25. Graham JP, Newell SM, Voges AK, et al: The dural tail sign in the diagnosis of meningiomas. *Vet Radiol Ultrasound* 39:297–302, 1998.

26. Dahme E: Meningome bei fleischfressern. *Berl Münch Teirärztl Wschr* 70:32–34, 1957.

27. Fusco JV, Hohenhaus AE, Aiken SW, et al: Autologous blood collection and transfusion in cats undergoing partial craniectomy. *JAVMA* 216:1584–1588, 2000.

28. Niebauer GW, Dayrell-Hart BL, Speciale J: Evaluation of craniotomy in dogs and cats. *JAVMA* 198:89–95, 1991.

29. Munson L, Nesbit JW, Meltzer DGA, et al: Diseases in captive cheetahs *(Acinonyx jubatus jubatus)* in South Africa: A 20-year retrospective survey. *J Zoo Wildl Med* 30:342–347, 1999.

30. Berry WL, Higgins RJ, LeCouteur RA, et al: Papillary ependymomas and hydrocephalus in three cats. *J Vet Intern Med* 12:243, 1998.

31. McKay JS, Targett MP, Jeffery ND: Histological characterization of an ependymoma in the fourth ventricle of a cat. *J Comp Pathol* 120:105–113, 1999.

32. Ingwersen W, Groom S, Parent J: Vestibular syndrome associated with an ependymoma in a cat. *JAVMA* 195:98–100, 1989.

33. Fox JG, Snyder SB, Reed C, Campbell LH: Malignant ependymoma in a cat. *J Small Anim Pract* 14:23–26, 1973.

34. Simpson DJ, Hunt GB, Tisdall PLC, et al: Surgical removal of an ependymoma from the third ventricle of a cat. *Aust Vet J* 77:645–648, 1999.

35. Tremblay C, Girard C, Quesnel A, et al: Ventricular ependymoma in a cat. *Can Vet J* 39:719–720, 1998.

36. Hayes Jr HM, Priester WA, Pendergrass TW: Occurrence of nervous-tissue tumors in cattle, horses, cats and dogs. *Int J Cancer* 15:39–47, 1975.

37. Smith DA, Honhold N: Clinical and pathological features of a cerebellar oligodendroglioma in a cat. *J Small Anim Pract* 29:269–274 1988.

38. Cooper ERA, Howarth I: Some pathological changes in the cat brain. *J Comp Pathol* 66:35–38, 1956.

39. Knowlton FP: A case of tumor of the floor of the fourth ventricle with cerebellar symptoms, in a cat. *Am J Physiol* 13:20–21, 1905.

40. Dickinson PJ, Higgins RJ, Keel MK, et al: Diagnostic and pathological features of caudal fossa oligodendrogliomas in two cats [abstract 197]. *J Vet Intern Med* 13:275, 1999.

41. Duniho S, Schulman FY, Morrison A, et al: A subependymal giant cell astrocytoma in a cat. *Vet Pathol* 37:275–278, 2000.

42. Chénier S, Quesnel A, Girard C: Intracranial teratoma and dermoid cyst in a kitten. *J Vet Diagn Invest* 10:381–384, 1998.

43. Ross J, Wyburn RS: A report on the clinical investigation of a paraplegic cat. *N Z Vet J* 17:251–253, 1969.

44. Jones BR: Spinal meningioma in a cat. *Aust Vet J* 50:229–231, 1974.

45. McGrath JT: Meningiomas in animals. *J Neuropathol Exp Neurol* 21:327–328, 1962.

46. Levy MS, Mauldin G, Kapatkin AS, Patnaik AK: Nonlymphoid vertebral canal tumors in cats: 11 cases (1987–1995). *JAVMA* 5:663–664, 1997.

47. Asperio RM, Marzola P, Zibellini E, et al: Use of magnetic resonance imaging for diagnosis of a spinal tumor in a cat. *Vet Radiol Ultrasound* 40:267–270, 1999.

48. Haynes JS, Leininger JR: A glioma in the spinal cord of a cat. *Vet Pathol* 19:713–715, 1982.

49. Milks HJ, Olafson P: Primary brain tumors in small animals. *Cornell Vet* 26:159–170, 1936.

50. Ruben JMS: Neurofibrosarcoma in a 19-year-old cat. *Vet Rec* 113:135, 1983.

51. Luttgen PJ, Braund Jr WR, Vandevelde M: A retrospective study of twenty-nine spinal tumors in the dog and cat. *J Vet Intern Med* 21:207–215, 1980.

52. Paul-Murphy J, Lloyd K, Turrel JM, et al: Management of a Schwannoma in the larynx of a lion. *JAVMA* 189:1202–1203, 1986.

MANAGEMENT OF SPECIFIC DISEASES

40

TUMORS OF THE AUDITORY AND VISUAL SYSTEMS

Antony S. Moore and Gregory K. Ogilvie

TUMORS OF THE EAR

CLINICAL BRIEFING

Common Presentation	Ceruminous adenocarcinomas are most common, although adenomas and other carcinomas are described. Signs of chronic otitis, odor, discharge, and pruritus are common regardless of histology. Vestibular signs may signal invasion of the middle ear. Tumors are occasionally bilateral.
Staging and Diagnosis	MDB, complete otic examination, lymph node palpation, and skull radiographs (including bullae) or CT scan to delineate bullae and tumor extension. Metastasis most commonly to deep parotid, retropharyngeal, and prescapular lymph nodes. Invasion of surrounding tissues is common.
Treatment	
Initial	Surgical resection of ear canal for benign tumors or noninvasive carcinomas. Most tumors are invasive, requiring ear ablation and bulla osteotomy.
Adjunctive	Radiation therapy for incompletely excised tumors. Chemotherapy unproven; may try carboplatin or doxorubicin.
Supportive	Analgesia, including local nerve blocks, as necessary. Otic or systemic antibiotics for secondary infection. Nutritional support may be necessary.

CERUMINOUS ADENOMA

Incidence, Signalment, and Etiology

Ceruminous adenomas are relatively common in cats. Benign tumors of the ceruminous glands are distinguished from their malignant counterparts by their relatively low mitotic index on biopsy. Adenomas have been seen in middle-aged to older cats (median age, 8 years; range, 3 to 15 years); in one study of 22 cats, only 2 were younger than 6 years.[1] All reported cats have been DSHs or DLHs. There does not appear to be a gender predisposition. Although 16 of 22 cats were male in one study,[1] 44% of 79 cats were male in another study, which is not significantly different from the general population.[2]

Clinical Presentation and History

Signs of otitis with odor, discharge, and pruritus that have been chronic (sometimes up to a year) should prompt investigation for an underlying tumor.[1] Pruritus and odor may be absent,[3] and cats may even be asymptomatic.[1] Most ceruminous adenomas arise from the wall of the au-

ditory meatus, although one arising on the pinna of a cat was described.[1]

Staging and Diagnosis

Preoperative incisional biopsy is necessary to distinguish benign tumors from early adenocarcinomas. Biopsy almost always requires general anesthesia. An ear cleaning, MDB, careful evaluation of regional lymph nodes, and skull radiographs (when indicated) are recommended.

Treatment

Concurrent otitis externa is often the predominating clinical presentation, and thus aggressive, appropriate treatment based on results of ear cytology and bacterial culture is warranted. Surgery is the treatment of choice. Surgical excision was performed in most reported cats,[3] although results of these surgeries were not provided. In most cats with ceruminous adenoma, surgical excision via a lateral ear resection should be sufficient to render the cat tumor free. More aggressive surgery, as outlined for ceruminous adenocarcinomas, may be required for larger tumors. Appropriate supportive care should be provided, including nerve blocks, oral or parenteral analgesia, and topical steroidal otic preparations, to alleviate discomfort caused by this condition and its treatment.

OTHER BENIGN EAR TUMORS

Benign otic polyps that may extend to involve the bullae or the nasopharynx are described in more detail in the section on nasal polyps in Chapter 47. Cutaneous papilloma of the pinna has been reported, without clinical details, in two cats,[1,3] one of which was a 10-year-old castrated male.

CERUMINOUS GLAND ADENOCARCINOMAS

Incidence, Signalment, and Etiology

Ceruminous gland adenocarcinoma is the most common malignancy involving the ear canal in cats and is equal in frequency to, or more common than, the benign variant.[2] Ceruminous gland adenocarcinoma accounted for approximately one third of all tumors (and 40% of all malignant tumors) of the ear canal in a large survey.[3]

Affected cats are older (average age, 11[2,3] to 13[4] years). Except for one Siamese,[1] all reported cats were DSHs or DLHs or the breed was not stated. There were no breed or gender predilections for this tumor in one study of 91 cats.[2] There is one report that describes a ceruminous gland tumor occurring in a female cat and "several" of its offspring,[5] but there are no other reports of familial tendency toward developing this tumor.

Clinical Presentation and History

Signs of otitis predominate; a discharge that is often malodorous, purulent, and occasionally bloody, pruritus, pain, and a mass are common signs (Figures 40-1 and 40-2). Neurologic signs such as facial nerve paralysis, head tilt, circling, anisocoria (Horner's Syndrome), and ataxia occur in 25% to 35% of cats[3,6] and are sometimes the only signs of disease.[6] Some cats may be presented for an ulcerated mass. A discharging abscess below the ear extending to the angle of the jaw may prove to be a cutaneous extension of an ear canal tumor.[1,4] Occasionally, a ceruminous gland carcinoma will extend further to involve the skin of the neck and even the shoulder.[1] In one study, 28 of 56 malignant ear canal tumors appeared invasive. Nine of the tumors invaded the subcutis while 19 invaded cartilage of the ear and canal.

> ### KEY POINT
>
> *Ceruminous gland carcinoma should be considered in older cats with chronic otitis that develop vestibular signs.*

To further complicate initial differentiation from chronic otitis, the clinical history may be long (up to 3 years in one cat); it is also possible that chronic otitis may predispose a cat to developing ceruminous gland carcinoma. Further support for this comes from the finding that tumors sometimes occur bilaterally.[7,8]

Staging and Diagnosis

Prior to planning or performing the definitive procedure, it is important to stage cats appropriately to detect potential tumor spread. Vascular invasion is noted in more than half the tumors, and lymph node metastases are seen in 20% to 50% of cats.[1,3,4,6] Lung metastases at the time of presentation have not been reported, but thoracic radiographs should be obtained as part of the MDB and as a baseline for future evaluations.

Metastases to the deep parotid, retropharyngeal, and prescapular lymph nodes occur most commonly,[1] but spread to salivary glands, skeletal muscle, lungs, kidney, thoracic

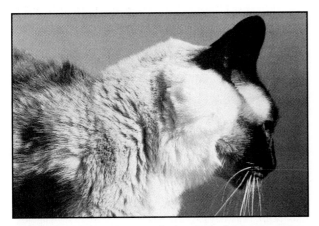

Figure 40-1: *A large ceruminous gland carcinoma showing extension out of the ear canal and into surrounding tissues. Aggressive surgical excision and radiation therapy is the appropriate treatment for this tumor. (Courtesy of G.H. Theilen)*

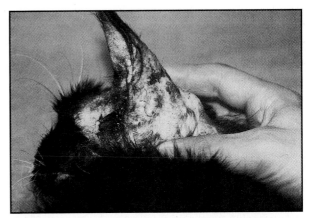

Figure 40-2: *Ceruminous gland carcinoma is often associated with pruritus and otitis externa, as in this 12-year-old cat. Persistent signs should alert the veterinarian to the possibility of a tumor.*

MANAGEMENT OF SPECIFIC DISEASES

lymph nodes, and pleura has been observed.[1,3,4] Enlarged lymph nodes should be examined by fine-needle aspiration cytology and the skin and subcutis carefully palpated for evidence of tumor extension. The tympanic bulla is frequently involved by direct tumor extension, and therefore clinical staging should include open-mouth radiographs to view the bullae as well as skull and thoracic radiographs.

KEY POINT

Radiographic examination of the bullae should be performed in cats with ceruminous gland carcinoma.

Histologically, these tumors show expansion of apocrine-type ceruminous glands that vary greatly in their histologic grade, mitotic index, and ability to invade surrounding stroma. The prognostic significance of the degree of differentiation has not been examined, although fewer than 50% of the tumors are classified as well differentiated.[7,9] In one study the mitotic rate was always high (range, 5 to 40 mitotic figures/high power field; average, 16).[1]

Treatment

Surgical resection of the ear canal may be sufficient in cats with a tumor that affects only the vertical ear canal and has no bulla involvement. Six cats that were treated in this manner had a median disease-free period of 10 months (range, 1 to 14 months), and two cats were alive and without tumor recurrence 1 year after surgery.[6] Most cats, however, have more invasive tumors, and recurrence of even apparently localized tumors is common after surgery. Surgical excision of these tumors is best accomplished by ear canal ablation and lateral bulla osteotomy. The median disease-free period for 16 cats treated in this manner was 42 months (range, 4 to 60 months). Recurrence, usually as di-

rect tumor extension into the parotid region, happened within the first year after surgery in 4 cats.[6] It would appear that more aggressive surgery should be performed even in cats with apparently localized tumors.

KEY POINT

Bulla osteotomy and ear canal ablation is warranted in most cats with ceruminous gland carcinoma.

Radiation therapy may also reduce recurrence in surrounding tissues (Figures 40-3 and 40-4). Six cats were treated with megavoltage radiation[7]; tumors recurred 3 months after treatment in one cat and 8 months after treatment in another, and two cats died of other causes. One cat was alive 36 months after treatment and another 66 months after treatment.

Radiation therapy following aggressive surgical excision appears to be the treatment of choice for ceruminous gland carcinomas that have not metastasized. In a large study, these modalities were used alone or in combination and the median survival for cats with ceruminous gland carcinoma was longer than 49 months.[3]

Chemotherapy with carboplatin or doxorubicin may be warranted in cats with metastatic lesions, although there are no reports about the efficacy of these drugs.

SQUAMOUS CELL/UNDIFFERENTIATED CARCINOMA

Incidence, Signalment, and Etiology

In a large study that included 56 cats with malignant tumors of the ear canal, 20 tumors were squamous cell carcinoma (SCC) and 13 were undifferentiated carcinoma. The behavior of these two tumor types was biologically similar, and it there-

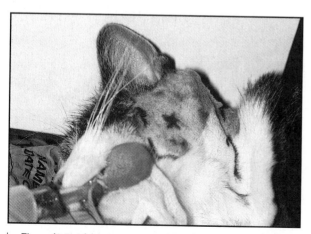

Figure 40-3: *A large, recurrent ceruminous gland adenocarcinoma in a 15-year-old cat after multiple surgeries.*

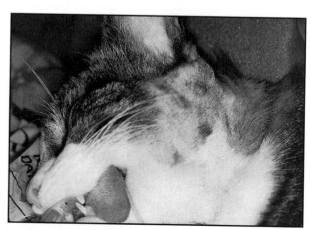

Figure 40-4: *Palliative radiation therapy for the cat in Figure 40-3 caused almost complete resolution of the tumor mass for 6 months. Radiation after an aggressive surgery is best performed early in the clinical course.*

fore makes sense to combine these cases.[3] Undifferentiated carcinoma and SCC have been reported primarily in older cats (5[1] to 13[10,11] years old), and all tumors were unilateral. There have been no reports of these tumors in purebred cats.

Clinical Presentation and History

Signs of chronic otitis are usually present; in this regard, ceruminous gland carcinomas are clinically indistinguishable from SCC and undifferentiated carcinoma of the ear canal.[3,12] Some cats have a long history of otitis prior to an acute onset of ataxia, anisocoria, and head tilt as well as occasional dysphagia, hypersalivation, and pain.[1,11,13,14] Clinical signs were not separated by tumor type in one large study, but cats with malignant tumors in general showed discharge (75%), a visible mass (47%), and pruritus (36%).[3]

Staging and Diagnosis

As is seen in cats with ceruminous gland carcinoma, cats with SCC or undifferentiated carcinoma usually have evidence of bulla involvement on radiographs or CT scan.[1,8,10–14] Lysis is often severe and may extend to involve the petrous temporal bone, zygomatic arch, skull, and mandible and may invade the brain.[1,13] Metastasis to retropharyngeal lymph nodes and lungs has been reported.

Staging should therefore encompass an MDB, complete otic examination, palpation of mandibular, prescapular, and, if possible, retropharyngeal lymph nodes, and radiographs of the skull, including an open-mouth view of the bullae.

Treatment

To date, treatment of these tumors has often been unrewarding when surgery was used alone. For example, bulla osteotomy was performed as the sole treatment for three cats that survived an average of 6 weeks from surgery,[12–14] which was not much longer than survival rates in untreated cats.[10,13] Most cats are euthanized due to worsening ataxia and neurologic signs related to tumor invasion.[10,14]

Cats with SCC of the pinna that extended to involve the ear canal fared better. Of four cats treated with ablation of the ear canal and bulla osteotomy, three were tumor free 6 months later.[8]

Overall, the median survival was 3.8 months for 20 cats with SCC of the ear canal and 5.7 months for 13 cats with undifferentiated carcinoma. Histologic evidence of stromal invasion was associated with a significantly shorter survival (4 months) than if invasion was not noted (21.7 months). These latter two survival times also included cats with ceruminous gland carcinomas.[3]

It appears that radiation therapy following aggressive surgical excision is appropriate for these carcinomas, as it is for cats with ceruminous gland carcinoma. For cats with metastatic lesions, chemotherapy with carboplatin or doxorubicin may be warranted, although there are no reports about the efficacy of these drugs.

Supportive care should include antibiotic treatment of any secondary infections, systemic and/or regional analgesia, and nutritional support.

TUMORS OF THE OCULAR GLOBE

▶ OCULAR MELANOMA

CLINICAL BRIEFING

Common Presentation	Uveal melanoma is more common than limbal. Unilateral chronic uveitis, pigment change, buphthalmos, and glaucoma are common. A mass, usually pigmented, may be seen.
Staging and Diagnosis	MDB, complete ocular examination, lymph node palpation, abdominal ultrasonography, ocular ultrasonography, and MRI or CT scan. Tumors may extend to involve retrobulbar space. Metastasis (typically to the lungs) is common and may be widespread.
Treatment Initial	Enucleation—particularly for locally unresectable tumors—is the treatment of choice and is best done early. Local excision of limbal tumors may be successful.
Adjunctive	Coarse fractional radiation therapy may be palliative in patients with unresectable tumors. Carboplatin or doxorubicin may be used for metastatic tumors or as an adjuvant to local therapies (unproven).
Supportive	Medical treatment of uveitis or glaucoma prior to surgery. Analgesia as necessary.

MANAGEMENT OF SPECIFIC DISEASES

UVEAL MELANOMA

Incidence, Signalment, and Etiology

In two large studies of ocular pathology, uveal melanoma was found in 85 of 694 globes examined.[15,16] Other conditions that resemble uveal melanoma include iris freckles, in which the iris is not thickened and there are indistinct margins to the area of pigmentation, and iridal cysts, which are usually at the pupillary margin and have smooth edges.[17]

Uveal melanomas occur in older cats (median age, 11 years).[1,16,18] Cats under 4 years of age have rarely been reported to have this tumor[19,20]; similarly, affected cats older than 18 years are rarely described.[1,18] Of 127 reported cats, the majority (95) have been DSHs, with DLHs (17), Persians (12),[1,6,18,21–24] and Siamese (3) less commonly affected. In contrast, there were no Persians reported to have cutaneous melanoma, suggesting a possible breed predisposition for the ocular form of this disease. There were 58 males and 41 females reported in the literature.

MDB = minimum database; includes CBC, biochemical profile, urinalysis, FeLV/FIV serology, T_4 testing, and thoracic radiographs (three views).

Intraocular inoculation of feline sarcoma virus (FeSV) in kittens may lead to rapid (5 to 6 months) development of uveal melanoma.[25,26] It is difficult to link experimental data with the etiology of the naturally occurring tumor. Only two cats with naturally occurring uveal melanoma have tested positive for FeLV, which is necessary for replication of FeSV.[20,21]

Clinical Presentation and History

Initial signs of uveal melanoma may be subtle, such as a resolving cloudy eye due to uveitis. Slight increase in iris pigmentation, starting as discrete spots and extending to cause a complete change in iris color, may be the first sign noted by an owner[18,21,22,24,27,28] (Figure 40-5). Pigment change may precede more serious changes (e.g., buphthalmos, glaucoma) by months[21,27] to years.[18,22,28] In a study of 128 cats with glaucoma, 38 had uveal melanoma causing obliteration of the trabecular meshwork.[29] Glaucoma may cause irritation and pruritus and lead to a corneal ulcer,[1,21,23] and the globe may rupture if glaucoma is untreated.[30] The eye may prolapse or show deviation from its normal position if the tumor extends into the retrobulbar space.[1,18,31]

Sometimes the iris may be thickened or irregular in addition to showing pigmentation[1,22,32]; however, pigmentation may be quite mild (not black).[18] Cats with uveal melanoma may also present with an obvious intraocular mass that has been noticed by the owners[1,19,24,28,33] (Figure 40-6). The mass may extend to involve the lens, ciliary body,[19] or cornea.[16] Other signs seen in association with ocular melanoma are hyphema,[1,20,24] panophthalmitis, and chemosis, which may be chronic for years.[1] One cat collapsed with a subdural hematoma and pathologic skull fracture due to invasive melanoma.[20] Ocular melanoma is rarely bilateral, although one such case was cited in an early study.[24]

Staging and Diagnosis

An MDB should be obtained and regional lymph nodes assessed prior to surgical intervention. Pulmonary metastases may be seen at the time of diagnosis in the absence of obvious lymph node metastases.[16,20,23] Abdominal radiographs may show organomegaly consistent with metastatic disease,[23] although abdominal ultrasonography is more accurate for staging these cats.

Metastases may be widespread and have been reported in the

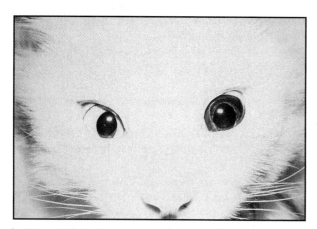

Figure 40-5: Uveal melanoma in a domestic cat. Note the iris hyperpigmentation and anisocoria. (Courtesy of M. Brown)

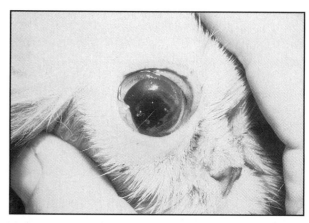

Figure 40-6: A large, intraocular melanoma in a Persian cat. (Courtesy of M. Brown)

brain, lungs, and liver as well as the mediastinum, pericardium, pleura, diaphragm, adrenals, peritoneum, spleen, stomach, intestine, tonsils, and regional and distant lymph nodes.

Ultrasonography of the eye may disclose the extent of tumor within the globe. CT or MRI may be useful in identifying cats that would not benefit from surgery because of large inoperable tumors extending beyond the globe. These imaging modalities have also been used to accurately guide preoperative biopsy.[34] Biopsy of the tumor prior to definitive surgery is often unnecessary, as enucleation is usually warranted due to the associated ocular pathology. The presence of metastatic disease or tumor invasion to involve the optic nerve as well as surrounding muscle, bone, and brain would obviously preclude surgery.[20]

More invasive tumors appear to have a more aggressive clinical course. In one study, survival appeared to be longer in cats with tumors limited to the iris and ciliary body.[18] Presurgical imaging may therefore assist clinicians in making prognostic predictions.

The number of mitotic figures on histopathologic sectioning has been shown to correlate with increasing tumor invasion of the surrounding sclera in one study.[35] However, mitotic index is not an absolute criterion for malignancy since tumor invasion has been reported when the mitotic rate is zero; no correlation has been made between mitotic index and survival.[16,19,22,27,32,35] It is important to submit the entire surgical specimen for accurate and complete histologic evaluation.

Treatment

Enucleation is the treatment of choice for cats with uveal melanoma and no evidence of metastases. Other less aggressive surgeries such as iridectomy or iridocyclectomy rarely provide long-term tumor control.[22] One study found that cats with tumors involving only the iris and ciliary body had a median survival of 383 days after enucleation, compared with 122 days for cats with tumors invading beyond these structures and 14 days for those with tumors involving the whole eye.[18] These findings imply that long-term survival following enucleation is possible, but surgery (preferably enucleation) should be performed early in the course of disease.

Excluding the larger study cited above,[18] survival times following enucleation for 17 other reported cats ranged from 5 months to 3 years (median, 1 year).[1,16,21–24,27,30,32,33,35,36] One cat was alive at 6 months,[33] one at 18 months,[22] and one at 2 years after surgery,[22] although a subsequent report implied that the latter two cats died due to metastases.[27] Many of these early reports concluded that ocular melanoma is rarely metastatic, but lack of follow-up and necropsy data weakens this conclusion. In fact, metastases appear to occur frequently but the onset may be delayed until long after the published follow up.[16,21,22,24,30,32,35] Nonspe-

cific signs of weight loss and lethargy, particularly if accompanied by dyspnea or abdominal enlargement, are likely to be associated with widespread metastatic disease.[1,16,23,24,36]

Radiation therapy has not been evaluated for the treatment of feline melanoma, although anecdotal reports exist. Coarse fractionation protocols may be palliative in cats with large, invasive intraocular melanoma.

Carboplatin and doxorubicin have not been evaluated for treatment of ocular melanoma. Anecdotally, these drugs appear to have some efficacy for the treatment of melanoma of other sites in cats. Human recombinant interferon alpha (1.5 million U SQ q48h for 6 weeks) and cimetidine (4–8 mg/kg PO q8h) have been used based on data from other species, but no efficacy data are available for these treatments.

Systemic analgesia and regional nerve blocks are often warranted in treatment of this disease prior to enucleation.

LIMBAL MELANOMA

Incidence, Signalment, and Etiology

The limbus is defined as the scleral-corneal interface, and tumors in this location should be differentiated from extraocular extension of an uveal melanoma. Melanoma of the ocular limbal tissue is less common than uveal melanoma. In a survey of eyelid neoplasia in 121 cats, only five tumors were melanoma,[37] and two of these were amelanotic.

Of 14 cats in which clinical details were reported, most (10) have been DSHs[10]; 1 Siamese was the only purebred described.[38] The ages of affected cats ranged from 1 to 17 years (median, 9 years). There was no obvious gender predilection.[18,35,38–42]

Clinical Presentation and History

The majority of cats were presented because owners had noticed a mass or swollen eyelid. Duration of signs ranged from 2 to 10 weeks, with some tumors measuring more than 2.5 cm in diameter.[35,39,41] The melanoma was found incidentally in one cat examined for poor vision due to taurine deficiency and in another cat with spinal lymphoma.[38] Although the mass overlaid the cornea in one cat, there was no intraocular invasion.[39]

Staging and Diagnosis

Prior to any treatment, a complete ocular examination should be performed in addition to an MDB. Most tumors appear to be locally infiltrative[35] and sometimes invade the surrounding muscle and lacrimal gland.[41] Aspiration cytology of regional lymph nodes (mandibular, retropharyngeal, and parotid) should be performed if possible since regional lymph node metastases have been reported at the time of diagnosis.[18,39,41] Thoracic radiographs and abdominal ultrasonography should be performed as widespread metastasis is possible.

Treatment

Lamellar sclerokeratectomy, alone or followed by cryosurgery, was performed in three cats. Neither tumor recurrence nor metastasis had occurred 30 months after surgery in any of these cats.[38,42] One developed widespread metastases (to bone, spleen, liver, lungs, heart, muscle, adrenal glands, and both eyes) 31 months after initial surgery, indicating that late onset of metastases may occur.[42] There was no tumor recurrence noted in one cat 11 months after and in another 18 months after local excision of conjunctival melanoma.[39,41] One cat with a limbal melanoma that appeared static was merely observed for 36 months, and there was no apparent change in the tumor[38]; despite the success of this approach in this cat, a "wait and watch" option should not be recommended to owners when surgical excision is possible.

Photocoagulation using a laser was performed in two cats with melanoma.[40] Follow-up times did not exceed 6 months, so the efficacy of this modality is difficult to compare with that of surgery.

In contrast to the success of localized surgery cited above, local excision of the tumor was unsuccessful in controlling multiple local recurrences in three cats. Enucleation was performed as the final surgical procedure in these cats. All three cats developed metastases, two at 3 months and one at 3 years after surgery.[18] Recurrence and distant metastases occurred 6 months after local excision in another cat.[35]

Aggressive local surgery, if performed early, may be sufficient to control limbal melanoma. If adequate surgical margins cannot be obtained, however, enucleation should not be delayed.

Coarse fractionation radiation protocols may be palliative in cats with uveal melanoma, although only anecdotal reports are available regarding the use of radiation therapy in the treatment of this disease. Carboplatin and doxorubicin have not been evaluated for treatment of ocular melanoma. Anecdotally, these drugs appear to have some efficacy in treating melanoma of other sites in cats. Systemic analgesia and regional nerve blocks may be warranted prior to definitive treatment.

▶ OCULAR SARCOMA

CLINICAL BRIEFING

Common Presentation	Change in pupil color, blindness, or glaucoma in an eye that experienced previous trauma or chronic inflammation. Many histologic variants of sarcoma occur.
Staging and Diagnosis	MDB, ocular ultrasonography, MRI or CT scan, and lymph node palpation. Metastases and/or extension to involve CNS is common.
Treatment Initial	Enucleation is the treatment of choice but is rarely curative.
Adjunctive	Radiation therapy for local control and chemotherapy (carboplatin or doxorubicin) are unproven potential adjuncts to surgery.
Supportive	Medical treatment of uveitis or glaucoma prior to surgery. Analgesia, including local nerve blocks, as necessary.

Incidence, Signalment, and Etiology

Ocular sarcoma following previous ocular trauma has been described in many cats. A similar mechanism has been postulated as contributing to the occurrence of vaccine-related sarcomas in this species (see Chapter 51).

Ocular sarcoma has been reported only in cats older than 7 years (median age, 12 years). A study of 13 cats found intact males to be most commonly affected (9 cats), which is consistent with these cats being more likely to experience trauma.[43] Most reported cats were DSHs, with only two Siamese reported.[43–47]

A history of ocular trauma or inflammation was established for 26 of 30 reported cats. Trauma was documented to have occurred 5 months to 12 years prior to tumor diagnosis[43,46]

and may have been severe enough to cause phthisis bulbi,[47] cataract,[44] a tear in the lens,[45] or hyphema.[46] Chronic uveitis was the most common inflammatory cause and had been seen 1 month to 4 years prior to tumor diagnosis.[43] Four cats with intraocular sarcoma had no history of ocular problems.[43,48]

Most cats were not tested for FeLV; those that were tested negative.

The specific histologic diagnosis of tumor types is variable. While fibrosarcoma is the most common diagnosis, osteosarcoma or undifferentiated sarcoma may occur. There does not appear to be any variation in biologic behavior for different histopathologic types, and the clinician should treat them all as variations of ocular soft tissue sarcoma.

Clinical Presentation and History

Any cat with a history of ocular trauma or chronic ocular disease should be evaluated if there are any changes to the eye. A change in iris color may be seen,[44,46] and one author noted that white discoloration (or loss of iris pigment) was most common.[48] Acute blindness has been reported when the tumor invaded the optic chiasm.[45] Other cats were presented because medical management of inflammatory disease was no longer effective, the size of the globe increased, or the owner noticed a mass (Figure 40-7).[43,46] Glaucoma may result from an obstruction to the pupillary angle. Ocular sarcoma was found in 4 of 128 cats with glaucoma.[29]

Staging and Diagnosis

Ocular sarcomas are highly invasive, often invading the posterior portion of the globe, the retina, the optic nerve, and posterior to the lenticular capsule. In one study of 13 cats, 8 had tumors that invaded the optic nerve.[48] In another study, 9 of 13 tumors occupied the whole globe while 4 were localized to the ciliary body.[43] Ocular ultrasonography may allow evaluation of the globe prior to surgery,[46] although CT and MRI are more accurate imaging modalities to help clinicians decide the most appropriate method of management and plan a surgical approach.

Aspiration cytology and biopsy of regional (mandibular, retropharyngeal, and parotid) lymph nodes should be performed if they are enlarged. Metastases to regional lymph nodes have been seen in some cats.[43,44] Thoracic radiography should be obtained as pulmonary metastases have also been described.[43]

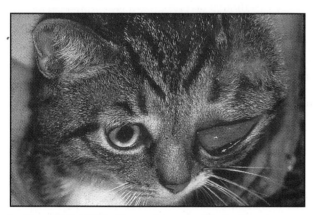

Figure 40-7: *A DSH with an ocular sarcoma following blunt trauma (car accident) years previously. (Courtesy of D. Ruslander)*

Treatment

Enucleation is the treatment of choice for ocular sarcoma. However, these are very invasive tumors, and cats with extension beyond the globe are unlikely to be helped by surgery. The imaging modalities described above will help the surgeon in identifying cats that are likely to benefit from surgery.

Follow-up information after enucleation was available for 21 cats.[43,44,46–48] Nineteen cats were dead within 8 months of surgery while 2 cats lived more than a year after surgery.[44,48] Metastasis with or without tumor recurrence was seen in 8 cats 2 to 17 months after surgery, and extension to involve the CNS was seen in 8 cats.[43,44,48]

Radiation therapy may have a role in advanced, invasive ocular sarcomas, although the high dosages that are necessary require sophisticated computer planning equipment to minimize damage to the CNS. Chemotherapy has not proven very helpful in the treatment of soft tissue sarcomas to date (see Chapter 51). Doxorubicin and carboplatin could be offered for palliation.

▶ OTHER OCULAR TUMORS

Uveal lymphoma was a cause of glaucoma in 8 of 128 cats with glaucoma.[29] More information can be found in Chapter 36.

In a study that looked at the pathology associated with 374 cat globes, 12 cats had ciliary epithelial neoplasia.[49] There is no information as to the treatment or prognosis for these tumors.

The eye is an occasional site of metastasis from other tumors, particularly carcinomas. Metastatic uterine carcinoma to the eye has been reported in 2 cats,[50,51] and metastatic carcinoma was a cause of glaucoma in 2 of 128 cats.[29] Glaucoma arose secondary to fibrinous uveitis and posterior synechiae.

NONDOMESTIC FELIDAE

A 5-year-old cheetah developed corneal SCC at the site of an apparently congenital corneal opacity. An orbital exenteration was performed, and there was no evidence of tumor recurrence or metastases 1 year after surgery.[63]

A 20-year-old Asiatic lion with SCC of the eye had local recurrence within 2 months of globe extirpation and died with pulmonary metastases 6 months after surgery.[64]

ORBITAL/RETROBULBAR TUMORS

CLINICAL BRIEFING

Common Presentation	SCC is most common, usually as an extension of a maxillary or nasal tumor. Other tumors include fibrosarcoma, plasma cell tumor, and lymphoma. Exophthalmos and anterolateral globe deviation are commonly seen. *(continued)*

Staging and Diagnosis	MDB, skull radiographs, CT, and lymph node palpation. Tumors are often very invasive and may metastasize.
Treatment	
Initial	Orbitectomy is rarely successful because of local recurrence. Radiation therapy may be more successful, but CT planning is mandatory.
Adjunctive	Chemotherapy as an adjunct to radiation may be helpful (unproven).
Supportive	Analgesia as needed; antibiotics if invasion into oral cavity with secondary infection is present.

RETROBULBAR SQUAMOUS CELL CARCINOMA

Incidence, Signalment, and Etiology

SCC is the most common retrobulbar tumor in cats. This tumor often originates in the oral cavity, nasal cavity, external auditory meatus, or conjunctiva.[52-55] As is seen with SCC of other sites, older cats are usually affected (median age in five reported cats, 11 years).[52-55]

Clinical Presentation and History

Exophthalmos and anterolateral globe deviation are most commonly described, although enophthalmos due to scar contracture was seen in four of nine cats in one study.[53] Associated signs of epiphora, pain and dysphagia, nasal discharge, and strabismus are also seen.

Staging and Diagnosis

Plain radiographs may show bony lysis of orbital structures or a soft tissue density; although in one study, four of nine cats with retrobulbar SCC had no radiographic changes.[53] If there is a clinical suspicion for a tumor, ultrasonography may be more helpful than radiography in identifying a soft tissue mass.[54] CT and MRI are the best methods to assess soft tissue and bony proliferation or lysis, which may be difficult to evaluate on plain radiography.[52,54] Not only are CT and ultrasonography helpful diagnostically, they are also essential to assist in planning surgery or radiation therapy and should be performed in addition to obtaining an MDB and assessing regional lymph nodes.

Treatment

In one study, surgical excision of orbital SCC in two cats was unsuccessful—tumors recurred within 4 months in both cats.[53] Radiation therapy was more successful in another cat; there was no local recurrence, but pulmonary metastases developed 12 months after treatment.[53] Regrowth and tumor extension occurred in another cat 2 months after radiation therapy, implying that the radiation treatment field was not large enough. CT scan prior to radiation therapy will ensure adequate treatment margins.

In addition to local therapies, chemotherapy with mitoxantrone, doxorubicin, or carboplatin may be an effective adjuvant to delay or treat metastatic disease (also see the sections on SCC in Chapters 41 and 50).

These tumors are highly invasive and treatment is often extensive, making systemic analgesia, regional nerve blocks, and nutritional support essential adjuncts to any treatment plan. In addition, antibiotics are often warranted as supportive care if invasion into the oral cavity with secondary infection occurs.

SCC of the oral cavity, nasal cavity, and ear canal are covered in more detail in the relevant chapters.

OTHER RETROBULBAR TUMORS

Fibrosarcoma is another common orbital tumor that, like SCC, may arise from the globe or invade from other sites. One cat treated with radiation therapy had tumor recurrence as well as pulmonary metastases 4 months later.[53]

An 11-year-old Abyssinian with a basal cell carcinoma showed orbital lysis and sclerosis on CT scan.[52]

Doxorubicin combined with immunotherapy was ineffective in treating a periorbital adenocarcinoma.[56]

A plasma cell tumor arose in the temporal muscles and extended to involve the retrobulbar space in a 13-year-old castrated male Abyssinian.[57] The cat also had a monoclonal gammopathy but no other evidence of multiple myeloma. Treatment was not attempted.

Lymphoma, frequently of nasal origin, may extend to the retrobulbar space and cause bony lysis of the orbit[52] (also see Chapter 47).

An orbital hemangioma was described in a 2-year-old cat but was not treated.[53]

TUMORS OF EYELID AND NICTITANS

In a study of 121 eyelid tumors in cats, the most common tumor type was SCC (69 cats[37]). SCC occurs mainly in older cats (Figure 40-8) and is associated with sunlight exposure (also see Chapter 50). Less common tumors were fibrosarcoma (7 cats), adenocarcinoma (3), adenoma (3), and mast cell tumor (7). Other skin tumors, such as basal cell tumors (Figure 40-9), hemangiosarcoma, melanoma, papilloma, lymphoma, neurofibroma, and trichoepithelioma,[37] were rarely reported.

Three Persians and one Himalayan, all older than 7 years, had multiple apocrine "cysts" of the eyelids.[58] These hidrocystomas ranged in size from 2 to 10 mm and caused blepharospasm, epiphora, or color change in the lid. Surgical removal in two cats and repeated drainage in another appeared curative, although a new hidrocystoma developed 5 years after initial surgery in one cat.

The nictitans is an uncommon site for tumors in cats. All reported tumors have been in DSHs older than 8 years. Tumor types include squamous cell carcinoma,[36] adenocarcinoma,[36,59] lymphoma,[36] and melanoma.[60]

Some tumors of the nictitans appear to be biologically aggressive. Although there were no metastases from two SCCs,[36] metastases were seen in one cat 1 month after surgery, in another cat 3 months after surgery, and in a third cat 7 months after surgery.[36,59] These metastases were widespread to the lungs, pleura, mediastinum, liver, and kidney in one cat.[59] The cat with melanoma of the nictitans presented with lung metastases as well as neurologic signs due to cortical metastases.[60]

Treatment options for SCC are discussed in Chapter 50. Orbitectomy for SCC of the eyelid was described in one report[61]; surgical margins were complete in only two of four cats so treated. Regardless of surgical margins, the tumor had not recurred in three cats 16 months to 5 years later. A cat with a hemangiosarcoma of the eyelid died soon after surgery.[61]

Another cat with SCC of the lower eyelid was treated with local current frequency hyperthermia, and the tumor was not present after necrosis and exudation had resolved 2 months later.[62]

Systemic analgesia and/or local nerve blocks can assist in reducing local discomfort and should be provided as part of the supportive care regimen. There are no reports of treatment for other eyelid tumors.

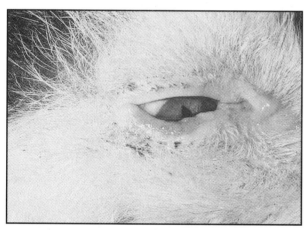

Figure 40-8: *The most common eyelid tumor in cats is the sunlight-induced squamous cell carcinoma. (Courtesy of W. Shapiro)*

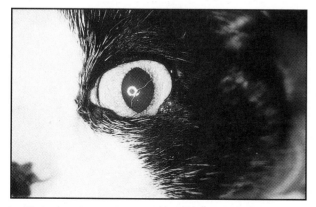

Figure 40-9: *Less common eyelid tumors, such as this basal cell tumor in a 10-year-old cat, are benign and surgically treatable.*

REFERENCES

1. Carpenter JL, Andrews LK, Holzworth J: Tumors and tumor-like lesions, in Holzworth J (ed): *Diseases of the Cat. Medicine and Surgery.* Philadelphia, WB Saunders, 1987, pp 407–596.
2. Goldschmidt MH, Shofer FS: *Skin Tumors of the Dog and Cat.* New York, Pergamon Press, 1992.
3. London CA, Dubilzeig RR, Vail DM, et al: Evaluation of dogs and cats with tumors of the ear canal: 145 cases (1978–1992). *JAVMA* 208:1413–1418, 1996.
4. Cotchin E: Skin tumours of cats. *Res Vet Sci* 2:353–361, 1961.
5. Holzwoth J: The ear, in Holzworth J (ed): *Diseases of the Cat. Medicine and Surgery.* Philadelphia, WB Saunders, 1987, pp 724–738.
6. Marino DJ, MacDonald JM, Matthiesen DT, Patnaik AK: Results of surgery in cats with ceruminous gland adenocarcinoma. *JAAHA* 30:54–58, 1994.
7. Theon AP, Barthez PY, Madewell BR, Griffey SM: Radiation therapy of ceruminous gland carcinomas in dogs and cats. *JAVMA* 205:566–569, 1994.
8. Williams JM, White RAS: Total ear canal ablation combined with lateral bulla osteotomy in the cat. *J Small Anim Pract* 33:225–227, 1992.
9. Miller MA, Nelson SL, Turk JR, et al: Cutaneous neoplasia in 340 cats. *Vet Pathol* 28:389–395, 1991.
10. Stone EA, Goldschmidt MH, Littman MP: Squamous cell carcinoma of the middle ear in a cat. *J Small Anim Pract* 24:647–651, 1983.
11. Fiorito DA: Oral and peripheral vestibular signs in a cat with squamous cell carcinoma. *JAVMA* 188:71–72, 1986.
12. Trevor PB, Martin RA: Tympanic bulla osteotomy for treatment of middle-ear disease in cats: 19 cases (1984–1991). *JAVMA* 202:123–128, 1993.
13. Indrieri RJ, Taylor RF: Vestibular dysfunction caused by squamous cell carcinoma involving the middle ear and inner ear in two cats. *JAVMA* 184:471–473, 1984.
14. Pentlarge VW: Peripheral vestibular disease in a cat with middle and inner ear squamous cell carcinoma. *Compend Contin Educ Pract Vet* 6:731–736, 1984.
15. Peiffer Jr RL, Wilcock BP: Histopathologic study of uveitis in cats: 139 cases (1978–1988). *JAVMA* 198:135–138, 1991.
16. Schäffer EH, Funke K: Das primär-intraokulare maligne melanom bei hund

and katze. *Tierärztl Prax* 13:343–359, 1985.

17. Peiffer Jr RL: The differential diagnosis of pigmented ocular lesions in the dog and cat. *California Vet* 5:14–18, 1981.

18. Patnaik AK, Mooney S: Feline melanoma: A comparative study of ocular, oral, and dermal neoplasms. *Vet Pathol* 25:105–112, 1988.

19. Souri E: Intraocular melanoma in a cat. *Feline Pract* 8:43–45, 1978.

20. Schulze Schleithoff N, Opitz M: Intraokuläres, metastasierendes, pigment armes melanom bei einer hauskatze. *Kleintierpraxis* 28:215–218, 1982.

21. Schwink K, Betts DM: Malignant melanoma of the iris in a cat. *Comp Anim Pract* 2:35–41, 1988.

22. Acland GM, McLean IW, Aquirre GD, Trucksa R: Diffuse iris melanoma in cats. *JAVMA* 176:52–56, 1980.

23. Schiller I, Spiess B, Pospischil A: Maligne melanome bei zwei katzen. *Schweiz Arch Tierheilk* 137:50–53, 1995.

24. Bellhorn RW, Henkind P: Intraocular malignant melanoma in domestic cats. *J Small Anim Pract* 10:631–637, 1970.

25. Shadduck JA, Albert DM, Niederkorn JY: Feline uveal melanomas induced with feline sarcoma virus: Potential model of the human counterpart. *J Natl Cancer Inst* 67:619–627, 1981.

26. Albert DM, Shadduck JA, Craft JL, Niederkorn JY: Feline uveal melanoma model induced with feline sarcoma virus. *Invest Ophthalmol Vis Sci* 20:606–624, 1981.

27. Bertoy RW, Brightman AH, Regan K: Intraocular melanoma with multiple metastases in a cat. *JAVMA* 192:87–89, 1988.

28. Wolfer J, Grahn B: Diagnostic ophthalmology. *Can Vet J* 32:440, 1991.

29. Wilcock BP, Peiffer Jr RJ, Davidson MG: The causes of glaucoma in cats. *Vet Pathol* 27:35–40, 1990.

30. Cardy RH: Primary intraocular malignant melanoma in a Siamese cat. *Vet Pathol* 14:648–649, 1977.

31. Grahn B, Wolfer J: Diagnostic opthalmology. *Can Vet J* 33:683, 1992.

32. Bjerkas E, Arnesen K, Peiffer Jr RL: Diffuse amelanotic iris melanoma in a cat. *Vet Comp Ophthalmol* 7:190–191, 1997.

33. Peiffer Jr RL, Seymour WG, Williams LW: Malignant melanoma of the iris and ciliary body in a cat. *Mod Vet Pract* 58:854–856, 1977.

34. Grahn BH, Stewart WA, Towner RA, Noseworthy MD: Magnetic resonance imaging of the canine and feline eye, orbit, and optic nerves and its clinical application. *Can Vet J* 34:418–424, 1993.

35. Day MJ, Lucke VM: Melanocytic neoplasia in the cat. *J Small Anim Pract* 36:207–213, 1995.

36. Schäffer EH, Pfleghaar S, Gordon S, Knödlseder M: Maligne nickhauttumoren bei hund und katze. *Tierärztl Prax* 22:382–391, 1994.

37. McLaughlin SA, Whitley RD, Gilger BC, et al: Eyelid neoplasms in cats: A review of demographic data (1979–1989). *JAAHA* 29:63–67, 1993.

38. Harling DE, Peiffer RL, Cook CS, Belkin PV: Feline limbal melanoma: Four cases. *JAAHA* 22:795–802, 1986.

39. Neumann W, Juchem R: Epibulbäres melanom bei einer katze. *Tierärztl Prax* 16:65–68, 1988.

40. Sullivan TC, Nasisse MP, Davidson MG, Glover TL: Photocoagulation of limbal melanoma in dogs and cats: 15 cases (1989–1993). *JAVMA* 208:891–894, 1996.

41. Cook CS, Rosenkrantz W, Peiffer RL, MacMillan A: Malignant melanoma of the conjunctiva in a cat. *JAVMA* 186:505–506, 1985.

42. Betton A, Healy LN, English RV, Bunch SE: Atypical limbal melanoma in a cat. *J Vet Intern Med* 13:379–381, 1999.

43. Peiffer RL, Monticello T, Bouldin TW: Primary ocular sarcomas in the cat. *J Small Anim Pract* 29:105–116, 1988.

44. Hakanson N, Shively JN, Reed RE, Merideth RE: Intraocular spindle cell sarcoma following ocular trauma in a cat: Case report and literature review. *JAAHA* 26:63–66, 1990.

45. Barrett PM, Merideth RE, Alarcon FL: Central amaurosis induced by an intraocular, posttraumatic fibrosarcoma in a cat. *JAAHA* 31:242–245, 1995.

46. Miller WW, Boosinger TR: Intraocular osteosarcoma in a cat. *JAAHA* 23:317–320, 1987.

47. Woog J, Albert DM, Gonder JR, Carpenter JJ: Osteosarcoma in a phthisical feline eye. *Vet Pathol* 20:209–214, 1983.

48. Dubielzig RR, Everitt J, Shadduck JA, Albert DM: Clinical and morphologic features of post-traumatic ocular sarcomas in cats. *Vet Pathol* 27:62–65, 1990.

49. Peiffer Jr RL, Wilcock BP, Yin H: The pathogenesis and significance of pre-iridal fibrovascular membrane in domestic animals. *Vet Pathol* 27:41–45, 1990.

50. Bellhorn RW: Secondary ocular adenocarcinoma in three dogs and a cat. *JAVMA* 160:302–307, 1972.

51. O'Rouke MD, Geib LW: Endometrial adenocarcinoma in a cat. *Cornell Vet* 60:598–604, 1970.

52. Calia CM, Kirschner SE, Baer KE: The use of computed tomography scan for the evaluation of orbital disease in cats and dogs. *Vet Comp Ophthalmol* 4:24–30, 1998.

53. Gilger BC, McLaughlin SA, Whitley RD, Wright JC: Orbital neoplasms in cats: 21 cases (1974–1990). *JAVMA* 201:1083–1086, 1992.

54. Murphy CJ, Koblik P, Bellhorn RW, et al: Squamous cell carcinoma causing blindness and ophthalmoplegia in a cat. *JAVMA* 195:965–968, 1989.

55. Hayden DW: Squamous cell carcinoma in a cat with intraocular and orbital metastases. *Vet Pathol* 13:332–336, 1976.

56. Brown NO, Hayes AA, Mooney S, et al: Combined modality therapy in the treatment of solid tumors in cats. *JAAHA* 16:719–722, 1980.

57. Ward DA, McEntee MF, Weddle DL: Orbital plasmacytoma in a cat. *J Small Anim Pract* 38:576–578, 1997.

58. Chaitman J, van der Woerdt A, Bartick TE: Multiple eyelid cysts resembling apocrine hidrocystomas in three Persian cats and one Himalayan cat. *Vet Pathol* 36:474–476, 1999.

59. Komaromy AM, Ramsey DT, Render JA, Clark P: Primary adenocarcinoma of the gland of the nictitating membrane in a cat. *JAAHA* 33:333–336, 1997.

60. Roels S, Ducatelle R: Malignant melanoma of the nictitating membrane in a cat (*Felis vulgaris*). *J Comp Path* 119:189–193, 1998.

61. O'Brien MG, Withrow SJ, Straw RC, et al: Total and partial orbitectomy for the treatment of periorbital tumors in 24 dogs and 6 cats: A retrospective study. *Vet Surg* 25:471–479, 1996.

62. Neumann SM: Palpebral squamous cell carcinoma in a cat. *Modern Vet Pract* 63:547–549, 1982.

63. Caliguri R, Carrier M, Jacobson ER, Buergelt CD: Corneal squamous cell carcinoma in a cheetah (*Acinonyx jubatus*). *J Zoo Anim Med* 19:219–222, 1988.

64. Kaul L, Kaul PL, Patel BJ, Sabapara RH: Squamous cell carcinoma of eye with pulmonary metastasis in an asiatic lion. *Int J Anim Sci* 9:219, 1994.

41

TUMORS OF THE ALIMENTARY TRACT

Antony S. Moore and Gregory K. Ogilvie

MALIGNANT ORAL TUMORS

Squamous cell carcinoma (SCC) accounts for 60% to 80% of all oral tumors in published surveys.[1-5] Fibrosarcoma, the only other commonly reported malignant tumor, accounts for 10% to 20% of oral tumors; all other individual tumor types comprise less than 3% of oral tumors.

In a survey of 24 cats with mandibular swelling, only 12 had malignancies.[6] Radiographic evidence of matrix calcification or pathologic fracture was more likely in malignant tumors; otherwise there was a wide overlap of radiographic signs between tumors and osteomyelitis due to dental disease.

SQUAMOUS CELL CARCINOMA

CLINICAL BRIEFING

Common Presentation	Most common oral tumor in cats (usually older cats); typically involves the tongue. Occasionally invades bone, causing large bony swelling. Dysphagia and ptyalism are common.
Staging and Diagnosis	MDB, lymph node palpation (normal-sized nodes can contain metastasis), skull radiographs, CT scan. Possibly ultrasonography for the tongue. Metastases rare to lungs, uncommon to regional nodes.
Treatment Initial	Because of inadequate margins, surgical excision is rarely curative unless tumor is confined to bone. Radiation therapy often gives excellent tumor response, but such response is short lived even after surgery. Chemotherapy alone is rarely effective. Best responses achieved via a combination of surgery, radiation therapy, and chemotherapy. Carboplatin or doxorubicin may be palliative (unproven).
Supportive	Antibiotics may reduce secondary bacterial infection, and corticosteroids may reduce inflammation. Esophagostomy/pharyngostomy or gastrostomy tube mandatory if further treatment is pursued. Dental care important following mandibulectomy.

Incidence, Signalment, and Etiology

SCC is the most common oral tumor reported in cats. In six surveys totaling 585 cats with oral tumors, 380 (65%) had oral SCC.[1-5,7] While cats with white coats appear to have an increased risk of developing cutaneous SCC, there is no influence of coat color, gender, or breed on the occurrence of oral SCC.[8]

Affected cats tend to be older (average age, 12 years), although cats as young as 5 months[1] and as old as 21 years[2] have been reported. The majority of reported cats have been DSHs or DLHs. Only 5 of 52 cats with oral SCC in one study were purebreds.[9] Persians and Himalayans are reported occasionally[5,10,11] and Siamese rarely.[4,12] There is no obvious gender predilection (186 male and 205 female cats in six studies),[1,2,5,9,13,14] and neutering had no effect in an epidemiologic study of this disease.[4] *Trichinella* larvae seen in one tumor were probably incidental, not causative.[15]

Recent evidence suggests that exposure to environmental tobacco smoke increases the risk of a cat developing oral SCC.[15a]

Clinical Presentation and History

SCC can affect any mucosal surface in the mouth, but the tongue is most commonly involved (Figure 41-1). The frenulum and ventral surfaces are often ulcerated; even though the tumor is deeply invasive, the dorsum of the tongue is rarely affected.[2,9,13,16] This site predilection has been suggested to be due to increased carcinogen exposure caused by coat grooming in cats. SCC of the oral cavity is, however, rare in other felids.[17,18]

The mucosa adjacent to the maxilla or mandible is the next most commonly affected site. Most tumors are found caudal to the canine teeth.[13] SCC may invade the underlying bone and extend to involve the palate, pharynx, or angle

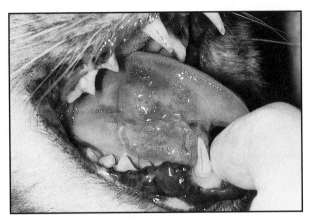

Figure 41-1: SCC is commonly seen on the lingual frenulum of older cats. The tumor interferes with food prehension and often causes ptyalism and oral bleeding.

of the jaw (Figure 41-2). Invasion of mandibular bone can cause a huge periosteal reaction that mimics a primary bone tumor both clinically and radiographically.[9,13,14,19,20] Occasionally, there will be no evidence of mucosal lesions despite a large underlying bony mass.[14] While oral SCC may progress to invade the tonsillar area, it is uncommon for the tonsil to be the primary site.[2,9,13,21]

KEY POINT

Squamous cell carcinoma is the most common oral tumor in cats.

The most common reason for an owner of a cat with an oral tumor to seek veterinary advice is that he or she has noticed a mass.[13] Ptyalism is often reported and is due to necrosis and ulceration, particularly of tongue lesions; dysphagia and even difficulty in swallowing water may be noted. The saliva may be ropey, bloody, and fetid.[9,12,13,15,16] Dysphagia may worsen gradually due to a slowly enlarging mass[13] or may occur acutely due to mandibular luxation[13] or a pathologic fracture.[6,22] Some cats may not be able to close their mouth due to a mass of tumor tissue and reactive stroma.[10,14] Ulceration and the suppurative inflammation associated with necrosis account for the halitosis that is often reported.

KEY POINT

A large bony mandibular mass is more likely to be SCC than osteosarcoma.

Large maxillary SCC may invade the periocular space and cause exophthalmos as well as nasal and ocular discharge.[14,15] In these cats it may be difficult to determine the site of tumor origin. Loose teeth noted during a dental examination may be the first signs of oral SCC.[14] Biopsy of any ulcerated

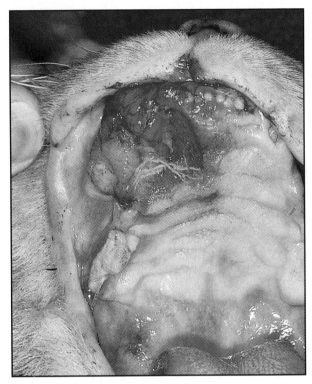

Figure 41-2: Mucosal tumors may erode the surrounding tissue as they grow, causing ulceration of the palate, destruction of bone, and loss of teeth, as in this 12-year-old cat.

mucosal tissue is warranted in old cats with dental disease. In one study the duration of clinical signs varied widely (1 week to 5 years); however, approximately half the cats show signs for 4 weeks or less.[13,22] Tumors may grow rapidly; one mandibular tumor quadrupled in size in 2 months.[10]

KEY POINT

Oral SCCs are highly invasive and are usually much larger than indicated by physical examination.

Staging and Diagnosis

Biopsy is the only method to definitively diagnose oral SCC. Clinically, this tumor is indistinguishable from benign lesions (e.g., eosinophilic granuloma) or odontogenic tumors, both of which have a better prognosis with appropriate treatment. Histologic differentiation of the tumor does not, however, predict biologic behavior[23] as all oral SCCs act aggressively.

The most common site of metastasis is the mandibular or retropharyngeal lymph nodes, which should be palpated at the time of physical examination. In one study, 15 of 52 cats (30%) had enlarged regional lymph nodes and 7 of these had evidence of SCC on cytology from a fine-needle aspirate.[13] Unfortunately, lymphadenopathy does not always occur with metastatic tumors; in one study, a cat with normal-sized mandibular lymph nodes had histologic evidence of tumor while 2 cats with lymphadenopathy did not.[22] In other studies that included treated cats, the incidence of lymph node metastases ranged from 8% to 30% (average, about 10%).[5,14,24] Lung metastases are rare. There have been no reports of metastatic disease on thoracic radiographs at the time of diagnosis, although 1 cat had pulmonary metastases on necropsy.[24]

Skull radiographs are helpful in developing a treatment plan. As described, oral SCC may invade underlying bone, thereby causing an intensely sclerotic, periosteal proliferation (Figure 41-3). This syndrome appears almost exclusively in the mandible.[14,19,20,25] Marked osteolysis may also occur because of tumor invasion and is seen in up to 70% of affected cats.[11,13,24,26] In one study, radiographs showed that osteolysis affected a much greater area than was clinically apparent in 24 of 52 cats, thereby changing the treatment plan. Tooth root resorption and ankylosis may indicate tumor progression beyond the apparent soft tissue borders.[27] Computed tomography (CT) is an even more accurate method to determine the extent of tumor and, if available, should be performed prior to surgery or radiation therapy to ensure that adequate treatment margins are obtained. Ultrasonography appears useful for delineating soft tissue margins of lingual SCC, and may play a role in monitoring response to treatment.[28]

Oral SCC is staged according to tumor size as well as the presence of bone invasion and metastatic disease. The ma-

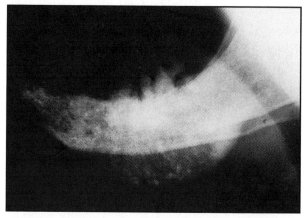

Figure 41-3: *Invasion of underlying bone may cause a severe proliferative bony reaction that may mimic a primary bone tumor both clinically and radiographically. (Courtesy of L. Kleine)*

jority of tumors in one study were clinical stage 2 or 3.[13]

Retroviruses do not seem to be associated with this disease; only 2 of 40 cats were FeLV positive in one study,[13] and one cat was FIV positive in another.[22]

A paraneoplastic hypercalcemia was described in a cat with oral SCC causing bony lysis of the maxilla.[29] Hypercalcemia was not associated with elevated serum parathyroid hormone levels and resolved after treatment of the tumor. Recurrence of hypercalcemia was concurrent with a lymph node metastasis. While uncommon, this finding underscores the importance of obtaining an MDB for all cats with suspected neoplasia.

Treatment

In some cats with oral SCC, palliation with antibiotics may improve quality of life but does not extend duration of survival. Cats treated this way rarely live more than 8 weeks.[12,15,24,30]

Surgery

Surgical removal of visible tumor is rarely successful as oral SCCs are deeply invasive into both soft tissue stroma and bone. Cats treated in this way rarely live longer than untreated cats. In one study, recurrence and metastases occurred in all cats 1 to 14 weeks after surgery.[23]

To ensure complete resection of an oral SCC, it is usually necessary to excise underlying or affected bone. Maxillectomy or mandibulectomy allows the surgeon to obtain tumor-free margins, but recurrences are still commonly reported 1 to 5 months after surgery.[11,13,26,31] More aggressive surgery (i.e., removing the entire mandible; Figures 41-4 and 41-5) delayed recurrence to 4 to 9 months after surgery.[11] Individual cats have lived a long time after maxillectomy[32] or mandibulectomy,[11] but the median survival is still less than 2 months.[13] Imaging with CT scanning prior to surgery may assist the surgeon in deciding on the extent of surgery needed to obtain appropriate margins.

The risk of surgical complications increases with more aggressive procedures. One cat died due to aspiration of a food particle,[31] and another cat was unable to swallow following bilateral mandibulectomy.[11] Less life-threatening problems include tongue lagging, which results in the owner needing to clean saliva from the chest and feet of cats that underwent mandibulectomy.[22] Mandibulectomy may also result in "mandibular drift" when the unattached bone

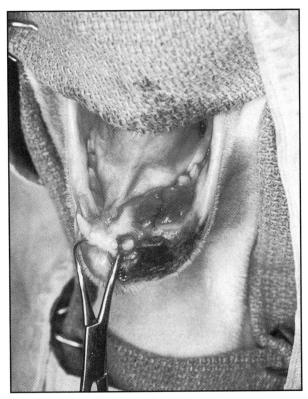

Figure 41-4: *A rostral mandibular SCC can be treated by hemimandibulectomy. Most SCCs in other oral locations are not amenable to surgery. (Courtesy of J. Berg)*

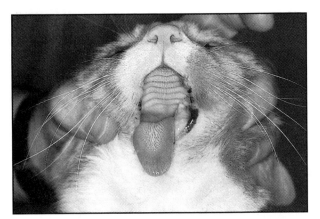

Figure 41-5: *Complete right and partial left mandibulectomy was performed 1 year previously in this 15-year-old cat. An enteral tube should be placed at the time of surgery to ensure nutritional support during the recovery phase.*

moves medially. If the canine tooth has not been removed or trimmed, a painful ulcer can develop at the point of contact with the hard palate. A similar problem can occur with molar teeth, and the surgeon should be prepared to file these teeth at the time of original surgery.

Gastrostomy tube placement is mandatory for all cats undergoing extensive oral surgery and should be performed at the time of surgery. In one study the gastrostomy tube was left in place 3 to 44 days after surgery, with half the cats requiring it for 2 weeks or less.[22]

KEY POINT

A gastrostomy tube is warranted for any cat undergoing treatment for oral SCC.

Radiation Therapy

Because recurrence is still a problem following even radical surgery, radiation therapy either alone or following surgery has been used to treat oral SCC. Megavoltage radiation therapy was used in 24 cats; median survival was 3 months.[13] Orthovoltage radiation (total dose of 52 Gy) was administered in conjunction with the hypoxic cell sensitizer etanidazole to 11 cats with oral SCC.[24] Nine cats completed

the treatment, but all had tumor recurrence a median of 4.5 months later. Complications due to radiation or tumor were seen in 5 cats, including ischemic necrosis of the tongue in 3 cats and osteonecrosis or tracheal obstruction in 2 others. Repeated radiation is unlikely to be successful and has a high complication rate in cats with oral SCC.[33] Tumor response to radiation is often dramatic initially (Figures 41-6 and 41-7) but is usually of short duration.

Hyperthermia has been thought to increase the response rate by sensitizing hypoxic tumor cells.[34] However, the average survival was only 2.5 months in 11 cats treated with radiation and hyperthermia.[13]

One cat treated with cobalt radiation did not develop tumor recurrence but had lymph node metastasis 3 months after treatment.[29] To address this problem, seven cats were treated with a combination of mandibulectomy, lymph node resection, and radiation that included the surgical site of regional lymph node resection.[22] The median disease-free period for these cats was 11 months (range, 2.5–34

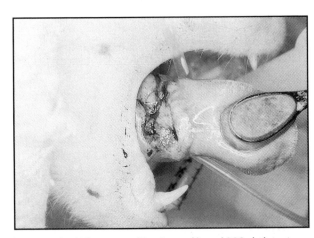

Figure 41-6: *This 11-year-old cat has a sublingual SCC; the lesion is seen prior to radiation therapy.*

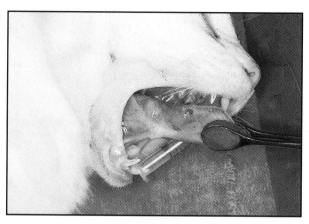

Figure 41-7: Radiation therapy provided rapid clinical improvement in the cat shown in Figure 41-6; the lesion has healed. Regrowth is usually rapid, however, and adjunctive chemotherapy may be warranted.

months). All cats developed recurrence, although the 1 year survival rate was 57%. It appears that aggressive combination therapy may be warranted in selected cats. A gastrostomy tube was placed in all cats.

KEY POINT

Single modality therapy, whether it be surgery, radiation, or chemotherapy, provides a median survival of 2 months for cats with oral SCC.

Chemotherapy

Chemotherapy alone or in combination with radiation therapy has done little to improve survival. Low doses of cisplatin did not cause toxicity but also did not improve efficacy of radiation therapy in treated cats.[13,26] Similarly, liposome-encapsulation of cisplatin resulted in abrogation of toxicity but caused no clinical responses in 14 cats with oral SCC.[35] Cisplatin should never be administered to cats at any dosage due to the risk of fatal pulmonary edema.[36]

Doxorubicin and cyclophosphamide were given to five cats with oral SCC.[37] Tumors progressed within 2 months

in four cats, and one cat had a partial response for 3 months. Four cats were anorectic and one cat lost weight, although whether this was due to chemotherapy or to the tumor is uncertain.

KEY POINT

Combinations of surgery and radiation or radiation and chemotherapy have provided the longest survival times in cats with oral SCC.

Mitoxantrone chemotherapy alone caused a complete tumor response in one cat for 60 days and partial responses in three cats for 21 to 60 days.[38] Mitoxantrone in combination with high doses of radiation caused responses for a median of 6 months, with two of seven cats alive a year after treatment.[39] Carboplatin has shown anecdotal efficacy in the treatment of oral SCC.[40] Other treatment modalities such as photodynamic therapy do not appear to be successful in part because of the increased sensitivity of oral mucosa to toxicity and also because the tumor invades bone or deep into tissue, thereby preventing adequate light penetration.[41] Cryosurgery is unlikely to be successful for the same reasons. Investigational treatments, such as benzaldehyde, have not been successful in cats with oral SCC.[42]

The best treatment for oral SCC has yet to be decided. In one study comparing surgical treatment with radiation alone or in combination with hyperthermia or chemotherapy, no influence of treatment modality on survival was noted[13]; tumor location, tumor stage, or duration of clinical signs also had no influence on survival. In contrast, some cats with oral SCC have long survival times and occasionally an animal is cured. Combination therapy using aggressive surgery, radiation therapy, and chemotherapy to treat both the local tumor and regional lymph nodes will probably result in the best survival times. Owners should be counseled about the required nursing care, and a gastrostomy tube should be placed for the duration of treatment and until the cat is able to eat on its own. The prognosis for this tumor, particularly when it is advanced and the cat is debilitated, remains poor.

FIBROSARCOMA

CLINICAL BRIEFING	
Common Presentation	Anywhere in the oral cavity; often invades bone, causing dysphagia and similar signs to SCC.
Staging and Diagnosis	MDB, lymph node palpation, CT scan prior to definitive treatment. Metastasis is rare.

(continued)

Treatment	
Initial	Surgical excision possible with wide excision that includes bone.
Adjunctive	Radiation therapy reduces recurrence rate for soft-tissue sarcoma at other sites and is probably also effective in oral sarcomas, although this use is unproven. Chemotherapy may reduce local recurrence as well, but metastatic rate is low and thus the value in improving survival is unproven. Carboplatin, doxorubicin, and vincristine have shown efficacy and could be considered if radiation is not available.
Supportive	Antibiotics and antiinflammatory drugs as well as analgesics as necessary for palliation. Enteral feeding tube mandatory if definitive treatment attempted.

Incidence, Signalment, and Etiology

In two large surveys of 429 oral tumors in cats, fibrosarcoma was the second most common malignancy described. Fifty-three cats (12.4%) had fibrosarcoma, and their ages ranged from 1 to 21 years (average, 10.3 years).[1,2] Males and females were equally represented. Case reports of oral fibrosarcoma fit into these same signalment criteria.[5,11,25,26,32,43] One cat was reported to have concurrent fibrosarcoma and SCC.[44] A tonsillar granular cell tumor in a 2-year-old cat[45] and one on the tongue of a 9-year-old cat[46] were described as having features of sarcoma.

MDB = minimum database; includes CBC, biochemical profile, urinalysis, FeLV/FIV serology, T_4 testing, and thoracic radiographs (three views).

Clinical Presentation and History

Unlike oral SCC, which seems to have a predilection for the sublingual tissues, there does not appear to be a site predilection for oral fibrosarcoma.[2] Fibrosarcoma is invasive in the oral cavity, just as it is at other sites in cats; advanced lesions may invade surrounding bone and muscle.[20] Lesions may be ulcerated, causing dysphagia and other signs similar to oral SCC,[25] and cats may be presented because an owner noticed swelling or a mass.[5,25]

Staging and Diagnosis

It is rare for metastases to be noted at the time of presentation, and no cat has been reported to have metastatic disease after surgery.[5,11,26,32,37,43] Many of these cats died soon after surgery due to tumor recurrence or surgical complications before any subclinical metastases became apparent, therefore the reported low metastatic rate may not be accurate. It is good practice to obtain thoracic radiographs and carefully evaluate mandibular and pharyngeal lymph nodes prior to attempting definitive surgery. CT scan may assist in planning surgery or radiation therapy.

Treatment

Surgical excision should be as aggressive as possible. If adequate postsurgical nursing care and nutritional support are provided as described for cats with oral SCC, cats tolerate procedures such as mandibulectomy and maxillectomy as well as dogs.

Maxillectomy needs to be aggressive in order to assure adequate surgical margins. Tumor recurrence was noted 3.5 months after maxillectomy in one cat with a lesion centered around the upper canine,[26] whereas another cat had no evidence of tumor 24 months after a unilateral premaxillectomy.[32] Mandibulectomy was reported in three cats. A cat that underwent hemimandibulectomy for a small fibrosarcoma had no evidence of tumor nearly a year later.[11] In contrast, an older cat treated via a rostral hemimandibulectomy and one that received a total hemimandibulectomy either had recurrence or did not eat postoperatively. Both were euthanized within 10 weeks of surgery.[11] Cats that undergo such procedures should have a gastrostomy tube placed at the same time.

Radiation therapy has a role in preventing recurrence after incomplete surgery for soft tissue sarcomas of other sites but is not reported for oral tumors.

Adjuvant chemotherapy may have a role in reducing the risk of recurrence. Carboplatin and doxorubicin have anecdotal efficacy against soft tissue sarcomas in cats. Two cats with a 2 to 4 cm fibrosarcoma of the maxilla and one with a similar-sized fibrosarcoma of the mandible received cyclophosphamide and 25 mg/m^2 of doxorubicin IV every 3 weeks.[37] One cat had a complete response for 5 months and another had more than 50% reduction in tumor size for 2 months, but tumors eventually recurred in both cats. The tumor in the third cat did not grow for 7 months.[37] Complete regression of an oral fibrosarcoma lasted for 10 months in a cat treated with vincristine.[47]

KEY POINT

A gastrostomy tube is mandatory for cats undergoing treatment of any oral tumor.

MELANOMA

Incidence, Signalment, and Etiology

While oral melanoma is common in dogs, it is rare in cats. Small dark mucocutaneous patches (lentigo simplex) around the oral cavity of orange cats do not progress to melanoma.[48]

In three surveys totaling 146 oral tumors in cats, only 4 were melanomas.[3-5] In the sole report that included signalment for affected cats, there were three females (one spayed) and two castrated males. Four cats were DSHs and one was Siamese; they ranged in age from 8 to 16 years.[49]

Clinical Presentation and History

The affected location within the oral cavity was provided for six cats.[5,49] Three tumors affected the maxilla, two occurred on the palate, and one on the mandible (Figure 41-8). The lesion was "crater-like" in one cat,[5] and another cat was presented for mucosal swelling and drooling of 2 weeks' duration.[49] An oral mass was noted by the owner in three cats.

Staging and Diagnosis

Of the six cats, four developed metastatic disease, one had no obvious metastases on necropsy,[5] and one was lost to follow-up.

The staging procedures for cats with oral melanoma should include MDB, abdominal ultrasonography, and cytologic or histologic examination of the mandibular and pharyngeal lymph nodes; these should be performed prior to definitive surgery.

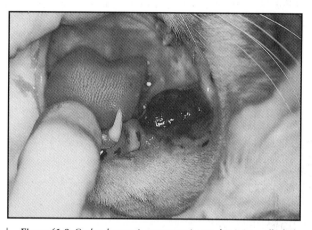

Figure 41-8: Oral melanoma is uncommon in cats, but it is usually dark pigmented and friable. Biopsy is warranted because a benign oral tumor (CEOT) can also be pigmented.

Treatment

Oral melanoma was surgically excised in three cats. All developed metastatic disease within 5 months of surgery, and metastases were diffuse throughout the body in two of these cats.[49]

Radiation therapy may be helpful in local tumor control, but the results are variable.[a] Carboplatin may have efficacy against metastases but is unproven.

[a]Moore AS, Ogilvie GK: Personal observations.

BENIGN ORAL TUMORS

Nonneoplastic lesions in the mouth, such as eosinophilic granuloma (Figure 41-9) or inflammatory polyps (Figure 41-10), may mimic malignant lesions. Biopsy should always be performed.

Multifocal, small, light pink, oral sessile warts have been seen on the ventral lingual surface of the tongue of a 6-month-old and a 9-year-old cat.[50] Papillomavirus was isolated from the tumors, but the role (if any) of these in progression to SCC is obscure.

▶ ODONTOGENIC TUMORS

A number of different terms have been used to describe tumors arising from the components of teeth. Some tumors retain the ability to induce reactive proliferation of connec-

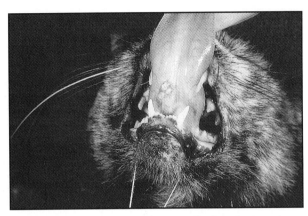

Figure 41-9: *Eosinophilic granuloma may affect the oral cavity and clinically mimic a malignant tumor. Biopsy is always warranted for a feline oral tumor.*

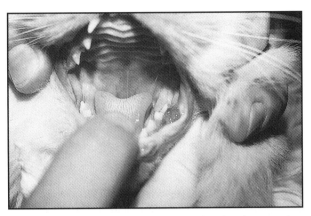

Figure 41-10: *Other inflammatory lesions, such as the polyp seen in this young cat, can resemble a malignant lesion. Biopsy of oral lesions is mandatory.*

tive tissue, and thus odontogenic tumors are often described as "inductive" or "noninductive."

Inductive tumors include fibroameloblastoma (adamantinoma), which often has histologic remnants of normal odontogenesis where cords of epithelium tend to form cuplike structures. The most common noninductive tumor in cats is the calcifying epithelial odontogenic tumor (CEOT), which contains amyloid deposits within its stroma.

Other tumor types include ameloblastic fibroma (which is usually encapsulated and, unlike fibroameloblastomas and CEOT, does not invade bone) and odontoma.[51]

Unfortunately, there is considerable and confusing overlap in the terminology used in veterinary references; however, the majority of odontogenic tumors are benign and most are not aggressively invasive, so the clinical distinction may not be critical.

Epulides, arising from the periodontal ligament, are rare in cats.

C L I N I C A L   B R I E F I N G

Common Presentation	Inductive fibroameloblastoma in cats less than 18 months old; CEOT and epulides in older cats. CEOT may be pigmented. Clinically indistinguishable from malignant oral tumors.
Staging and Diagnosis	Biopsy mandatory. MDB; thoracic radiographs particularly important in older cats. Metastasis not recorded. Skull radiographs and CT scan before surgery or radiation therapy.
Treatment Initial	Both surgery and radiation therapy are likely to be curative.
Adjunctive	Chemotherapy not indicated; radiation therapy for recurrence after surgery or postoperatively for incomplete excision.
Supportive	As for malignant oral tumors.

INDUCTIVE FIBROAMELOBLASTOMA

Incidence, Signalment, and Etiology

The tumors may be confused clinically with epulides.[9,52] Inductive fibroameloblastomas have been almost exclusively described in cats 18 months of age or younger. Of 20 affected cats reported, the youngest were 7 months old (median age, 9 months).[2,52–59] Most of these tumors have occurred in DSH cats; 2 Siamese have been reported.[57,59] There does not appear to be a gender predilection.

KEY POINT

An oral tumor in a cat younger than 1 year of age is likely to be a fibroameloblastoma.

Clinical Presentation and History

Cats may be presented because the owner has noticed a rapidly growing mass,[53,55] although occasionally it may be present for some time. A cat with an oral mass of 3 months' duration had a painful tumor that was 3 cm in diameter on presentation.[54] One cat had problems prehending food.[53] Tumor location was identified in 15 cats; it occurred in the maxilla in 9 cats and the mandible in the other 6.[2,52-57] Seven of the maxillary tumors were located around or cranial to the canine tooth. The tumor had been noticed in 1 cat at the time of permanent teeth eruption.[57]

Staging and Diagnosis

Skull radiographs should be obtained; lysis of the underlying bone is common, and areas of mineralization within the tumor may occasionally be seen.[53-55,57] Teeth may be missing when larger lesions are present (Figure 41-11),[57] and the tumor may invade the nasal cavity.[57]

Treatment

Surgery is the treatment of choice, particularly for small inductive fibroameloblastomas. Localized excision may not be successful because of the high probability of bony invasion. In 5 of 10 cats treated surgically, there was no recurrence 6 to 36 months after surgery.[52,54,56,57] Local recurrence was seen within 2 to 6 weeks of surgery in 3 of the remaining cats[56,57] and at 42 months after surgery in a fourth.[52] The 3 cats with early recurrence were treated a second time by surgery, either alone or in conjunction with radiation therapy. One cat had no recurrence 5 years later; another had a second recurrence 6 months later, but the tumor then remained static for 3.5 years.[56] A very low dose (15 Gy) of ra-

KEY POINT

Long survival times are possible when cats with fibroameloblastoma are treated aggressively.

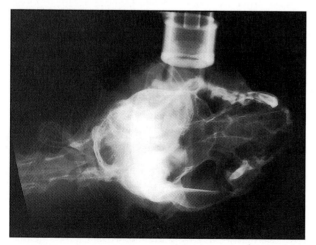

Figure 41-11: *Inductive fibroameloblastoma is an invasive odontogenic tumor seen in young cats. This large oral lesion in a 12-month-old cat had eroded bone and caused loss of teeth. It was successfully treated with surgery and radiation, and the cat was alive 5 years later.*

diation failed to prevent a second recurrence 10 months later in the third cat.[57]

Radiation therapy at appropriate doses does appear to be effective when combined with surgery.[60]

MDB = minimum database; includes CBC, biochemical profile, urinalysis, FeLV/FIV serology, T_4 testing, and thoracic radiographs (three views).

CALCIFYING EPITHELIAL ODONTOGENIC TUMOR (CEOT)

Incidence, Signalment, and Etiology

These tumors are characterized by their production of amyloid. They have been reported in 12 older DSH cats between 7 and 15 years of age (median, 9 years). All but one[61] occurred in male cats.[2,51,52,56,62-64]

Clinical Presentation and History

Reported CEOTs have been between 1 and 3 cm in diameter; six of eight tumors for which location was provided were in the maxilla (Figure 41-12).[51,52,56,61-64] Most clinical descriptions indicate that the tumor appears very much like an SCC: They are friable, ulcerated, and often bleed easily. Interestingly, some CEOTs are darkly pigmented,[56,64] making them difficult to distinguish clinically from oral melanoma.

Staging and Diagnosis

Biopsy is required for definitive diagnosis and differentiation from more common oral tumors. Radiographs should be obtained (osteolysis may be marked) and will allow the surgeon to better prepare for definitive excision.[61] Metastasis has not been reported.

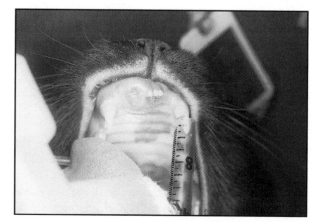

Figure 41-12: *CEOT in an older cat. This benign tumor may be cured by surgery or, as was used in this cat, radiation therapy.*

Treatment

The prognosis following surgery appears to be cautiously optimistic. In four of the six cats treated surgically and for which adequate follow-up information was available, there was no evidence of disease 7 months to 2.5 years after surgery.[56,64] Tumor recurrence was seen after surgery in the other two cats, at 13 months in one and 17 months in the second.[52,63]

KEY POINT

Cats with epulides or CEOT may be cured with surgical excision.

Surgical excision should include underlying bone and be as aggressive as possible. Radiation therapy appears to be an effective treatment modality in cats with CEOT and should be considered for recurrent tumors or following incomplete surgery.[60]

EPULIDES

Incidence, Signalment, and Etiology

Epulides are much less common in cats than in dogs, accounting for 3 of 89 oral neoplasms in one study[9] and 29 of 371[2] in a second study. All epulides described in cats have been fibromatous or ossifying. Acanthomatous epulis has not been reported. Signalment of affected cats has rarely been reported, but Siamese and Persians have been affected[9] in addition to DSH cats.[32] Affected cats have ranged in age from 5 to 17 years.[9,32]

Clinical Presentation and History

There is considerable morphologic variation of these tumors, ranging from pedunculated to sessile. They may also contain varying amounts of osseous material.[2] They may occur in the mandible[9] or maxilla[2] and are usually less than 1.5 cm in diameter.

Staging and Diagnosis

Biopsy is the only definitive method of diagnosis, and staging should be performed as described for the more common oral SCC. Epulides are benign, but skull radiographs should be obtained to check for bony lysis.

Treatment

Surgery should be curative. These tumors arise from the periodontal ligament, and thus the tooth with its socket must be removed to prevent recurrence. A cat that had a unilateral premaxillectomy for an epulis had no recurrence 7 months later.[32] Radiation therapy appears effective in preventing recurrence after incomplete surgery.[60]

OTHER ODONTOGENIC TUMORS

Incidence, Signalment, and Etiology

Tumors described in 11 cats were called ameloblastic fibroma,[25,52,55] keratinizing ameloblastoma,[2] complex odontoma,[56] odontogenic fibroma and odontogenic fibrosarcoma,[2] and odontoblastoma.[25] Affected cats were between 3 and 14 years of age and primarily DSHs (except for 1 Siamese[2]); 8 were males. The histologic distinction among these tumors, CEOT, and inductive fibroameloblastoma may be clinically artificial.

Clinical Presentation and History

These tumors have occurred equally in the upper and lower dental arcade and usually appear as a small fleshy mass.[55] They are therefore clinically indistinguishable from other oral tumors in older cats.

Staging and Diagnosis

Radiographs of the skull should be obtained, as tumors may cause considerable osteolysis and may affect both the oral and nasal cavities.[25]

Treatment

Surgical excision was performed in seven cats, and two had no evidence of tumor 2 years after surgery.[25,52] Recurrence was noted in the other cats 2 months to 2 years after surgery (median, 16 months).[2,25,56] These treatment data are very similar to those obtained for cats with other odontogenic tumors.

▶ OTHER BENIGN ORAL TUMORS

Sebaceous adenomas, presumably of alveolar origin, were described in two cats (5 and 7 years old). These tumors were less than 1 cm in diameter. Surgical excision was presumably curative.[65]

Multiple gingival fibropapillomas were described in two cats. Resection appeared to be curative in one cat, but lesions recurred 2 months later in the other. The authors postulated that these may be virally induced,[66] but there were no identifiable viral antigens in two other oral fibropapillomas in cats.[67]

A 12-month-old male DLH had an odontogenic cyst of the posterior mandible diagnosed on biopsy.[52] Although it appeared firm and fleshy, periodic drainage was sufficient to control it for nearly 6 years.

NONDOMESTIC FELIDAE

Oral SCC in domestic cats has been suggested to be due to the feline practice of coat-grooming, which exposes the oral cavity to environmental carcinogens. Despite similar grooming habits in nondomestic cats, only one oral SCC has been reported in a Canadian lynx (Felis lynx canadensis).[17]

A hemangioma of the tongue was recorded in a cheetah (*Acinonyx jubatus*).[17]

Small, multifocal, pink, sessile warts have been identified on the ventral surface of tongues in various Felidae. Species-specific papillomaviruses were identified in such lesions from two Florida panthers (*Felis concolor*), two bobcats (*Fe-lis rufus*), four Asiatic lions (*Panthera leo*), and a clouded leopard (*Neofelis nebulosa*). All cats were adults.[50] Similar lesions containing papillomavirus were seen in three snow leopards (age range, 5 to 16 years). These cats had lesions on the tip and dorsal surface of the tongue as well as the buccal mucosa.[50]

TUMORS OF THE SALIVARY GLANDS

CLINICAL BRIEFING

Common Presentation	Most commonly affect major salivary glands, causing swelling and signs similar to those described for other oral tumors. Most tumors are malignant but are clinically indistinguishable from benign tumors.
Staging and Diagnosis	MDB and lymph node palpation (up to 80% have metastases here). Palpate surrounding skin as tumors may be invasive. CT scan prior to definitive treatment.
Treatment	
Initial	Surgical excision curative for adenoma. Carcinomas are invasive and thus are rarely completely removed.
Adjunctive	Radiation therapy gives best chance of local control following incomplete surgical excision. Chemotherapy with doxorubicin, or possibly carboplatin, is recommended due to high rate of metastases. A combination of surgery, radiation, and chemotherapy is recommended for these tumors.
Supportive	As for oral tumors. Consider gastrostomy tube rather than pharyngostomy tube due to tumor location.

Incidence, Signalment, and Etiology

The salivary glands can be broadly divided into major glands (parotid, mandibular, sublingual, molar, and zygomatic) and minor glands (lip, cheek, palate, gingiva, tongue, and floor of the mouth). Salivary gland tumors most commonly affect the major glands. All six case reports prior to the 1960s were of parotid carcinomas,[68,69] and the majority of cats in recent surveys also have involvement of the major salivary glands, mainly the mandibular glands.[9,70]

Most tumors are adenocarcinomas, accounting for 89 of 106 tumors.[70,71] Other carcinomas are less common, and adenomas comprise approximately 5% of salivary tumors.[9,70-72] Mixed tumors (carcinosarcomas) are rare[73,74] and may occasionally be benign.[71] Some carcinomas appear to arise from the salivary duct rather than the glandular tissue.[75]

The average age of affected cats is 10.5 years but ranges from 2 months[71] to 20 years.[9] There does not appear to be a gender predilection.[2,70,71,75] Most affected cats have been DSHs, although 14 of 53 affected cats were Siamese in one study.[71] Other purebred cats in that study included Tonkinese (1) and Persians (2).

Clinical Presentation and History

Some cats are presented for an enlarging mass on the side of the face or below the ear. Less commonly, ulcerated mucosal gingiva or other affected oral sites may lead to a diagnosis of salivary adenocarcinoma (Figure 41-13). Oral tumors that are "undifferentiated" adenocarcinomas are probably of salivary derivation (Figure 41-14).[37]

Ulceration of the overlying skin is common, possibly due to pruritus, which may be exacerbated by secondary otitis externa from parotid tumors; deeper invasion may result in facial nerve damage[9] or vestibular signs.[72] Signs of hypersalivation, dysphagia, and weight loss are common, as is the case with other oral tumors such as SCC. Tumors can be very large, reaching more than 8 cm in diameter.[9,73,74] In one series of cats, 2 of 13 had secondary aspiration pneumonia and both had been force-fed by their owner.[9] It is not possible to distinguish a salivary adenoma from an adenocarcinoma on the basis of clinical signs.

Staging and Diagnosis

In addition to performing a careful physical examination of the primary tumor, regional lymph nodes, particularly mandibular lymph nodes, should be palpated. If the nodes

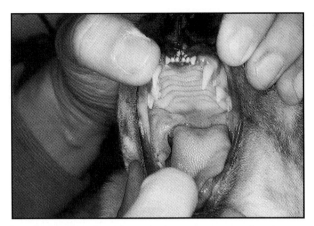

Figure 41-13: A large salivary gland carcinoma is seen in the right caudal oropharynx of a 9-year-old Siamese. This tumor was not accessible for surgery and was treated with radiation therapy. Metastasis to the regional lymph nodes occurred within 1 year.

are enlarged, aspiration cytology or biopsy should be performed as this is a common site of metastasis even at the time of first diagnosis. Up to 80% of cats have regional lymph node metastases.[9,68,71,72,75,76]

KEY POINT

Salivary adenocarcinomas have a high rate of lymph node metastasis.

Pulmonary metastases are less commonly seen. One cat developed lung metastases within 5 months of surgery,[71] and widespread metastases to lung,[9,77] heart, brain, and abdominal viscera were seen in two other cats. In one study of 31 cats, 5 had evidence of distant metastasis at the time of diagnosis.[78] Thoracic radiographs should be obtained prior to treatment. Salivary adenocarcinomas can be very invasive into surrounding musculature[76] and may even extend along the skin of the neck to involve the thoracic wall and scapula.[9]

Clinical stage was not prognostic in a study[78] of 31 cats with salivary carcinomas, although the multiple treatment methods used could confuse the issue. This implies that the finding of metastasis should not preclude treatment.

MDB = minimum database; includes CBC, biochemical profile, urinalysis, FeLV/FIV serology, T$_4$ testing, and thoracic radiographs (three views).

Treatment

Surgical treatment of salivary adenomas is usually successful. Of three cats treated by surgery alone, two had no recurrence, although one was euthanized due to concurrent lymphoma.[9]

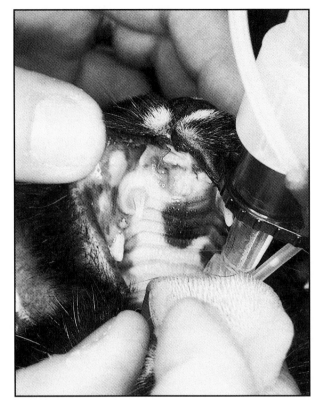

Figure 41-14: An adenocarcinoma of the minor salivary glands affecting the rostral maxilla of a 16-year-old cat.

Another cat with salivary adenoma had two recurrences over a period of several months before an aggressive surgery was performed. No follow-up information was provided.[72]

In contrast to salivary adenomas, salivary adenocarcinomas are more difficult to treat due to deep invasion around the jugular vein and associated structures.[69] Cats with adenocarcinoma[71] or malignant mixed tumors[73] that were not treated lived between 5 and 6 months and were euthanized due to weight loss and enlargement of the tumor. Rapid recurrence occurred in two cats, one of which was euthanized because of dysphagia.[69,71]

Radiation therapy for these tumors has been reported,[78] albeit with few details. Similar treatment protocols to those used for ceruminous gland tumors may be helpful in slowing tumor progression. Anecdotal local control has been achieved with these tumors using radiation therapy. We have treated several with good results for local control.[a]

Doxorubicin chemotherapy resulted in greater than 50% reduction in the size of a salivary adenocarcinoma for 9 months.[37] Combination therapy using surgery, radiation therapy, and chemotherapy with doxorubicin (or possibly carboplatin) is the most likely to be successful in cats with salivary adenocarcinomas. A median survival of 516 days was achieved in 31 cats treated with any combination of these modalities.[78]

ESOPHAGEAL TUMORS

Common Presentation	Most are carcinomas and cause regurgitation of solid foods and gagging. Common locations are thoracic inlet or intrathoracic, but tumors can be anywhere in the esophagus.
Staging and Diagnosis	MDB, lymph node palpation, contrast esophagography, and endoscopic biopsy. Metastasis is common, and tumor may extend to involve stomach.
Treatment	
Initial	Surgery unlikely to be curative due to extent of tumor.
Adjunctive	None reported; radiation may be palliative but unlikely to be successful.
Supportive	Gastrostomy tube will allow feeding. Analgesics mandatory, but treatment not recommended for this tumor type.

Incidence, Signalment, and Etiology

Epithelial tumors of the esophagus are more common than mesenchymal tumors but are still considered very rare, at least in the United States. Earlier reports by Cotchin described 10 of 33 GI tumors in cats as esophageal carcinomas,[79] and another report from the 1930s stated that the "cat is most prone to cancer of the esophagus of all the domestic species."[80] The British reports contrast with U.S. reports, where only 6 cases have been identified,[9,81,82] the Netherlands (2 cats),[83] Italy (2 cats),[84] France (1 cat),[85] and Australia (1 cat).[86]

Affected cats range in age from 5[80] to 14[82] years, and most cats have been male.[79–82,85] Only one purebred cat, a Siamese, has been reported.[82] SCC is the most common histologic type reported.

Clinical Presentation and History

Most cats appear eager to eat but regurgitate soon after. Often liquids are not regurgitated. As the tumor progresses, postprandial regurgitation may precede regurgitation unrelated to eating.[84] Affected cats may show excessive swallowing or gagging, particularly after palpation of the neck.[81,82] Vomitus may be streaked with blood.[80,81] Most affected cats are described as thin to emaciated, although regurgitation has often been noticed by the owner for only 2 to 3 weeks. One cat had a hiatal hernia presumably due to an ulcerated stenotic tumor in the caudal esophagus.[9]

Staging and Diagnosis

Most tumors are at the thoracic inlet or intrathoracic.[80] Esophageal carcinoma in the neck may be palpable.[80] Plain radiography may demonstrate a soft tissue opacity if the lesion is intrathoracic[83] or may show an air-filled and dilated esophagus.[81,84,85] Fluoroscopy may demonstrate a roughened mucosal pattern with intramural filling defects and may show a completely obstructive mass.[81–84] Esophagoscopy is useful for visualizing the mass and obtaining a biopsy sample, but superficial biopsies may be insufficient to obtain a diagnosis as a result of severe ulceration and inflammatory changes.[82,83] It is important to obtain multiple biopsy samples to ensure a diagnosis. In one report,[84] cytologic examination of samples obtained by endoscopic brushing diagnosed a neoplastic epithelial process.

Metastasis to regional lymph nodes has been frequently reported,[81–83,85] and extension to involve the gastric mucosa has also been seen. Most cats, however, are euthanized due to the primary lesion rather than metastases. One cat developed aspiration pneumonia, possibly following attempts at force-feeding by the owner.[83]

Treatment

No treatment has been reported for the majority of these rare tumors. Esophagectomy of 3 cm of the cervical portion was attempted on one cat, but the animal died 3 days after surgery.[84]

GASTRIC TUMORS

Common Presentation	Lymphoma is the most common tumor and is likely to involve other systems. Carcinomas are very rare, and adenomas are uncommon. Other tumors are also seen. Vomiting and weight loss are common with all tumor types.

(continued)

Staging and Diagnosis	MDB, abdominal ultrasonography, and gastroscopy. Biopsy mandatory owing to multiple tumor types.
Treatment	
Initial	Surgery curative for benign tumors; uncertain for carcinomas but would require partial gastrectomy.
Adjunctive	Chemotherapy for lymphoma (see Chapter 36); unproven for other tumor types.
Supportive	Analgesia as necessary. Jejunostomy tube should be placed at time of laparotomy to allow postoperative alimentation. Alternatively, could use parenteral nutrition.

Lymphoma is by far the most common gastric tumor in cats other tumors are rare (see Chapter 36 for details). Gastric polyps are mainly an incidental finding. One cat with a duodenal adenomatous polyp also had a gastric polyp.[87] Three "aged," purebred cats—a Siamese, a Burmese, and an Angora-Manx—had gastric polyps, but only one showed any clinical signs.[9] This cat had a 1 month history of vomiting and weight loss.

Gastric carcinoma or gastric adenoma has been reported without details or in conjunction with intestinal tumors. These reports account for 10 such neoplasms.[88-92] A possible gastric carcinoma had metastasized to the lungs in another cat.[93] Peritoneal effusion was noted in one cat with gastric carcinoma.[94]

A gastric extramedullary plasmacytoma was seen in a 10-year-old DSH that was presented for chronic vomiting.[95] Partial gastrectomy was performed, and because lymph node biopsies showed metastasis, chemotherapy (prednisone, cyclophosphamide, vincristine, and chlorambucil) was given for 11 months. The cat died when the tumor recurred 13 months after surgery.[95]

A 3-year-old cat with a ruptured gastric mast cell tumor (MCT) appeared to recover well after surgery but died suddenly 1 month later with widespread metastatic disease.[96] Other rare gastric tumors are cited without detail.[9]

Ultrasonography and contrast radiography may be used to image gastric tumors and to direct ultrasound-guided biopsy; gastric endoscopy or laparotomy is required for definitive diagnosis.

INTESTINAL TUMORS

Lymphoma is the most common intestinal tumor of cats. Epithelial tumors, MCTs, and mesenchymal tumors are described less commonly. Lymphoma of the alimentary system is reviewed in Chapter 36.

ADENOMATOUS POLYPS

CLINICAL BRIEFING

Common Presentation	Benign polyps are much less common than carcinomas and may be premalignant. Vomiting is common. Hematemesis or hematochezia may be seen.
Staging and Diagnosis	MDB, abdominal ultrasonography, contrast radiography, and endoscopy (duodenal or colonic tumors); patient should be cross-matched for blood transfusion.
Treatment	
Initial	Surgical excision of affected bowel segment should be curative, but some cats may have a second (unrelated?) malignancy. Control of hemorrhage is important.
Adjunctive	None required after complete excision.
Supportive	Parenteral nutrition if postoperative recovery is prolonged. Have blood transfusion available. Analgesia is necessary.

Incidence, Signalment, and Etiology

Polypoid growths have been described in every segment of the feline intestinal tract but are much less common than intestinal adenocarcinoma. Affected cats are mostly older (5 to

18 years of age; median, 12 years).[9,87,97] The notable exceptions were two 2-year-old Siamese (mother and daughter) with ileal polyps.[98] Of 32 cats with polypoid intestinal growths, 5 were Siamese and 8 more were classified as Oriental breeds. In addition, 2 Himalayans, 1 Persian, and 1 Russian Blue were reported. Fifteen were DSHs, and 21 were male.[9,87,97,98] All tested cats were FeLV and FIV negative.[87] One cat had a jejunal adenocarcinoma in addition to a duodenal polyp.[87]

Clinical Presentation and History

Signs at presentation depended greatly on tumor location within the intestinal tract. In one series of 18 cats, all polyps were located in the duodenum[87] and vomiting was the most common clinical sign. Vomiting was acute in 6 cats and contained blood in 5 of the 6. Chronic vomiting for 2 months to 4 years was seen in 9 cats and was associated with hematemesis in 2 of the 9. Blood loss caused anemia in 8 cats, and a further 2 cats collapsed without showing any prior signs due to acute intestinal blood loss from a necrotic ulcerated polyp.[87] In another series of 11 cats, only 1 had a duodenal tumor[9]; three tumors affected the jejunum, and 1 of these cats had an intussusception.[9] Ileal polyps occurred in 2 related cats that both started vomiting 8 to 12 weeks after parturition. One of these cats had a palpable abdominal mass.[98] A cecal tumor,[9] four colonic tumors,[9,97] and three rectal polyps[9] were seen in cats that were mostly asymptomatic. Hematochezia was noticed for 10 months in 1 cat with a rectal tumor and in 1 with a colonic mass.[97]

Most polyps were less than 2 cm in diameter, but one was more than 3 cm.[97] Three of 11 cats had multiple polyps in one series,[9] and 4 cats with a duodenal polyp also had two or three other polyps in the duodenum or stomach.[97]

Staging and Diagnosis

Contrast radiography (via oral ingestion or enema) was useful in outlining an intestinal abnormality in most cats. Of 12 cats with duodenal polyps, contrast radiography showed a mass in 10 cats, thickened intestine in 1, and possible ulceration in another.[87] An obstructive pattern was seen in a cat with a large ileal tumor,[98] and a colonic mass was seen following a barium enema in another cat.[97]

Endoscopy was used to identify duodenal polyps in three cats that were vomiting.[87] Endoscopy is useful for gastric, duodenal, and colonic exploration but cannot provide information about lesions in other parts of the intestinal tract. Ultrasonography may be an excellent noninvasive method of examining the intestinal tract[99] and may allow biopsy of larger lesions.[100,101]

Two of the 18 cats with duodenal polyps had concurrent intestinal lymphoma or jejunal adenocarcinoma, and a further 2 had a history of cutaneous or systemic MCTs.[87] This serves to emphasize the importance of complete staging even when a tumor is thought to be benign.

> ### KEY POINT
>
> *Surgical excision of intestinal polyps should be curative; however, multiple polyps may be present.*

Treatment

Surgical excision of a colonic polyp with only 1 to 1.5 cm margins appeared to be curative in one cat that died without evidence of tumor 8 months later.[97] Unless the surgeon is very certain that an intestinal tumor is a polyp, a minimum of 5 to 10 cm of macroscopically normal bowel should be resected on either side of the lesion to ensure complete excision.

Surgical excision of duodenal polyps was performed in 17 cats.[87] Despite the use of blood transfusions in 6 cats, 3 of these cats died due to blood loss. Of the remaining cats for which follow-up information was available, 12 had no evidence of tumor 1 to 49 months after surgery.

INTESTINAL ADENOCARCINOMA

C L I N I C A L B R I E F I N G	
Common Presentation	Most tumors affect the small intestine (ileum). The colon is the most common large bowel location. Siamese account for 70% of cases. Anorexia is common; other signs, such as vomiting or diarrhea, melena, and tenesmus, depend on tumor location. Mass is usually palpable.
Staging and Diagnosis	MDB, abdominal ultrasonography, contrast radiography, endoscopy for duodenal or colonic tumors. Biopsy by endoscopy, ultrasound guidance, or exploratory laparotomy. Lymph node biopsy at time of surgery. Metastases may arise long after definitive treatment.

(continued)

Treatment	
Initial	Surgical excision should include a minimum 5 cm of normal bowel on either side of the tumor. Rectal "pull through" for colonic tumors. Watch for postoperative infection/peritonitis due to dehiscence. Prognosis good even if nodal metastases present.
Adjunctive	Postoperative chemotherapy with doxorubicin improves survival for colonic tumors and probably other sites as well. Carboplatin is unproven but may have efficacy.
Supportive	Postoperative analgesia; parenteral nutrition if postoperative recovery is prolonged.

Incidence, Signalment, and Etiology

There are numerous reports detailing the clinical course of cats with intestinal carcinomas, but there has been little attempt to differentiate between tumors of the small intestine and those of the large intestine. Prognostically there may not be a difference, but signalment appears to vary between cats with tumors in the cecum, colon, and rectum and those with tumors in other intestinal sites.

When combined, the clinical reports of 283 intestinal tumors in cats show that 194 were in the small intestine (duodenum = 15; jejunum = 64; ileum = 99; not specified = 16) and 89 were from the large intestine (cecum = 22; colon = 58; rectum = 9). A number of case series have shown that Siamese are overrepresented as a breed, accounting for approximately 70% of cats in three surveys.[9,88,102] It is difficult, however, to decide if Siamese are at increased risk of developing any intestinal carcinoma or just those in the small intestine. One study that divided tumor location into small and large intestine found that 64 of 91 cats with small intestinal carcinomas were Siamese but all 22 cats with carcinoma of the large intestine were DSHs.[9] It is interesting that Oriental breeds are also overrepresented in reports of small intestinal adenomas,[98] suggesting a breed susceptibility. Other breeds reported in series of all intestinal carcinomas include Russian Blue,[88] Persian,[102] and Manx[103]; in addition, 2 Persians were reported to have large intestinal carcinomas.[5,104]

The ages of cats with intestinal carcinoma ranged from 1[104] to 20[103] years (average in larger studies, 10 to 11 years).[9,88,89,105–107] Of cats identified as having large intestinal carcinoma, the youngest was 5 years of age[108] while a series of 22 cats ranged in age from 14 to 18 years.[9] There does not appear to be a strong gender predilection, although 102 (59%) of the 173 cats for which these data were recorded were males.

Clinical Presentation and History

Clinical signs depend largely on the location of the tumor within the intestinal tract. Regardless of tumor location, however, anorexia is the most common sign and is seen in about 50% of reported cats.[8,102,107] Anorexia may be due to intestinal ileus[109] and is often chronic; in one study cats had signs of anorexia and weight loss for an average of 83 days prior to presentation and signs had been present for up to 1 year in some animals.[107] Weight loss can be severe, and many cats are debilitated and cachectic.[89,107,110] This problem may be exacerbated by vomiting. Vomiting was reported in 27 of 32 cats (84%) with small intestinal tumors and tends to be seen in these cats more than in those with large intestinal tumors.[89,105]

Hematochezia, diarrhea, and occasionally melena are described in cats with carcinomas of the large intestine.[59,89,102] Cats with rectal carcinoma may show signs of constipation or tenesmus, and the stool may be "thin" in diameter due an obstructive mass.[89,105,111]

Abdominal distension caused by ascites due to peritoneal carcinomatosis is seen in some cats.[94,105] Abdominal pain has rarely been recorded, although cats with strictures of the small intestine may have ileus.[109] One cat was described as pulling out its flank hair in addition to vomiting and may have had abdominal pain.[112]

KEY POINT

A small intestinal tumor should be considered in any cat with chronic anorexia and vomiting.

An abdominal mass was palpated in 30% to 60% of cats, and palpable tumors ranged in size from 1 cm to large strictures extending many centimeters. Both large and small intestinal tumors were palpable.[59,89,102–105,107,113] Tumors smaller than 1 cm may be palpated on digital rectal examination.[104]

Staging and Diagnosis

Radiographs may demonstrate gas-filled loops of intestine in an "obstructive pattern" outlining a prestenotic dilation of the bowel rostral to an intestinal stricture. This pattern was seen in up to 50% of cats with intestinal carcinoma in one study[89] but was noted in less than 10% of cats in another study.[102] A mass was detected radiographically in 15% to 40% of cats,[102,103,107] while some cats may appear normal or have decreased radiographic detail that obscures any definitive finding.[103]

Contrast radiography appears to be more successful in

outlining either an obstructive pattern or an intestinal mass. Orally administered barium increased the diagnostic efficacy of radiographs over plain radiography in most studies,[89,102,107,114] and a barium enema was very effective in outlining a mass in cats with colorectal carcinomas.[89,111,115] Small intestinal carcinomas often involve the intestinal wall circumferentially, causing a stenotic stricture. When outlined by contrast media, this lesion creates an "apple-core" sign.[105,116] Other contrast techniques than can show abnormal GI transport include barium impregnated polyethylene sphere (BIPS) markers.[112]

One study found that barium contrast upper GI radiographs lacked the ability to differentiate between inflammatory and neoplastic lesions,[117] and thus care should be taken in interpreting these studies. It is important to remember that barium will interfere with the diagnostic accuracy of ultrasonography. Thus ultrasonography is best performed before barium is administered.

KEY POINT

Ultrasonography should not be performed after barium studies.

Ultrasonography is often superior to contrast radiography in identifying a mass involving the intestinal wall, although it may be difficult to locate the lesion to a specific area of the bowel. In one study, only one of five cats was found to have a mass on radiography and three cats were considered normal; on ultrasonography, all five were found to have an intestinal mass and one was found to have liver metastases that were not suspected based on radiography.[103] Ultrasonography may identify enlarged regional lymph nodes and guide a needle biopsy for definitive diagnosis.[99] An ultrasound-guided automated 18-ga "tru-cut" needle is available in 23 and 11 mm lengths, enabling biopsy of thickened intestinal wall with little risk of perforation.[100] Limitations of ultrasonography include a poor ability to visualize peritoneal tumor seeding even in the presence of ascites.[103] In addition, specimens obtained may not be correctly interpreted on cytology.[101] Despite these limitations, ultrasonography is probably the imaging modality of choice for intestinal tumors (Figure 41-15).

Endoscopy may provide a less invasive method of obtaining a diagnosis than laparotomy. Endoscopy is limited to the stomach, duodenum, and colon and does not allow visualization of regional lymph nodes or other abdominal organs for accurate staging.

KEY POINT

It is important to obtain deep biopsies when endoscopy is used.

Thoracic radiographs rarely show metastatic disease at the time of tumor diagnosis.[103,107,111,112] However, the finding of pulmonary metastases occasionally on radiography[102] and commonly on autopsy indicates that thoracic radiographs should be included in staging procedures.

In one study, 40% of 112 intestinal tumors metastasized to regional lymph nodes, peritoneum, mesentery, and omentum, while 31% metastasized to visceral sites such as liver, lung, spleen, stomach, bladder, and uterus.[9] In other series, up to 70% of cats had metastases from an intestinal tumor.[88] When the data from all reports is combined, the most common metastatic site is the regional lymph nodes (65 of 132 cats; 50%), with carcinomatosis occurring in 53 (40%), hepatic metastases in 11 (8%), and pulmonary metastases in 6 (5%); splenic, renal, pancreatic, and uterine metastases were rarely noted.[59,88,90,102,104–106,110] Most of these case series did not separate out carcinomas of the large intestine. Of 31 cats known to have carcinomas of the cecum, colon, or rectum, 13 (42%) had metastasis to regional lymph nodes and 10 (33%) had carcinomatosis. Other sites of metastasis included the liver (7; 23%), lung (5; 17%) and spleen; the kidney and duodenum were rarely affected. Some colonic tumors extended to involve the bladder and urethra.[59,90,104,105,118,119]

Ascitic fluid from cats with carcinomatosis was found to contain malignant cells on cytology approximately 20% of the time.[9]

Definitive biopsy may require exploratory surgery, and it is important to carefully examine all areas of the intestinal tract. Multiple carcinomas of the jejunum and ileum have occasionally been found.[9] Excisional biopsy is warranted if there is an obstruction.

Treatment

In one series of cats, those that were not treated died between 1 and 6 days after diagnosis.[102]

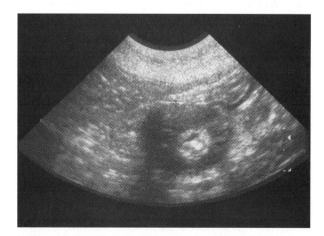

Figure 41-15: *Ultrasonography is the imaging modality of choice for intestinal tumors. In addition to identifying an asymmetric lesion, as is this image, a needle biopsy can be guided and other abdominal orgns assessed for metastasis prior to surgery. (Courtesy of D. Penninck)*

Surgical excision of a small intestinal carcinoma is best accomplished by resecting a minimum of 5 cm of normal appearing bowel on either side of the lesion. If there has been a stricture (Figure 41-16), the dilated prestenotic area may be ulcerated, particularly if the lesion is in the colon,[105,110] and may occasionally be filled with debris such as grass.[110] In one study, all 4 large intestinal lesions and 7 of 18 small intestinal lesions had marked mucosal ulceration.[105] A rectal "pull-through" has been recommended for treatment of rectal carcinoma (Figure 41-17).[111]

Postoperative mortality can be high. In a series of cats that had undergone surgical resection of the mass, death due to peritonitis, metastatic disease, or other complications ranged from 27% to 50%.[89,107,109] Other reports listed short survival times for some cats,[88,102,114] often due to postsurgical complications. This serves to emphasize the importance of postoperative care in these patients.

Those cats that survive the postoperative period can have an excellent prognosis. Cats with intestinal tumors have been reported with no evidence of tumor 6 to 54 months after surgery.[9,59,88,90] Long survival does not mean that metastases will not occur. Cats have been reported to develop recurrence and/or metastases 1 to 2 years after surgery.[9,89,107,109,113,116,118] Average survivals vary among studies. In one series of 12 cats with small intestinal tumors that survived the postoperative period, average survival was 15 months (range, 1.5 to 50 months).[107] Survival in other series averaged between 4 and 6 months.[9,89] All these studies had some long-term survivors, including cats that had evidence of metastatic disease or even carcinomatosis at the time of surgery.[107]

KEY POINT

Despite a high rate of metastasis, survival times may be long following surgery for intestinal carcinoma.

In a series of 21 cats with colonic adenocarcinoma, both the type of surgery and the presence of lymph node metastases was prognostic for a cat's survival.[118] The median survival for cats that had a subtotal colectomy was 20 weeks, compared with 10 weeks for those that had a simple mass resection. Cats in both groups survived a year after surgery. Similarly, cats that had lymph node metastases at the time of surgery lived an average of 7 weeks, compared to 37 weeks for cats without metastases. Again, some cats in both groups lived for 1 year after surgery.

KEY POINT

Aggressive surgery extends survival for cats with colonic carcinoma, particularly those without lymph node metastases.

A second resection was performed in one cat when a small intestinal tumor recurred.[107] This cat lived an additional 14 months before metastases developed.

Additional therapy has rarely been described in cats with intestinal adenocarcinoma. One cat that had a surgical resection was treated with levamisole (5 mg/kg PO three times per week) as a nonspecific immunomodulator.[116] This cat lived more than 2 years before developing widespread abdominal metastases. Given the long survival times for some cats treated with surgery alone, it is difficult to assess the impact of this additional treatment.

KEY POINT

Doxorubicin chemotherapy improves survival after surgery for cats with colonic carcinoma.

In a series of 16 cats with colonic adenocarcinoma, 4 received postoperative doxorubicin and survived a median of

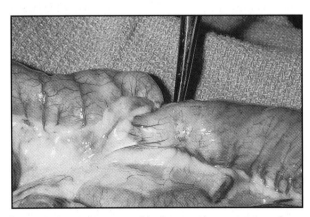

Figure 41-16: *A carcinoma of the ileum caused a constrictive annular lesion in this cat. (Courtesy of J. Berg)*

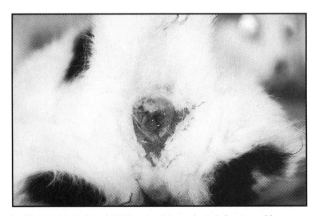

Figure 41-17: *Rectal SCC causing hematochezia is best treated by aggressive surgical excision (rectal "pull through").*

40 weeks while 12 cats that did not receive doxorubicin survived a median of 8 weeks after surgery.[118] Other chemotherapeutics such as carboplatin have yet to be evaluated for this disease.

Wide surgical excision of the primary tumor should be performed and resection of enlarged lymph nodes attempted. Postoperative doxorubicin (1 mg/kg or 25 mg/m² IV every 3 weeks for five to six cycles) should be considered in all cats, particularly if there is evidence of metastasis or vessel invasion on histopathology.

INTESTINAL MAST CELL TUMORS

CLINICAL BRIEFING	
Common Presentation	Most common in small intestine, causing vomiting, inappetence, and weight loss.
Staging and Diagnosis	MDB, buffy coat smear, abdominal ultrasonography, contrast radiography, and bone marrow aspiration. Metastasis very common.
Treatment	
Initial	Wide surgical excision including 5 to 10 cm of normal bowel.
Adjunctive	None described, but consider chemotherapy with prednisone or possibly CCNU. Other drugs may have anecdotal success (vincristine, L-asparaginase). Prognosis is poor.
Supportive	As for other intestinal tumors. Prednisone may be palliative after wounds have healed

Incidence, Signalment, and Etiology

MCTs are the third most common intestinal tumor in cats.[9] Of 38 cases in which signalment data was available, the age of affected cats ranged from 7[9,120] to 21[9] years of age (average, 13 years). There is no gender predilection, and purebred cats have not been reported to be affected. Obsolete terms for these tumors include *argentaffin cell tumors* or *argentaffinomas*.

KEY POINT

More than half the cats with intestinal MCT have other organ involvement.

Clinical Presentation and History

Intestinal MCTs are most commonly found in the small intestine. In one series of 28 cats,[9,120] 24 had MCTs affecting the small intestine. There have been only 8 tumors reported to occur in the colon and only 1 in the cecum.[9,118,120,121] One cat had multiple affected sites in the intestinal tract as well as other organ involvement.[122] Peritoneal effusion may be marked.[94]

Signs may relate to the primary tumor (e.g., vomiting, inappetence, diarrhea, weight loss).[96,120,123] In other affected cats, weight loss and mild inappetence were the only GI signs.[122] Vomiting is most likely due to mechanical factors rather than histamine-induced ulceration, as the latter has not been reported in affected cats.[120] Signs are often chronic, usually protracted over 3 months or more, but intestinal MCTs can also be an incidental finding at necropsy.[120] Most cats have a pal-pable tumor on physical examination.[120] The palpable mass may be discrete, although it is often a poorly demarcated, firm, segmental thickening that can be up to 7 cm wide.[120]

Staging and Diagnosis

Intestinal MCTs commonly metastasize; in one study, 18 of 28 affected cats had other organ involvement.[9] In another study that included 24 of the same 28 cats, the mesenteric lymph nodes were the most common metastatic site.[120] Other metastatic sites that are less commonly reported are liver and spleen,[118,121,122] lung, other lymph nodes (hepatic, thoracic, cecal, and colonic), and rarely the bone marrow (1 of 24 affected cats).[120]

One cat with intestinal MCTs also had mastocythemia,[121] and two others had eosinophilia and basophilia (92,000 eosinophils/µl in one animal).[59,122] These cats had increases in eosinophilic precursors in their bone marrow but no evidence of mast cell infiltration.

Intestinal MCTs are not always easily recognizable on histopathology; cytoplasmic granules may be very fine or absent, and special staining with toluidine blue may be necessary for definitive diagnosis.[59] These tumors may occasionally be misdiagnosed as eosinophilic cellulitis[123] or lymphoma.[122] In one study, 5 of 24 cats had other unrelated tumors in addition to an intestinal MCT.[120]

Staging should be performed as for systemic MCTs (see Chapter 42), including abdominal ultrasonography and bone marrow aspiration in addition to the MDB. Contrast radiography or ultrasonography will help localize the tumor and may guide a preoperative biopsy (Figure 41-18).

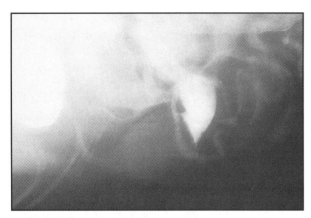

Figure 41-18: A barium contrast study shows an obstruction due to an intestinal MCT. Ultrasonography is better able to examine other organs for metastases than radiography and may guide a preoperative biopsy. (Courtesy of J. Berg)

Treatment

Intestinal MCTs are behaviorally aggressive, and there are few reports of successful treatment. In many cats, the tumor may be unresectable due to adhesions and lymph node enlargement.[59,122,123] Treatment with prednisone has had variable, but overall poor, success in controlling the tumor in these cats,[122,123] even at dosages of up to 3 mg/kg.[123] Dexamethasone and azathioprine caused a 50% reduction in tumor size for 3 months in one cat[123] and a transitory reduction in tumor size followed chemotherapy with vincristine and L-asparaginase in another cat.[122] Prednisone had little impact on disease progression in four cats with colonic MCTs.[118]

One author has recommended that at least 5 to 10 cm of normal bowel be resected on either side of the tumor because of the infiltrative nature of intestinal MCT (Figures 41-19 and 41-20).[9] Clinical signs were palliated in one cat so treated until metastatic disease caused its death 5 months later.[9]

▶ OTHER INTESTINAL TUMORS

EPITHELIAL TUMORS

Two neuroendocrine carcinomas of the colon were found to have metastasized to the colonic lymph nodes and throughout the peritoneal cavity, causing carcinomatosis.[118] One of the cats also had hepatic metastases. Other details were not available. A duodenal carcinoid in a 9-year-old cat caused anorexia and frequent vomiting for a month.[124] The carcinoid had massive adhesions that made it unresectable; metastasis to the lungs as well as regional and sternal lymph nodes had also occurred. A 7 cm carcinoid of the ileum in a 13-year-old cat caused constipation and signs of pruritus, possibly due to release of active amines.[125] A ganglioneuroma of the jejunum in a 6-week-old Siamese was resected, but the cat died of peritonitis and esophagitis soon after surgery.[126]

MESENCHYMAL TUMORS

Fibrosarcomas were described in the duodenum of a 13-year-old male and the colon of a 2-year-old female; both were DSHs.[88,104] The duodenal tumor was an incidental finding in a cat with a bladder tumor and no GI signs.[104] A neurofibroma in the jejunum of a 9-year-old cat with mammary carcinoma also did not cause GI signs.[104] A liposarcoma in the jejunum of an 18-year-old cat had metastasized to the mesenteric lymph nodes and kidney.[106]

SMOOTH MUSCLE TUMORS

Leiomyosarcomas of the duodenum (two cats),[59] ileum (one cat),[106] jejunum (two cats),[59,88] ileocecocolic junction (one cat),[127] and rectum (one cat)[106] have been described in cats ranging from 5 to 17 years of age. Five of seven cats were 12 years of age or older. Only one of the seven was Siamese.

A leiomyoma was described in a 13-year-old cat with an intussusception.[9] A cat with a leiomyosarcoma of the ileum

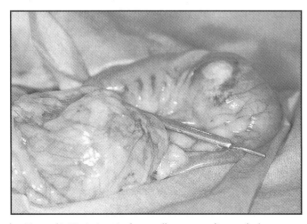

Figure 41-19: An intestinal mast cell tumor was discovered when surgery was performed on the cat in Figure 41-18. (Courtesy of J. Berg)

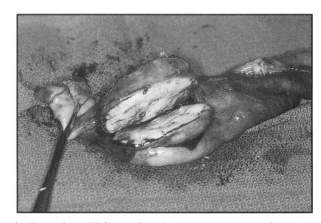

Figure 41-20: Wide surgical margins were necessary to excise the intestinal MCT seen in Figures 41-18 and 41-19. Despite the apparently localized nature of this tumor grossly, tumor infiltration may occur along the intestinal tract. (Courtesy of J. Berg)

had GI tract obstruction and was anorectic.[106] Another cat with ileocecocolic leiomyosarcoma had nonspecific malaise, inappetence, and weight loss for 2 to 3 weeks.[127]

Leiomyosarcomas may be palpable if they are large,[127] but ultrasonography is necessary to detect smaller lesions. Ultrasonography in one cat showed a 2.5 × 2.0 cm comma-shaped inhomogeneous mass that was an intestinal leiomyosarcoma.[99] A rectal leiomyosarcoma had metastasized to regional lymph nodes,[106] but metastases were not described in other reports.

Surgical excision of a large ileocecocolic leiomyosarcoma was unsuccessful; the tumor recurred 15 weeks after surgery.[127] Another cat treated surgically was normal 14 months after excision.[59] This implies that wide margins are important in the surgical treatment of intestinal smooth muscle tumors.

PLASMA CELL TUMORS

An abdominal mass encompassed the ileocecal region of a 14-year-old DSH. Malignant cells had plasmacytoid features.[128] Another cat had a duodenal plasma cell tumor that invaded abdominal viscera. This cat had a monoclonal gammopathy due to IgA but did not have any other signs of multiple myeloma.[129]

NONDOMESTIC FELIDAE

Although gastric carcinomas are rare in domestic cats, three have been reported in other felids. A 10-year-old male lion (Panthera leo) died due to gastric perforation and peritonitis. An SCC of the gastric cardia was found to have necrosed and had metastasized to the lungs and cardiac muscle.[130] An emaciated 23-year-old male jungle cat (Felis chaus) had an ulcerated, 1.5 cm adenocarcinoma of the greater curative of the stomach in addition to three other malignancies.[131] A 9-year-old female cougar (Felis concolor) was vomiting and losing weight for 9 months before it died. On autopsy, a diffusely invasive gastric adenocarcinoma was found in the antrum to body region of the stomach. It had not metastasized.[132]

> *MDB = minimum database; includes CBC, biochemical profile, urinalysis, FeLV/FIV serology, T_4 testing, and thoracic radiographs (three views).*

In a large survey, intestinal carcinomas of the jejunum in a male tiger (Panthera tigris) and the rectum of a male lion were described.[133] A 6-year-old male clouded leopard (Neofelis nebulosa) was anorectic for 6 weeks before it died. On necropsy, a 5 cm neuroendocrine tumor was found in the small intestine. The tumor had metastasized widely.[134]

A 9-month-old male cougar (Felis concolor) was presented for vomiting and anorexia and was found to have a painful abdominal mass on palpation.[135] Radiographs showed a pyloric mass. A gastrojejunostomy was performed to remove a 15 cm pyloric MCT, but surgical margins were incomplete. The cat was treated with prednisone (2 mg/kg PO) and cimetidine for 6 months and was free of tumor 6 months after surgery.

PERINEAL APOCRINE GLAND CARCINOMA

Incidence, Signalment, and Etiology

This is a rare tumor that has been reported in detail for only three cats (9 to 17 years of age).[9,136,137] Two were males, and one was a female.

Clinical Presentation and History

A perineal swelling below or to the side of the anus may be noticed by the owner. The swelling may be ulcerated, pruritic, and bleeding. Rectal examination may reveal a localized swelling, but there is often invasion into the surrounding tissue.[9,137]

Staging and Diagnosis

Metastases to the sublumbar lymph nodes has been reported to occur in some cats at the time of diagnosis,[9] as have pulmonary and hepatic metastases.[9]

Prior to surgical resection of the affected gland, careful rectal palpation should be performed, preferably under anesthesia. Abdominal ultrasonography and thoracic radiography should also be performed. Serum calcium is included in the MDB, but unlike the situation in dogs with anal sac apocrine adenocarcinoma, hypercalcemia has not been reported in affected cats.

Treatment

Treatment was not described for the three case reports.[9,136,137] In a series of 10 cats, the median survival was 5 months (range, 2 to 8 months). These cats died due to local or regional recurrences.[b] Perhaps adjuvant radiation or chemotherapy may have some efficacy in this tumor. Anecdotally, there was no response to carboplatin but a long-term partial response to doxorubicin was noted in a cat with sublumbar lymph node metastases from a perineal apocrine gland carcinoma.[c]

[b]Cronin K: Personal communication, 1998.
[c]Moore AS: Personal observation.

REFERENCES

1. Vos JH, van der Gaag I: Canine and feline oral-pharyngeal tumours. *J Vet Med A* 34:420–427, 1987.

2. Stebbins KE, Morse CE, Goldschmidt MH: Feline oral neoplasia: A ten year survey. *Vet Pathol* 26:121–128, 1989.

3. Cotter SM: Oral pharyngeal neoplasms in the cat. *JAAHA* 17:917–920, 1981.

4. Dorn CR, Priester WA: Epidemiologic analysis of oral and pharyngeal cancer in dogs, cats, horses and cattle. *JAVMA* 169:1202–1206, 1976.

5. Brodey RS: The biological behavior of canine oral and pharyngeal neoplasms. *J Small Anim Pract* 11:45–53, 1970.

6. Kapatkin AS, Marretta SM, Patnaik AK, et al: Mandibular swellings in cats: Prospective study of 24 cats. *JAAHA* 27:580, 1991.

7. Gorlin RJ, Barron CN, Chaudhry AP, Clark JJ: The oral and pharyngeal pathology of domestic animals. A study of 487 cases. *Am J Vet Res* 20:1032–1061, 1959.

8. Dorn CR, Taylor DON, Schneider R: Sunlight exposure and risk of developing cutaneous and oral squamous cell carcinomas in white cats. *J Natl Cancer Inst* 46:1073–1078, 1971.

9. Carpenter JL, Andrews LK, Holzworth J: Tumors and tumor-like lesions, in Holzworth J (ed): *Diseases of the Cat. Medicine and Surgery.* Philadelphia, WB Saunders, 1987, pp 407–596.

10. Miller AS, McCrea MW, Rhodes WH: Mandibular epidermoid carcinoma with reactive bone proliferation in a cat. *Am J Vet Res* 30:1465–1468, 1969.

11. Bradley RL, MacEwen EG, Loar AS: Mandibular resection for removal of oral tumors in 30 dogs and 6 cats. *JAVMA* 184:460–463, 1984.

12. Bond E, Dorfman HD: Squamous cell carcinoma of the tongue in cats. *JAVMA* 154:786–789, 1969.

13. Postorino Reeves NC, Turrel JM, Withrow SJ: Oral squamous cell carcinoma in the cat. *JAAHA* 29:438–441, 1993.

14. Quigley PJ, Leedale A, Dawson IMP: Carcinoma of mandible of cat and dog simulating osteosarcoma. *J Comp Pathol* 82:15–20, 1972.

15. Moisan PG, Lorenz MD, Stromberg PC, Simmons HA: Concurrent trichinosis and oral squamous cell carcinoma in a cat. *J Vet Diagn Invest* 10:199–202, 1998.

15a. Moore AS: Unpublished dta.

16. Young PL: Squamous cell carcinoma of the tongue of the cat. *Aust Vet J* 54:133–134, 1978.

17. Effron M, Griner L, Benirschke K: Nature and rate of neoplasia found in captive wild mammals, birds and reptiles at necropsy. *J Natl Cancer Inst* 59:185–198, 1977.

18. Martin HE: The zoologic distribution of intra-oral cancer. *Scientific Monthly* 62–266, 1939.

19. Madewell BR, Ackerman N, Sesline DH: Invasive carcinoma radiographically mimicking primary bone cancer in the mandibles of two cats. *Cancer* 17:213–215, 1976.

20. Liu S-K, Dorfman HD, Patnaik AK: Primary and secondary bone tumours in the cat. *J Small Anim Pract* 15:141–156, 1974.

21. Cotchin E: Further examples of spontaneous neoplasms in the domestic cat. *Br Vet* 112:263–272, 1956.

22. Hutson CA, Willauer CC, Walder EJ, et al: Treatment of mandibular squamous cell carcinoma in cats by use of mandibulectomy and radiotherapy: Seven cases (1987–1989). *JAVMA* 201:777–781, 1992.

23. Bostock DE: The prognosis in cats bearing squamous cell carcinoma. *J Small Anim Pract* 13:119–125, 1972.

24. Evans SM, LaCreta F, Helfand S, et al: Technique, pharmacokinetics, toxicity, and efficacy of intratumoral etanidazole and radiotherapy for treatment of spontaneous feline oral squamous cell carcinoma. *Int J Radiat Oncol* 20:703–708, 1991.

25. Quigley PJ, Leedale AH: Tumors involving bone in the domestic cat: A review of fifty-eight cases. *Vet Pathol* 20:670–686, 1983.

26. Emms SG, Harvey CE: Preliminary results of maxillectomy in the dog and cat. *J Small Anim Pract* 27:291–306, 1986.

27. Verstraete FJM, Kass PH, Terpak CH: Diagnostic value of full-mouth radiography in cats. *Am J Vet Res* 59:692–695, 1998.

28. Solano M, Penninck DG: Ultrasonography of the canine, feline and equine tongue: Normal findings and case history reports. *Vet Radiol Ultrasound* 37:206–213, 1996.

29. Klausner JS, Bell FW, Hayden DW, et al: Hypercalcemia in two cats with squamous cell carcinomas. *JAVMA* 196:103–105, 1990.

30. Plotnick A, Brunt JE, Reitz BL: What is your diagnosis? *JAVMA* 202:991–994, 1993.

31. Penwick RC, Nunamaker DM: Rostral mandibulectomy: A treatment for oral neoplasia in the dog and cat. *JAAHA* 23:19–25, 1987.

32. Salisbury SK, Richardson DC, Lantz GC: Partial maxillectomy and premaxillectomy in the treatment of oral neoplasia in the dog and cat. *Vet Surg* 15:16–26, 1986.

33. Turrel JM, Théon AP: Reirradiation of tumors in cats and dogs. *JAVMA* 193:465–469, 1988.

34. Dewhirst MW, Sim DA, Wilson S, et al: Correlation between initial and long-term responses of spontaneous pet animal tumors to heat and radiation or radiation alone. *Cancer Res* 43:5735–5741, 1983.

35. Fox LE, Levine PB, King RR, et al: Use of cis-bis-neodocanoato-trans-R,R-1,2-diaminocyclohexane platinum (II), a liposomal cisplatin analogue, in cats with oral squamous cell carcinoma. *Am J Vet Res* 61:791–795, 2000.

36. Knapp DW, Richardson RC, BeNicola DB, et al: Cisplatin toxicity in cats. *J Vet Intern Med* 1:29–35, 1987.

37. Mauldin GN, Matus RE, Patnaik AK, et al: Efficacy and toxicity of doxorubicin and cyclophosphamide used in the treatment of selected malignant tumors in 23 cats. *J Vet Intern Med* 2:60–65, 1988.

38. Ogilvie GK, Moore AS, Obradovich JE, et al: Toxicoses and efficacy associated with the administration of mitoxantrone to cats with malignant tumors. *JAVMA* 202:1839–1844, 1993.

39. LaRue SM, Vail DM, Ogilvie GK, et al: Shrinking-field radiation therapy plus mitoxantrone for the treatment of oral squamous cell carcinoma in the cat. *Vet Cancer Soc Newsl* 15:4–7, 1991.

40. Wood CA, Moore AS, Frimberger AE, et al: Phase I evaluation of carboplatin in tumor bearing cats. *Proc Vet Cancer Soc 16th Annu Conf* 39–40, 1996.

41. Frimberger AE, Moore AS, Cincotta L, et al: Photodynamic therapy of naturally occurring tumors in animals using a novel benzophenothiazine photosensitizer. *Clin Cancer Res* 4:2207–2218, 1998.

42. MacEwen EG: Anti-tumor evaluation of benzaldehyde in the dog and cat. *Am J Vet Res* 47:451–452, 1986.

43. Bradley RL, Sponenberg DP, Martin RA: Oral neoplasia in 15 dogs and 4 cats. *Semin Vet Med Surg Small Anim* 1:33–42, 1986.

44. Warrlich A: Gleichzeitiges vorkommen eines fibrosarkoms und eines plattenepithelkarzinoms der mundschleimhaut im oberkiefer bei einer katze. *Praktische Tierarzt* 76:213–214, 1995.

45. Wilson RB, Holscher MA, Casey TT, Berry KK: Tonsillar granular cell tumour in a cat. *J Comp Pathol* 101:109–112, 1989.

46. Patnaik AK: Histologic and immunohistochemical studies of granular cell tumors in seven dogs, three cats, one horse, and one bird. *Vet Pathol* 30:176–185, 1993.

47. Hahn KA: Vincristine sulfate as single-agent chemotherapy in a dog and a cat with malignant neoplasms. *JAVMA* 197:796–798, 1990.

48. Scott DW: Lentigo simplex in orange cats. *Compan Anim Pract* 1(2):323–325, 1987.

49. Patnaik AK, Mooney S: Feline melanoma: A comparative study of ocular, oral, and dermal neoplasms. *Vet Pathol* 25:105–112, 1988.

50. Sundberg JP, Van Ranst M, Montali R, et al: Feline papillomas and papillomaviruses. *Vet Pathol* 37:1–10, 2000.

51. Gardner DG: An orderly approach to the study of odontogenic tumours in animals. *J Comp Pathol* 107:427–438, 1992.

52. Poulet FM, Valentine BA, Summers BA: A survey of epithelial odontogenic tumors and cysts in dogs and cats. *Vet Pathol* 29:369–380, 1992.

53. Hawkins CD, Jones BR: Adamantinoma in a cat. *Aust Vet J* 59:54–55, 1982.

54. Dernell WS, Hullinger GH: Surgical management of ameloblastic fibroma in the cat. *J Small Anim Pract* 35:35–38, 1994.

55. Mills JHL, Lewis RJ: Adamantinoma—Histogenesis and differentiations from the periodontal fibromatous epulis and squamous cell carcinoma. *Can Vet J* 22:126–129, 1981.

56. Walsh KM, Denholm LJ, Cooper BJ: Epithelial odontogenic tumours in domestic animals. *J Comp Pathol* 97:503–521, 1987.

57. Dubielzig RR, Adams WM, Brodey RS: Inductive fibroameloblastoma, and unusual dental tumor of young cats. *JAVMA* 174:720–722, 1979.

58. Dubielzig RR: Proliferative dental and gingival diseases of dogs and cats. *JAAHA* 18:577–584, 1982.

59. Brodey RS: Alimentary tract neoplasms in the cat: A clinicopathologic survey of 46 cases. *Am J Vet Res* 27:74–80, 1966.

60. Moore AS, Wood CA, Engler SJ, Bengston AE: Radiation therapy for long term control of odontogenic tumors and epulis in three cats. *J Feline Med Surg* 2:57–60, 2000.

61. Ohmachi T, Taniyama H, Nakade T, et al: Calcifying epithelial odontogenic tumours in small domesticated carnivores: Histological, immunohistochemi-

cal and electron microscopical studies. *J Comp Pathol* 114:305–314, 1996.

62. Breuer W, Geisel O, Linke RP, Hermanns W: Light microscopic, ultrastructural, and immunohistochemical examinations of two calcifying epithelial odontogenic tumors (CEOT) in a dog and a cat. *Vet Pathol* 31:415–420, 1994.

63. Langham RF, Bennett R, Koestner A: Amyloidosis associated with a calcifying ameloblastoma (calcifying epithelial odontoma) in a cat. *Vet Pathol* 21:549–550, 1984.

64. Abbott DP, Walsh K, Diters RW: Calcifying epithelial odontogenic tumours in three cats and a dog. *J Comp Pathol* 96:131–136, 1986.

65. Levene A: Sebaceous gland differentiation in tumours of the feline oral mucosa. *Vet Rec* 114:69, 1984.

66. Rest JR, Gumbrell RC, Heim P, Rushton-Taylor P: Oral fibropapillomas in young cats. *Vet Rec* 141:528, 1997.

67. Sironi G, Caniatti M, Scanziani E: Immunohistochemical detection of papillomavirus structural antigens in animal hyperplastic and neoplastic epithelial lesions. *J Vet Med A* 37:760–770, 1990.

68. Koestner A, Buerger L: Primary neoplasms of the salivary glands in animals compared to similar tumors in man. *Path Vet* 2:201–226, 1965.

69. Bosselut R, Samso A, Cattanei J: Cancer des glandes salivaires chez le chat. *Bull Algerien Carcinologie* 4:407–408, 1951.

70. Spangler WL, Culbertson MR: Salivary gland disease in dogs and cats: 245 cases (1985–1988). *JAVMA* 198:465–469, 1991.

71. Carberry CA, Flanders JA, Harvey HJ, Ryan AM: Salivary gland tumors in dogs and cats: A literature and case review. *JAAHA* 24:561–567, 1988.

72. Case MT, Simon J: Oncocytomas in a cat and a dog. *Vet Med Small Anim Clin* 61:41–43, 1966.

73. Wells GAH, Robinson M: Mixed tumour of salivary gland showing histological evidence of malignancy in a cat. *J Comp Pathol* 85:77–85, 1975.

74. Carpenter JL, Bernstein M: Malignant mixed (pleomorphic) mandibular salivary gland tumors in a cat. *JAAHA* 27:581–583, 1991.

75. Sozmen M, Brown PJ, Eveson JW: Salivary duct carcinoma in five cats. *J Comp Pathol* 121:311–319, 1999.

76. Burek KA, Munn RJ, Madewell BR: Metastatic adenocarcinoma of a minor salivary gland in a cat. *J Vet Med A* 41:485–490, 1999.

77. Karbe E, Schiefer B: Primary salivary gland tumors in carnivores. *Can Vet J* 8:212–215, 1967.

78. Hammer A, Getzy D, Ogilvie G, et al: Salivary gland neoplasia in the dog and cat: Survival times and prognostic factors. *Proc 17th Annu Vet Cancer Soc*:87, 1997.

79. Cotchin E: Neoplasms in small animals. *Vet Rec* 63:67–72, 1951.

80. Gray H: Cancer of the oesophagus in the cat. *Vet Rec* 15:532–533, 1935.

81. Fernandes FH, Hawe RS, Loeb WF: Primary squamous cell carcinoma of the esophagus in a cat. *Compan Anim Pract* 1(2):16–22, 1987.

82. Vernon FF, Roudebush P: Primary esophageal carcinoma in a cat. *JAAHA* 16:547–550, 1980.

83. Happe RP, Gaag Ivd, Wolvekamp WThC, Van Toorenburg J: Esophageal squamous cell carcinoma in two cats. *Tijdschr Diergeneesk* 103:1080–1086, 1978.

84. Gualtieri M, Monzeglio MG, Di Giancamillo M: Oesophageal squamous cell carcinoma in two cats. *J Small Anim Pract* 40:79–83, 1999.

85. Dargent F, Gau M-L, Olivie J: Primary oesophageal epidermoid carcinoma in a cat. *7th Annu Conf ESVIM*:119, 1997.

86. Johnson K: Oesophageal carcinoma in a cat. *Aust Vet Pract* 6:228, 1976.

87. MacDonald JM, Mullen HS, Moroff SD: Adenomatous polyps of the duodenum in cats: 18 cases (1985–1990). *JAVMA* 202:647–651, 1993.

88. Turk MAM, Gallina AM, Russell TS: Nonhematopoietic gastrointestinal neoplasia in cats: A retrospective study of 44 cases. *Vet Pathol* 18:614–620, 1981.

89. Cribb AE: Feline gastrointestinal adenocarcinoma: A review and retrospective study. *Can Vet J* 29:709–712, 1988.

90. Lingeman CH, Garner FM, Taylor DON: Spontaneous gastric adenocarcinomas of dogs: A review. *J Natl Cancer Inst* 47:137–153, 1971.

91. Patnaik AK, Liu S-K, Hurvitz AI, McClelland AJ: Nonhematopoietic neoplasms in cats. *J Natl Cancer Inst* 54:855–860, 1975.

92. Cotchin E: Neoplasia, in Wilkinson GT (ed): *Diseases of the Cat and Their Management.* Melbourne, Blackwell Scientific Publications, 1983.

93. Breese CE: What is your diagnosis? *JAVMA* 197:908–909, 1990.

94. Wright KN, Gomph RE, DeNovo Jr RC: Peritoneal effusion in cats: 65 cases (1981–1997). *JAVMA* 214:375–381, 1999.

95. Zikes CD, Spielman B, Shapiro W, et al: Gastric extramedullary plasmacytoma in a cat. *J Vet Intern Med* 12:381–383, 1998.

96. Bortnowski HB, Rosenthal RC: Gastrointestinal mast cell tumors and eosinophilia in two cats. *JAAHA* 28:271–275, 1992.

97. Olin FH, Lea RB, Kim C: Colonic adenoma in a cat. *JAVMA* 153:53–56, 1968.

98. Orr CM, Gruffydd-Jones TJ, Kelly DF: Ileal polyps in Siamese cats. *J Small Anim Pract* 21:669–674, 1980.

99. Penninck DG, Nyland TG, Kerr LY, Fisher PE: Ultrasonographic evaluation of gastrointestinal diseases in small animals. *Vet Radiol* 31:134–141, 1990.

100. Penninck DG, Crystal MA, Matz ME, Pearson SH: The technique of percutaneous ultrasound guided fine-needle aspiration biopsy and automated microcore biopsy in small animal gastrointestinal diseases. *Vet Radiol Ultrasound* 34:433–436, 1993.

101. Crystal MA, Penninck DG, Matz ME, et al: Use of ultrasound-guided fine-needle aspiration biopsy and automated core biopsy for the diagnosis of gastrointestinal diseases in small animals. *Vet Radiol* 34:438–444, 1993.

102. Birchard SJ, Couto CG, Johnson S: Nonlymphoid intestinal neoplasia in 32 dogs and 14 cats. *JAAHA* 22:533–537, 1986.

103. Rivers BJ, Walter PA, Feeney DA, Johnston GR: Ultrasonographic features of intestinal adenocarcinoma in five cats. *Vet Radiol Ultrasound* 38:300–306, 1997.

104. Loupal G, Pfeil C: Tumoren im darmtrakt der katze unter besonderer Berücksightigung der nicht-hämatopoetischen Geschwülste. *Berl Münch Teirärztl Wschr* 97:208–213, 1984.

105. Patnaik AK, Liu SK, Johnston GF: Feline intestinal adenocarcinoma: A clinicopathologic study of 22 cases. *Vet Pathol* 13:1–10, 1976.

106. Head KW, Else RW: Neoplasia and allied conditions of the canine and feline intestine. *Vet Annu* 21:190–208, 1981.

107. Kosovsky JE, Matthiesen DT, Patnaik AK: Small intestinal adenocarcinoma in cats: 32 cases (1978–1985). *JAVMA* 192:233–235, 1988.

108. Schneider HE: Therapieversuch bei rectomsarkom einer katz mittels enteroanastomase. *Kleintierpraxis* 6:23–24, 1961.

109. Böhmer E, Matis U, Zedler W, Hänichen T: Dünndarmileus bei katze und hund–Katamnestische betrachtungen von 704 patienten. *Tierärztl Prax* 18:171–183, 1990.

110. Taylor PF, Kater JC: Adenocarcinoma of the intestine of the dog and cat. *Aust Vet J* 30:377–379, 1954.

111. Gerosa RM, de Esrada MMM: Colorectal resection in a cat with adenocarcinoma. *Feline Pract* 12:6–15, 1982.

112. Stewart C: Jejunal adenocarcinoma in a cat. *Aust Vet Pract* 27:131–136, 1997.

113. Palumbo NE, Perri SF: Adenocarcinoma of the ileum in a cat. *JAVMA* 164:607–608, 1974.

114. Theran P, Thornton GW: Case records of the Angell Memorial Animal Hospital. *JAVMA* 152:1017–1022, 1968.

115. Mayrhofer E: Enddarmneoplasma und chronische obstipation bei einem kater. *Wien Tierärztl Mschr* 71:103–104, 1984.

116. Patnaik AK, Johnson GF, Greene RW, et al: Surgical resection of intestinal adenocarcinoma in a cat, with survival of 28 months. *JAVMA* 178:479–481, 1981.

117. Weichselbaum RC, Feeney DA, Hayden DW: Comparison of upper gastrointestinal radiographic findings to histopathologic observations: A retrospective study of 41 dogs and cats with suspected small bowel infiltrative disease (1985 to 1990). *Vet Radiol Ultrasound* 35:418–426, 1994.

118. Slawienski MJ, Mauldin GE, Mauldin GN, Patnaik AK: Malignant colonic neoplasia in cats: 46 cases (1990–1996). *JAVMA* 211:878–881, 1997.

119. Mulligan RM: Spontaneous cat tumors. *Cancer Res* 11:271, 1951.

120. Alroy J, Leav I, DeLellis A, Weinstein RS: Distinctive intestinal mast cell neoplasms of domestic cats. *Lab Invest* 33:159–167, 1975.

121. Garner FM, Lingeman CH: Mast-cell neoplasms of the domestic cat. *Path Vet* 7:517–530, 1970.

122. Peaston AE, Griffey SM: Visceral mast cell tumour with eosinophilia and eosinophilic peritoneal and pleural effusions in a cat. *Aust Vet J* 71:215–217, 1994.

123. Howl JH, Petersen MG: Intestinal mast cell tumor in a cat: Presentation as eosinophilic enteritis. *JAAHA* 31:457–461, 1995.

124. Carakostas MC, Kennedy GA, Kittleson MD, Cook JE: Malignant foregut carcinoid tumor in a domestic cat. *Vet Pathol* 16:607–609, 1979.

125. Lahellec M, Joncourt L, Dhennin L: Étude clinique et histologique d'une tumeur carcinoïde du grêle chez un chat. *Bull Acad Vet* 45:363–365, 1972.

126. Patnaik AK, Lieberman PH, Johnson GF: Intestinal ganglioneuroma in a kitten—A case report and review of literature. *J Small Anim Pract* 19:735–742, 1978.

127. Barrand KR, Scudamore CL: Intestinal leiomyosarcoma in a cat. *J Small An-*

im Pract 40:216–219, 1999.

128. Rowland PH, Linke RP: Immunohistochemical characterization of lambda light-chain-derived amyloid in one feline and five canine plasma cell tumors. *Vet Pathol* 31:390–393, 1994.

129. Hawkins EC, Feldman BF, Blanchard PC: Immunoglobulin A myeloma in a cat with pleural effusion and serum hyperviscosity. *JAVMA* 188:876–878, 1986.

130. El-Sergany M: Magenkarzinom bei eineum löwen. *Berliner-und-Munchener-Tierarztliche-Worchenschrift* 21:410–412, 1966.

131. Sagartz JW, Garner FM, Sauer RM: Multiple neoplasia in a captive jungle cat *(Felis chaus)*—Thyroid adenocarcinoma, gastric adenocarcinoma, renal adenoma, and Sertoli cell tumor. *J Wildl Dis* 8:375–380, 1972.

132. Yanai T, Masegi T, Hosoi M, et al: Gastric adenocarcinoma in a Cougar *(Fe-*

lis concolor). J Wildl Dis 30:603–606, 1994.

133. Lombard LS, Witte EJ: Frequency and types of tumors in mammals and birds of the Philadelphia Zoological Garden. *Cancer Res* 19:127–141, 1959.

134. Wada Y, Kondo H, Bando G, et al: Intestinal adenocarcinoma with neuroendocrine cells in a clouded leopard *(Neofelis nebulosa). J Comp Pathol* 115:305–310, 1996.

135. Martin HD, Lewis DD, Lin SL, Jacobson ER: Gastric mast cell tumor in a cougar. *JAVMA* 187:1258–1260, 1985.

136. Chun R, Jakovljevic S, Morrison WB, et al: Apocrine gland adenocarcinoma and pheochromocytoma in a cat. *JAAHA* 33:33–36, 1997.

137. Weissman S, Pulley LT: Perianal gland adenocarcinoma. *Feline Pract* 4:26, 1974.

SPLENIC, HEPATIC, AND PANCREATIC TUMORS

Antony S. Moore and Gregory K. Ogilvie

42

This chapter has been separated into two sections. Because many tumors of the spleen also affect the liver and vice versa, these diseases have been grouped together. In addition, miscellaneous sites for tumors such as visceral mast cell tumors and angiosarcomas are included in this chapter for convenience. The second section discusses exocrine tumors of the pancreas (endocrine pancreatic tumors are discussed in Chapter 44).

TUMORS OF THE SPLEEN AND LIVER

In a survey that included 455 feline splenic biopsies, four tumor types accounted for one third of all tumors: mast cell tumor (15%), lymphoma (9%), myeloproliferative disease (6%), and hemangiosarcoma (3%). Other tumors found in more than one cat but accounting for less than 1% of tumors included undifferentiated sarcoma, plasmacytosis, and myeloma. Other tumors were considered incidental findings.[1] In another study, lymphoma was the most common malignancy to involve the spleen and extramedullary hematopoiesis was the most common nonneoplastic cause of splenic tumor.[2] In a German study of 61 splenic tumors, lymphoma (41%), mast cell tumor (29%), hemangiosarcoma (15%), and myeloid tumors (7%) were the most commonly diagnosed malignancies.[3] Lymphoma nearly always occurs in the spleen as part of multisystemic disease.

Lymphoma is covered in Chapter 36, and myeloproliferative disease and myeloma are discussed in Chapter 37.

The most common hepatic tumors (benign and malignant) are those derived from the biliary tracts. Tumors of the liver parenchyma are less common. As noted, many of the tumors that affect the spleen also involve the liver, either via metastasis or as part of a systemic disease.

▶ VISCERAL MAST CELL TUMORS

<table>
<tr><td colspan="2" align="center">C L I N I C A L   B R I E F I N G</td></tr>
<tr><td>Common Presentation</td><td>Most common in older nonpurebred cats. Usually splenic. Signs include nonspecific illness or chronic vomiting due to histamine release and resultant gastroduodenal ulceration.</td></tr>
<tr><td>Staging and Diagnosis</td><td>Liver, lymph nodes, and bone marrow are also commonly affected. Staging includes MDB, abdominal ultrasonography, bone marrow aspiration, and fine-needle aspiration cytology or biopsy of the spleen. Diagnosis is sometimes made from ascitic fluid or blood smear.</td></tr>
<tr><td>Treatment
Initial
Adjunctive
Supportive</td><td>Splenectomy normalizes other disease within 5 weeks. Median survival, 12 months.
Use of corticosteroids is controversial. Chemotherapy (CCNU, vinblastine) not reported.
Preoperative H_1 and H_2 antihistamines may reduce risk of GI damage and shock, especially during surgery. The same drugs may be palliative for clinical signs (variable results). Antiserotonin drugs (e.g., cyproheptadine) may be better for symptomatic relief. Analgesia and nutritional support as needed.</td></tr>
</table>

Incidence, Signalment, and Etiology

The principle site for visceral mast cell tumor (MCT) is the spleen. In a survey of 41 cats with this disease, 35 had splenic MCT, 4 had mediastinal MCT, and 2 had MCT that primarily affected the peripheral lymph nodes.[2] While it is possible for cutaneous MCT to spread systemically, this is considerably less likely to occur in cats than in dogs and the viscera usually appear to be the primary site (also see Chapter 50). Unlike cutaneous MCT, visceral MCT occurs most commonly in DSH and DLH cats and is rarely re-

MANAGEMENT OF SPECIFIC DISEASES

ported in Siamese,[4] Maine Coon cats,[5] or other purebreds. This disease has been reported in cats as young as 3 years of age[6] but usually occurs in older cats (average age, 8 to 10 years).[2,5,7]

MDB = minimum database; includes CBC, biochemical profile, urinalysis, FeLV/FIV serology, T_4 testing, and thoracic radiographs (three views).

Clinical Presentation and History

Cats with visceral mast cell disease may present for non-specific malaise, inappetence, weight loss, or vomiting.[5,8,9] Vomiting may be occasional but may also have persisted for up to 6 weeks prior to presentation.[5] In one study, chronic vomiting was a sign in seven of seven cats[5] and was presumably due to gastroduodenal ulceration following the release of vasoactive amines (e.g., histamine, serotonin) that cause gastric parietal cell hyperplasia and increased gastric acid production. These ulcerations can be extensive and may eventually perforate, causing sudden death due to hemorrhage[10,11] or peritonitis.[12] Splenic rupture may also occur.[2] Sudden increase in the frequency of vomiting in a cat that has been vomiting intermittently, particularly when accompanied by anorexia, may be a sign that ulceration has worsened.[8]

Abdominal distention may be noticed by the owner and may be a chronic condition in some cats.[13] Abdominal distension may be due to ascites (present in up to one third of all affected cats[2,14]) or possibly a massively enlarged spleen. A spleen that is infiltrated by neoplastic mast cells may be 28 cm long, 8 cm wide, and up to 2 cm in thickness and may have a white fibrinous capsule (Figures 42-1 and 42-2).[4,5,11] Abdominal discomfort may also occur as a consequence of organomegaly.[15]

Involvement of the liver and less commonly the lungs, kidneys, and bone marrow may be noted when the spleen is very enlarged.[7] Rarely, a cat with multiple cutaneous metastases noticed by the owner will be found by the veterinarian to have a primary visceral MCT (Figure 42-3).[6,12]

KEY POINT

Cats with splenomegaly are more likely to have MCT or lymphoma than any other tumor.

Cats with mediastinal MCT will present with dyspnea due to either pleural effusion or a large mass that causes an incompressible anterior thorax.

Staging and Diagnosis

While the spleen is the most common primary site for visceral MCT, the liver is involved in up to 90% of affected cats.[2] Other common sites of involvement (listed in de-

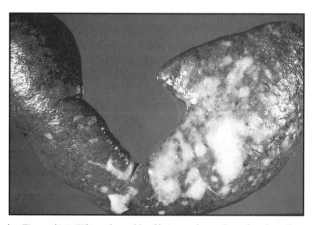

Figure 42-2: White, plaque-like, fibrin pseudocapsule on the spleen of a cat with splenic MCT.

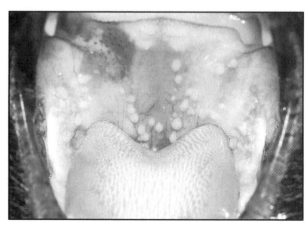

Figure 42-3: Multiple cutaneous and mucosal MCTs arose in this cat 5 years after splenectomy for visceral MCT. The cat was asymptomatic despite hundreds of similar lesions and circulating mast cells.

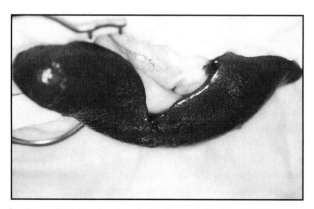

Figure 42-1: Grossly enlarged spleen in a cat with visceral MCT. (Courtesy of K.M. Rassnick)

creasing order) are the visceral lymph nodes, bone marrow, lung, intestine, and kidney.[2,7] Thus complete staging should include an MDB, abdominal radiographs or ultrasonography, and bone marrow aspiration. Aspiration cytology or a preoperative biopsy of the spleen may also be helpful.

Abdominal radiographs may demonstrate enlargement of the spleen and liver or even a mass effect, although the picture is often obscured by the presence of ascites.[13] Ultrasonography allows detailed visualization of abdominal organs and is unaffected by the presence of ascites. It is the imaging method of choice for these cats and may confirm a mass lesion or infiltrative pattern.[13,15] Thoracic radiographs may demonstrate pleural effusion or an anterior mediastinal mass; however, pulmonary infiltrates may be mild and difficult to distinguish from nonneoplastic processes (Figures 42-4 and 42-5).

Ascitic fluid may be reactive and not contain mast cells, and thus cytologic examination may not be diagnostic.[13] Fine-needle aspiration cytology from the spleen can often provide a diagnosis with minimal patient trauma.[6,8,13] To re-

duce the risk of bleeding or degranulation, a 25-ga needle may be used to obtain a sample.

A complete blood count will provide valuable information. Up to one third of cats with visceral MCT are anemic.[2,5] Anemia may be due to chronic blood loss from GI ulceration or to suppression of erythrocyte production by the bone marrow following infiltration by neoplastic cells. Erythrophagocytosis by malignant splenic mast cells was described in four cats with visceral MCT.[16] Circulating mast cells may be seen on routine blood smears and often account for 5% to 25% of circulating white blood cells.[4,6,9,17,18] Interestingly, the number of circulating mast cells has been reported to fluctuate in individual cats.[2] Basophilia may accompany mastocythemia. If systemic mast cell disease is suspected, a buffy-coat preparation from a microhematocrit tube may improve chances of tumor cell detection (Figure 42-6).

KEY POINT

Cats with splenic MCT often have liver and bone marrow involvement and may have skin metastases.

A bone marrow aspirate should be performed as part of the staging procedure. Bone marrow involvement occurs in 20% to 40% of cats with visceral MCT.[2,7–9]

If there is concern regarding gastric or duodenal ulceration, endoscopy may provide a definitive diagnosis but will not be therapeutic. Conversely, if ulcerations are noted in a chronically vomiting cat, the other staging procedures outlined above may help to diagnose an underlying MCT (Figure 42-7).

Treatment

Palliative medical treatment of visceral MCTs does not seem to result in significant clinical improvement. Corti-

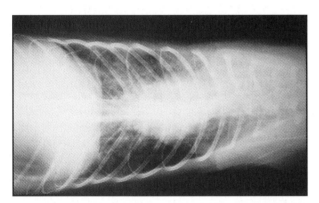

Figure 42-4: Systemic mastocytosis is common with visceral splenic MCT. Liver, blood, and bone marrow may be affected. Rarely, even the lungs may be affected, as in this 5-year-old cat. (Courtesy of K.M. Rassnick)

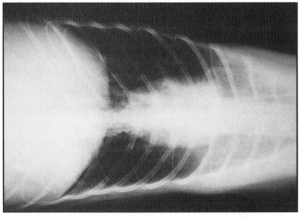

Figure 42-5: Splenectomy alone may cause regression of systemic mast cell disease. Following splenectomy, the pulmonary masses seen in Figure 42-4 regressed, as shown in this radiograph. (Courtesy of K.M. Rassnick)

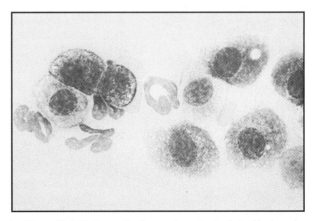

Figure 42-6: Finely granulated mast cells seen in circulating blood may be concentrated by spinning a microhematocrit tube and smearing the white cell layer (buffy coat smear). This buffy coat smear is from a 10-year-old cat with splenic MCT and circulating mast cells. (Courtesy of S.M. Cotter)

MANAGEMENT OF SPECIFIC DISEASES

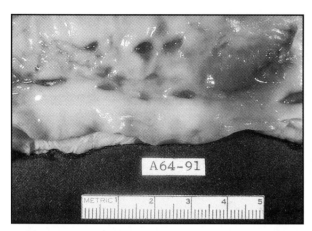

Figure 42-7: Gastroduodenal ulceration is a secondary effect of histamine release from visceral MCTs. This sample was taken from a 5-year-old cat with chronic vomiting due to a splenic MCT. (Courtesy of S.M. Cotter)

costeroids and antihistamines (specifically the H1-blocker diphenhydramine) do not seem to reduce the incidence of vomiting or result in tumor regression,[8] although one cat remained stable for 20 months before it died of concurrent lymphoma.[18]

Splenectomy is the treatment of choice, even in cats with other evidence of systemic involvement. Cats with circulating mastocythemia may have complete normalization of their hemogram 4 to 5 weeks after surgery.[6,17] Of 21 reported cats undergoing splenectomy, survival ranged from 2 months to 34 months (median, approximately 12 months).[2,4–6,13,15,17] There was still gross evidence of disease in some cats that survived a long time. One cat developed cutaneous and mucosal MCTs 6 months after surgery. The tumors continued to increase in number, but there were no signs of systemic illness 30 months after surgery.[4] Owner tolerance obviously plays a role in survival, because another cat was euthanized 2.5 months after surgery because its cutaneous lesions did not regress.[6]

KEY POINT

Splenectomy may result in long-term remission even in cats with other organ or system involvement.

Recurrence of GI signs (vomiting, diarrhea) that had ceased after splenectomy was the reason for euthanasia in most other cats,[5,17] and this occurred 6 to 25 months after surgery.

Concern over the release of vasoactive amines due to surgical manipulation during splenectomy has led to the recommendation that cats be treated with corticosteroids and both H_1 and H_2 blocking antihistamines for 48 hours prior to surgery. It appears that serotonin may be a more impor-

tant vasoactive substance in cat mast cells, so it is possible that cyproheptadine may prove a better drug for symptomatic relief and preoperative GI protection.[19]

The role of corticosteroids and antihistamines after splenectomy is uncertain. Because some investigators believe that regression of disease following splenectomy may be immune mediated, the use of corticosteroids is often discouraged because of their potential immunosuppressive effects. In contrast, a cat that collapsed with bloody ascites after splenectomy was maintained for an additional 2 years on prednisone despite persistence of the ascites.[13] Antihistamines led to resolution of vomiting in another cat,[5] and the author of that report recommended the use of cimetidine postoperatively. The efficacy of H_2 receptor antagonists remains unknown.

The usefulness of chemotherapy has not been reported for visceral MCTs in cats. In dogs, CCNU, vinblastine, L-asparaginase, and chlorambucil have at least anecdotal activity against cutaneous MCTs and thus may be worth considering in cats with MCTs.

Supportive care is essential, particularly postoperative analgesia and nutritional support. Antiemetics can be helpful in decreasing nausea and vomiting if chemotherapy is used but are unlikely to affect tumor-induced vomiting.

NONDOMESTIC FELIDAE

An adult female cheetah (*Acinonyx jubatus*) became inappetent following chronic weight loss. A liver mass was palpated, and radiographs revealed a large liver and spleen. The cat was found to have circulating mast cells and mast cell infiltration of the bone marrow and was therefore euthanized. The spleen and liver were also infiltrated with mast cells. This cat also had a ruptured duodenal adenocarcinoma.[20]

▶ OTHER TUMORS OF THE SPLEEN

Incidental findings (one case of each of the following among 455 feline spleens) include fibrosarcoma, malignant fibrous histiocytoma, rhabdomyosarcoma, lipoma, and myelolipoma.[1] In a series of 61 splenic tumors, 3 undifferentiated sarcomas and 1 leiomyosarcoma were diagnosed, mainly in older cats.[3] Myelolipomas, which have been described in the spleen of cheetahs, are more commonly seen in the liver than the spleen of domestic cats and, are discussed later in this chapter.

MDB = minimum database; includes CBC, biochemical profile, urinalysis, FeLV/FIV serology, T_4 testing, and thoracic radiographs (three views).

► HEMANGIOSARCOMA

HEMANGIOSARCOMA OF THE SPLEEN

Incidence, Signalment, and Etiology

While some surveys found the skin to be the most common site for hemangiosarcoma in cats,[21] the spleen is also a reported primary site.[2,22]

Clinical Presentation and History

Tumors in the spleen may be solitary or multiple[2,22] They ranged in size from 3 to 15 cm^3 in one study.[22]

Collapse and dyspnea due to rupture of the tumor and blood loss may be acute,[2,23] or the cat may show episodic weakness with no acute signs.[2] The abdomen may be swollen due to hemoabdomen, and chylous peritoneal effusion has been seen in some cats.[2] In other cats the effusion has been a transudate.[14]

Staging and Diagnosis

Staging for splenic vascular tumors includes an MDB, abdominal ultrasonography, and often an excisional biopsy. It is rare to see neoplastic cells in peritoneal effusion, and hemorrhage may obscure cytologic diagnosis and may even be life threatening when fine-needle aspiration or needle biopsies of the tumor are collected. Ultrasonography is the imaging modality of choice, particularly in cats in which peritoneal effusion obscures radiographic details. The ultrasonographic appearance is most often that of multiple cavernous splenic nodules as well as metastases to intraabdominal organs.

Metastasis appears common and has been reported in 15 of 21 cats with splenic hemangiosarcoma.[2,21–23] In one series

of 6 cats, only 1 had metastases at diagnosis but 3 more cats developed hepatic metastasis within 35 weeks of surgery.[21] The liver is the most common metastatic site, although metastases to the regional lymph nodes, heart, lung, kidney, and brain have been reported.[2,21]

Fragmented red blood cells seen in dogs with hemangiosarcoma have not been reported in cats.[2]

A coagulation profile should be obtained prior to any surgery in cats with hemangiosarcoma.

Treatment

Splenectomy has been reported in five cats.[21,23] Four of these cats died between 8 and 35 weeks after surgery, and one did not die and was alive 19 weeks after surgery.

Adjuvant chemotherapy with doxorubicin alone or in combination with other cytotoxic drugs has improved survival in dogs with hemangiosarcoma; its efficacy has not been reported in cats.

Analgesia, antiemetic therapy, and appropriate nutritional support should be provided as needed to reduce postoperative discomfort and chemotherapy-induced anorexia.

HEMANGIOSARCOMA OF THE LIVER

Incidence, Signalment, and Etiology

The liver is another common site for abdominal hemangiosarcoma, although splenic or mesenteric hemangiosarcomas are reported more commonly.

Clinical Presentation and History

Cats with hepatic hemangiosarcoma are usually found to

have a large solitary mass with multiple smaller tumors in the liver parenchyma.[2,22] The large size attained by these tumors (70 to 155 cm³) makes them highly susceptible to rupture and bleeding.[22] Clinical presentation is therefore similar to cats that have splenic hemangiosarcoma. One cat had hepatomegaly for a year and vomiting for a month before being diagnosed with multiple hepatic hemangiosarcomas.[24]

Staging and Diagnosis

Staging for hepatic vascular tumors is the same as for splenic vascular tumors. Ultrasonography is the imaging modality of choice and may reveal multiple small and/or solitary large cavernous lesions in the liver parenchyma.[24] Free peritoneal fluid seen on ultrasonography may be blood or chyle.

Metastasis is less commonly reported for cats with hepatic hemangiosarcoma than for cats with splenic tumors; however, because cats are often euthanized without treatment or necropsy, the true incidence of metastases is difficult to ascertain. Metastases to lungs, spleen, mesentery, or regional lymph nodes were seen in 6 of 16 cats.[2,22,24,25]

KEY POINT

There is a high rate of metastasis from hemangiosarcoma of any visceral site.

Treatment

Surgical resection of a solitary ruptured hepatic hemangiosarcoma was performed in one cat, which was still alive 5 months after surgery.[26] Another cat was lost to follow up 4 months after surgical excision of a hepatic hemangiosarcoma.[27]

Chemotherapy using doxorubicin and cyclophosphamide was reported, but efficacy was not documented beyond questionable prolongation of survival in one report.[28]

Supportive care should be provided as described for splenic vascular tumors.

HEMANGIOSARCOMA OF OTHER SITES

Abdominal Cavity

Mesenteric hemangiosarcoma is probably the second most common site of involvement after the skin (Figure 42-8). In one study, 11 of 56 hemangiosarcomas occurred in the mesentery.[2] Close association with the duodenum, colon, or pancreas can make the site of origin difficult to determine in some cats [22]; in one series, tumors of the mesentery, intestine, and peritoneum were grouped together. Bleeding is a common complication, resulting in abdominal swelling due to hemoabdomen[22] and dyspnea.[23] Tumors may be large, reaching 18 cm in diameter in one cat.[22] Chylous ascites may be seen, presumably due to oc-

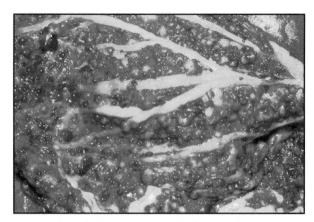

Figure 42-8: *The skin is the most common site for hemangiosarcoma in cats; mesenteric, hepatic, and splenic locations are much less common. This cat has mesenteric hemangiosarcoma. (Courtesy of W. Dernell)*

clusion of lymphatic drainage at the root of the mesentery. Ultrasonography in these cats may reveal a mass originating from the mesentery and allow ultrasound-guided needle core biopsy.[29]

As for other sites of hemangiosarcoma, metastasis is common. Metastases, most commonly to the liver but also to regional lymph nodes, omentum, diaphragm, spleen, pancreas, lung, and heart, were seen in 19 of 24 cats (Figure 42-9).[2,21–23,30]

Little information on treatment has been reported, although one cat died soon after receiving doxorubicin. This lack of information probably reflects the paucity of options for primary treatment of the mass. Three cats were found to have unresectable tumors in one study.[29]

Thoracic Cavity

Mediastinal hemangiosarcoma was diagnosed in six cats, and hemothorax was a cause of dyspnea in five of these cats.[2,22,23] Metastases to pleural surfaces were common, and the tumor had infiltrated the thoracic skeletal musculature.[2,22] In

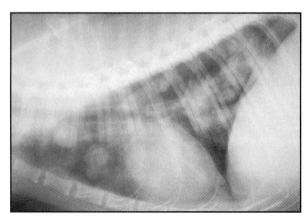

Figure 42-9: *Visceral hemangiosarcoma is a highly metastatic tumor in cats. Pulmonary metastases from a hemangiosarcoma are seen in this cat. (Courtesy of K.M. Rassnick)*

one cat, metastasis was noted outside the pleural cavity (i.e., affecting the liver, spleen, lung, and regional lymph nodes). Treatment has not been reported. A hemangiosarcoma of the thoracic wall has been reported,[21] as has primary pulmonary hemangiosarcoma that involved all lung lobes and metastasized to the spleen, brain, and bones of the skull.[22]

Nasal

Four cats with nasal hemangiosarcoma have been reported. One cat, in which the tumor aggressively invaded the palate and nasal bones, had been sneezing for a year.[21] None of the tumors had metastasized.[2,21]

Tongue and Oral Cavity

Hemangiosarcoma of the tongue in two cats was reported to be locally invasive and recurred after surgical excision (Figure 42-10). Metastases were not reported.[2] Hemangiosarcoma may also occur at other sites in the mouth.

NONDOMESTIC FELIDAE

Abdominal masses were found on palpation and radiographs in a 12-year-old male cheetah *(Acinonyx jubatus)* that had been depressed and inappetent with inter-

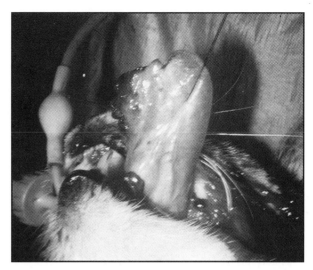

Figure 42-10: Oral hemangiosarcoma, particularly of the tongue, may appear as a bleeding mass. (Courtesy of S.M. Cotter)

mittent vomiting for 2 months.[31] Surgery disclosed a large, unresectable splenic hemangiosarcoma that had metastasized to the liver, kidneys, and abdominal musculature and was causing hemorrhage.

▶ LYMPHANGIOMA AND LYMPHANGIOSARCOMA

CLINICAL BRIEFING

Common Presentation	Similar to hemangiosarcoma; distinction probably unimportant clinically. Most common site is skin, but liver, mesentery, mediastinum, and oral cavity are also affected.
Staging and Diagnosis	As for hemangiosarcoma. May be multicentric or highly metastatic.
Treatment	None reported; probably as for hemangiosarcoma.

Incidence, Signalment, and Etiology

This is a rare tumor that seems to have a similar biologic behavior to hemangiosarcoma in cats. The most common primary site is the skin (Figure 42-11; also see Chapter 50). Lymphangiomas and lymphangiosarcomas have been reported to affect the liver,[32] mediastinum,[33,34] abdominal serosa,[29] cranial mesentery,[34] oral cavity,[32] and tongue.[32] Lymphatics (unspecified locations) were the primary site in six cats.[32]

Males may be overrepresented, although the small number of cases makes this determination difficult. A Norwegian forest cat is the only purebred reported with this tumor.[34]

Clinical Presentation and History

Chylous ascites was associated with multiple punctate

lymphangiosarcomas involving the abdominal wall and serosal surface of the small intestine in one cat.[29] Similarly, chyloperitoneum was seen in two cats with lymphangiosarcoma of the cranial mesentery. One of these cats was anorectic and vomiting.[34] Chylothorax was associated with a mediastinal lymphangiosarcoma and caused dyspnea in another two cats, one of which also had tumor involvement of the pericardium, mesentery, and omentum.[33,34] Neither this cat nor one with two hepatic lymphangiomas and necrotizing orchitis had chylous ascites.[32]

Staging and Diagnosis

As for hemangiosarcoma, staging should include an MDB, abdominal ultrasonography, and possibly an excisional biopsy. Ultrasonography is the imaging modality of

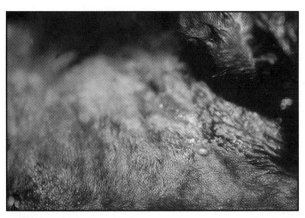

Figure 42-11: *Lymphangiosarcoma may be difficult to distinguish, even histologically, from hemangiosarcoma and occurs as a rare tumor in similar locations. This lymphangiosarcoma infiltrates the abdominal skin and subcutis. (Courtesy of A. Evans)*

choice, and lymphangiosarcoma may appear as a cystic tumor.[33] Biopsy differentiation between hemangiosarcoma and lymphangiosarcoma may be difficult,[35] and the distinction may not be clinically important.

Treatment

Attempted surgical resection was unsuccessful in the only four cats reported.[29,33,34] The tumor has appeared to be multicentric if not strictly metastatic in the majority of reported cats. Supportive care should be provided as described for hemangiosarcomas.

NONDOMESTIC FELIDAE

A lymphangioma of the omentum was reported in a jaguar *(Panthera onca)*. In the same survey, a mesenteric lymphangioma was reported in a leopard *(Panthera pardus)*.[36]

▶ MYELOLIPOMAS

C L I N I C A L B R I E F I N G	
Common Presentation	Uncommon liver tumor in older domestic cats; rarely affects the spleen. Tumors may be solitary and large or multiple. Usually asymptomatic, incidental finding. Cheetahs appear predisposed to splenic myelolipomas.
Staging and Diagnosis	Benign tumor. MDB and abdominal ultrasonography to assess size and number of masses. Fine-needle aspiration cytology shows adipocytes and marrow elements.
Treatment Initial Supportive	Surgical excision, if symptoms are present, should be curative. Analgesia and nutritional support postoperatively.

Incidence, Signalment, and Etiology

These benign tumors are composed of adipocytes and normal hematopoietic cells in all stages of development. In other species they are thought to be a secondary development in response to chronic hematologic stress. The tumor has been reported in detail in the liver of only seven cats. A congenital or acquired diaphragmatic hernia was suggested to be the cause of myelolipoma development in an incarcerated and chronically hypoxic liver in three cats.[37–39] Another two cats had leukocytosis, which was thought to be a consequence of the tumor rather than an indication of chronic hematologic stress.[40,41] Myelolipomas will occasionally occur in the spleen.[1]

All affected cats have been DSHs (six cats) or DLH (one cat).[40] The cats ranged in age from 7 to 16 years (median, 13 years), and there was no gender predilection.

Clinical Presentation and History

Dyspnea due to diaphragmatic hernia was the presenting sign in three cats,[37–39] and nonspecific signs led to palpation

of an abdominal mass in three other cats.[2,40,41] Hepatic myelolipomas were an incidental finding in conjunction with a large hepatocellular carcinoma in one emaciated older cat.[2]

Masses may be multiple, vary in size, and affect all liver lobes[40] or a single lobe,[37] or they may be solitary and discrete. Two cats had two solitary myelolipomas, each situated in a different liver lobe.[2,41]

Staging and Diagnosis

Fine-needle aspiration of a myelolipoma will disclose adipocytes and normal marrow elements. Radiographs may demonstrate liver masses, some of which have been reported to be mineralized.[41] Ultrasonography will allow more thorough investigation of liver and splenic parenchyma than radiography. Metastasis is unlikely.

Treatment

Surgical resection of an affected liver lobe[37] or removal of large hepatic nodules[2,41] was associated with long-term survival in two cats. One cat was alive with no evidence of disease more than a year after surgery,[37] while the other died due to unknown causes 27 months after surgery.[41] Treatment may not be necessary in animals without clinical signs. It is important to obtain a diagnosis to differentiate from other tumor types.

NONDOMESTIC FELIDAE

Incidence, Signalment, and Etiology

Myelolipomas are rare in domestic cats and uncommon in nondomestic Felidae other than cheetahs *(Acinonyx jubatus)*. In a survey of 109 wild Felidae that were autopsied, myelolipomas were described in 6 cheetahs and a male tiger *(Panthera tigris).*[42] Overall, myelolipomas have been described in 26 cheetahs. Signalment was available for 8 of these cats: There were 5 males and 3 females ranging in age from 4 to 14 years.[42–44] In another survey, all affected cheetahs were older than 6 years.[45] Eleven of 35 cheetahs examined by ultrasonography were found to have myelolipomas ("nodular lipomatosis"). Interestingly, 9 of 14 European cheetahs[46] but only 2 of 21 Namibian cheetahs[46] and 5 of 30 South African cheetahs[45] were found to be affected.

Chronic stress was discussed as a possible mechanism for the development of these tumors.

Clinical Presentation and History

Myelolipomas occur in the liver but may concurrently affect the spleen or affect the spleen alone.[43,46] There may be no clinical signs, or signs may be nonspecific (e.g., anorexia) or unrelated (e.g., ataxia, hematuria).[44,47]

Staging and Diagnosis

These benign tumors usually occur as multiple lesions that are 1 to 2 cm in diameter[43] but can be quite large.[44] Ultrasonography proved to be an excellent screening method for this disease; myelolipomas appear as well-demarcated echogenic splenic nodules.[46] Serology for FeLV, FIV, and FIP was negative for all affected cheetahs in one study.[46]

Treatment

Treatment has not been described in exotic Felidae, but surgical excision in domestic cats has been associated with long survival times.[37,41]

▶ TUMORS OF THE LIVER PARENCHYMA

C L I N I C A L B R I E F I N G	
Common Presentation	Hepatoma and hepatocellular carcinoma may be part of a disease spectrum rather than distinct entities. Uncommon in older cats. Mostly nonspecific signs; abdominal mass may be palpable. Hypoglycemia reported in association with very large tumors.
Staging and Diagnosis	MDB and abdominal ultrasonography. Metastasis uncommon but usually to lymph nodes. Biopsy samples should be collected from hepatic nodes at surgery. Other tumors may be present.
Treatment Initial Supportive	 Surgery if solitary. Analgesia postoperatively and nutritional support as needed.

HEPATOCELLULAR CARCINOMA

Incidence, Signalment, and Etiology

Tumors of the liver parenchyma are less common in cats than tumors of the biliary tree. This means that the signal-

ment and outcome for cats with hepatocellular carcinoma is often obscured in large studies due to lack of discrimination between cases.

The median age of 11 cats for which information was available was 11 years (range, 2–18 years). Using reported data, there were

11 males; 16 cats were DSHs and 2 were Siamese.[2]

Toxicity trials using diethylnitrosamine in cats induced multiple types of liver tumors, including hepatocellular carcinoma, 1 to 2 years after exposure.[48]

Clinical Presentation and History

Signs are mostly nonspecific, such as anorexia and weight loss, but ascites, polydipsia, and palpable abdominal masses have been reported.[2,27] In another study, signs of vomiting, diarrhea, weight loss, and an abdominal mass were absent in two cats with hepatocellular carcinoma[49]; hemorrhage from a ruptured tumor caused sudden death in one cat.[2] The tumor may appear as a solitary large mass or as multiple nodules.

KEY POINT

Surgical excision of a large solitary liver tumor is warranted regardless of the histology.

Staging and Diagnosis

The histopathologic appearance of hepatocellular carcinoma does not appear to correlate with metastatic behavior.[2] Metastases were seen in 7 of 26 cats with hepatocellular carcinoma.[2,25] The hepatic lymph nodes were the most common metastatic site (4 cats), but the spleen (2 cats) and lungs (2 cats) were also affected.

Unrelated tumors of the liver were common in one group of 18 cats with hepatocellular carcinoma; 3 cats had biliary cystadenomas, 1 had a myelolipoma, and 1 had an MCT.[2] Another cat with hepatocellular carcinoma had a biliary cystadenoma.[49] Staging for a cat with hepatocellular carcinoma should therefore include abdominal ultrasonography (and/or CT or MRI) in addition to an MDB. Biopsy specimens should be collected from enlarged hepatic lymph nodes at the time of surgery.

Treatment

Surgery should be the treatment of choice for solitary hepatocellular carcinomas, but survival data is not available for cats treated in this way. Supportive care is important; postoperative analgesia and nutritional support should be considered.

HEPATOMA OR HEPATOCELLULAR ADENOMA

Incidence, Signalment, and Etiology

This is an uncommon tumor and difficult to distinguish histologically from low-grade hepatocellular carcinoma. Hepatomas were not reported in two studies that included 57 cats with liver tumors.[2,25] In another study, 9 cats with hepatoma were included with cats that had other benign liver tumors. This group of cats tended to be older than those with malignant tumors, and there was no gender predilection.[27] Multiple hepatomas are occasionally reported.[50]

Clinical Presentation and History

One cat with hepatoma had marked weight loss over several months as well as muscle weakness and fasciculations due to severe hypoglycemia.[51] This cat had a very large palpable liver mass (5.5 cm in diameter). Another cat died suddenly due to rupture of a hepatoma 8 months after it was initially diagnosed.[52]

Hepatocellular adenomas can also be quite small. In one series, only one of nine cats had a palpable abdominal mass; hepatomas were incidental findings at necropsy in the other eight cats

Staging and Diagnosis

Staging is as for other liver tumors. Hypoglycemia in the face of decreased serum insulin was seen in a cat with a large hepatoma. Liver enzymes were increased, although serum bilirubin was normal.[51]

Treatment

The large hepatoma in the aforementioned cat was believed to be unresectable, so the cat was maintained on multiple small meals daily for 6 months. No other treatment for these tumors has been reported. Presumably, surgery should be curative for solitary tumors.

▶ TUMORS OF THE BILIARY SYSTEM

CLINICAL BRIEFING

Common Presentation	Adenomas and carcinomas usually affect older cats; possibly increased prevalence of carcinomas in Siamese. Signs often are nonspecific, although ascites or a palpable mass may occur. Icterus is common with extrahepatic carcinomas. Carcinomas may develop from biliary adenomas.
Staging and Diagnosis	MDB and abdominal ultrasonography. Guided biopsy for diagnosis. Check for other abdominal tumors. Although adenomas are benign tumors, malignant transformation

Staging and Diagnosis *(continued)*	is common. Carcinomas may often be multiple. Metastasis from carcinomas is common, usually to peritoneum, lungs, and mesenteric lymph nodes.
Treatment Initial	Surgical excision of solitary or few tumors because of the risk of malignant transformation. Recurrence (or new tumors) usually develops after 2 years or more. Surgical resection of carcinomas may be briefly palliative in cats with solitary tumors.
Adjunctive	Not reported.
Supportive	Analgesia postoperatively. If surgery not an option for carcinoma, disease is rapidly fatal. Nutritional support as needed.

BILIARY ADENOMAS

Incidence, Signalment, and Etiology

Other nomenclature for these tumors includes bile duct adenoma, biliary cystadenoma, biliary adenoma, and cholangiocellular adenoma.

These tumors occur almost exclusively in older cats (12 to 18 years of age),[2,53,54] although two 6-year-old cats, including a Persian, have been described.[2,54] Otherwise, the majority of affected cats have been DSHs or DLHs.[2,53,54] There does not appear to be a gender predilection, although 17 of 23 cats in two studies were males.[53,55] Adenomas may show anaplastic or dysplastic changes that signal transformation to adenocarcinoma.[25]

Three young cats in Hong Kong developed biliary adenoma after infection with a liver fluke *(Chonorchis sinensis)*. One of the cats was experimentally infected and developed a tumor within 4 months.[56]

Clinical Presentation and History

Biliary cystadenomas may be multiple[49] and occasionally can be very large (up to 9 cm in diameter).[2] An abdominal mass was palpable in 29 of 51 cats with this tumor type,[27,49,53–55,57] although biliary adenomas were still an incidental finding in many cats.[53]

Clinical signs such as lethargy, vomiting, and polydipsia may not be specific for biliary adenomas.[54] Abdominal swelling due to ascites or a mass may be noticed by owners.[54] While jaundice is rare for benign tumors,[27] it may still be a sign that leads to a diagnosis of biliary adenomas, depending on tumor location.[53]

Staging and Diagnosis

Transformation of biliary adenoma to biliary adenocarcinoma may be a common event,[25] and both tumor types may be found in the same cat.[49,56] Hepatocellular carcinoma was also present in 3 of 18 cats with biliary adenoma.[49]

As for other liver tumors, radiography may disclose a hepatic mass but ultrasonography will allow the clinician to decide if surgery is an option (solitary large lesion) or not

(multiple diffuse lesions; Figure 42-12). Ultrasonography is excellent for detecting tumors larger than 2 to 3 mm, although larger tumors may be missed because their ventral

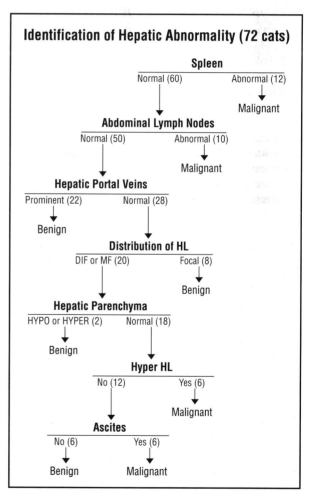

Figure 42-12: *A schematic for ultrasonographic appearance of 72 liver lesions and potential for benign vs. malignant disease. As with all schematics, some exceptions occur; however, this schematic correctly identified 64 of the 72 lesions (89%). HL = hepatic lesion; DIF = diffuse; MF = multifocal; HYPO = hypoechoic; HYPER = hyperechoic. (From Newell SM, Selcer BA, Girard E, et al: Correlations between ultrasonic findings and specific hepatic diseases in cats: 72 cases (1985–1997). JAVMA 213:94–98, 1998; with permission)*

MANAGEMENT OF SPECIFIC DISEASES

location can be obscured by "near-field" reverberations.[55] Ultrasound-guided needle core biopsy is mandatory for definitive diagnosis. Unrelated tumors have been reported in some cats. In one study, 8 of 34 cats with biliary adenoma also had lymphoma or MCTs.[2,25] In another study, 2 of 10 cats had pancreatic carcinoma and one had carcinomatosis in association with biliary cystadenoma.[55] This means that the clinician should fully evaluate all organ systems by performing complete staging, including an MDB, abdominal ultrasonography, and biopsy, prior to treating the adenoma.

KEY POINT

Surgical excision of biliary adenoma should be performed early in the course of disease as malignant transformation is common.

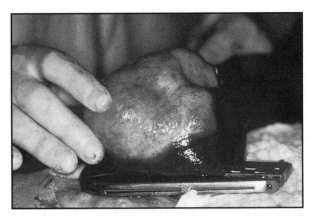

Figure 42-13: *A solitary hepatobiliary cystadenoma may be resected using stapling equipment. Early removal is encouraged as these tumors may undergo malignant transformation. (Courtesy of J. Berg)*

Treatment

Surgical excision appears to be successful in the majority of cats with biliary adenomas. Removal of focal lesions in eight cats[2,27,53,54] and multiple lesions in two cats[54,57] via a lobectomy achieved complete surgical margins in all but one animal. The tumor in this animal was attached to the gallbladder, and the cat still lived 12 months before tumor recurrence was clinically noted.[54] Survival times for the remaining nine cats ranged from 1 to 42 months (median, 22 months), with recurrence noted in only one cat 25 months after surgery.[27,53,54,57] Adjunctive therapy is not warranted in cats with resectable tumors, and even cats with multiple tumors have a good prognosis following resection (Figure 42-13).

Since these tumors may transform to biliary adenocarcinoma, surgical resection is best done early in the course of disease. It would not be good practice to simply monitor a cat with a solitary biliary adenoma.

Supportive care, including analgesia and nutritional support, should be considered postoperatively.

BILE DUCT CARCINOMA

Incidence, Signalment, and Etiology

Other terms for this tumor include cholangiocarcinoma, bile duct or biliary adenocarcinoma, and biliary carcinoma. Some authors distinguish between intrahepatic and extrahepatic tumors. Bile duct carcinomas have been reported in cats ranging in age from 11 months[58] to 21 years,[2] although most affected cats are older than 9 years. Of 27 cats for which the breed was reported, there were 18 DSHs, 8 Siamese, and 1 Burmese.[2,58–62] More females than males are reported, but there does not appear to be a strong predilection except in one study, in which 15 of 20 affected cats were female.[2] Natural and experimental infestation with the fluke *Clonorchis sinensis* has led to bile duct carcinoma in-

duction,[56] as has experimental administration of the carcinogen diethylnitrosamine.[48] Residual benign and precancerous lesions were found concurrently with bile duct carcinoma in 10 of 15 carcinomas affecting the intrahepatic (9 cats) or extrahepatic (4 cats) biliary tree or gallbladder (2 cats).[25]

Clinical Presentation and History

Abdominal distension noted by the owner or a palpable abdominal mass on physical examination led to a diagnosis of hepatic bile duct carcinoma in 18 of 23 cats.[27,49,58–62] Other less specific signs such as anorexia, depression, vomiting, and weight loss were also reported, although the tumor was occasionally an incidental finding at necropsy.[27,58]

Icterus appears to be more common with tumors involving the extrahepatic bile ducts[2,59] than with those involving the intrahepatic biliary tree. One cat was presented for severe symmetric generalized alopecia; histologically, the skin had follicular atrophy with minimal inflammation and was identical to a paraneoplastic alopecia seen in some cats with pancreatic carcinoma.[62]

Staging and Diagnosis

Staging for this disease focuses on evaluating for abdominal disease and metastasis using an MDB and abdominal ultrasonography. Radiographs may disclose an anterior abdominal mass that is associated with the liver, but ultrasonography is the imaging modality of choice.[27,63] Ultrasonographically, the liver is often diffusely mottled or has multiple small masses throughout the parenchyma (Figures 42-14 and 42-15).

Ascites is rare and may be due to peritonitis.[59] Evaluations in serum liver enzyme activity may be seen,[2,58,60] but this is not a consistent finding.[59] Increases in bilirubin are similarly inconsistent, although all cats that were icteric in one study had a malignant tumor.[27]

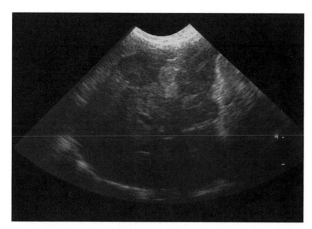

Figure 42-14: An ultrasonogram of the liver of a 3-year-old cat. The liver was normal sized with irregular borders and multiple echogenic masses. The diagnosis was anaplastic carcinoma.

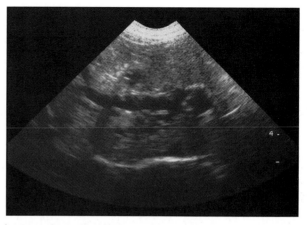

Figure 42-15: This ultrasonogram shows a cholangiocarcinoma invading the common bile duct and causing dilation of the biliary tree in a 13-year-old Siamese.

Metastasis is common and does not seem to alter with the tumor's site of origin. In two studies that distinguished between intrahepatic, extrahepatic, and gallbladder carcinomas, metastasis was detected in 17 of 23 cats with intrahepatic tumors, 5 of 8 cats with extrahepatic tumors, and 4 of 4 cats with gallbladder tumors.[2,25] A primary gallbladder tumor metastasized widely in one other cat, causing pleural effusion and dyspnea.[64] The pattern of metastasis did not seem to differ among the three sites of origin; the most common sites of metastasis were the peritoneum, lungs, and regional lymph nodes,[2,25] while metastases to the diaphragm, spleen, kidney, eye, pancreas, and stomach wall were less commonly reported.[2,25,58,65]

Treatment

Therapy for these aggressive tumors is rarely reported. One cat with ascites that was palliated with prednisone was euthanized 10 days later due to progressive disease.[59]

Surgery was attempted in four cats with biliary carcinoma.[27] Three died immediately postoperatively, and the surviving cat was euthanized due to tumor recurrence 2 weeks after surgery.

▶ OTHER TUMORS OF THE LIVER

A hepatic embryonal sarcoma (rhabdomyosarcoma) has been described in a 2-year-old cat.[66] The tumor had metastasized to the spleen.

▶ NONDOMESTIC FELIDAE

Three of 81 necropsies over a 20 year period revealed carcinomas of the biliary tract in captive Felidae,[67] accounting for nearly 40% of tumors in that family. A further survey found bile duct carcinomas in both a black leopard *(Panthera pardus)* and a margay *(Felis wiedii)*[68] and a biliary cystadenoma in a cheetah.[45] The only hepatic tumor reported in a third survey was a fibroadenoma of the biliary ducts in a leopard *(Panthera onca)*.[36] An 18-year-old female cougar *(Felis concolor)* was reported to have a bile duct carcinoma,[69] and a margay died suddenly due to hemorrhage from a cholangiocarcinoma that had metastasized to the perihilar lymph nodes and lungs.[70] A hepatoma in conjunction with hepatic myelolipomas was seen in a cheetah *(Acinonyx jubatus)*.[42]

CARCINOMA OF THE EXOCRINE PANCREAS

CLINICAL BRIEFING

Common Presentation	Seen in older cats and causes severe weight loss and anorexia; vomiting is rare. Paraneoplastic alopecia is often reported. Abdominal mass is rarely palpable. Benign tumors are rare.
Staging and Diagnosis	MDB. Ascites is common, so abdominal ultrasonography is useful. Hepatic metastases are common, as is peritonitis. Pancreatic enzyme elevations are inconsistent.

(continued)

Treatment	
Initial	Surgery not an option if metastases are present but may be palliative if not. Gastrojejunostomy or enteral feeding (jejunostomy) tube placement is required.
Adjunctive	Not reported.
Supportive	Enteral or parenteral feeding postoperatively. Analgesia both peri- and postoperatively.

Incidence, Signalment, and Etiology

This neoplasm is rarely reported in cats. Pancreatic carcinomas have been reported in cats ranging from 8 to 18 years of age; in 20 cats for which the data were available, only 3 cats were younger than 10 years of age.[62,71–78] There does not appear to be a gender predilection, as 14 females and 17 males were reported in these studies. Of 13 cats for which breed information was available, 11 were DSHs and 2 were DLHs.[62,71–76]

MDB = minimum database; includes CBC, biochemical profile, urinalysis, FeLV/FIV serology, T_4 testing, and thoracic radiographs (three views).

Clinical Presentation and History

Nonspecific findings of anorexia, weight loss (which can be severe), lethargy, and listlessness are often the only systemic signs in cats with pancreatic carcinoma.[71–76] A distinctive syndrome of feline paraneoplastic alopecia has been described in many of the cats with pancreatic carcinoma. It has also been described in cats with biliary carcinomas,[62] and a similar syndrome has been seen in some cats with thymoma. The alopecia is symmetric and associated with excessive grooming and easily epilated hair.[62,73] The face, ventrum, and medial surfaces of the limbs are most commonly affected, and the feet may be painful due to crusting lesions of the foot pads and caseous paronychia characterized by erythema.[62,72,73,79] The skin is also often erythematous and has been described as "glistening alopecia," presumably due to loss of the stratum corneum (Figure 42-16).[62]

The skin changes are characterized histologically by an absent stratum corneum, minimal inflammatory infiltrate, and severe follicular atrophy with a characteristic finding of miniaturized hair bulbs.[62,73] The skin is not pruritic unless complicated by secondary infections such as *Malasezzia*.[72] Only rarely is an abdominal mass palpable during physical examination.[71,76,78] If pancreatic carcinoma is resected, alopecia resolves within 3 months.[78]

Two reported cats were diabetic for many months prior to diagnosis of pancreatic carcinoma.[74]

Staging and Diagnosis

Staging involves an MDB and abdominal ultrasonography, CT, or MRI. Abdominal radiographs are often of limited value because of ascites[75,80] or interpretation difficulties, although a barium study may show a displaced duodenum if the mass is sufficiently large.[71] One review found that the tumor occurred more often in the head of the pancreas than in the tail.[77] Ultrasonography is a more useful imaging modality; although the pancreatic tumor may be visualized,[55,74] it is often the metastatic spread, which appears ultrasonographically as "target lesions" within the liver parenchyma, that is noted.[62,75]

> **KEY POINT**
>
> *Paraneoplastic skin disease may be common in cats with pancreatic carcinoma.*

Screening blood work may be normal, although increases in serum activity of liver enzymes may indicate metastatic spread.[73] Serum activity of lipase was elevated in one cat with pancreatic carcinoma, although the elevation was only 2.5 times the normal upper limit.[74] Obstruction of the common bile duct will cause jaundice (Figure 42-17).

Metastasis is common in these tumors and often occurs before any clinical signs are obvious.[81] Metastases to the liver (Figure 42-18), peritoneum, and regional lymph nodes are most commonly described,[62,71,74,75,77] although lung,

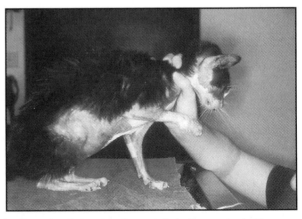

Figure 42-16: An unique dermatopathy has been associated with pancreatic carcinoma in cats. The skin lesions resolve if the tumor can be resected. (Courtesy of R. Meuller)

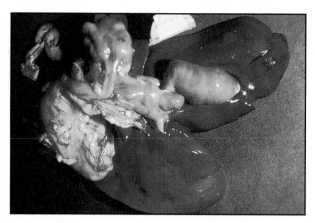

Figure 42-17: Necropsy specimen showing pancreatic carcinoma invading the duodenum, causing fibrosis and biliary stasis in a 9-year-old cat.

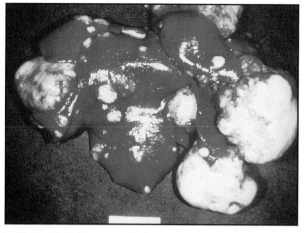

Figure 42-18: Metastases to the liver, as in this 9-year-old cat, are a common sequela to pancreatic carcinoma.

spleen, diaphragm, GI tract, ovary, kidney, and pleura are all reported sites of metastatic spread.[62,73,75,77,78] One cat developed retractile peritonitis, presumably secondary to enzyme leakage from a large pancreatic carcinoma.[80] On occasion, a cat with pancreatic carcinoma will have no evidence of metastasis on necropsy.[74,76]

Treatment

Surgical resection is usually impossible due to the presence of metastases.[71,75] Resection of a localized but poorly differentiated pancreatic carcinoma in one cat led to resolution of alopecia and weight gain before metastases became clinically evident 18 weeks after surgery.[78] If aggressive surgery such as a gastrojejunostomy is attempted, placement of a jejunostomy tube[78,82] is warranted to maintain alimentation in the postoperative period. Palliation with prednisone was not helpful in one cat.[73]

OTHER PANCREATIC TUMORS

Insulinomas are discussed in Chapter 44. Benign pancreatic tumors are sometimes diagnosed as an incidental finding in cats with other problems.[83]

NONDOMESTIC FELIDAE

An adenoma of the intrapancreatic ducts was recorded in a Palestine jungle cat *(Felis chaus furax).*[84]

REFERENCES

1. Spangler WL, Culbertson MR: Prevalence and type of splenic diseases in cats: 455 cases (1985–1991). *JAVMA* 201:773–776, 1992.
2. Carpenter JL, Andrews LK, Holzworth J: Tumors and tumor-like lesions, in Holzworth J (ed): *Diseases of the Cat. Medicine and Surgery.* Philadelphia, WB Saunders, 1987, pp 407–596.
3. Kessler M, Fickenscher Y, von Bomhard D: Zum vorkommen primärer tumoren der milz bei der katze. *Kleintierpraxis* 43:601–608, 1998.
4. Confer AW, Langloss JM, Cashell IG: Long-term survival of two cats with mastocytosis. *JAVMA* 172:160–161, 1978.
5. Liska WD, MacEwen EG, Zaki FA, Gavery M: Feline systemic mastocytosis: A review and results of splenectomy in seven cases. *JAAHA* 15:589–579, 1979.
6. Madewell BR, Gunn CR, Gribble DH: Mast cell phagocytosis of red blood cells in a cat. *Vet Pathol* 20:638–640, 1983.
7. Goto N, Ozasa M, Takahashi R, et al: Pathological observations of feline mast cell tumor. *Jpn J Vet Sci* 36:483–494, 1974.
8. Weller RE: Systemic mastocytosis and mastocytemia in a cat. *Mod Vet Pract* 59:41–43, 1978.
9. Kobayashi Y, Usuda H, Ochiai K, Itakura C: Malignant mesothelioma with metastasis and mast cell leukaemia in a cat. *J Comp Pathol* 111:453–458, 1994.
10. Hasler UC, van den Ingh TSGAM: Malignant mastocytosis and duodenal ulceration in a cat. *Schweiz Arch Tierheilk* 120:263–268, 1978.
11. Lillie RD: Mast myelocyte leukemia in a cat. *Am J Pathol* 713–721, 1931.
12. Seawright AA, Grono LR: Malignant mast cell tumour in a cat with perforating duodenal ulcer. *J Path Bact* 87:107–111, 1964.
13. Crawford MA: Challenging cases in internal medicine: What's your diagnosis? *Vet Med* 84:1126–1143, 1989.
14. Wright KN, Gomph RE, DeNovo Jr RC: Peritoneal effusion in cats: 65 cases (1981–1997). *JAVMA* 214:375–381, 1999.
15. Schulman A: Splenic mastocytosis in a cat. *Calif Vet* 41:17–18, 1987.
16. Madewell BR, Munn RJ, Phillips LK: Ultrastructure of canine, feline and bovine mast cell neoplasms. *Am J Vet Res* 45:2066–2073, 1984.
17. Guerre R, Millet P, Groulade P: Systemic mastocytosis in a cat: Remission after splenectomy. *J Small Anim Pract* 20:769–772, 1979.
18. Jeraj KP, O'Brien TD, Yano BL: Systemic mastocytoma associated with lymphosarcoma in an aged cat. *Can Vet J* 24:20–23, 1983.
19. Padrid PA, Mitchell RW, Ndukwu IM, et al: Cyproheptadine-induced attenuation of type-I immediate-hypersensitivity reactions of airway smooth muscle from immune-sensitized cats. *Am J Vet Res* 56:109–115, 1995.
20. Winter VH, Caarund C, Göltenboth R: Mastzellenleukose und duodenumkarzinom bei einem gepard (Azinonyx jubatus schräber). *Kleinterpraxis* 25:499–504, 1980.
21. Scavelli TD, Patnaik AK, Mehlaff CJ, Hayes AA: Hemangiosarcoma in the cat: Retrospective evaluation of 31 surgical cases. *JAVMA* 187:817–819, 1985.
22. Patnaik AK, Liu S-K: Angiosarcoma in cats. *J Small Anim Pract* 18:191–198, 1977.
23. Kraje AC, Mears EA, Hahn KA, et al: Unusual metastatic behavior and clinicopathologic findings in 8 cats with cutaneous or visceral hemangiosarcoma (1981–1997). *JAVMA* 214:670–672, 1999.
24. Ring RD, Godshalk CP, Smith TA: What is your diagnosis? *JAVMA* 205:423–424, 1994.
25. Patnaik AK: A morphologic and immunocytochemical study of hepatic neoplasms in cats. *Vet Pathol* 29:405–415, 1992.
26. Carb AV: What is your diagnosis? *JAVMA* 153:556–558, 1978.
27. Lawrence HJ, Erb HN, Harvey HJ: Nonlymphomatous hepatobiliary masses in cats: 41 cases (1972 to 1991). *Vet Surg* 23:365–368, 1994.
28. MacEwen EG, Mooney S, Brown NO, Hayes AA: Management of feline neoplasms: Surgery, immunotherapy and chemotherapy, in Holzworth J (ed): *Diseases of the Cat. Medicine and Surgery.* Philadelphia, WB Saunders, 1987, pp 597–606.
29. Gores BR, Berg J, Carpenter JL, Ullman SL: Chylous ascites in cats: Nine cases

(1978–1993). *JAVMA* 205:1161–1164, 1994.

30. Mulligan RM: Spontaneous cat tumors. *Cancer Res* 11:271, 1951.

31. Ervin AM, Junge RE, Miller RE, Thornburg LP: Hemangiosarcoma in a cheetah *(Acinonyx jubatus)*. *J Zoo Anim Med* 19:143–145, 1988.

32. Lawler DF, Evans RH: Multiple hepatic cavernous lymphangiomas in an aged male cat. *J Comp Pathol* 109:83–87, 1993.

33. Stobie D, Carpenter JL: Lymphangiosarcoma of the mediastinum, mesentery and omentum in a cat with chylothorax. *JAAHA* 29:78–80, 1993.

34. Hinrichs U, Puhl S, Rutteman GR, et al: Lymphangiosarcomas in cats: A retrospective study of 12 cases. *Vet Pathol* 36:164–167, 1999.

35. Swayne DE, Mahaffey EA, Haynes SG: Lymphangiosarcoma and haemangiosarcoma in a cat. *J Comp Pathol* 100:91–96, 1989.

36. Ratcliffe HL: Incidence and nature of tumors in captive wild mammals and birds. *Am J Cancer* 17:116–135, 1933.

37. Gourley IM, Popp JA, Park RD: Myelolipomas of the liver in a domestic cat. *JAVMA* 158:2053–2057, 1971.

38. Tani K, Goryo M, Okada K: Hepatic myelolipoma in a cat. *J Fac Agric Iwate Univ* 22:177–180, 1996.

39. Schuh JCL: Hepatic nodular myelolipomatosis (myelolipomas) associated with a peritoneo-pericardial diaphragmatic hernia in a cat. *J Comp Pathol* 97:231–235, 1987.

40. Ikede BO, Downey RS: Multiple hepatic myelolipomas in a cat. *Can Vet J* 13:160–163, 1972.

41. McCaw DL, da Silva Curiel JMA, Shaw DP: Hepatic myelolipomas in a cat. *JAVMA* 197:243–244, 1990.

42. Lombard LS, Fortna HM, Garner FM, Brynjolfsson G: Myelolipomas of the liver in captive wild felidae. *Pathol Vet* 5:127–134, 1968.

43. Cardy RH, Bostrom RE: Multiple splenic myelolipomas in a cheetah *(Acinonyx jubatus)*. *Vet Pathol* 51:556–558, 1978.

44. Wadsworth PF, Jones DM: Myelolipoma in the liver of a cheetah *(Acinonyx jubatus)*. *J Zoo Anim Med* 11:75–76, 1980.

45. Munson L, Nesbit JW, Meltzer DGA, et al: Diseases in captive cheetahs *(Acinonyx jubatus jubatus)* in South Africa: A 20-year retrospective survey. *J Zoo Wildl Med* 30:342–347, 1999.

46. Walzner C: Noduläre lipomatose—"Myelolipome"—in der Mitz des gepards *(Acinonyx jubatus)*. *Wien Tierärztl Mschr* 81:24, 1994.

47. Parihar NS, Charan K, Charkravarty IB: Lipomatosis in a hunting cheetah *(Acinonyx jubatus)*. *Indian J Vet Pathol* 1:4–5, 1976.

48. Schmähl D, Habs M, Ivankovic S: Carcinogenesis of N-nitrosodiethylamine (DENA) in chickens and domestic cats. *Int J Cancer* 22:552–557, 1978.

49. Post G, Patnaik AK: Nonhematopoietic hepatic neoplasms in cats: 21 cases (1983–1988). *JAVMA* 201:1080–1082, 1992.

50. Capellaro CEMPDM, Ribeiro LOC, Mueller SBK, Alencar Filho RA: Hepatoma em gato doméstico. Descricáo de um caso. *O Biológico* 41:108–110, 1975.

51. Thompson JC, Hickson PC, Johnstone AC, Jones BR: Observations on hypoglycemia associated with a hepatoma in a cat. *N Z Vet J* 43:186–189, 1995.

52. Rees CA, Goldschmidt MH: Cutaneous horn and squamous cell carcinoma in situ (Bowen's disease) in a cat. *JAAHA* 34:485–486, 1998.

53. Adler R, Wilson DW: Biliary cystadenoma of cats. *Vet Pathol* 32:415–418, 1995.

54. Trout NJ, Berg RJ, McMillan MC, et al: Surgical treatment of hepatobiliary cystadenomas in cats: Five cases (1988–1993). *JAVMA* 206:505–507, 1995.

55. Nyland TG, Koblik PD, Tellyer SE: Ultrasonographic evaluation of biliary cystadenomas in cats. *Vet Radiol Ultrasound* 40:300–306, 1999.

56. Hou PC: Primary carcinoma of bile duct of the liver of the cat *(Felis catus)* infested with *Chonorchis sinesis*. *J Path Bact* 87:239–244, 1964.

57. Peterson SL: Intrahepatic biliary cystadenoma in a cat. *Feline Pract* 14:29–32, 1984.

58. Feldman BF, Strafuss AC, Gabbert N: Bile duct carcinoma in the cat: Three case reports. *Feline Pract* 1:33–39, 1976.

59. Sechet B, Regnier A, Diquelou A, et al: Tumeur hépatique primaire chez un chat: Discussion a propos d'un cas de cholangiocarcinome. *Revue Méd Vét* 142:877–880, 1991.

60. Pastor J, Majo N, Arbona C, et al: Sclerosing adenocarcinoma of the extrahepatic bile duct in a cat. *Vet Rec* 140:367–368, 1997.

61. Chooi KF, Little PB: Immunoblastic lymphoma and cholangiocarcinoma in a cat. *Vet Rec* 120:578–579, 1987.

62. Pascal-Tenorio A, Olivry T, Gross TL, et al: Paraneoplastic alopecia associated with internal malignancies in the cat. *Vet Dermatol* 8:47–52, 1997.

63. Newell SM, Selcer BA, Girard E, et al: Correlations between ultrasonographic findings and specific hepatic diseases in cats: 72 cases (1985–1997). *JAVMA* 213:94–98, 1998.

64. Foley P, Miller L, Graham K, Bellamy J: Cholecystadenocarcinoma in a cat. *Can Vet J* 39:373–374, 1998.

65. Rehmtulla AJ: Occurrence of carcinoma of the bile ducts: A brief review. *Can Vet J* 15:289–292, 1974.

66. Minkus G, Hillemanns M: Botryoid-type embryonal rhabdomyosarcoma of liver in a young cat. *Vet Pathol* 34:618–621, 1997.

67. Lombard LS, Witte EJ: Frequency and types of tumors in mammals and birds of the Philadelphia Zoological Garden. *Cancer Res* 19:127–141, 1959.

68. Hubbard GB, Schmidt RE, Fletcher KC: Neoplasia in zoo animals. *J Zoo Anim Med* 14:33–40, 1983.

69. Kennedy GA, Strafuss AC: Multiple neoplasia in an aged cougar. *J Zoo Anim Med* 7:24–26, 1976.

70. McClure HM, Chang J, Golarz MN: Cholangiocarcinoma in a Margay *(Felis wiedii)*. *Vet Pathol* 14:510–512, 1977.

71. Banner BF, Alroy J, Kipnis RM: Acinar cell carcinoma of the pancreas in a cat. *Vet Pathol* 16:543–547, 1979.

72. Godfrey DR: A case of feline paraneoplastic alopecia with secondary *Malassezia*-associated dermatitis. *J Small Anim Pract* 39:394–396, 1998.

73. Brooks DG, Campbell KL, Dennis JS, Dunstan RW: Pancreatic paraneoplastic alopecia in three cats. *JAAHA* 30:557–563, 1994.

74. Kipperman BS, Nelson RW, Griffey SM, Feldman EC: Diabetes mellitus and exocrine pancreatic neoplasia in two cats with hyperadrenocortism. *JAAHA* 28:415–418, 1992.

75. Love NE, Jones C: What is your diagnosis? *JAVMA* 195:1285–1286, 1989.

76. Ditchfield J, Archibald J: Carcinoma of the pancreas in small animals. A report of two cases. *Small Anim Clin* 1:173–176, 1961.

77. Rowlatt U: Spontaneous epithelial tumours of the pancreas of mammals. *Br J Cancer* 21:82–107, 1967.

78. Tasker S, Griffon DJ, Nuttall TJ, Hill PB: Resolution of paraneoplastic alopecia following surgical removal of a pancreatic carcinoma in a cat. *J Small Anim Pract* 40:16–19, 1999.

79. McEwan NA: Nail disease in small animals. *Vet Dermatol Newsl* 11:18–19, 1987.

80. Rothwell TLW: Retractile mesenteritis in a cat. *Vet Rec* 130:492, 1992.

81. Kircher CH, Nielsen SW: Tumours of the pancreas. *Bull WHO* 53:195–202, 1992.

82. Swann HM, Sweet DC, Michel K: Complications associated with use of jejunostomy tubes in dogs and cats: 40 cases (1989–1994). *JAVMA* 210:1764–1767, 1997.

83. Van Der Riet FdStJ, McCully RM, Keen GA, Forder AA: Lymphosarcoma in a cat. *J South Afr Vet Assoc* 57–59, 1983.

84. Effron M, Griner L, Benirschke K: Nature and rate of neoplasia found in captive wild mammals, birds and reptiles at necropsy. *J Natl Cancer Inst* 59:185–198, 1977.

43

TUMORS OF THE URINARY TRACT

Antony S. Moore and Gregory K. Ogilvie

RENAL TUMORS[a]

RENAL TRANSITIONAL CELL CARCINOMA

Incidence, Signalment, and Etiology

There are 11 detailed reports of renal transitional cell carcinoma (TCC) in cats.[1,2] In one report, 7 cats were DSHs and 1 was Siamese.[2] Another group of 3 cats that was discussed in a combined report with bladder TCC included 1 Siamese.[1] The age range of these cats was 4 to 15 years (average, 9 years). There does not seem to be a gender predilection for this tumor in cats.

Clinical Presentation and History

Hematuria and abdominal enlargement appear to be rare findings, and cats may be diagnosed with metastatic lesions (one cat with muscle metastases was lame) while showing no urinary tract signs.[2] An enlarged kidney on routine physical examination may be the first sign of a tumor.[2] Nonspecific signs of lethargy, anorexia, and weight loss are seen most commonly.

Staging and Diagnosis

These tumors are infiltrative and readily invade the cap-

sule to involve perirenal tissue (Figure 43-1).[1,2] In two series of 11 cats, all developed metastases.[2,3] Metastatic sites in these two studies included the adrenals, omentum, ureter, other kidney, sublumbar lymph nodes, spleen, lung, pleura, tracheobronchial lymph nodes, heart, meninges, eye, and skeletal muscle.

Ultrasonography is more easily performed than a contrast

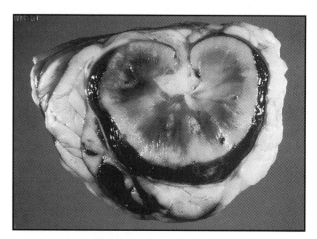

Figure 43-1: *Renal TCC in a 15-year-old spayed female DSH showing marked hemorrhage localized beneath the renal capsule.*

[a]Lymphoma commonly involves the kidneys but is covered separately in Chapter 36. All other renal tumors are included here.

renogram, allows examination of all renal parenchyma (Figure 43-2), and should be performed in addition to an MDB and urine culture and sensitivity testing.

Treatment

There are no reports of treatment for this highly aggressive tumor. Supportive therapy may be the only option. In this situation, ensure adequate hydration, possibly via fluid therapy. Appetite stimulants, antiemetics, and analgesics should be provided as needed.

RENAL CELL CARCINOMA

Incidence, Signalment, and Etiology

Signalment was reported for nine cats with renal carcinomas or adenocarcinomas.[2,4–6] All cats were DSHs and ranged in age from 4 to 17 years. Two cats were spayed females and one was a castrated male; information was unavailable for the others.

Clinical Presentation and History

In the three cats for which history was available, anorexia, weight loss, and lethargy predominated. Reports of azotemia are inconsistent. Two cats with bilateral primary or metastatic renal involvement were azotemic,[4,6] and hypertension had led to blindness 9 months previously in one of these animals.[4] Another cat with bilateral tumors was not azotemic,[5] and azotemia did not appear to be present in the other six cats with unilateral tumors.[2] In another study, however, azotemia was a clinical feature in eight cats with unilateral renal tumors,[3] and one cat was polycythemic.[3]

Staging and Diagnosis

In published reports of six cats with unilateral tumors, tumor size ranged from 1.5 to 6 cm (Figure 43-3).[2] Another cat had a unilateral renal carcinoma and a contralateral metastatic adrenal carcinoma.[4] Two other cats had bilateral

tumors that could have arisen de novo[6] or possibly spread by extension.[5] Metastases (to the pleura and renal fat) were noted in only one cat. In a series of 13 cats with renal carcinoma, 5 cats had metastases to the distant viscera but not the lymph nodes.[3] Metastases were most commonly to the lung, but the liver and adrenal gland were also affected.[3]

Ultrasonography provided a view of the contralateral kidney and enabled a guided percutaneous biopsy or fine-needle aspiration in two cats.[4,6] Ultrasonography and CT have been used to evaluate other renal disorders[7,8] and appear to be the imaging modalities of choice. In one study, ultrasonography disclosed renal lesions that had not been seen on radiographs in 6 of 24 cats.[9] Urine culture and sensitivity testing are indicated in addition to the MDB.

Treatment

The lower rate of metastases for renal cell carcinoma compared with TCC may mean that surgical excision of a unilateral renal cell carcinoma could prolong survival, but the prognosis is still guarded. One cat was alive after surgery for a low-grade carcinoma.[3] The tumor recurred 3 months after surgery in another cat with a high-grade carcinoma. Doxorubicin did not alter disease progression in this patient.[3]

Postoperative analgesics are essential. Fluid therapy may be necessary, along with antiemetics and other supportive care, if renal function is compromised.

> **KEY POINT**
>
> *Renal cell carcinoma may metastasize less frequently than renal TCC.*

NEPHROBLASTOMA

Incidence, Signalment, and Etiology

Five DSH cats have been reported with this tumor type. One male and two females were between 1 and 2 years of

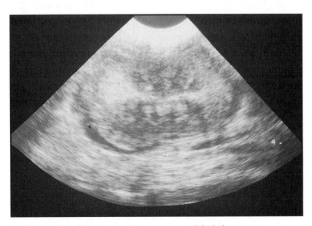

Figure 43-2: *Ultrasonographic appearance of the kidney prior to euthanasia of the cat in Figure 43-1.*

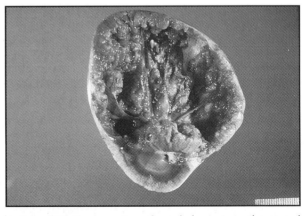

Figure 43-3: *Necropsy specimen of a renal adenocarcinoma that appeared cystic on ultrasonography.*

age,[2,10,11] and one affected cat was an 8-year-old castrated male.[12] The tumor in the older cat was bilateral and was identified as an embryonal sarcoma rather than a nephroblastoma. The fifth cat was also an adult.[3]

Clinical Presentation and History

Weight loss without anorexia was a common sign for all cats. Abdominal distension noted by owners or an easily palpable mass was also seen in all cats, and one cat had experienced 3 months of pain on urination.[2]

Staging and Diagnosis

Ultrasonography is the imaging modality of choice, although radiographs showing ventral, caudal, and unilateral displacement of intestinal loops would be highly suspicious for nephroblastoma in a young cat.[10] Metastases were not seen in four of the cats at the time of diagnosis; one cat, however, did have peritoneal metastases.[3] Complete staging as outlined for other renal tumors should be performed.

Treatment

Surgery is the treatment of choice provided the remaining kidney has adequate functional reserve. Two cats were treated by unilateral nephrectomy. One cat recovered well from surgery, and the implication was that it continued to "do well," although a time period was not stated.[2] The other cat had a thoracotomy to remove lung metastases 5 months after nephrectomy; another surgery was performed to remove both abdominal and thoracic metastases 3 months later, and a third finding of metastases led to euthanasia 1 year after the initial surgery.[11] Adjuvant chemotherapy has not been reported for cats with nephroblastoma, but doxorubicin, vincristine, and actinomycin-D are efficacious in canine and human patients.

RENAL ADENOMA

Renal adenoma may be a misnomer, as it is difficult to distinguish this lesion from an early or low-grade renal carcinoma. In one study, tumors originally diagnosed as renal adenoma were later reclassified as low-grade carcinomas in two cats.[3]

Incidence, Signalment, and Etiology

Four cats with renal adenoma have been reported. No signalment was provided for one.[3] Two were DSHs (a 10-year-old castrated male and a 15-year-old spayed female), and one was Persian.

Clinical Presentation and History

One cat was polycythemic, presumably due to unregulated erythropoietin production by the adenoma.[9] Another cat that had swollen limbs and was reluctant to rise had hypertrophic osteopathy, presumably due to the renal adenoma as thoracic radiographs were normal.[13] The periosteal changes affected all long bones and the ilea. A third cat was lethargic and had lost weight. It was not azotemic but had an 8 cm palpable abdominal mass.[14]

Staging and Diagnosis

An excretory urogram disclosed a lesion in the right renal pole of a cat with an adenoma.[13] Ultrasonography is equally effective in disclosing renal lesions and allows examination of other abdominal organs. Complete staging as outlined for other renal tumors should be performed.

Treatment

Surgery is the treatment of choice; however, the remaining kidney must have adequate functional reserve. Unilateral nephrectomy was performed in two cats. There was no follow-up reported for one cat.[9] The other cat did well for 7 months but was then found to be azotemic and to have a pulmonary adenocarcinoma.[14]

OTHER RENAL TUMORS

A renal squamous cell carcinoma in a DSH had metastasized to the perirenal fat, adjacent muscles, lumbar vertebrae, omentum, adrenals, sublumbar lymph nodes, diaphragm, and lung. Its behavior and histologic appearance were similar to TCCs.[2]

Poorly differentiated sarcomas (10 cm in diameter) were described in a 2-year-old and a 9-year-old DSH.[2] No metastases were seen in either cat. It is possible the tumor in the younger animal was a nephroblastoma. No treatment was reported.

A primary renal hemangiosarcoma that had not metastasized was seen in an adult cat.[3]

URINARY BLADDER TUMORS

C L I N I C A L   B R I E F I N G

Common Presentation	TCCs are the most common malignancy; SCC occurs less commonly. Leiomyoma is the most common benign tumor; leiomyosarcoma is also seen occasionally. Hematuria, pollakiuria, and stranguria occur with both malignant and benign tumors.

(continued)

Staging and Diagnosis	MDB, abdominal ultrasonography, and urine culture and sensitivity testing. Tumors are often apical rather than trigonal but are widely invasive. Iliac lymph nodes, regional extension, and rarely lungs are sites of metastasis for carcinomas. Metastasis appears to be rare for leiomyosarcomas.
Treatment Initial	Partial cystectomy for carcinoma usually fails owing to local recurrence and/or metastases. Surgery for leiomyoma or leiomyosarcoma may be curative.
Adjunctive	Chemotherapy with carboplatin or mitoxantrone could be considered for carcinoma.
Supportive	Antiinflammatories; antibiotics for concurrent urinary tract infection. Appetite stimulants and analgesia as needed.

TRANSITIONAL CELL CARCINOMA OF THE BLADDER

Incidence, Signalment, and Etiology

TCC is the most common bladder tumor in cats. Of 43 reported cases, 22 occurred in females (15 spayed) and 21 in males (16 castrated). Thirty-four were DSHs or DLHs, and 4 were Siamese.[1,2,15] Ages ranged from 4[16] to 20[1] years (mean age in one group of 23 cats, 13 years).[2]

Two castrated male cats with a bladder tumor (presumably TCC) underwent perineal urethrostomy prior to diagnosis of the tumor. It is uncertain whether inflammation due to obstruction or surgery may have induced the tumors.[17]

Clinical Presentation and History

The clinical signs of bladder cancer are indistinguishable from those seen with feline urologic syndrome (FUS) or urinary tract infection. Hematuria was a feature of all reported cases, and other signs of cystitis such as pollakiuria and stranguria were common.[2,15,16,18–22] One cat was constipated, but no reported signs were referable to the urinary tract.[23] Another cat presented with uroperitoneum due to bladder rupture at the site of an unresectable tumor.[24]

Other less specific signs such as straining and anorexia may occur, and some cats may have a palpable caudal abdominal mass. Tenesmus due to an extensive bladder TCC caused rectal prolapse in one cat.[25]

Staging and Diagnosis

The location of the tumor was not reported in all papers. In a series of 17 cats, 10 tumors were in the fundus, 4 in the dorsal wall, and 1 in the ventrolateral wall. Only 1 tumor in the trigone and 1 in the urethra were described.[2] Although there are other case reports of TCC occurring in the trigone and urethra,[16,18,23] these appear to be rare locations, in contrast to dogs with TCC. The bladder wall was mineralized in 2 cats with TCC.[21] Bladder tumors were concurrent with cystic calculi in 3 cats, although it is uncertain what type of tumor these cats had.

Staging for bladder tumors includes an MDB, abdominal imaging, urine culture and sensitivity testing, and bladder imaging via contrast radiography, ultrasonography, CT, or MRI. Endoscopy is rarely possible due to the small diameter of the urethra. Urinalysis rarely discloses cells with cytologic characteristics of malignancy[18,22]; in one survey, only 2 of 15 urine samples indicated a diagnosis of neoplasia.[21] Fine-needle aspiration using ultrasound guidance is a less invasive alternative to laparotomy[22] but is not always diagnostic.[26] Ultrasonography is the imaging modality of choice for bladder tumors as contrast cystography is difficult to perform without anesthesia for catheterization (Figure 43-4).

Metastases seem to be rare at the time of diagnosis; in two series of 31 cats with TCC, however, metastases to the iliac lymph nodes occurred in 9 cats and the tumor extended to involve the uterine stump and omentum in 2 cats. Metastases to the lung occurred in 2 cats that also had lymph node metastases.[2,21] Another cat with TCC also developed lung metastases.[15] Other sites of reported metastasis include the spleen, stomach, small intestine, diaphragm, skeletal muscle, and liver.[20,21] Metastases to the spleen were seen in a cat with TCC of the bladder or the kidney.[1] A

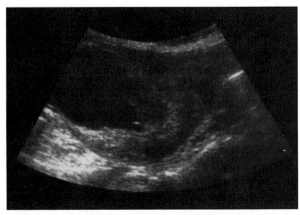

Figure 43-4: *Abdominal ultrasonography can be performed without anesthesia and allows visualization of other abdominal structures for potential metastases. This ultrasonogram of a 14-year-old cat shows a large concave mass filling the entire caudal portion of the bladder.*

KEY POINT

Wide surgical resection of leiomyoma in the urinary bladder may be curative.

A fibroma of the bladder apex in an 8-year-old spayed female Burmese was treated by partial cystectomy, and the cat had no evidence of disease 18 months later.[21] Similarly, an apical hemangioma in a 15-year-old castrated male was removed, and the cat died of cardiomyopathy 22 months later with no tumor recurrence.[21]

NONDOMESTIC FELIDAE

Two benign renal lesions reported in exotic Felidae appear to be incidental findings. A 23-year-old male jungle cat *(Felis chaus)* had a 7 mm renal adenoma, adenocarcinomas of the thyroid and stomach, and a Sertoli cell tumor.[37] A renal cystadenoma was found in an 18-year-old male tiger *(Panthera tigris)* that hemorrhaged to death from a retroperitoneal paraganglioma.[83] An infiltrative cell carcinoma of the bladder caused bladder rupture and death due to peritonitis in a middle-aged male fishing cat *(Felis viverrina).*[39]

REFERENCES

1. Wimberly HC, Lewis RM: Transitional cell carcinoma in the domestic cat. *Vet Pathol* 16:223–228, 1979.
2. Carpenter JL, Andrews LK, Holzworth J: Tumors and tumor-like lesions, in Holzworth J (ed): *Diseases of the Cat. Medicine and Surgery.* Philadelphia, WB Saunders, 1987, pp 407–596.
3. Henry CJ, Turnquist SE, Smith A, et al: Primary renal tumors in cats: 19 cases (1992–1998). *J Feline Med Surg* 1:165–170, 1999.
4. Carlson RA, Badertscher RR: Feline renal pseudocyst with metastatic carcinoma of the contralateral kidney. *Feline Pract* 21:23–27, 1993.
5. Britt JO, Ryan CP, Howard EB: Sarcomatoid renal adenosarcoma in a cat. *Vet Pathol* 22:514–515, 1985.
6. Steinberg H, Thomson J: Bilateral renal carcinoma in a cat. *Vet Pathol* 31:704–705, 1994.
7. Biller DS, Bradley GA, Partington BP: Renal medullary rim sign: Ultrasonographic evidence of renal disease. *Vet Radiol Ultrasound* 33:286–290, 1992.
8. Yamazoe K, Ohashi F, Kadosawa T, et al: Computed tomography on renal masses in dogs and cats. *J Vet Med Sci* 56:813–816, 1994.
9. Walter PA, Johnston GR, Feeney DA, O'Brien TD: Applications of ultrasonography in the diagnosis of parenchymal kidney disease in cats: 24 cases (1981–1986). *JAVMA* 192:92–98, 1988.
10. Moon ML, Davenport DJ: What is your diagnosis? *JAVMA* 191:1491–1492, 1987.
11. Potkay S, Garman R: Nephroblastoma in a cat: The effects of nephrectomy and occlusion of the caudal vena cava. *J Small Anim Pract* 10:345–369, 1969.
12. Fitts RH: Bilateral feline embryonal sarcoma. *JAVMA* 136:616, 1960.
13. Nafe LA, Herron AJ, Burk RL: Hypertrophic osteopathy in a cat associated with renal papillary adenoma. *JAAHA* 17:659–662, 1981.
14. Clark WR, Wilson RB: Renal adenoma in a cat. *JAVMA* 193:1557–1559, 1988.
15. Kohno T, Matsuda H: Transitional-cell carcinoma of the urinary bladder in a cat. *Mod Vet Pract* 68:286–287, 1987.
16. Anderson WI: Transitional cell carcinoma encasing the distal ureter in a cat. *Mod Vet Pract* 67:824, 1986.
17. Buffington CAT, Chew DJ, Kendall MS, et al: Clinical evaluation of cats with nonobstructive urinary tract diseases. *JAVMA* 210:46–50, 1997.
18. Barrett RE, Nobel TA: Transitional cell carcinoma of the urethra in a cat. *Cornell Vet* 66:14–26, 1976.
19. Brearley MJ, Thatcher C, Cooper JE: Three cases of transitional cell carcinoma in the cat and a review of the literature. *Vet Rec* 118:91–94, 1986.
20. Dill Jr GS, McElyea Jr U, Stookey JL: Transitional cell carcinoma of the urinary bladder in a cat. *JAVMA* 160:743–745, 1972.
21. Schwarz PD, Greene RW, Patnaik AK: Urinary bladder tumors in the cat: A review of 27 cases. *JAAHA* 21:237–245, 1985.
22. Walker DB, Cowell RL, Clinkenbeard KD, Turgai J: Carcinoma in the urinary bladder of a cat: Cytologic findings and a review of the literature. *Vet Clin Pathol* 22:103–108, 1993.
23. Arnal C, Badiola JJ, García de Jalón JA, Juste R: Carcinoma de células de transición de la uretra en un gato. *Med Vet* 2:239–243, 1985.
24. Aumann M, Worth LT, Drobatz KJ: Uroperitoneum in cats: 26 cases (1986–1995). *JAAHA* 34:315–324, 1998.
25. Barrand KR: Rectal prolapse associated with urinary bladder neoplasia in a cat. *J Small Anim Pract* 40:222–223, 1999.
26. Sellon RK, Rottman JB, Jordan HL: Hypereosinophilia associated with transitional cell carcinoma in a cat. *JAVMA* 201:591–593, 1992.
27. Guptill L, Scott-Moncrieff CR, Janovitz EB: Response to high-dose radioactive iodine administration in cats with thyroid carcinoma that had previously undergone surgery. *JAVMA* 8:1055–1058, 1995.
28. Magunna C, Spellmeyer O, Hund M, Nickel R: Augmentation der harnblase nach radikaler resektion: erste klinische erfahrungen mit einem lyophilisierten xenoimplantat aus der Dünndarmsubmukosa des Schweins bei Hund und Katze. *Kleinterpraxis* 44:809–821, 1999.
29. Ogilvie GK, Moore AS, Obradovich JE, et al: Toxicoses and efficacy associated with the administration of mitoxantrone to cats with malignant tumors. *JAVMA* 202:1839–1844, 1993.
30. Dorn AS, Harris SG, Olmstead ML: Squamous cell carcinoma of the urinary bladder in a cat. *Feline Pract* 8:14–17, 1978.
31. Burk RL, Meierhenry EF, Schaubhut Jr CW: Leiomyosarcoma of the urinary bladder in a cat. *JAVMA* 167:749–751, 1975.
32. Sent U, Pothmann M, von Bomhard D: Felines urologisches syndrom: Hervorgerufen durch ein leiomyosarkom der harnblase. *Kleintierpraxis* 42:663–668, 1997.
33. Speakman CF, Pechman RD, D'Andrea GH: Aortic thrombosis and unilateral hydronephrosis associated with leiomyosarcoma in a cat. *JAVMA* 182:62–63, 1983.
34. Swalec KM, Smeak DD, Baker AL: Urethral leiomyoma in a cat. *JAVMA* 195:961–1119, 1989.
35. Patnaik AK, Greene RW: Intravenous leiomyoma of the bladder in a cat. *JAVMA* 175:381–383, 1979.
36. Patnaik AK, Schwarz PD, Greene RW: A histopathologic study of twenty urinary bladder neoplasms in the cat. *J Small Anim Pract* 27:433–435, 1986.
37. Sagartz JW, Garner FM, Sauer RM: Multiple neoplasia in a captive jungle cat *(Felis chaus)*–Thyroid adenocarcinoma, gastric adenocarcinoma, renal adenoma, and Sertoli cell tumor. *J Wildl Dis* 8:375–380, 1972.
38. Hruban Z, Carter WE, Meehan T, et al: Retroperitoneal paraganglioma in a tiger *(Panthera tigris).* *J Zoo Anim Med* 19:231–234, 1988.
39. Rewell RE, Willis RA: Some tumours of wild animals. *J Pathol Bacteriol* 62:450–452, 1950.

MANAGEMENT OF SPECIFIC DISEASES

ENDOCRINE TUMORS

44

Antony S. Moore and Gregory K. Ogilvie

THYROID TUMORS

THYROID ADENOMA

	CLINICAL BRIEFING
Common Presentation	Thyroid adenomas are hyperfunctional. Common in older DSH cats; Siamese and Himalayan cats are at low risk. Factors that increase risk include feeding canned food as a majority of the diet and living indoors. Clinical signs relate to increased metabolic rate, such as weight loss with normal to increased appetite. Hypertrophic cardiomyopathy is common. Thyroid nodule is often palpable in the neck.
Staging and Diagnosis	Serum T_4 level is the most useful component of the MDB. Thyroid scintigraphy will help rule out a functional carcinoma. Complete cardiac evaluation (thoracic radiographs, echocardiogram, and ECG) is necessary. Stabilize cardiac disease and assess renal function before surgery or ^{131}I treatment.
Treatment	
Medical	Methimazole, carbimazole, or ipodate associated with high rate of control. Intrathyroid injection of 95% ethanol investigational only for unilateral disease.
Surgical	Staged modified extracapsular thyroidectomy. Bilateral disease is common; temporary postoperative hypocalcemia due to parathyroid damage mandates monitoring serum calcium; supplementation may be necessary.
Radiation	IV, SQ, or PO administration of ^{131}I is very effective, specific, and the treatment of choice if available.
Supportive	Stabilize cardiac disease medically (could include short-term medical management of hyperthyroidism) prior to definitive treatment. Treatment of hyperthyroidism will worsen concurrent renal disease; consider methimazole trial. Provide adequate nutrition to increase weight.

Incidence, Signalment, and Etiology

Reports of histologic thyroid atypia occurring without vascular or capsular invasion were made prior to 1980.[1-4] These cats were diagnosed with adenomas that were occasionally bilateral[3] and rarely associated with signs of hyperthyroidism.[1,4] One study noted an increased incidence of functional tumors in the late 1970s.[1] In the past two decades, the incidence of hyperthyroidism due to thyroid adenomas has increased in many developed countries[5] except Japan.[6] There is unlikely to be a single etiologic reason for this increase.

The median age of 524 hyperthyroid cats was 13 years (range, 6 to 20 years); 300 were female. All but 15 cats were neutered.[7] Most cats (456 [87%]) were DSHs or DLHs. There were 20 Siamese, 10 Burmese, 10 Maine Coon, 9 Persian, 8 American Shorthaired, 3 Himalayan, 3 Manx, 3 Russian Blue, 1 Balinese, and 1 Tonkinese.

The etiology of hyperthyroidism remains obscure. It does not appear to be an immune-mediated disease (as it is in Grave's disease in humans),[8] although thyroid autoantibodies were detected in some affected cats.[9] The pathologic change in thyroid tissue truly appears to be neoplastic, and one study showed consistent overexpression of the *c-ras* oncogene in thyroid adenomas.[10] It is unclear, however, why these tumors rarely, if ever, progress to carcinoma.

Two studies have examined risk factors for hyperthyroidism in cats.[11,12] Himalayans[12] and Siamese[11,12] were found to be at decreased risk of developing hyperthyroidism, which is consistent with breed descriptions in large series of hyperthyroid cats.[7] Relatives of hyperthyroid cats were more likely to be hyperthyroid,[12] as were cats that lived in the same household.[11] Cats that ate more than 50% of their diet as canned cat food had an increased risk,[11,12] as did cats that used kitty litter.[12] Being an indoor cat also appeared to increase risk.[11] Neutering, number of cats in the household, use of dietary supplements, medications, or vaccination frequency did not affect the risk. Factors that increased risk but were not independent of those listed above included high levels of smoking by owners and the use of flea control products. Although use of flea products was found to increase risk in one study,[11] the other study indicated that this risk was not related to frequency of usage (or "dosage"). Supplementing the diet with beef or poultry decreased the risk of disease, but again this was not an independent factor.[11] Viral causes appear unlikely, and one study found no association between FIV infection and hyperthyroidism.[13]

Clinical Presentation and History

Classically, signs of an increased metabolic rate (due to elevated levels of circulating thyroid hormones) predominate. The majority of affected cats show weight loss despite a normal to increased appetite. Less frequently, increases in activity, defecation frequency, and/or vocalization, vomiting, or a poor hair coat may prompt owners to seek veterinary advice. Other reported signs include panting, nervousness, heat intolerance, diarrhea, and hair loss.[14]

Neuromuscular signs may be due to thyroid hormone binding to muscle receptor sites, thereby increasing skeletal muscle heat production and mitochondrial oxygen consumption, which in turn leads to muscle fatigue.[15] Cats with hyperthyroidism may therefore show generalized weakness, fatigue, muscle atrophy, breathlessness, or collapse. More specific signs include ataxia, incoordination, poor jumping, and even marked ventroflexion of the neck.

Thyroid hormones also cause an increase in cerebral blood flow and oxygen and glucose consumption. Hyperactivity may be a result of increased adrenergic activity and synergistic interaction with catecholamines. Increases also occur in levels of serotonin and substance P and in dopaminergic activity. Clinically, these changes are perceived as restlessness, irritability, hyperexcitability, hyperresponsiveness to stimuli, and even aggression. In addition, insomnia, aimless wandering, pacing, circling, apathy, lethargy, or depression may occur. More specific signs such as motor seizures appear to be rare[15] and may be due to thyroid hormones causing a decrease in the seizure threshold in the CNS. Acute focal neurologic deficits may be due to cerebrovascular accident rather than the direct action of thyroid hormones. Stupor due to "thyroid storm" appears to be very rare in cats.[15]

A palpable thyroid nodule is usually present in hyperthyroid cats and can best be felt when the cat's chin is elevated and the thumb and forefinger are gently run down the trachea. A small thyroid nodule will be felt as a "blip" as it slips beneath the moving digits. Bilateral involvement is common, and it is important to remember that an apparently normal-sized lobe (even at surgery) may be affected (Figure 44-1).[16] Most tumors are small but can exceed 1 cm in diameter.[17] A thyroid adenoma may occasionally be cystic and become very large, causing dyspnea as a result of displacement of the trachea and/or laryngeal hemiplegia due to damage to the recurrent laryngeal nerve.[18]

Increased food intake elevates fat excretion in hyperthyroid cats. This elevation may be up to 15 times normal and appears to correlate with T_4 level.[19]

Hyperthyroidism appears to be causing less severe disease in recent years. Studies comparing populations of cats diagnosed in the 1980s with cats diagnosed in the 1990s show that the percentage of cats exhibiting clinical signs is decreasing (Table 44-1). There was no change in the average age at which cats were diagnosed with hyperthyroidism and no difference in the percentage of cats with elevated T_4 levels. Cats diagnosed in the 1990s were less likely to have elevated ALT and T_3 serum levels. The difference was probably related to earlier testing for hyperthyroidism as a result of increased awareness about the disorder rather than an essential change in the disease itself.[5]

Cardiac muscle hypertrophy is a common consequence of prolonged hyperthyroidism. The most common clinical finding is tachycardia ($\geq$240 bpm), which appears to correlate directly with thyroid hormone levels.[20] Dysrhythmias and changes in the ECG are less common. Physically, the effect of hyperthyroidism on the heart results in increased thickness of the ventricular septum as well as both the left

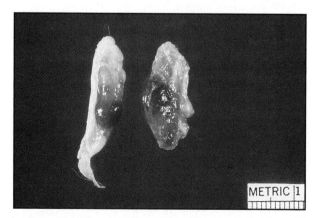

Figure 44-1: *Thyroid adenomas are often bilateral, as in this 16-year-old cat. A tumor may be present even in a gland that appears normal externally.*

TABLE 44-1
Comparison of 131 Hyperthyroid Cats Diagnosed Between 1979 and 1982 with 202 Cats Diagnosed Between 1992 and 1993[5]

Clinical Sign	Percent Affected 1979–1982	Percent Affected 1992–1993
Weight loss	98	87
Polyphagia	81	49
Hyperactivity	76	31
Polyuria/ Polydipsia	60	36
Diarrhea	33	15
Muscle weakness	25	12
Panting	25	9
Increased fecal volume	31	8
Anorexia	25	7

MDB = minimum database; includes CBC, biochemical profile, urinalysis, FeLV/FIV serology, T_4 testing, and thoracic radiographs (three views).

and right ventricular free walls.[21] Cardiomyopathy may lead to congestive heart failure and dyspnea[1,4] and may cause a secondary pleural pseudochylous effusion.[22]

Cardiac disease in cats with hyperthyroidism appears to be less severe in the 1990s than the 1980s.[23] There has been a decrease in the percent of cats with sinus tachycardia (66% to 34%) and ECG changes (29% to 8%). In addition, the incidence of congestive heart failure dropped from 20% to 8% over these two decades. However, there was no difference in cardiomegaly between the two populations, again implying that improved veterinary awareness has lead to earlier diagnosis of cats with less severe clinical signs.[23]

KEY POINT

Hypertrophic cardiomyopathy is a common sequela to hyperthyroidism.

Staging and Diagnosis

Measurement of serum T_4 levels provides the highest probability of confirming hyperthyroidism in cats. Measurement of serum T_3 is less useful. In a study from the 1980s, serum levels of T_4 and T_3 ranged from 4 to 54.1 µg/dl and 54 to 1,000 ng/dl, respectively.[19] In a comparison of cats diagnosed in the 1980s with those diagnosed in the 1990s, elevations in T_3 were seen in 97% and 71% of affected cats, respectively, showing a significant decrease in the reliability of this test,[5] probably as a result of earlier diagnosis of the disease. In the same study, the percentage of cats with elevated T_4 decreased from 100% in 1983 to 98% in 1993. Serum T_4 determination is still the best screening test available, but it should be remembered that T_4 levels fluctuate by up to 50% throughout the day.[24,25] In one study, the highest levels of feline T_4 were found at 9:00 AM,[25] and the stress of venipuncture did not affect levels. For cats with advanced hyperthyroidism, the fluctuation in thyroid hormones is insufficient to drop levels into the normal range; a cat with mild or early hyperthyroidism, however, may have a normal serum T_4 at the time of sample collection. Serum T_4 was normal, sometimes on more than one occasion, in 26 cats with thyroid adenoma; the majority of these animals also had clinical signs of hyperthyroidism.[26] Thus hyperthyroidism should not be excluded on the basis of a single normal T_4 result.

A further confounding factor in measuring serum T_4 and T_3 is the influence of other nonthyroid illness on these hormones. Several diseases, including diabetes mellitus (DM), renal failure, and inflammatory bowel disease, may cause low serum T_4 levels.[27] The implication is that concurrent illness may decrease serum T_4 levels into the normal range in hyperthyroid cats. Clinicians should carefully evaluate all test results in cats with suspected hyperthyroidism.

If hyperthyroidism is suspected but serum T_4 is normal, the first step is to repeat the T_4 measurement on a different day (rather than at a different time on the same day).[28] If the second T_4 level is normal, free T_4 and free T_3 levels should be measured. In theory, these levels reflect the hormone available for entry into cells and thus are not as affected by other nonthyroid diseases; in practice, however, free T_4 and T_3 may have little advantage over total T_4 and T_3.

If free T_3 and T_4 levels are normal, a T_3 suppression test is performed. The rationale for this test is that administration of T_3 will cause a feedback suppression of thyroid-stimulating hormone (TSH), which will lead to a rapid decrease in T_4. If the cat is hyperthyroid, TSH is already suppressed and T_4 levels will not change. Oral T_3 (liothyronine, 25 µg) is given three times/day for seven treatments, and serum for T_3 and T_4 testing is collected 4 hours after the last dose is administered.[29,30] A comparison is made to pretesting basal levels (posttesting T_3 should be high if the owner has administered the medication and T_4 will be markedly decreased in a normal, nonhyperthyroid cat).

If a definitive diagnosis still cannot be made, a TSH response test may be performed. Serum T_4 is measured before and 4 hours after IV administration of TSH (1.0 µg/kg).[31] If the cat is normal, T_4 should be increased by more than twofold. Hyperthyroid cats are less responsive to TSH, and a subnormal response is suggestive of the disease.

A thyrotropin-releasing hormone (TRH) response test may also be performed. This test involves the administration of 0.02 mg/kg TRH, which should increase TSH levels in normal cats but not hyperthyroid cats. Because there is no validated assay for measurement of TSH in cats, serum T_4 is measured 4 hours after TRH administration; the increase in T_4 will be less than twofold in hyperthyroid cats.[28] TRH administration is often associated with vomiting and hypersalivation, and the validity of this test for identifying hyperthyroidism in critically ill cats has been questioned.[32]

A complete cardiac evaluation is warranted in cats with hyperthyroidism prior to definitive treatment for the disease. In addition to careful cardiac auscultation, an ECG, thoracic radiographs, blood pressure measurement, and cardiac ultrasonography are indicated. Thoracic radiographs may show cardiomegaly but should be examined for other signs of congestive heart failure or pleural effusion.[22,23] An ECG may confirm a suspected dysrhythmia or disclose one in a cat with tachycardia that is difficult to auscultate. The most common abnormality is an increased amplitude in the R wave.[21,23,34] Atrial or ventricular premature contractions and atrioventricular block have been noted less frequently.[21] More than half of the cats have more than one abnormality on an ECG.[34]

Echocardiography is the most reliable indicator of cardiac function. The most common abnormalities, occurring in approximately 70% of hyperthyroid cats, are an increase in left ventricular caudal wall thickness and left atrial diameter.[21,33] Most significantly, the left ventricular end diastolic diameter is greater than in normal cats, indicating ventricular dilation. Cardiac contractility improves with treatment within an average of 10 months in the majority of cats; some cats do not improve, however, which may indicate permanent structural damage.[35]

KEY POINT

Renal disease may worsen when hyperthyroidism is treated. A therapeutic trial of medical management should be used in cats with mild renal disease.

Blood pressure measurements using an indirect Doppler-shift ultrasonic sphygmomanometer on the proximal hock showed an increase in either systolic or diastolic pressures in 87% of hyperthyroid cats; both were elevated in 50% of affected cats.[36] Blood pressure changes did not correlate with T_4 levels. In this study, normal systolic and diastolic pressures were 108 to 130 and 70 to 95 mmHg, respectively.[36] There was no evidence of retinal detachment in affected cats, although elevated blood pressure should be treated to prevent this possible sequela.

A serum biochemical profile may disclose evidence of other diseases, but the most common abnormalities are in the levels of "liver enzymes." Increases in ALP, AST, and ALT may best be explained by altered hepatic blood flow as a consequence of cardiac disease. In a comparison of hyperthyroid cats diagnosed in the 1980s and 1990s, elevations in serum ALT levels were less common in the 1990s,[5] paralleling the decreased severity of cardiac disease.[23]

Elevations in serum creatinine indicate renal disease and are not secondary to hyperthyroidism.[37] In fact, increased renal perfusion may mask renal disease by decreasing serum creatinine.[38] This is important when treatment is contemplated, as seemingly mild azotemia may progress rapidly following control of hyperthyroidism. Even cats with normal serum creatinine prior to treatment for hyperthyroidism may become azotemic after treatment. In one study, only 9 of 58 hyperthyroid cats had an elevated serum creatinine prior to treatment. This rose to 22 cats after 1 month and to 30 cats after 3 months of treatment.[38] For cats suspected to have subclinical or mild renal disease, treatment with methimazole prior to definitive surgery or ^{131}I therapy may help identify at-risk cats. Medical management to achieve a balance between hyperthyroidism and renal disease may be the best option for cats that become azotemic after treatment with methimazole.

Prior to surgery, it is important to identify the location of the thyroid adenoma, particularly if it cannot be palpated. It is likewise crucial to know whether one or both thyroids are hyperfunctional. The dose of ^{131}I is often based on the size of affected gland(s). Ultrasonography of the neck may be used to detect and measure a thyroid adenoma but is not as sensitive as pertechnetate ($^{99m}TcO_4^-$) nuclear scintigraphy imaging.[39]

$^{99m}TcO_4^-$ is used to obtain nuclear functional images of thyroid adenomas (Figure 44-2). It is particularly useful in identifying nonpalpable ectopic tumors, such as those in the thoracic inlet.[40] $^{99m}TcO_4^-$ (20–45 megabecquerels [MBq], or 0.5–1.2 mCi, per cat) is given 20 minutes prior to nuclear scanning.[41,42] In a series of 135 cats, 38 had unilateral disease (7 with nonpalpable tumors) and 97 had bilateral disease (9 with nonpalpable tumors).[41] All 16 cats with nonpalpable adenomas had intrathoracic tissue that was disclosed by $^{99m}TcO_4^-$ imaging. In the United Kingdom, bilateral disease (based on $^{99m}TcO_4^-$ scans) occurs in 65% of hyperthyroid cats.[42] Radioiodine tracer (^{123}I or ^{131}I) has been given orally, but the quality of images is inferior to those obtained with $^{99m}TcO_4^-$.[14,41] The half-life of $^{99m}TcO_4^-$ is 6 hours (compared with 4 hours for ^{123}I and 24 hours for ^{131}I), and its uptake is not affected by concurrent antithyroid medications.

$^{99m}TcO_4^-$ scans do have limitations. In a series of 28 cats treated surgically for hyperthyroidism, $^{99m}TcO_4^-$ scans cor-

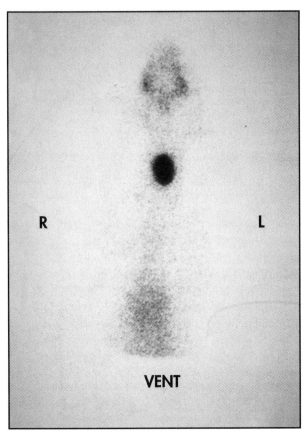

Figure 44-2: A $^{99m}TcO_4^-$ scan may demonstrate unilateral hypertrophy because the contralateral thyroid has become hypoplastic under influence of circulating thyroid hormones. (Courtesy of A. Tidwell)

rectly identified the number and site of 18 tumors.[43] In 7 cats the scan indicated unilateral disease that was bilateral at surgery, and in 3 cats the wrong side was identified. Nuclear scans may be limited in their ability to accurately diagnose small functional adenomas, since measurements are taken as an average over time, making it difficult to differentiate a normal gland from early adenoma. A normal thyroid gland should atrophy when an adenoma is present in the contralateral gland due to feedback on TSH; therefore any $^{99m}TcO_4^-$ uptake in the "normal" side should be considered as evidence for bilateral adenomas.

Treatment

Multiple treatment options are available for cats with functional thyroid adenoma. The choice of which to use may depend on availability, owner resources, or the coexistence of other nonthyroid illness, particularly renal disease.[38] Treatment of hyperthyroidism may worsen subclinical or low-grade renal disease, and a therapeutic trial of medical management for 1 month followed by a repeat serum biochemical profile is recommended for cats with suspected renal disease prior to undertaking more definitive surgery or radioiodine treatment.

Medical Management (Figure 44-3)

The most common medical treatment for hyperthyroidism in the early 1980s was propylthiouracil (PTU), which inhibits both organification of iodine and conversion of T_4 into the more metabolically active T_3. PTU has poor bioavailability in cats[44] and is associated with a high risk of side effects. At a dose of 50 mg every 8 hours (reduced to every 12 hours for maintenance), vomiting and inappetence were common, occurring in up to 30% of cats.[1,45] Response was rapid, and T_4 was in the normal range in all cats within 3 weeks.[45] Further clinical use of the drug disclosed a nearly 10% rate of serious immune-related drug reactions occurring an average of 25 days after starting PTU therapy. Affected cats were all severely anemic and thrombocytopenic (but not granulocytopenic) and had a positive direct antiglobulin test (DAT, Coombs' test) and often a positive antinuclear antibody (ANA) test.[46] Clinically, all cats were lethargic or weak and many experienced bleeding or bruising. Cats treated with blood transfusions and immunosuppressive drugs (prednisone ± cyclophosphamide) recovered within 2 weeks after PTU was discontinued.

When PTU was given to normal cats, more than half (9 of 17) developed immune-mediated disease.[20,47] A positive ANA or DAT was seen an average of 4.5 weeks after starting the drug; clinical signs developed about 2 weeks later. Clinical signs resolved within 2 weeks and ANA returned to normal within 4 weeks, but readministration of PTU led to more rapid onset of signs. A similar drug without the sulfur atom (i.e., propyluracil) did not cause these signs.

Methimazole is the most commonly used drug for medical management of hyperthyroidism in the United States. It is highly bioavailable, and oral administration of a 5 mg dose leads to a peak plasma level within hours. Hyperthyroid cats appear to metabolize methimazole more rapidly than normal cats, but the frequency of dosing makes this clinically insignificant.[44] Cessation of drug administration leads to elevations in serum T_4 within 48 hours.[48] Methimazole and the related drug carbimazole act to inhibit organification of iodine in the thyroid. In a clinical study of 262 cats treated with methimazole either preoperatively (n = 181) or as sole treatment (n = 81), the most common dose was 10 to 15 mg divided into two or three daily doses.[48] Dose adjustments were made in 2.5 or 5 mg increments (half or whole tablet, respectively). The average course of therapy in cats that received methimazole preoperatively was 21 days, and the daily dose ranged from 10 to 20 mg (median, 15 mg). Cats treated solely with methimazole received it for up to 3 years. Daily doses ranged from 5 to 20 mg (median, 10 mg), except in one cat in which hyperthyroidism was controlled with a daily dose of 2.5 mg.[48]

After 3 weeks of methimazole treatment, serum T_4 was normal in 52% of cats and low in 35%. Daily methimazole doses were increased in the remaining 33 cats to either 15

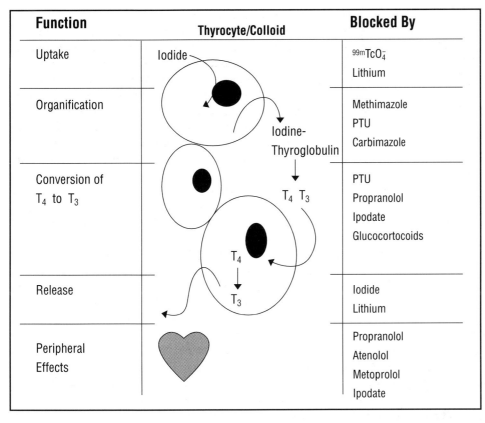

Function	Thyrocyte/Colloid	Blocked By
Uptake	Iodide	$^{99m}TcO_4^-$ Lithium
Organification	Iodine-Thyroglobulin	Methimazole PTU Carbimazole
Conversion of T_4 to T_3	T_4 T_3	PTU Propranolol Ipodate Glucocortocoids
Release	T_4 T_3	Iodide Lithium
Peripheral Effects		Propranolol Atenolol Metoprolol Ipodate

Figure 44-3: *This schematic diagram shows the mechanism of action of different drugs used to treat hyperthyroidism due to adenomatous hyperplasia. Drugs may act at different levels of uptake, organification, and release of thyroid hormones, and some drugs act to interfere with their peripheral effects.*

mg (25 cats) or 20 mg (8 cats), which resulted in normal to low serum T_4 in 31 of these cats after an additional 3 weeks of treatment. The remaining 2 cats were refractory to treatment. Those cats with low serum T_4 after methimazole treatment had a normal serum T_3 and did not show clinical signs of hypothyroidism.

Side effects of methimazole treatment, most commonly anorexia, vomiting, or lethargy, were seen in 48 cats (18.3%) and occurred within 2 to 3 weeks of starting treatment. These signs resolved in most cats despite continued methimazole treatment.

Hematologic changes were often mild (leukopenia, eosinophilia, lymphocytosis), were not associated with clinical disease, and resolved despite continued treatment. More severe changes of thrombocytopenia were seen in about 3% of cats and agranulocytosis in 1.5% of cats. These presumably immune-mediated signs resolved within a week of drug cessation. A positive DAT was seen in only 2% of cats. A positive ANA was more likely to be seen after prolonged (>6 months) methimazole administration. There were no clinical effects of a positive ANA test and none of the cats with positive DAT became anemic, so the significance of these findings is difficult to determine.

Hepatopathy was rare (1.5% of cats) and associated with serum liver enzyme elevations, icterus, vomiting, and anorexia. Histologic changes included hepatic degeneration and necrosis but resolved within 1 to 7 weeks after cessation

of methimazole treatment. When methimazole is used presurgically, there does not appear to be any effect on coagulation parameters.[49]

Carbimazole, which metabolizes to methimazole,[50] is the most commonly used drug in the United Kingdom and Europe for medical control of hyperthyroidism. One advantage of carbimazole is that it is tasteless, while methimazole has a bitter flavor.

Carbimazole was administered to 45 cats either preoperatively or as sole treatment for hyperthyroidism.[50] Dosages were similar to those described for methimazole. Preoperatively, all cats received 15 mg/day given at 12 or 8 hour dosing intervals. Serum T_4 was normal within 2 weeks of starting treatment in 31 of 34 cats dosed on an 8 hour schedule but was normal in only 1 of 5 cats treated at 12 hour intervals. This emphasizes the importance of an 8 hour dosing schedule at least initially; cats treated long-term with carbimazole were able to be maintained on a 12 hour treatment schedule. Of the appropriately treated cats, 2 initially responded then appeared resistant and 1 never responded; inadequate dosing was due to vomiting in 1 cat and poor owner compliance in another. The most common side effect was vomiting (5 cats), which was accompanied by anorexia in 3 cats. Vomiting resolved in some cats despite continued treatment. A mild transient leukopenia and lymphocytosis was seen in some cats.[50]

Long-term maintenance of cats on methimazole and carbimazole requires dose adjustments as the disease progresses. Periodic thyroid hormone level checks are required to fine-tune the dose to maintain euthyroidism.

Calcium ipodate inhibits 5'-deiodinase, thus blocking the conversion of T_4 to T_3; it also decreases release of thyroid hormones and their peripheral effects. Twelve cats were treated with ipodate that had been reformulated as 50 mg capsules.[51] Ten of these cats had been treated with methimazole, which had been discontinued due to vomiting, anorexia, self-excoriation, or thrombocytopenia. Seven cats responded to an initial ipodate dose of 50 mg every 12 hours; one additional cat responded 2 weeks after the dose was increased to 150 mg/day. As would be predicted, serum T_4 levels did not decrease but serum T_3 decreased in all cats. The two cats that did not respond had the highest T_3 levels, implying that cats with more severe hyperthyroidism are less likely to respond. Recurrence of signs was seen within 4 months in two cats; other cats had longer control. Ipodate may be a good choice for cats that cannot tolerate methimazole or carbimazole and are not good candidates for other therapies.

Percutaneous injection of 95% ethanol into the affected thyroid gland has been recently used in cats refractory to other forms of treatment.[52–54] This technique is best performed using ultrasonographic guidance and a 27 ga needle in an anesthetized cat.[53] Use of a larger needle may increase the risk of laceration of the recurrent laryngeal nerve.[52] It is recommended to treat only cats with unilateral disease as determined by $^{99m}TcO_4^-$ scans, as one cat died after both lobes were treated and control of bilateral disease was inferior to other treatment methods.[53] Reduction in thyroid size[52] and normalization of T_4 levels within 72 hours[53] have been reported, and resultant euthyroidism appears to be long-lasting.[52,54] Side effects of dysphonia, Horner's syndrome, and gagging appear to be transient, typically resolving within 8 weeks.[53,54]

Management of Peripheral Effects

Critically ill patients may require supportive therapeutic measures in addition to definitive treatment for thyroid hyperplasia. Patients should be stabilized prior to definitive therapy. If cardiac manifestations, such as significant hypertrophy of the myocardium or supraventricular tachycardia, are clinically apparent, a β-adrenergic antagonist (propranolol, atenolol, metoprolol) or diltiazem may stabilize tachyarrhythmias and improve cardiac performance. Furosemide and other drugs may be indicated for cats in overt cardiac failure. Treatment of cats with concurrent cardiovascular abnormalities with PTU, digoxin, and furosemide may result in rapid clinical improvement within 1 month.[55]

Seizures rarely occur due to hyperthyroidism. If they do, propranolol and methimazole have been suggested to be better than phenobarbital.[15]

Surgical Management

Surgical excision of the affected gland(s) is the most common definitive treatment for hyperthyroidism in cats; because of the high rate of bilateral disease, most authors recommend bilateral thyroidectomy. Ideally, medical management of hyperthyroidism and stabilization of existing cardiac disease should be undertaken prior to surgery. Surgery may not be indicated if renal insufficiency, previously "masked" by the hyperthyroidism, is discovered.

In one study, six of eight cats that died during surgery had not been "conditioned" with antithyroid medication prior to surgery.[56] A presurgical conditioning protocol using propranolol, a β-adrenergic antagonist, for 20 days with the addition of potassium iodate for the last 10 days was proposed for cats that could not tolerate methimazole or carbimazole.[57] Prorpanolol was given at 2.5 mg/cat every 8 hours. If the heart rate was over 200 bpm after 4 days of treatment, the dose was increased to 5.0 mg every 8 hours; if the heart rate was still over 200 bpm after 7 days, the dose was increased to 7.5 mg every 8 hours. After 10 days, potassium iodate was started at a dose of 21.25 mg every 8 hours. Higher doses of potassium iodate (42.5 mg) were associated with anorexia, vomiting, and depression.

KEY POINT

Hypocalcemia may occur due to removal of parathyroid glands when bilateral thyroidectomy is performed. Serum calcium levels should be monitored after surgery.

Intracapsular removal of the thyroid gland was initially favored to preserve the parathyroid gland (which is closely adhered to the thyroid capsule) and thus reduce the likelihood of postoperative hypocalcemia. In one study, however, 8 of 53 cats that received bilateral intracapsular thyroidectomy developed hypocalcemia; 4 of these cats required treatment with calcium and vitamin D for 2 to 6 months.[56] In fact, bilateral intracapsular excision was not significantly less likely than bilateral extracapsular excision to cause hypocalcemia: Decreases in ionized calcium occurred in 82% of cats treated by extracapsular excision and 47% treated by intracapsular excision.[58,59] The duration of hypocalcemia averaged 2 weeks but lasted as long as 29 weeks in some patients. When hypocalcemic tetany occurred, it was most commonly seen within 3 days of surgery but was noted in one cat 6 days after surgery; tetany corresponded with a serum calcium of less than 6.9 mg/dl. Intracapsular excision is more likely to result in a relapse of hyperthyroidism, occurring in over 20% of cats in one study.[60]

In contrast, cats treated with a modified intracapsular technique in which most of the capsule was removed except anteriorly near the parathyroid gland or a modified extracapsular technique in which electrocautery was used to decrease blunt dissection near the parathyroid had very low rates (<2%) of disease recurrence.[60] The incidence of hypocalcemia was similar (approximately 25%) for both techniques. Recurrence of hyperthyroidism was seen a median of 23 months after surgery (range, 8–63 months). Repeated surgery in three cats led to severe clinical hypocalcemia. Thus a second surgery is not recommended[60]; instead, cats with recurrent disease should be treated medically or with radioactive iodine. Similar long-term control has been seen with both modified techniques,[1,14,61] and recurrence rates appear to be between 10% and 15%.[9,43] Recurrences develop 7 to 40 months after surgery.

A "staged" modified intracapsular technique in which each thyroid was removed during separate surgeries 4 weeks apart appeared superior in preventing hypocalcemia; only 1 of 11 cats developed this complication.[58] Treatment with calcium lactate (350 mg PO q8h) and dihydrotachysterol (0.03 mg/kg PO q8h) was required for short-term supplementation in most cats, although one required permanent supplementation. The 4 week interval appears to allow sufficient time for the parathyroid gland to revascularize before the contralateral gland is removed. A staged modified intracapsular or extracapsular surgery is considered to be the method of choice, with the final choice of technique a matter of surgeon preference.[62]

Another surgical technique involved an extracapsular bilateral thyroid resection and autotransplantation of the parathyroid gland. The parathyroid was dissected into pieces and placed in the sternohyoideus muscle.[63] All cats became depressed and anorectic due to hypocalcemia within 48 hours and one showed signs of tetany, but all recovered within 2 weeks. If the parathyroid was not transplanted, the median time until ectopic parathyroid activity was 10 weeks. This technique is not currently recommended

Radioiodine

Incorporation of ^{131}I into the thyroid adenoma creates a localized high-dose brachytherapy specific to the hyperfunctional thyroid. Because methimazole inhibits organification of iodine, most authors have recommended stopping its administration 1 to 2 weeks before ^{131}I therapy is initiated.[7] However, a study that used concurrent methimazole and ^{131}I found no apparent decrease in efficacy,[64] which is clinically important when scheduling treatment for an unstable hyperthyroid cat that requires methimazole to stabilize disease. Again, as for surgical excision, medical management of hyperthyroidism prior to radioiodine treatment is desirable to reveal renal insufficiency that may be masked in patients with unmanaged hyperthyroidism. It should be remembered that these cats are often systemically compromised, and cardiac disease may result in death in an unstable patient treated with [131]I.[65,66] Methimazole or a "conditioning"

protocol, as described in conjunction with surgical excision, may help to stabilize patients prior to ^{131}I therapy.[64]

Following ^{131}I administration, cats present a potential radiation exposure risk when handled. To minimize the risk to owners, cats are hospitalized until the surface radiation over the thyroid is at a safe level. Depending on the dose of iodine given, this can range from 7 to 25 days (average, 8 to 10 days).[7,67] Decreasing the definition of a safe surface dose from 45 mR/hour to 1.5 mR/hour increased the median stay from 8 days to 23 days.[65,67] Hospital stays were 10 to 14 days when oral ^{131}I was given.[68]

The route of administration does not seem to influence outcome. No difference in control rates was seen in studies that directly compared IV versus SQ administration.[69,70] However, sedation was needed for some cats receiving IV ^{131}I, and exposure duration for the handlers was increased with IV administration. Oral administration requires slightly higher doses but is less stressful to the cat. An increased risk of spillage following rupture of ^{131}I capsules is a disadvantage of oral administration.[68]

The dose of ^{131}I is determined by the use of a "tracer" dose. Peak radioiodine uptake is then measured and the thyroid mass estimated to determine the appropriate therapeutic dose.[69,71] Estimating the weight of the thyroid gland is the largest potential source of error in this technique. Some investigators estimated size by digital palpation or by $^{99m}TcO_4^-$ scans.[67,72]

Another system to determine a dose of radioiodine uses a "score" based on severity of clinical signs, serum T_4, and size of thyroid gland (Figure 44-4).[7,70] Three dosing levels are used: low (<130 MBq), intermediate (130–167 MBq), or high (>167 MBq). Other investigators have used a fixed dose of ^{131}I per cat: 150 MBq IV[64–66] or 200 to 300 MBq PO.[68,73]

In the largest study of the efficacy of radioiodine, 524 cats were treated with SQ ^{131}I based on the three-level scoring system described above.[7] Serum T_4 levels decreased in all cats after ^{131}I treatment, but 8 cats remained persistently hyperthyroid (Table 44-2). T_4 in these 8 cats was above 250 µg/dl before treatment, and 7 received the high dose. A second course of treatment in 4 of these cats resulted in euthyroidism; the remaining 4 cats were treated with methimazole.[7] Repeated treatment with ^{131}I seemed to be successful in other cats that were still hyperthyroid 6 months after treatment.[65,68,72]

Transient dysphagia was seen in 8 cats immediately following administration of ^{131}I, possibly due to radiation-induced inflammation.[7] Side effects have rarely been reported in other studies,[65,69,70] although administration of a fixed oral dose resulted in one cat dying due to seizures within 48 hours of administration[73] and agitation and collapse (which resolved within 3 minutes) were seen at the time of IV administration in two other cats.[66] Of 927 cats, some sort of toxicosis associated with ^{131}I administration was seen in 11 cats but resulted in death in only 1.[7,65–70,72,73]

Factor	Classifications	Score
Clinical signs[a]	Mild	1
	Moderate	2
	Severe	3
Serum T_4 concentration	<125 nmol/L	1
	125–250 nmol/L	2
	>250 nmol/L	3
Thyroid tumor size[b]	<1.0 × 0.5 cm	1
	1.0 × 0.5 to 3.0 × 1.0 cm	2
	>3.0 × 1.0 cm	3

[a]Severity of clinical signs determined on the basis of number and magnitude of clinical signs and duration of illness.

[b]Thyroid tumor size estimated from digital palpation of the thyroid gland; if both thyroid lobes were enlarged, the sizes of both lobes were added together to determine the score.

Cats with a total score of 3, 4, or 5 were treated with a low dose (2.0–3.4 mCi; 74–130 megabecquerels [MBq]), cats with a total score of 6 or 7 were treated with a moderate dose (3.5–4.4 mCi; 130–167 MBq), and cats with a total score of 8 or 9 were treated with a high dose (4.5–6.0 mCi; 167–222 MBq) of radioiodine.

Figure 44-4: *A scoring system has been devised to estimate a therapeutic dose of [131]I. This system accounts for the size of the tumor, serum T_4 level, and severity of clinical signs (From Peterson MG, Becker DV: Radioiodine treatment of 524 cats with hyperthyroidism. JAVMA 207: 1422–1428, 1995; with permission.*

TABLE 44-2
Serum T_4 Levels Following SQ ^{131}I in 524 Cats[7,a]

Time	Hypothyroid Cats (No.)	Euthyroid Cats (No.)	Hyperthyroid Cats (No.)
Upon release	26	448	80
3 months after treatment	84	422	13
6–12 months after treatment	57	437	8

[a]Numbers do not add up per original reference.

Hypothyroidism, as measured by serum T_4, was common in one large study (Table 44-2),[7] but only 11 cats developed clinical signs of lethargy, dullness, weight gain, and seborrhea sicca. Decreased grooming, hypothermia, and bradycardia were less commonly seen. Of 11 cats, 2 became anemic and 3 became azotemic. All of these signs resolved after thyroid supplementation. The occurrence of hypothyroidism could not be predicted on the basis of pretreatment serum T_4.[7] The overall incidence of hypothyroidism in reported studies was 109 of 927 cats (12%); associated clinical signs were rare, occurring in only 14 of 927 cats.[7,66–70,72,73]

The prognosis for long-term survival following ^{131}I treatment is excellent. In one large study, the median survival was 2 years[7]; 89% of cats were alive 1 year after treatment, 72% at 2 years, 52% at 3 years, and 34% at 4 years. In two studies totaling 755 cats,[7,74] renal disease was the most common cause of death (132 of 755 cats); 109 cats died of a malignant, nonthyroid tumor. This emphasizes the importance of pretreatment screening of cats and using a 1 month methimazole trial to determine whether control of hyperthyroidism will worsen renal disease.[38]

Prognostic factors for long-term survival were studied in 231 cats treated with [131]I.[74] The median survival was 25 months. Male gender and increasing age were predictors of poor survival, but health problems such as cardiac disease at diagnosis did not influence survival. Survival times have been similar in other studies in which cats received IV or SQ ^{131}I, regardless of whether the dose was based on a dosing formula or fixed dose administration.[66,69]

Recurrence of hyperthyroidism after ^{131}I treatment is uncommon. Only 13 of 524 (2.5%) cats had a recurrence between 1 and 6 years (median, 3 years) after initial ^{131}I treatment.[7] Five of these 13 cats were successfully retreated with ^{131}I, and the others were treated with methimazole. Recurrence was not predictable based on initial serum T_4 levels. Similar low recurrence rates (occurring 16 to 28 months after treatment) have been reported in cats treated with IV,[66,69] and presumably oral, administration, although details were not available.[68,73]

Supportive care for cats with thyroid adenomas and secondary thyrotoxicosis should include nutritional support because of the frequent prevalence of cachexia. Postsurgical analgesia should also be used, as should antiemetics when needed. Specific therapy for hypertrophic cardiomyopathy, renal disease, and hypertension may be vital for long-term survival and must be considered in addition to definitive therapy for the hyperthyroidism.

THYROID CARCINOMA

CLINICAL BRIEFING

Common Presentation	Less common than adenoma; presenting signs are similar (hyperfunctional thyroid) and difficult to distinguish clinically. Biopsy samples should be collected if multiple or large masses are found when staging for adenoma. Large masses may cause dyspnea or dysphagia.

Staging and Diagnosis	Biopsy of suspicious mass after MDB, thoracic radiographs, and cardiac evaluation as for thyroid adenoma. Regional lymph nodes (tracheal) and lungs most common metastatic sites. Could use neck ultrasonography as well as scintigraphy.
Treatment	
Initial	Surgical excision usually not possible; ^{131}I may be successful and may accumulate in functional metastasis.
Adjunctive	Chemotherapy untried, but carboplatin or doxorubicin most likely to be effective. External beam radiation may be helpful in controlling incompletely excised, localized tumors.
Supportive	Palliative medical management of hyperthyroidism and secondary cardiac disease. Nutritional support if cachectic. Medical management of thyroid disease may not be successful due to high tumor burden.

Incidence, Signalment, and Etiology

Thyroid carcinoma is considerably more rare than thyroid adenoma. In a large study of 588 hyperthyroid cats, only 6 had a thyroid carcinoma[7]; likewise, in two series totaling 177 hyperthyroid cats treated surgically for presumed adenoma, 5 had a carcinoma.[60] In one study, however, there were two carcinomas in only 23 hyperthyroid cats.[37]

The signalment for cats with thyroid carcinoma is similar to that for cats with thyroid adenoma. Of 32 cats for which signalment was available, ages ranged from 4 to 20 years (median, 13 years).[4,39,75–82] All were DSHs or DLHs (with the exception of one Siamese[81]), and all were neutered.

The most common histologic type is functional papillary carcinoma,[83] which may occur concurrently with a contralateral thyroid adenoma.[1,78] Nonfunctional tumors are rare.[78,79] Thyroid carcinoma is rarely bilateral.[4,84]

Clinical Presentation and History

The most common presentation of a cat with a functional thyroid carcinoma is essentially identical to that of a cat with a functional thyroid adenoma, which accounts for the "unexpected" discovery of a carcinoma at thyroidectomy.[60] Some carcinomas are encapsulated[76] and may go undiagnosed if the resected tissue is not submitted to pathology. A large mass may surround the trachea and esophagus, causing dyspnea and dysphagia in addition to signs of hyperthyroidism.[75]

The majority of cats have at least one palpable mass in the neck region.[78] The index of suspicion for a thyroid carcinoma increases if the gland is fixed or invasive into surrounding tissue[75,76] or if it rapidly increases in size.[81] Similarly, a cat that fails to respond to treatment with [131]I[78] or that has multiple masses[78,79] (palpable or detected via a [99m]TcO$_4^-$ scan) should be suspected of having thyroid carcinoma.

Staging and Diagnosis

The finding of an irregular tumor or multiple neck mass-

es in a hyperthyroid cat should increase suspicion for a carcinoma. As for cats with thyroid adenoma, concurrent renal disease may be exacerbated by definitive treatment and should be considered when evaluating a serum chemistry profile.[79]

MDB = minimum database; includes CBC, biochemical profile, urinalysis, FeLV/FIV serology, T$_4$ testing, and thoracic radiographs (three views).

Ultrasonography of the neck has been used to detect thyroid carcinoma and may be useful for detecting multiple masses.[39]

Cardiomyopathy is equally likely to occur in cats with functional carcinoma or adenoma,[75,78–80] and complete cardiac evaluation including thoracic radiographs, careful auscultation, ECG, and echocardiography should be performed prior to definitive treatment.

Thoracic radiographs may show that the carcinoma extends into the cranial mediastinum.[14,41,78,79] Similarly, a [99m]TcO$_4^-$ scan may show multiple cervical masses, extension of tumor into the thoracic inlet, mediastinal masses, or even functional lung metastases (Figure 44-5).[78,79] Thyroid carcinoma is highly metastatic. Metastasis, most commonly to the regional lymph nodes, was found in 15 of 31 cats; the tracheal nodes and those adjacent to the thyroid were involved in 11 of these 15 cats at diagnosis.[77,78,81] Miliary pulmonary metastases were seen at the time of diagnosis in 7 cats,[4,75,77,78,81,82] and metastases involved other organs in 3 cats.[77,78,82]

Paraneoplastic hypercalcemia was seen in two cats, one of which also had pulmonary metastases.[78,79] In one cat with a nonfunctional tumor, hypercalcemia resolved after surgical excision of the tumor, which was most likely a parathyroid carcinoma. Clinicians are cautioned that a parathyroid ade-

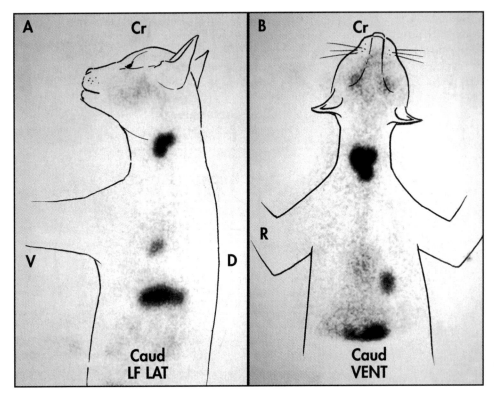

Figure 44-5: *A* $^{99m}TcO_4^-$ *scan (lateral [**A**] and dorsal ventral [**B**] views) that demonstrates a large irregular thyroid mass (or multiple irregular masses) is highly suggestive of a thyroid carcinoma. This cat had a thyroid carcinoma and a functional lung metastasis. (Scan courtesy of A. Tidwell; artwork by Beth Mellor)*

nocarcinoma may be clinically indistinguishable from a nonfunctional thyroid carcinoma, and immunohistochemical staining of the biopsy specimen for parathormone should be requested if hypercalcemia is present.

KEY POINT

Thyroid carcinoma is an uncommon cause of hyperthyroidism but may respond to ^{131}I treatment.

Treatment

Surgical excision of a carcinoma is often impossible due to extension into surrounding tissue, the thoracic inlet, or even the mediastinum.[14,75,78] Surgical excision, even if incomplete, may result in euthyroidism and clinical improvement within a few weeks; even cats that remain hyperthyroid may show clinical improvement. This is advantageous if ^{131}I treatment is being considered.[78,79] However, the high rate of metastases at diagnosis makes surgery alone a less than ideal option.

Radioiodine was used to treat 20 cats with thyroid carcinoma. One cat died soon after treatment,[14] one died because of metastases, and two died as a result of severe debility.[78] Six cats were not suspected to have carcinoma and received 60 and 200 MBq of ^{131}I as treatment for presumed

adenoma.[78] Survival in these cats ranged from 8 to 39 months (average, 19 months). Three cats were treated a second time, one after 2 years of euthyroidism; 2 of these cats failed to respond to a second treatment with ^{131}I and were treated surgically.[78]

The remaining 10 cats were treated with a high dose of ^{131}I (20–30 mCi [750–1,000 MBq]), and survival times ranged from 10 to 41 months (median, 20 months).[78,79] Other diseases, such as renal disease, were a common cause of mortality. It is possible that radioiodine may accumulate in functional metastases, accounting for the paucity of metastatic disease in these cats. Four cats required L-thyroxine supplementation for clinical signs of hypothyroidism.

External beam radiation may reduce the risk of local recurrence in cats with localized, nonfunctional thyroid carcinoma that cannot be completely excised.[78]

Chemotherapy for this uncommon tumor has not been reported. Carboplatin and doxorubicin are the most active agents in dogs.

Palliation with antithyroid medication has not been reported as a sole method of treatment. Methimazole or PTU was used prior to ^{131}I treatment in five cats but failed to control the hyperthyroidism.[14,78,79] Medical management will likely be unsuccessful in these cats because of the large volume of hyperfunctional tissue. Very high doses may be required for control but increase the risk for drug-related toxicity.

Supportive care for cats with thyroid carcinomas is the same as for cats with thyroid adenomas. Nutritional support, analgesia, and specific therapy for hypertrophic cardiomyopathy, renal disease, and hypertension should be considered as important as definitive treatment for the tumor.

NONDOMESTIC FELIDAE

Thyroid carcinomas have been diagnosed in three leopards (*Panthera pardus*); no clinical details were provided,[85,86] although one study implied an apparent increasing incidence over time.[86] Bilateral thyroid carcinoma was diagnosed in a puma that had died suddenly; it also had lung metastases.[87] Another puma had a functional thyroid adenoma with cardiomyopathy.[88] The animal continued to deteriorate after surgical resection of the primary tumor, and a $^{99m}T_cO_4^-$ scan showed multiple areas of uptake in the mediastinum. A thyroid carcinoma with pulmonary metastases was noted on autopsy in addition to the adenoma. Although the overall incidence of thyroid tumors is rare in nondomestic Felidae,[89] the majority appear to be carcinomas.

PANCREATIC ISLET CELL TUMORS

CLINICAL BRIEFING

Common Presentation	Insulinomas cause hypoglycemia and neurologic signs in older cats. Gastrinomas, which are very rare, are associated with chronic vomiting.
Staging and Diagnosis	Confirm diagnosis with MDB. Normal to high insulin with concurrent low glucose (insulinoma) or serum gastrin (gastrinoma) levels. Abdominal ultrasonography may show pancreatic mass. Metastatic rate is unknown but probably high for both insulinoma and gastrinoma; metastasis is usually to the liver or other abdominal organs.
Treatment	
Initial	Surgical excision of a benign tumor may be curative, but most tumors are probably malignant and there may be multiple primary pancreatic tumors.
Adjunctive	Chemotherapy not reported. Somatostatin or streptozotocin could be helpful but are untried.
Supportive	Medical palliation of signs of hypoglycemia using prednisone may be successful. Diazoxide use not reported. H_2 antihistamines may be effective to reduce gastric acid secretion associated with gastrinoma.

INSULINOMA

Insulin is produced by pancreatic islet cells, and unregulated secretion by an insulinoma leads to hypoglycemia (often severe) that may be worse just before a meal or, paradoxically, just after a meal due to postprandial insulin release.

Incidence, Signalment, and Etiology

Not all reports of islet cell tumors in cats are accompanied by clinical histories, and the functional nature of these tumors is often speculative. Insulin secretion was confirmed or inferred in seven cats.[90–95] Signalment data were unavailable for two cats[93]; ages in the other cats ranged from 5 to 16 years (median, 14 years). Three were Siamese, one was Persian, and one was a DLH. Three were castrated males.

Clinical Presentation and History

Signs of hypoglycemia ranged from nervousness[94] and inappetence[95] to episodic staggering and twitching of the leg, skin, and facial muscles[90,91] and even grand mal seizures.[90,94]

These signs had been present for several months in most cats[90,91,95] and were noted either before or within 30 minutes after a meal. Seizures lasted up to 2 hours in one cat,[90] and one cat died because of uncontrolled seizure activity.[94] An abdominal mass is occasionally palpable on physical examination, but most insulinomas are small.[95]

Staging and Diagnosis

Presumptive diagnosis of an insulinoma may be made in a cat that shows Whipple's triad (i.e., hypoglycemia with neurologic signs that respond to glucose administration). The presence of hypoglycemia in the face of a normal to increased serum insulin level is much stronger evidence for an insulinoma. Serum determinations for glucose and insulin must be made at the same time to be diagnostic; this is because serum insulin levels should be low when serum glucose is low. Direct stimulation of insulin release from tumor cells using a glucagon tolerance test has been used to diagnose insulinoma,[90] but this test is not recommended due to the risk of inducing severe hypoglycemia.

More definitive diagnosis may be made based on either ultrasonography or exploratory laparotomy. Ultrasonography is often superior to radiography in identifying a mass involving the pancreas, although it may be difficult to locate the lesion to a specific area. Thoracic radiographs should be made in addition to the MDB in cats with suspected insulinoma.

Tumors have been described as adenomas in some cats[94] and may reach up to 2 cm in diameter,[91,94] although most are smaller.[90] Adenocarcinomas presumably occur as well. Although none of the reported cats had detectable metastases, prolonged or recurrent hypoglycemia following surgical removal of an insulinoma implies that metastases may occur. Multiple islet cell tumors have been reported,[95] so the pancreas should be carefully examined at surgery or by ultrasonography prior to surgery.

MDB = minimum database; includes CBC, biochemical profile, urinalysis, FeLV/FIV serology, T_4 testing, and thoracic radiographs (three views).

Treatment

Surgical excision of an apparently solitary insulinoma was unsuccessful in controlling seizures in one cat. It is possible that this cat developed CNS damage as a result of seizures that had lasted as long as 2 hours.[90] Prednisone at doses up to 2 mg/kg/day did not control seizures either, and the cat died. The rationale for prednisone use is that it acts to antagonize the effects of insulin and thus increases serum glucose levels. In another cat, surgical excision was followed by transient diabetes and then 7 months of normality before twitching and staggering recurred.[91] At that point prednisolone treatment was initiated and controlled signs for a further 2 years, at which time the cat died of unknown causes.

Diazoxide, an inhibitor of insulin secretion, has been shown to be effective in controlling signs of hypoglycemia in dogs with insulinoma, but its use has not been reported in cats. The efficacy of other antineoplastic agents, such as somatostatin or streptozotocin, has not been explored in cats with insulinoma, although they appear to have some efficacy in dogs with insulinoma.

GASTRINOMA

Incidence, Signalment, and Etiology

Gastrin is produced by pancreatic islet cells and acts to directly stimulate gastric parietal cells and hydrochloric acid production by the stomach. Gastrinomas have been described in two 12-year-old DSH cats. One was a spayed female[96] and the other a castrated male.[97]

Clinical Presentation and History

Chronic vomiting (2 years in one cat and 3 months in the other) was associated with weight loss in these two cats. One cat was also listless.[97] The tumor was a palpable 2 cm mass in the ventral cranial abdomen in one of the cats[97] but was much smaller in the other.[96]

Staging and Diagnosis

An MDB should be obtained for any cat with chronic vomiting. Endoscopy may reveal gastroduodenal ulceration. Both reported cats had duodenal ulceration but neither was anemic at presentation; one cat did develop anemia later, presumably due to hemorrhage from these ulcers.[96] Serum gastrin levels may be measured and should confirm the diagnosis. Serum gastrin level in one cat was 1,000 pg/ml; in comparison, levels ranged from 28 to 135 pg/ml in three control cats.[96] In both cats with gastrinoma, immunohistochemical staining of the tumor cells confirmed gastrin secretion; in one cat, tumor cells also secreted glucagon and cholecystokinin. Both cats had widespread hepatic metastases as well as thickening and ulceration of the duodenum.

More definitive diagnosis may be made based on ultrasonography, which is the imaging modality of choice for identifying a pancreatic mass; it may also be able to locate lesions in the liver or other abdominal sites. Thoracic radiographs should be obtained for a cat with suspected gastrinoma.

Treatment

Treatment was not attempted, although exploratory laparotomy was performed in one cat. Medical management using H_2 antihistamines has not been reported, nor has the efficacy of chemotherapeutic agents such as somatostatin or streptozotocin.

PARATHYROID TUMORS

CLINICAL BRIEFING

| Common Presentation | Rare in cats. Typically occurs in older animals. Siamese may be predisposed. Signs are usually nonspecific. Mass is frequently palpable in neck and often large. |

Staging and Diagnosis	Usually parathyroid adenoma, but can be adenocarcinoma. MDB shows hypercalcemia. High parathormone levels are supportive; multiple samples may be needed to reveal abnormal values. Neck mass often palpable; ultrasonography may detect nonpalpable masses.
Treatment	
Initial	Surgical excision of adenoma may be curative. Check other parathyroid glands as multiple adenomas and concurrent adenocarcinomas are reported. Monitor serum calcium for hypocalcemia or return of hypercalcemia after surgery.
Adjunctive	Chemotherapy not reported and may not be necessary. Cyclophosphamide and doxorubicin may be useful.
Supportive	Corticosteroids and fluid therapy may reduce serum calcium levels prior to surgery. Appetite stimulants as necessary.

Incidence, Signalment, and Etiology

Hyperparathyroidism due to a primary parathyroid tumor is rare in cats. Of 20 reported cases, bilateral "hyperplasia" was seen in 1 cat,[98] adenomas were seen in 17 cats,[99,100] and adenocarcinomas were seen in 3 cats.[100,101] One of the cats with adenoma developed adenocarcinoma 19 months after initial surgery,[100] and another had both an adenoma and a carcinoma.[95] Bilateral adenomas were seen in 2 of the cats.[95,100] Affected cats ranged in age from 8 to 15 years, and 6 were males and 5 were females. Six cats were Siamese,[95,100] 13 were DSHs or DLHs, and 1 was Persian.[95] Other cats reported as having nonfunctional thyroid carcinoma, often with hypercalcemia, may have actually had a parathyroid tumor.[78,79]

Clinical Presentation and History

In a study of 9 cats, only 2 were considered to have functional tumors; the rest of the tumors were incidental findings at autopsy.[95] Of 13 cats reported to have functional parathyroid tumors (including these 2), nonspecific signs of lethargy and anorexia for one to several months were commonly seen, presumably associated with hypercalcemia. Vomiting was seen in 6 cats[95,99–101] and polyuria/polydipsia in 3 cats.[98,100] Reluctance to move and weakness were seen occasionally. One cat with a parathyroid adenocarcinoma was obtunded and ataxic and had muscle tremors,[100] and another had muscular twitches.[95] One cat had no clinical signs despite significant hypercalcemia.[100]

Seven cats had a palpable mass in the neck, ranging from 2 to 6 cm in diameter (Figure 44-6). The largest tumor was a carcinoma.[101] The palpable mass was cystic in two cats.[100] A cat with bilateral adenomas,[100] one with bilateral hyperplasia,[98] and one with a parathyroid tumor within the thyroid gland[99]; all had nonpalpable tumors.

Staging and Diagnosis

Serum calcium was elevated in 12 of 13 cats with clinical signs but not in the cat with hyperplasia[98]; levels ranged

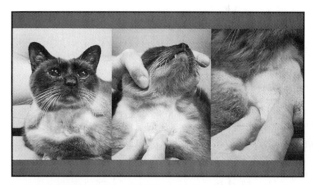

Figure 44-6: This 13-year-old Siamese was inappetent and hypercalcemic. A large irregular mass was palpable in the right cervical area. (Courtesy of M. Kent)

from 13.3 to 22.8 mg/dl, well above the upper normal limit of 11 mg/dl.[95,100,101] If multiple samples are obtained from a cat with a parathyroid tumor, some of the samples may have normal serum calcium levels. This implies that multiple samples should be obtained over time if a parathyroid tumor is suspected but the calcium level is normal in an initial sample.[100] Serum phosphorus was low to normal in all cats.[98–101] Most cats were azotemic, and some were isosthenuric. Calcium oxalate uroliths were seen in one cat.[101]

Serum parathormone (PTH) levels were elevated (range, 8–19.5 pmol/L; normal range, 2–13 pmol/L[100] or 8–32 ng/L[99]) in the three cats for which this information was available. Several serum samples were analyzed for one cat, and PTH levels were sometimes in the normal range,[99] again emphasizing the need to obtain multiple samples.

Immunohistochemical staining of biopsy specimens for parathormone is warranted if a carcinoma is resected from the thyroid area and yet the cat is not hyperthyroid. This is particularly true if the cat is also hypercalcemic.

Thoracic radiographs did not show evidence of pulmonary metastasis in any cat, although a decrease in bone density was seen in one[101] and there were multifocal polyostotic lesions in the axial skeleton of another.[98] Bone scintigraphy was performed in one cat with normal radiographs, and no evidence of increased bone activity was found.[99] Cervical ultrasonography disclosed a mass with cystic foci in four cats with parathyroid neoplasia.[101-102] Ultrasonography may be a useful imaging technique when there is no palpable mass but a parathyroid tumor is suspected (Figure 44-7A). Metastases were not reported in any of the three cats with parathyroid adenocarcinoma.[100,101] Exploratory surgery is diagnostic and therapeutic in most cats.

KEY POINT

Hypercalcemia may occur due to a solitary parathyroid adenoma, multiple adenomas, or concurrent adenoma and carcinoma.

Treatment

Surgical excision of a parathyroid adenoma should result in rapid clinical improvement (Figure 44-7B). Postoperative hypocalcemia was uncommon and was not associated with clinical signs in nine treated cats.[95,99,100]

Surgery was successful in nine of nine cats with parathyroid adenoma. No cats with carcinoma were treated. In one cat with an adherent tumor, transient Horner's syndrome developed after surgery.[100] Five cats were normal at least 6 to 7 months after surgery,[99,100] and three cats were lost to follow-up 1 to 4 months after surgery.[95,99,100] One cat had recurrent hypercalcemia 19 months after surgical excision of an adenoma; necropsy revealed a recurrent adenoma and parathyroid adenocarcinoma.[100]

The use of chemotherapy as an adjunct to surgery has not been reported and, due to the apparent low likelihood of metastasis, may not be necessary. Cyclophosphamide and doxorubicin are likely the most useful agents to prevent tumor recurrence.

Supportive care prior to surgery for parathyroid adenomas may include the use of fluid therapy and/or corticosteroids to reduce serum calcium levels. Nutritional support may also be necessary, particularly postoperatively.

NONDOMESTIC FELIDAE

A 20-year-old male snow leopard *(Panthera vinca)* had a chronic history of weight loss with more recent onset of epistaxis and depression. A 1 cm parathyroid adenoma was identified on necropsy.[103] It was apparently nonfunctional as the serum calcium level was normal. Parathyroid hyperplasia was seen in two nondomestic felids in a survey, but no parathyroid neoplasms were recorded.[89]

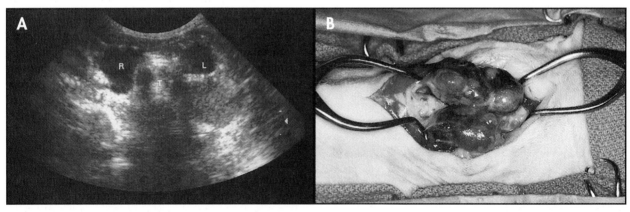

Figure 44-7: (A) Ultrasonography of the neck of the cat in Figure 44-6 demonstrates a large parathyroid mass and a previously undetected contralateral smaller mass, seen as dark structures labeled "R" (right) and "L" (left). (B) At surgery the large mass was identified as a parathyroid carcinoma and the smaller one as a parathyroid adenoma. Hypercalcemia resolved after surgical excision. (Courtesy of M. Kent)

PITUITARY TUMORS

CLINICAL BRIEFING

Common Presentation	Most commonly secrete growth hormone (GH), causing acromegaly, or ACTH, causing hyperadrenocorticism. Pituitary tumors are rarely large enough to cause CNS signs (blindness, disorientation).
Staging and Diagnosis	MDB and other specific tests as discussed in each relevant section below. CT scan or MRI for large pituitary tumors. Thoracic radiographs and abdominal ultrasonography,

Treatment	
Initial	Radiation therapy should be definitive. Monitor CT scan for macroadenomas. Cryoablation is experimental.
Supportive	Secondary renal or cardiac disease requires treatment, as does DM.

as second endocrine neoplasia is common. Secondary diabetes mellitus (DM) is common with acromegaly and hyperadrenocorticism.

Incidence, Signalment, and Etiology

Pituitary tumors are usually adenomas and, in cats, most commonly affect the anterior lobe of the pituitary (pars distalis and pars intermedia). These tumors are further classified on the basis of granule staining as basophil, acidophil, or chromophobe. Tumors of the posterior lobe (pars nervosa) are rare in cats. Acidophil adenomas are presumed to secrete growth hormone (GH), and basophilic tumors may secrete TSH. It is probably more helpful to use immunohistochemical staining techniques to distinguish between tumors that secrete ACTH, TSH, or GH, but this is not possible antemortem.

In a series of 18 cats with pituitary tumors diagnosed at necropsy, 15 were DSHs or DLHs and there was 1 each Siamese, Persian, and Maine Coon.[95] Ages ranged from 5 to 20 years (average, 13 years). Fourteen cats were male.

Clinical Presentation and History

Signs due to a space-occupying mass are comparatively rare among cats with pituitary tumors. The majority of cats in one survey (12 of 18 cats with pituitary tumors) had microscopic tumors, and 4 of the remaining 6 had very small visible tumors.[95]

Clinical signs related to space-occupying lesions seem to occur when the tumor is larger than 1 cm in diameter.[95,104–106] The most common sign is loss of vision, which may be reported by the owner as aimless wandering, inappropriate elimination, or dilated pupils. Systemic signs such as anorexia, depression, lethargy, vomiting, or diarrhea may occur following loss of vision.[106] Seizures are less common.[107]

Staging and Diagnosis

Blindness in a cat with normal funduscopy[106] or other neurologic deficits[105] should prompt a CT scan following a complete neurologic evaluation. Many cats with a pituitary adenoma have other endocrine abnormalities. In a series of 18 cats diagnosed at autopsy with pituitary tumors, 13 had thyroid adenomas and 13 had hyperplasia of the adrenal gland; 5 cats were diabetic and 5 had congestive heart failure (both diseases presumably due to secretion of GH). One cat had a microscopic pheochromocytoma. In another study of 14 cats, 6 had parathyroid hyperplasia.[107] In addition to the MDB, echocardiography, ECG, thoracic radiography, and abdominal ultra-

sonography are indicated in cats with a suspected pituitary tumor. Any other disease should be stabilized prior to anesthesia for CT scan.

KEY POINT

Blindness in a cat with normal funduscopy should be investigated with a CT scan.

CT scan and MRI are the most sensitive methods for imaging the pituitary.[106–110] For large tumors, measurements made on CT are helpful for planning definitive radiation treatment. Tumors may also be imaged by radioscintigraphy.[109] Plain skull radiography may show secondary skeletal changes if the tumor is secreting GH but will not allow identification of the pituitary mass.

Most tumors are adenomas. Although large adenomas may be invasive,[107] they will not metastasize. A pituitary carcinoma did not have evidence of metastasis.[106]

Treatment

Large pituitary tumors have rarely been treated, but the treatment of choice is megavoltage radiation therapy. Minimal shrinkage has been documented by repeating CT scans after megavoltage radiation,[107,108] but this has been enough to reduce hormonal effects of the tumor and improve neurologic function. Tumor volume in one cat was reduced by more than 50% over 2 months,[107] but another cat with an invasive tumor did not respond.[107]

One study used a transsphenoidal surgical approach to remove a pituitary adenoma in seven cats with pituitary-dependent hyperadrenocorticism.[111] Two cats died within 2 weeks of surgery (one had concurrent lymphoma), one cat died of anemia 6 months after surgery, and one cat died due to complications including soft palate necrosis 8 months after surgery. The tumor was incompletely excised in another cat, and hyperadrenocorticism recurred 19 months after surgery. One cat was still in remission 15 months after surgery and another at 46 months after surgery.[111] This surgery should be performed at specialized institutions, and careful staging for concurrent diseases is warranted.

NONDOMESTIC FELIDAE

Pituitary adenomas are rare,[89] and surveys do not include clinical signs or laboratory finding that could indicate their histogenesis.

POSTERIOR LOBE OF THE PITUITARY GLAND

Only one tumor of the pars nervosa, a pituicytoma, has been reported. A 7-year-old spayed female Siamese had systemic signs of vomiting and diarrhea as well as slow, uncertain movement. It was found to have no menace reflex in the right eye and decrease patellar reflexes.[105,112] No treatment was attempted, and on necropsy the tumor was over 1 cm in diameter and cystic, causing a space-occupying effect.

ACROMEGALY

C L I N I C A L B R I E F I N G	
Common Presentation	GH secretion causes weight gain, organomegaly, prognathia inferior, and arthropathy. Usually occurs in male DSH cats.
Staging and Diagnosis	MDB, echocardiography, ECG, thoracic radiographs, and GH or somatomedin-C serum levels. CT scan or MRI for large pituitary tumors. Secondary DM, renal failure, and hypertrophic cardiomyopathy are common.
Treatment Initial	Radiation therapy should be definitive. Monitor serum profile and GH levels or perform CT scan for macroadenomas. Somatostatin analogues and cryoablation are experimental.
Supportive	Secondary renal or cardiac disease requires treatment, as does DM.

Incidence, Signalment, and Etiology

Acidophil tumors of the anterior pituitary appear to secrete GH in cats (Figure 44-8). Of 22 cats reported to have confirmed GH-secreting tumors, all were neutered and all but 3 were males. Twenty-one cats were DSHs and 1 was a DLH. Ages ranged from 6 to 14 years (average, 10 years).[107–110,113–115] Due to increases in body mass secondary to GH, the average weight of affected cats (5.4 kg) was high.[107]

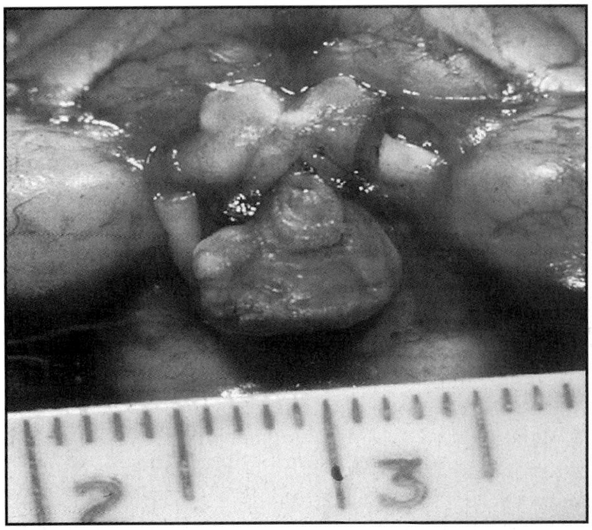

Clinical Presentation and History

GH is diabetogenic, and this is reflected in the history and clinical signs, which include polydipsia, polyuria, and polyphagia due to DM. Ketoacidosis is rare.[107,110] Most cats are presented due to insulin-resistant diabetes and may be receiving very high dosages of exogenous insulin. The average daily insulin requirement for these cats was 58 U (range, 20 to 130 U) in one study.[107] Similarly high doses were reported for other cats.[108,109,114] Average duration of treatment for diabetes exceeded 1 year in one study[107] and 2.5 years in another cat.[109,116] In some cats, the diabetic episodes may initially resolve spontaneously[110] or with intermittent insulin treatment[113] before becoming resistant to therapy.

Most cats are heavy due to an increase in body mass (not body fat), and weight gain may be reported. Increase in other organs, such as hepatomegaly, cardiomegaly, and renomegaly, are common. Organomegaly may lead to an enlarged abdomen.[107,109,115] Many cats have a large head and obvious protrusion of the lower jaw (prognathia inferior; Figure 44-9), and some cats may have an enlarged tongue.[107]

Figure 44-8: GH-secreting pituitary adenoma in a cat with acromegaly. These tumors may be very small and cause hormonal effects only; larger tumors may cause neurologic signs. (Courtesy of D. Greco)

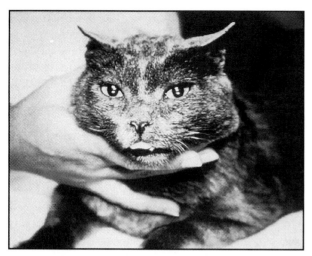

Figure 44-9: A cat with acromegaly. Note the protruding lower jaw (prognathia inferior) and generally "heavy" features. (Courtesy of D. Greco)

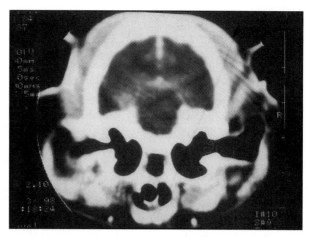

Figure 44-10: A CT image showing a large pituitary tumor in a cat with acromegaly and neurologic signs. (Courtesy of A. Tidwell)

Arthropathy was seen in 6 of 14 cats in one study[107] and affected the shoulder, elbow, carpus, stifle, or digit, either alone or in combination. Some cats may appear to have enlarged paws.[109] Cataracts may be seen in cats with prolonged, poorly controlled DM.[114]

Staging and Diagnosis

A serum chemistry profile is most consistent with DM, although half of the cats in one study also had renal failure.[107] Renal failure has also been reported in other cats with acromegaly.[113] Mild erythrocytosis may be caused by excess GH.

Cardiomegaly may result in hypertrophic cardiomyopathy and in turn may lead to congestive heart failure, as was seen in 6 of 14 affected cats in one study.[107] Complete cardiac evaluation including thoracic radiographs, ECG, and echocardiography should be performed, and cardiac disease should be stabilized prior to anesthesia or invasive procedures.

Thoracic radiographs may also reveal spondylosis, presumably due to excess GH. Limb radiographs may be warranted in cats clinically affected by arthropathy.[107,114] Skull radiographs will not help diagnose a pituitary mass, but the finding of prognathia inferior or thickening of the bony ridges of the calvarium is circumstantial evidence of acromegaly.

CT scan demonstrates a pituitary mass in the majority of cats (Figure 44-10). Tumors as small as 3 mm in height can be detected,[108,117] but smaller tumors may not be visible on CT scanning.[107] CT scanning is mandatory in cats with insulin-resistant diabetes that also exhibit CNS signs. CT findings of 16 cats with insulin-resistant diabetes were compared with findings in cats that had controlled diabetes; all resistant cats had a pituitary mass.[117] As stated, neurologic signs are rarely seen with adenomas smaller than 10 mm in

diameter. MRI is an alternative imaging method[110] and may be better able to image smaller tumors and provide greater detail (Figure 44-11). Radioscintigraphy (meglumine iothalamate) has rarely been reported, and results may be equivocal.[107,109]

Because a pituitary tumor may secrete other hormones, evaluation of other endocrine functions is warranted; however, serum T_4 was normal in 19 cats with GH-secreting tumors. Similarly, an ACTH stimulation test or dexamethasone suppression test was normal in all tested cats.[107,108,115] A diagnosis of acromegaly is confirmed by measurement of serum GH levels. Normal levels have been reported as 1.5 to 7.9 ng/ml[108] or 1.21 ± 0.14 ng/ml,[115] and affected cats have levels of 22 to 131 ng/ml.[107,108,115] A disadvantage of hormonal measurements may be the length of time (6 months or more) that it takes to receive results. In one study, a CT scan was found to be a more rapid way to identify cats that would benefit from treatment for acromegaly.[117]

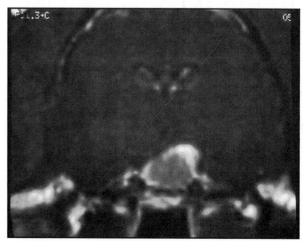

Figure 44-11: An MRI of the large pituitary mass in the cat in Figure 44-10 shows greater detail. (Courtesy of A. Tidwell)

Somatomedin-C mediates the growth-promoting effects of GH, and serum levels are therefore GH dependent. Normal cats have been reported to have levels of 150 to 600 U/L,[110,113] while two affected cats had levels of 1,200 to 5,000 U/L.[110,113] Serum somatomedin levels may be measured if GH assays are not available. If a biopsy is obtained prior to treatment,[110] definitive diagnosis can be made on the basis of immunohistochemical staining for GH.[113,114]

Treatment

The pituitary is surrounded by an arteriolar plexus in cats, making surgery very difficult.[95,111] Radiation therapy using a megavoltage source is the treatment of choice for this disease.

Radiation (total dose, 48 Gy) was used to treat five cats, two of which showed CNS signs prior to treatment.[107,108] A repeat CT scan was performed in three cats; one cat had minimal tumor shrinkage,[108] while the tumor in another shrank by 50% over 2 months. The tumor progressed in the third cat.[107] Of the remaining two cats, GH levels reduced to almost normal in one cat after 12 months but rose in the other.[108] Serum GH levels also dropped in the two cats with tumor shrinkage, to normal in one and almost normal in the other.[107,108] With the exception of the cat that did not re-spond at all, insulin requirements were reduced or completely abolished within 8 to 10 months. Recurrence of neurologic signs was seen within 6 months in one cat,[107] and the other three cats lived 16 to 26 months.[108]

Somatostatin analogues may have effects that can reduce pituitary GH production, although daily divided doses ranging from 20 to 200 μg SQ had no effect on GH levels in five cats so treated.[107,115]

One cat was treated by cryoablation of the tumor via a transsphenoidal approach. Somatomedin levels rose dramatically 6 weeks after treatment, and the cat experienced seizures before the tumor shrank and somatomedin levels fell to normal 15 months later. The cat was euthanized because of aggression, presumably due to hypothalamic vacuolation and lymphoplasmacytic meningitis resulting from treatment.[110]

Overall median survival in 14 cats, including those not treated, was 20 months (range, 4 to 42 months). Three cats were still alive between 5 and 30 months after diagnosis.[107] Death was due to renal and/or cardiac disease in 6 cats and DM in 1 cat. CNS signs were the cause of death in 2 others. Symptomatic control of concurrent disease is very important to prolong survival in cats with acromegaly, regardless of whether it is treated.

HYPERADRENOCORTICISM

CLINICAL BRIEFING

Common Presentation	Mostly affects DSH and DLH cats. Pituitary adenoma that secretes ACTH (PDH) is more common than adrenal tumor (AT). Most ATs are adenomas. Common signs are PU/PD due to secondary, often insulin-resistant, DM. Skin is thin and tears easily. Wound healing is poor. Large pituitary tumors may cause CNS signs.
Staging and Diagnosis	MDB to detect concurrent disease, ACTH response test, dexamethasone suppression tests, and determination of ACTH level. Abdominal radiographs and ultrasonography if AT suspected, CT scan if large pituitary tumor suspected. Adrenal carcinoma may metastasize to other abdominal sites.
Treatment Initial	Adrenalectomy is treatment of choice for both AT and PDH. Radiation is treatment for PDH with large tumor. Monitor adrenal function to avoid hypoadrenal crisis.
Adjunctive	Mitotane, ketoconazole, or metapyrone prior to surgery may improve symptoms and wound healing. Medical management alone not as successful as in dogs.
Supportive	Management of diabetes and secondary infections. Mineralocorticoid and glucocorticoid supplements mandatory after surgery.

Incidence, Signalment, and Etiology

Excess secretion of cortisol may occur due to an adrenal cortical adenoma or adenocarcinoma or bilateral adrenal hypertrophy caused by excess secretion of ACTH by a pituitary adenoma. In the latter situation, the disorder is termed *pituitary dependent hyperadrenocorticism* (PDH).

Hyperadrenocorticism is uncommon in cats. Of 48 cases cited in the literature, 37 cats had PDH,[118–129] 7 cats had an adrenal adenoma,[95,123,126,127,130,131] and 4 had an adrenocortical carcinoma.[123,126,128,132]

Some cats were reported as a series of cases, and thus individual signalment was not available; however, there does not seem to be any difference in signalment between cats with adrenal tumor (AT) and those with PDH. Affected cats ranged in age from 4[126] to 15[127] years (average, 10 years). The majority of cats were DSHs or DLHs; of 48 cats, the only purebreds were 3 Persians,[119,123,128] 3 Siamese,[126,129] 1 Abyssinian,[129] and 1 Devon Rex.[128] There were 25 males and 23 females.

Clinical Presentation and History

The clinical signs of hyperadrenocorticism do not differ between cats with PDH and those with AT, with the possible rare exception of central blindness due to a large pituitary tumor encroaching on the optic chiasm.[108] In 48 reported cases, the most common sign was polydipsia, which was accompanied by polyuria in 36 cats. These signs may be due to the hyperadrenocorticism or the secondary DM. Other commonly reported signs or conditions included polyphagia (30 cats), DM, which was usually resistant to exogenous insulin (28), pendulous abdomen (29), and alopecia (23) of the trunk or sometimes the limbs. Thin skin was reported in 22 cats, and spontaneous tearing of the skin occurred in 13 of these animals.[108,126–128,130,133,134] This increased skin fragility combined with insulin-resistant diabetes often led to nonhealing wounds (Figure 44-12).

KEY POINT

Thin, fragile skin and insulin-resistant diabetes increase the risk of infected, nonhealing wounds in cats with hyperadrenocorticism.

Lethargy was a presenting sign in 15 cats. Obesity or weight gain was reported in 16 cats and weight loss in 14 cats, presumably dependent on the stage of DM. Atrophy

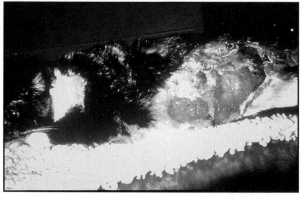

Figure 44-12: Thin skin in a cat with hyperadrenocorticism may be easily torn, heals poorly, and is prone to subsequent infections, as in this calico. (Courtesy of D. Greco)

of musculature causing weakness or abnormal gait in some cats was less commonly reported. Rarely, a cat was ataxic.[123] Hepatomegaly was noted on physical examination in 8 cats. Increased susceptibility to infections was seen in 6 cats that were septic or had abscesses. A further 4 cats had urinary tract infections, and others had oral or cutaneous infections. One cat with pancreatitis had no clinical signs consistent with hyperadrenocorticism. Pancreatitis was seen in 6 other cats,[122,123,126,130] and 2 cats had pancreatic adenocarcinoma in addition to hyperadrenocorticism.[121] Rarely, an AT may be detectable via abdominal palpation.[121]

MDB = minimum database; includes CBC, biochemical profile, urinalysis, FeLV/FIV serology, T_4 testing, and thoracic radiographs (three views).

Staging and Diagnosis

Some of the abnormalities seen in CBC and serum chemistry profiles for dogs with hyperadrenocorticism are not as reliable in cats. Lymphocyte counts and circulating eosinophils may be normal or elevated in cats with hyperadrenocorticism, so these are unreliable screening tests.[127,128] Cats with hyperadrenocorticism rarely have elevations in serum ALP.[127] The diagnostic plan for cats with clinical signs consistent with hyperadrenocorticism should include an ACTH response test, low- and high-dose dexamethasone suppression tests (0.015 and 1.0 mg/kg IV, respectively), and a determination of ACTH levels, if available. Each of these tests is described in the Box on page 338.[108,118–123,126–131,134–145]

Radiographs of the abdomen may show hepatomegaly and will occasionally reveal an adrenal mass,[126–128,132] particularly in cats with an AT (Figure 44-13). Mineralization of the adrenal gland does not imply an AT and may occur bilaterally.[119,125] Adrenal mineralization may also occur in other disease processes and can be an incidental finding in cats without hyperadrenocorticism.[146,147]

Abdominal ultrasonography may be helpful in diagnosing an AT or bilateral hyperplasia, but its accuracy is highly operator dependent. Bilateral enlargement may be missed completely or may only be noted unilaterally.[121,127] Normal adrenal ultrasonography has provided measurements of approximately $10 \times 4 \times 4$ mm,[138,148] which somewhat underestimates their actual size. A transverse image may be very difficult to obtain. Bilateral hyperplasia may cause adrenals to be as large as 40 mm in all dimensions,[119] but 10 to 15 mm in all dimensions is more common.[126] ATs are often similar in size[149] but are unilateral. Remember, it may be difficult to visualize both sides, and thus other supportive testing should be completed prior to making a di-

Testing for Hyperadrenocorticism in Cats[108,118–123,126–131,134–145]

ACTH Response Test

The ACTH response test is a good screening test; results supported a diagnosis of hyperadrenocorticism in 14 of 18 cats.[126–128] The use of synthetic ACTH (cosyntropin or tetracosactrin) is preferred for this test. In normal cats, IV administration of 0.125 mg (125 µg) per cat should result in a 200% to 1400% increase in cortisol over baseline.[121,135–138]

IV administration gives greater stimulation and a longer duration of response (6 hours) than IM injection (2 hours), and IM injection of synthetic ACTH is painful.[139] A basal serum cortisol level should be obtained, and a second sample is collected 2 to 3 hours after IV administration of synthetic ACTH.[139] Lower doses of cosyntropin (1.25 or 12.5 µg/cat) will also cause a response, but the peak is earlier and short lived.[140] Likewise, dosages higher than 125 µg have no real advantage.[141] Cosyntropin can be diluted to a concentration of 5 µg/ml of saline and stored refrigerated for more than 4 months.[140]

ACTH gel (2.2 U/kg IM) has a similar effect.[142] ACTH gel induces an earlier peak that may return to baseline quickly.[136,142]

Dexamethasone Suppression Tests

Dexamethasone administered as an IV bolus should cause "negative feedback" suppression of ACTH secretion by the pituitary and a reduction in serum cortisol. Dexamethasone is chosen because it will not cross-react with cortisol measurements.

In dogs, the low-dose dexamethasone suppression test (LDDST) is a good method of screening for hyperadrenocorticism. In cats, a dose of 0.01 mg/kg suppresses serum cortisol for 1 to 12 hours after administration, but levels return to baseline by 24 hours.[141,143,144] Samples are collected prior to dexamethasone administration and 6 to 10 hours afterward.[141] Lack of suppression does not confirm hyperadrenocorticism, as some

normal cats will not experience a reduction in serum cortisol, possibly due to stress associated with concurrent diseases.[141,144] Despite limitations, this is still a preferred screening method.[108,119–121,123,126,127] Some authors suggest that a dose of 0.015 mg/kg is more useful.[144]

An even higher dose of dexamethasone (0.1 mg/kg), with samples collected on the same schedule, was not completely consistent in suppressing cortisol secretion in all normal cats.[141] This test, however, has been widely used to distinguish ATs from pituitary tumors. While suppression of cortisol secretion should occur with pituitary tumors, the autonomous secretion of cortisol by ATs should allow the cortisol to rise again after initial suppression ("escape").[118,126,127] This test is not always diagnostic in cats,[120,121] leading some authors to recommend a dexamethasone dose of 1.0 mg/kg (i.e., the high-dose dexamethasone suppression test [HDDST]) in cats.[131,134,142,145] This dose consistently causes cortisol suppression in all normal cats.[141,145]

Determination of ACTH Levels

ACTH levels can be measured, although samples need to be chilled immediately and handled carefully, thus reducing the practicality of this test in many private practices. In normal cats, endogenous ACTH levels range from 10 to 60 pg/ml.[121,141] In cats with PDH, ACTH levels have ranged from 90 to over 1,000 pg/ml.[108,118,119,121,122,126,127] Cats with ATs should have low or normal serum ACTH levels.[130]

Urinary Cortisol

In cats, most cortisol is excreted in the bile. Therefore the urinary cortisol:urinary creatinine ratio is quite low (13×10^{-6}),[129] making it a potentially useful screening test. In one study, all six cats with hyperadrenocorticism had a urinary cortisol:creatinine ratio above the reference range (median, 122×10^{-6}).[129]

---

agnosis of an AT based on a unilateral ultrasonographic finding.

CT is warranted if a large pituitary adenoma is suspected, such as in a cat with neurologic signs.[108,126] The pituitary adenoma may be very small in some cats and not recognized on CT scan.[108]

Adrenal and pituitary adenomas do not metastasize. An adrenal carcinoma metastasized to the liver and mesenteric lymph nodes in one cat.[126]

Treatment

Symptomatic treatment with or without control of DM was the only therapy in 15 cats. While some cats lived more than 9 months,[118,120,124] most did not.[126–128,133] The reasons for death or euthanasia were pulmonary embolic disease[127]

or such infections as abscessation, sepsis, or pyothorax.[120,127,133] Abscessation often followed skin tearing and poor wound healing.

Medical management has been used as the sole form of treatment for cats with hyperadrenocorticism but is not as successful as it is in dogs. Medical management may play a role, however, in better preparing cats for surgery.[134]

Mitotane is specifically toxic to the adrenal cortex and may improve symptoms and wound healing if used prior to surgery. It has been used at doses ranging from 25 to 50 mg/kg/day in two divided doses. In normal cats, the higher dose (administered for a week) caused vomiting, lethargy, inappetence, and diarrhea that persisted for 2 weeks after mitotane was discontinued.[120] However, the same dose had no reported side effects in a cat with PDH.[145] It may be

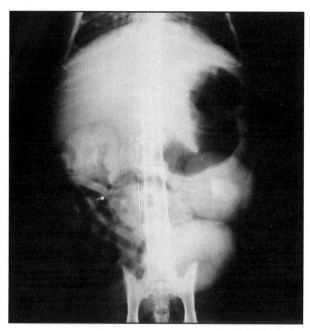

Figure 44-13: An abdominal radiograph showing a mineralized left adrenal mass in a cat with a cortisol-secreting AT. (Courtesy of D. Greco)

advisable to start with a lower dose (25 mg/kg/day) and increase it if the cat tolerates the lower dose.[119,127] After a "loading dose" is administered daily for 1 week, maintenance therapy (50 mg/kg/week in two divided daily doses) is used.[119,145] Some authors suggest the concurrent administration of the mineralocorticoid fludrocortisone (0.01 mg/kg daily) and the glucocorticoid prednisone (0.3 mg/kg daily),[119] although this is by no means a universal recommendation.

KEY POINT

Medical management may be used to improve the clinical signs in a cat prior to surgical adrenalectomy.

The success of mitotane is variable. Clinical signs abated and insulin dosage was able to be decreased in one cat after 3 months of mitotane therapy, and disease was controlled for a year with a mitotane dose of 12.5 mg/kg/week.[119] Disease control had been excellent in another cat until a hypoadrenal crisis occurred after 10 months of mitotane treatment (50 mg/kg/week).[145] Mitotane doses should be adjusted following periodic adrenal testing. Other authors found mitotane to have little success in treating cats with hyperadrenocorticism.[126,127]

Ketoconazole interferes with steroid hormone production; the recommended dose is 15 mg/kg every 12 hours. Toxicity (dry hair coat and weight loss) has been seen in some cats,[150] and control of the symptoms has been vari-

able.[126,130,150] Clinical signs improved in one cat with an adrenal adenocarcinoma after 4 to 5 months of ketoconazole treatment, but there was no improvement in adrenal response.[132]

Metyrapone inhibits 11β-hydroxylase, resulting in inhibition of cortisol production. Metyrapone (65 mg/kg q12h) resulted in decreased ACTH response within 5 days and clinical improvement (thicker skin, decreased insulin requirement) within 2 weeks.[134,151] One cat became hypocortisolemic when a higher dose (65 mg/kg q8h) was used; depression, tremors, and ataxia developed within 2 days.[134] As with mitotane and ketoconazole, responses to metyrapone are variable.

KEY POINT

Adrenalectomy, bilateral for PDH and unilateral for AT, is probably the treatment of choice for hyperadrenocorticism.

When medial management is used, it is important to monitor adrenal function to avoid precipitating a hypoadrenal crisis. An alternative approach is to use concurrent mineralocorticoids and glucocorticoids (as outlined above) which should avoid a hypoadrenal crisis. In addition, it is important to monitor DM in cats receiving exogenous insulin. Control of hyperadrenocorticism may result in reduced insulin resistance and thus a reduced insulin requirement. Continuation of insulin therapy without adjustment may precipitate a hypoglycemic crisis.[130,134]

Surgical excision of the adrenal glands, bilaterally for PDH or unilaterally for an AT, is probably the treatment of choice (Figure 44-14). Surgical success is often compromised by poor wound healing due to thin, easily torn skin as well as secondary infections.[126,129] It may be advisable to gain some degree of medical control prior to surgery.

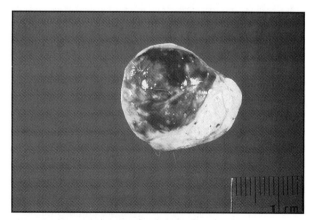

Figure 44-14: Excision of this adrenal adenoma in a hyperadrenocorticoid cat resulted in reduction of insulin requirement for concurrent diabetes and improvement in clinical signs.

Metyrapone was used successfully in one cat to reverse skin changes prior to surgery.[134]

Many different protocols have been used to prevent hypoadrenal crisis in the perioperative period. One study recommended continuous IV infusion of hydrocortisone at a rate of 625 µg/kg/hour during and for 48 hours after surgery.[126] Following surgery, cats must receive supplemental mineralocorticoid (e.g., fludrocortisone, 0.1 mg/day) and corticosteroid (e.g., prednisone, 2.5 mg/day) for life. These doses may need to be adjusted based on serum potassium levels, which should be measured daily for the first 48 hours after surgery and then monthly until the cat is stable. Similarly, reevaluation of diabetes should be made periodically as insulin requirements should reduce. Insulin can be discontinued in many cats 2 to 8 months after surgery.[126] Acute hypokalemia occurred within 24 hours of surgery in seven of eight cats that underwent adrenalectomy in one study[126]; this was followed by a rebound hyperkalemia in four of these cats 4 to 8 days later, emphasizing the need for close monitoring in the first 2 weeks after surgery.

Bilateral adrenalectomy for PDH has been reported for 14 cats.[126-128,152] Five cats died within the first 2 weeks after surgery due to skin slough,[126,127] pancreatitis and peritonitis,[126] embolic diseases,[126] and possible hypoadrenal crisis.[128] Survival for the remaining 9 cats ranged from 3 months to 60 months. Three cats died of unrelated disease; two other cats died of adrenal insufficiency, presumably due to poor owner compliance in administering replacement hormones. Median survival for these 9 cats was 9 months.

Adrenal adenoma was treated via unilateral adrenalectomy in three cats. One was treated with cortisone postoperatively, but no further follow-up information was provided.[131] An adrenal adenoma occurred on the contralateral side in the other two cats, one at 10 months and the other at 12 months after the first surgery.[126,127] One of these cats lived another 15 months but was lost to follow-up.[126] No further information was provided for the third cat. Unilateral adrenalectomy for an adrenal carcinoma was successful in another cat until metastases developed 12 months after surgery.[126]

Pituitary surgery is very difficult in cats because of the high vascularity around the pituitary fossa; however, a technique using a transsphenoidal approach has been described[111] (see the Pituitary Tumors section). The complication and mortality rates for both this surgery and adrenalectomy require that only experienced surgeons attempt these procedures.

Radiation of the pituitary may control ACTH production, but results are variable. Two cats died within 2 months of radiation therapy.[126,127] Another cat that had become resistant to mitotane and developed CNS signs due to a large pituitary tumor had a complete remission to radiation therapy by 10 months after treatment.[145] This cat died due to DM 2 years after radiation therapy. Further information on radiation therapy is found in the section on pituitary tumors.

ADRENAL TUMORS[a]

CLINICAL BRIEFING

Common Presentation	Aldosterone-secreting tumors, which cause severe hypokalemia, are very rare. Pheochromocytoma, which causes epinephrine release, is also rare. Progesterone-secreting adrenal tumors have been reported.
Staging and Diagnosis	Specific tests to confirm diagnosis are included in each section. Serum aldosterone and progesterone can be measured; serum epinephrine levels are unreliable. MDB and abdominal ultrasonography to image tumor and potential metastases are indicated. Fine-needle aspiration is probably unwise.
Treatment	
Initial	Adrenalectomy is curative for benign tumors and will palliate signs in all cats. Extra care needed with anesthesia and postoperative monitoring in cats with pheochromocytoma.
Adjunctive	Chemotherapy has not been described for these tumors.
Supportive	Symptomatic medical treatment with potassium chloride, amlodipine, and spironolactone for aldosterone-secreting tumors may be palliative. Presurgical stabilization is important for pheochromocytoma.

[a]Cortisol-secreting adrenal tumors are discussed in the Hyperadrenocorticism section.

ALDOSTERONE-SECRETING TUMORS

Incidence, Signalment, and Etiology

Although more cases are suggested in the literature,[153] there are only four case reports of aldosterone-secreting tumors. Three occurred in DSHs (ages: 10, 17, and 20 years old) and one in a 5-year-old DLH. Two tumors were adenocarcinomas,[154,155] and one was an adenoma (Figure 44-15).[156]

Clinical Presentation and History

One affected cat had been anorectic and depressed for 3 weeks but on presentation was collapsed with flaccid muscular weakness and decreased reflexes secondary to severe hypokalemia. There was no evidence of renal, gastrointestinal, or endocrine pancreatic disease.[154] A second cat showed ventroflexion of the neck and generalized weakness, both of which were episodic.[156] There was no evidence of muscle weakness in the other two cats, but they had lost weight and were blind due to retinal detachment[155]; both were polydipsic and polyuric.

Staging and Diagnosis

Hyperaldosteronism causes sodium retention and hence increased intravascular volume and hypertension. Blood pressure measurements were high in both cats in one report.[155]

The MDB, which should be part of staging, showed very low serum potassium and normal to high sodium in all four cats reported with aldosterone-secreting tumors. Potassium remained low after supplementation, and the urinary fractional excretion of potassium (FE_K) was very high (>50%) in one cat; a low FE_K (<6%) would be expected in hypokalemic cats.[155] Secondary muscle damage was indicated by a very high serum creatine kinase (CK) in one cat.[156]

Serum aldosterone was 181 ng/dl in one cat (normal, 22.7 ng/dl), over 3,000 pg/ml in two cats (normal, 194–388 pg/ml),[155,157] and 39,000 pmol/L in the fourth cat (normal, 150–430 pmol/L).[156]

Radiographs showed an irregular area cranial to the left kidney in one cat, but ultrasonography is superior for imaging the adrenal gland.[156] Abdominal ultrasonography detected a 1 cm adrenal mass in one cat and 3 cm masses in two others.[155,156] In two cats, a fine-needle aspirate from the mass showed evidence of a neuroendocrine tumor.[155] Thoracic radiographs should also be performed as part of a thorough staging protocol, as metastases to the lung have been reported.[154]

Treatment

Surgical excision of the AT was performed in one cat.[155] All hypertensive medications were discontinued when serum potassium became normal 5 days after surgery. Serum aldosterone normalized approximately 1 month after surgery. The cat died 1 year later (at 22 years of age), and no necropsy was performed. Biochemical abnormalities resolved in a second cat with an adrenal adenoma within 6 days of surgery to remove the tumor; the cat was still normal 20 months after surgery.[156]

Medical management of aldosterone-secreting tumors involves interference with the potassium-wasting effects of aldosterone. Spironolactone is an aldosterone antagonist that binds to renal tubular aldosterone receptors. If spironolactone is used, supplementation with potassium gluconate may be unnecessary. The recommended dose for spironolactone is 2 to 4 mg/kg/day and for potassium gluconate is 2 to 6 mEq/day. Amlodipine blocks sodium available for the Na/K pumps, thereby decreasing kaliuresis.

In one of the cats treated medically, initial symptomatic treatment with potassium chloride (24 mmol/day PO) maintained normal serum potassium until treatment with spironolactone (12.5 mg/day PO) was started. Potassium supplementation was able to be discontinued until the cat's condition deteriorated 3 months later. On necropsy, the primary tumor was 4 × 5 × 3 cm in size, and pulmonary and hepatic metastases were present.[154] Normal serum potassium was maintained in a second cat treated medically with potassium gluconate (4 mEq at each meal) and spironolactone (2.5 mg/kg q12h) Repeat ultrasonography showed an increase in tumor dimensions from 3 to 4.7 cm with invasion and thrombus formation in the caudal vena cava. Aspirin and amlodipine (0.18 mg/kg/day) were added, but the cat died of embolic disease 7 months later.

PHEOCHROMOCYTOMA

Incidence, Signalment, and Etiology

Pheochromocytoma is rarely reported in cats and is often an incidental finding. *Paraganglioma* is another term used for this epinephrine-secreting tumor.

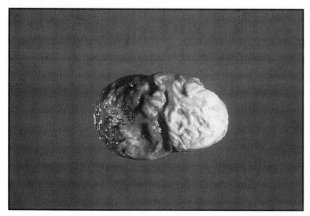

Figure 44-15: *An aldosterone-secreting adrenal adenocarcinoma that was removed from an 18-year-old castrated male DSH.*

The age range in eight reported cats was 8[95] to 18[158] years (median, 15 years). All cats for which breed information was available were DSHs.[158–161] There was no apparent gender predilection.

One cat with pheochromocytoma, thyroid adenoma, and parathyroid hyperplasia fulfills the criteria for MEN-II (multiple endocrine neoplasia-II),[160] which is the only report of this condition in a cat.

> *MDB = minimum database; includes CBC, biochemical profile, urinalysis, FeLV/FIV serology, T₄ testing, and thoracic radiographs (three views).*

Clinical Presentation and History

Pheochromocytoma was an apparently incidental finding in a cat with a perianal apocrine adenocarcinoma[159] and in a hyperthyroid diabetic cat.[160] In other cats, clinical signs were nonspecific but included polydipsia and polyuria (four cats), intermittent vomiting (two cats), listlessness, seizures, and oily hair coat. Signs consistent with epinephrine release were not obvious, although plasma epinephrine levels were high in one cat.[161] Pheochromocytomas ranged greatly in size; tumors 2 cm in diameter or larger were palpable adjacent to the kidney.[158,161] The tumor was 7 cm in diameter in one cat.[95]

Staging and Diagnosis

Staging for pheochromocytoma should include an MDB, abdominal ultrasound, and thoracic radiographs. Radiographs of the abdomen were not always helpful in delineating a mass,[158] even when it was palpable. Ultrasonography was more reliable in imaging the tumor[161] and allowed the clinician to determine its exact location prior to surgical intervention. In one cat, abdominal ultrasonography as part of staging for an unrelated tumor disclosed an adrenal mass[159] and allowed a guided biopsy. Ultrasonography may also allow visualization of the vena cava for evidence of tumor invasion.

The finding of an adrenal mass on ultrasonography should be further pursued with screening tests for hyperadrenocorticism (see the Hyperadrenocorticism section), which will be normal if the tumor is a pheochromocytoma.[161] Plasma epinephrine was 0.592 ng/ml in one cat and between 0.03 and 0.029 ng/ml in two normal cats. This test is probably not useful to practitioners because of difficulties in sample processing and interpretation. Other tests used in human patients are not widely available in veterinary medicine.[162]

Metastases were not reported in any of the recent cases. Carpenter and colleagues[95] cite a report by Vlaovitch of pulmonary metastases from a pheochromocytoma.

Treatment

Surgical excision is the treatment of choice for pheochromocytoma, but anesthetic management is critical during the procedure. Recommendations include α-adrenergic blocking agents to reduce the risk of severe hypertension during handling of the tumor and β-adrenergic blocking agents only if tachycardia or dysrhythmia occurs. Preanesthetic narcotic agents with glycopyrrolate followed by an opioid for anesthetic induction and isoflurane for maintenance have been recommended.[162] Phenothiazines, such as acepromazine, should be avoided as they may precipitate a hypotensive crisis. Because of the risk of hypotension, central venous pressure should be continually monitored during surgery in addition to ECG and arterial blood pressure. Dysrhythmias may occur during tumor manipulation but should resolve quickly.[158] If hypotension occurs, volume expansion should be rapidly undertaken; dopamine (2 μg/kg/min) has been used, but crystalloid fluids are a better choice.[161]

Pheochromocytomas may be highly vascularized, and postoperative monitoring of the cat's hematocrit is important. A rapid drop in hematocrit should be treated by transfusion.[159] Of the four cats treated surgically, one died of unknown causes postoperatively,[95] one died of progressive anemia 3 days after surgery,[158] and one died of pulmonary edema and thrombus formation soon after surgery.[159] The fourth cat required prednisone (1 mg/kg PO sid) for 6 weeks after adrenalectomy but then became clinically normal. At a recheck, the plasma epinephrine level had fallen from 0.592 ng/ml to 0.048 ng/ml.[161] Surgical excision should not be attempted without anesthetic monitoring and postoperative critical care capabilities.

Nondomestic Felidae

A 21-year-old male jaguar *(Panthera onca)* died after a period of lameness, anorexia, depression, and ataxia. In addition to multiple myeloma and an adrenocortical carcinoma, a pheochromocytoma with lymph node and hepatic metastases was found.[163] The clinical signs in this cat were not thought to be related to either adrenal neoplasm.

RETROPERITONEAL PARAGANGLIOMA

Two such tumors have been described.[95] One was found as a benign tumor in an asymptomatic 15-year-old cat. A second 14-year-old cat had "episodes" consistent with epinephrine release (salivation, rapid abdominal breathing, panting, and tail twitching) during which time the pupils dilated, hair stood on end, and heart rate increased.[95] A palpable abdominal mass was surgically removed from an area ventral to the caudal vena cava, and although the "episodes" did not recur over a 4 year period, splenic metastases were found on necropsy.[95]

Nondomestic Felidae

An 18-year-old tiger *(Panthera tigris)* collapsed suddenly and died due to a massive retroperitoneal hemorrhage. A retroperitoneal paraganglioma was identified at necropsy but had not been suspected clinically.[164]

PROGESTERONE-SECRETING ADRENAL TUMORS

Incidence, Signalment, and Etiology

Progesterone may cause insulin resistance in addition to alopecia, thinning of the skin, and poor wound healing. The signs are very similar to those caused by hyperadrenocorticism.

Clinical Presentation and History

Two 7-year-old castrated male cats, a Himalayan and a DSH, had chronic alopecia of the trunk and were polydipsic and polyuric. One cat had become increasingly aggressive,[149] and the other was a poorly regulated diabetic.[165]

Staging and Diagnosis

Adrenal testing (outlined in the section on hyperadrenocorticism) should be performed in cats with clinical signs consistent with hyperadrenocorticism. Other diagnostic tests should include an MDB, thoracic radiographs, and abdominal ultrasonography.

In the two cats reported, an ACTH stimulation test and a dexamethasone-suppression test showed that these animals were not hyperadrenocorticoid despite the ultrasonographic finding of a unilaterally enlarged adrenal gland. The resting serum progesterone was high (3.62 ng/ml in one and 13.2 ng/ml in the other) in both cats and was further elevated after ACTH administration (27.6 and 15.5 ng/ml, respectively). Normal cats had values between 0.03 and 0.35 ng/ml.[149,165] One cat also had an elevated serum testosterone concentration (0.71 ng/ml; normal, <0.04 ng/ml).[165]

Treatment

Surgical excision of a well-differentiated adrenal cortical carcinoma led to resolution of clinical signs and hyperprogesteronemia in one cat.[149] The cat required long-term prednisone therapy (1.25 mg/day PO) but had a normal hair coat within 12 months.

The second cat was treated medically with aminoglutethimide, an inhibitor of enzymatic cleavage during synthesis of multiple adrenal steroid hormones. The drug was administered at 6 mg/kg PO every 12 hours, and the cat improved clinically for 2 weeks but then deteriorated and died.[165]

OTHER ADRENAL TUMORS

A 12-year-old female DSH was inappetent and lame due to hypertrophic osteopathy of all four limbs. Removal of an apparently nonfunctional adrenal carcinoma caused resolution of both the hypertrophic osteopathy and retinal hemorrhages within 4 months of surgery.[166]

Nondomestic Felidae

Adrenal adenoma or adenocarcinoma was diagnosed in two nondomestic felids in a survey at the San Antonio Zoo.[89] In addition, an adrenal adenocarcinoma that had metastasized to the kidney was reported in a tiger *(Panthera tigris)*.[85]

A 14-year-old male cougar *(Felis concolor)* was inappetent, vomiting, polyuric, and polydipsic and had diarrhea. It was azotemic for 18 months before a 6 cm adrenal adenoma was palpated in the dorsocranial abdomen.[167] No treatment was attempted.

REFERENCES

1. Holzworth J, Theran P, Carpenter JL, et al: Hyperthyroidism in the cat: Ten cases. *JAVMA* 176:345–353, 1980.
2. O'Brien SE, Riley JH, Hagemoser WA: Unilateral thyroid neoplasm in a cat. *Vet Rec* 107:199–200, 1980.
3. Jones BR, Johnstone AC: Hyperthroidism in an aged cat. *N Z Vet J* 29:70–72, 1981.
4. Lucke VM: An histological study of thyroid abnormalities in the domestic cat. *J Small Anim Pract* 5:351–358, 1964.
5. Broussard JD, Peterson ME, Fox PR: Changes in clinical and laboratory findings in cats with hyperthyroidism from 1983–1993. *JAVMA* 206:302–305, 1995.
6. Miyamoto T, Kato M, Kuwamura M, et al: A first feline case of cardiomyopathy associated with hyperthyroidism due to thyroid adenoma in Japan. *Feline Pract* 26:6–9, 1998.
7. Peterson ME, Becker DV: Radioiodine treatment of 524 cats with hyperthyroidism. *JAVMA* 207:1422–1428, 1995.
8. Peterson ME, Livingston P, Brown RS: Lack of circulating thyroid stimulating immunoglobulins in cats with hyperthyroidism. *Vet Immunol Immunopathol* 16:277–282, 1987.
9. Kennedy RL: Autoantibodies in feline hyperthyroidism. *Res Vet Sci* 45:300–306, 1988.
10. Merryman JI, Buckles EL, Bowers G, et al: Overexpression of *c-ras* in hyperplasia and adenomas of the feline thyroid gland: An immunohistochemical analysis of 34 cases. *Vet Pathol* 36:117–124, 1999.
11. Scarlett JM, Moise NS, Rayl J: Feline hyperthyroidism: A descriptive and case control study. *Prev Med* 6:295–309, 1988.
12. Kass PH, Peterson ME, Levy J, et al: Evaluation of environmental, nutritional, and host factors in cats with hyperthyroidism. *J Vet Intern Med* 13:323–329, 1999.
13. Jones BR, Hodge H, Davies E: The prevalence of feline immunodeficiency virus infection in hyperthyroid cats. *N Z Vet J* 23–24, 1995.
14. Hoenig M, Goldschmidt MH, Ferguson DC, et al: Toxic nodular goitre in the cat. *J Small Anim Pract* 23:1–12, 1982.
15. Joseph RJ, Peterson ME: Review and comparison of neuromuscular and central nervous system manifestations of hyperthyroidism in cats and humans. *Prog Vet Neurol* 3:114–119, 1998.
16. Kintzer PP, Peterson ME: Thyroid scintigraphy in small animals. *Semin Vet Med Surg Small Anim* 8:131–139, 1991.
17. Lenarduzzi RF, Jones L: Feline hyperthryoidism: Curing the condition, understanding the cause. *Vet Med* 81:242–244, 1986.
18. Rozanski EA, Stobie D: Laryngeal paralysis secondary to a cystic thyroid adenoma in a cat. *Feline Pract* 23:6–7, 1995.
19. Peterson ME, Kintzer PP, Cavanagh PG, et al: Feline hyperthyroidism: Pretreatment clinical and laboratory evaluation of 131 cases. *JAVMA* 183:103–110, 1983.

20. Aucoin DP, Rubin RL, Petereson ME, et al: Dose-dependent induction of anti-native DNA antibodies in cats by propylthiouracil. *Arthritis Rheum* 31: 688–692, 1988.

21. Liu S-K, Peterson ME, Fox PR: Hypertrophic cardiomyopathy and hyperthyroidism in the cat. *JAVMA* 185:52–57, 1984.

22. Cowell RL, Cowell AK: Pseudochylous thoracic effusion and hyperthyroidism in a cat. *Mod Vet Pract* 80:309–312, 1985.

23. Fox PR, Petereson ME, Broussard JD: Electrocardiographic and radiographic changes in cats with hyperthyroidism: Comparison of populations evaluated during 1992–1993 vs. 1979–1982. *JAAHA* 35:27–31, 1999.

24. Peterson ME, Graves TK, Cavanagh I: Serum thyroid hormone concentrations fluctuate in cats with hyperthyroidism. *J Vet Intern Med* 1:142–146, 1987.

25. Broome MR, Feldman EC, Turrel JM: Serial determination of thyroxine concentrations in hyperthyroid cats. *JAVMA* 192:49–51, 1988.

26. Chaitman J, Hess R, Senz R, et al: Thyroid adenomatous hyperplasia in euthyroid cats [abstract 67]. *J Vet Intern Med* 13:242, 1999.

27. Peterson ME, Gamble DA: Effect of nonthyroidal illness on serum thyroxine concentrations in cats: 494 cases (1988). *JAVMA* 197:1203–1208, 1990.

28. Graves TK, Peterson ME: Diagnosis of occult hyperthyroidism in cats. *Prob Vet Med* 2:683–692, 1990.

29. Peterson ME, Graves TK, Gamble DA: Triiodothyrine (T3) suppression test. An aid in the diagnosis of mild hyperthyroidism in cats. *J Vet Intern Med* 4: 233–238, 1990.

30. Refsal KR, Nachreiner RF, Stein BE, et al: Use of the triiodothyronine suppression test for diagnosis of hyperthyroidism in ill cats that have serum concentration of iodothyronines within normal range. *JAVMA* 199:1594–1601, 1991.

31. Hoenig M, Ferguson DC: Assessment of thyroid functional reserve in the cat by the thyrotropin-stimulation test. *Am J Vet Res* 44:1229–1232, 1983.

32. Tomsa K, Glaus TM, Kacl GM, et al: Thyrotropin-releasing hormone stimulation test to assess thyroid function in severely sick cats. *J Vet Intern Med* 15: 89–93, 2001.

33. Moise NS, Dietze AE: Echocardiographic, electrocardiographic, and radiographic detection of cardiomegaly in hyperthyroid cats. *Am J Vet Res* 47: 1487–1494, 1986.

34. Peterson ME, Keene B, Ferguson DC, et al: Electrocardiographic findings in 45 cats with hyperthyroidism. *JAVMA* 180:934–937, 1982.

35. Bond BR, Fox PR, Peterson ME, et al: Echocardiographic findings in 103 cats with hyperthyroidism. *JAVMA* 192:1546–1549, 1988.

36. Kobayashi DL, Peterson ME, Graves TK, et al: Hypertension in cats with chronic renal failure or hyperthyroidism. *J Vet Intern Med* 4:58–62, 1990.

37. Venzin I, Vannini R: Feline hyperthyreose. *Kleintierpraxis* 35:183–188, 1990.

38. DiBartola SP, Broome MR, Stein BS, et al: Effect of treatment of hyperthyroidism on renal function in cats. *JAVMA* 208:875–878, 1996.

39. Wisner ER, Théon AP, Nyland TG, et al: Ultrasonographic examination of the thyroid gland of hyperthyroid cats: Comparison to $^{99m}TcO_4^-$ scintigraphy. *Vet Radiol Ultrasound* 35:53–58, 1994.

40. Noxon JO, Thornburg LP, Dillender MJ, et al: An adenoma in ectopic thyroid tissue causing hyperthyroidism in a cat. *JAAHA* 19:369–372, 1983.

41. Peterson ME, Becker DV: Radionuclide thyroid imaging in 135 cats with hyperthyroidism. *Vet Radiol* 25:23–27, 1984.

42. Mooney CT, Thoday KL, Nicoll JJ, et al: Qualitative and quantitative thyroid imaging in feline hyperthyroidism using technetium-99M as pertechnetate. *Vet Radiol Ultrasound* 33:313–320, 1992.

43. Swalec KM, Birchard SJ: Recurrence of hyperthyroidism after thyroidectomy in cats. *JAAHA* 26:433–437, 1990.

44. Trepanier LA, Peterson ME: Pharmacokinetics of methimazole in normal cats and cats with hyperthyroidism. *Res Vet Sci* 50:69–74,1991.

45. Peterson ME: Propylthiouracil in the treatment of feline hyperthyroidism. *JAVMA* 179:485–487, 1981.

46. Peterson ME, Hurvitz AI, Leib MS, et al: Propylthiouracil-associated hemolytic anemia, thrombocytopenia and antinuclear antibodies in cats with hyperthyrodism. *JAVMA* 184:806, 1984.

47. Aucoin DP, Peterson ME, Hurvitz AI, et al: Propylthiouracil-induced immune-mediated disease in the cat. *J Pharm Exp Therap* 234:13–18, 1985.

48. Peterson ME, Kintzer PP, Hurvitz AI: Methimazole treatment of 262 cats with hyperthyroidism. *J Vet Intern Med* 2:150, 1988.

49. Reine NJ, Peterson ME, Hohenhaus AE: Effects of methimazole on hemostatic parameters in cats with hyperthyroidism [abstract 76]. *J Vet Intern Med* 13: 245, 1999.

50. Mooney CT, Thoday KL, Doxey DL: Carbimazole therapy of feline hyperthyroidism. *J Small Anim Pract* 33:228–235, 1992.

51. Murray LAS, Peterson ME: Ipodate treatment of hyperthyroidism in cats. *JAVMA* 211:63–67, 1997.

52. Walker MC, Schaer M: Percutaneous ethanol treatment of hyperthyroidism in a cat. *Feline Pract* 26:10–12, 1998.

53. Wells AL, Long CD, Hornof WJ, et al: Use of percutaneous ethanol injection for treatment of bilateral nodules in cats *JAVMA* 218:1293–1297, 2001.

54. Goldstein RE, Long C, Swift NC, et al: Percutaneous ethanol injection for treatment of unilateral hyperplastic thyroid nodules in cats. *JAVMA* 218:1298–1302, 2001.

55. Jacobs G, Hutson C, Dougherty J, et al: Congestive heart failure associated with hyperthyroidism in cats. *JAVMA* 188:52–56, 1986.

56. Birchard SJ, Peterson ME, Jacobson A: Surgical treatment of feline hyperthyroidism: Results of 85 cases. *JAAHA* 20:705–709, 1984.

57. Foster DJ, Thoday KL: Use of propranolol and potassium iodate in the presurgical management of hyperthyroid cats. *J Small Anim Pract* 40:307–315, 1999.

58. Flanders JA: Surgical treatment of hyperthyroid cats. *Mod Vet Pract* 67: 711–715, 1986.

59. Flanders JA, Harvey HJ, Erb HN: Correspondence. *Vet Surg* 17:59, 1988.

60. Welches CD, Scavelli TD, Matthiesen DT, et al: Occurrence of problems after three techniques of bilateral thyroidectomy in cats. *Vet Surg* 18:392–396, 1989.

61. Liptak JM: Unilateral extracapsular thyroidectomy for a non-functional cystic thyroid adenoma. *Aust Vet Pract* 26:174–177, 1996.

62. Flanders JA: Surgical options for the treatment of hyperthyroidism in the cat. *J Feline Med Surg* 1:127–134, 1999.

63. Padgett SL, Tobias KM, Leathers CW, et al: Efficacy of parathyroid gland autotransplantation in maintaining serum calcium concentrations after bilateral thyroparathyroidectomy in cats. *JAAHA* 34:219–224, 1998.

64. Smith TA, Bruyette DS, Hoskinson JJ, et al: Radioiodine treatment outcome in hyperthyroid cats: Effect of prior methimazole treatment. *J Vet Intern Med* 9:183, 1995.

65. Meric SM, Rubin SI: Serum thyroxine concentrations following fixed-dose radioactive iodine treatment in hyperthyroid cats: 62 cases (1986–1989). *JAVMA* 197:621–623, 1990.

66. Craig A, Zuber M, Allan GS: A prospective study of 66 cases of feline hyperthyroidism treated with a fixed dose of intravenous ^{131}I. *Aust Vet Pract* 23:2–6, 1993.

67. Meric SM, Hawkins EC, Washabau RJ, et al: Serum thyroxine concentrations after radioactive iodine therapy in cats with hyperthyroidism. *JAVMA* 188: 1038–1040, 1986.

68. Malik R, Lamb WA, Church DB: Treatment of feline hyperthyroidism using orally administered radioiodine: A study of 40 consecutive cases. *Austr Vet J* 70:218–219, 1993.

69. Theon AP, VanVechten MK, Feldman E: A prospective randomized comparison of intravenous versus subcutaneous administration of radioiodine for treatment of feline hyperthyroidism: A study of 120 cats. *Am J Vet Res* 55: 1734–1738, 1994.

70. Mooney CT: Radioactive iodine therapy for feline hyperthyroidism: Efficacy and administration routes. *J Small Anim Pract* 35:289–294, 1994.

71. Broome MR, Turrel JM, Hays MT: Predictive value of tracer studies for ^{131}I treatment in hyperthyroid cats. *Am J Vet Res* 49:193–197, 1988.

72. Turrel JM, Feldman EC, Hays M, et al: Radioactive iodine therapy in cats with hyperthyroidism. *JAVMA* 184:554–559, 1984.

73. Klausner JS, Johnston GR, Feeney DA, et al: Results of radioactive iodine therapy in 23 cats with hyperthyroidism. *Minn J Vet Med* 27:28–32, 1987.

74. Handelsman H, Broder LE, Slavik M, et al: Streptozotocin NSC-85998. Clinical brochure. Invest Drug Branch Cancer Ther Eval Div Cancer Treatment. National Cancer Inst, pp 1–68, 1974.

75. Patnaik AK, Lieberman PH: Feline anaplastic giant cell adenocarcinoma of the thyroid. *Vet Pathol* 16:687–692, 1979.

76. Cowen PN, Jackson P: Thyroid carcinoma in a cat. *Vet Rec* 114:521–522, 1984.

77. King JM: Thyroid adenocarcinoma. *Vet Med* 89:1113, 1994.

78. Turrel JM, Feldman EC, Nelson RW, et al: Thyroid carcinoma causing hyperthyroidism in cats: 14 cases (1981–1986). *JAVMA* 193:359–364, 1988.

79. Guptill L, Scott-Moncrieff CR, Janovitz EB, et al: Response to high-dose radioactive iodine administration in cats with thyroid carcinoma that had previously undergone surgery. *JAVMA* 8:1055–1058, 1995.

80. Holzworth J, Husted P, Wind A: Arterial thrombosis and thyroid carcinoma in a cat. *Cornell Vet* 45:487–496, 1955.

81. Johnson KH, Osborne CA: Adenocarcinoma of the thyroid gland in a cat. *JAVMA* 156:906–912, 1970.

82. Clark ST, Meier H: A clinico-pathological study of thyroid disease in the dog and cat. *Zentralbl Veterinärmed* 5:17–32, 1958.

83. von Sandersleben J, Hänichen T: Tumours of the thyroid gland. *Bull WHO* 50:35–42, 1974.

84. Leav I, Schiller AL, Rijnber Rijnberk A, et al: Adenomas and carcinomas of the canine and feline thyroid. *Am J Pathol* 83:61–93, 1976.

85. Hubbard GB, Schmidt RE, Fletcher KC: Neoplasia in zoo animals. *J Zoo Anim Med* 14:33–40, 1983.

86. Lombard LS, Witte EJ: Frequency and types of tumors in mammals and birds of the Philadelphia Zoological Garden. *Cancer Res* 19:127–141, 1959.

87. Kennedy GA, Strafuss AC: Multiple neoplasia in an aged cougar. *J Zoo Anim Med* 7:24–26, 1976.

88. Li X, Steinburg H, Wallace C, et al: Functional thyroid follicular adenocarcinoma in a captive mountain lion *(Felis concolor)*. *Vet Pathol* 29:549–551, 1992.

89. Schmidt RE, Hubbard GB, Fletcher KC: Systematic survey of lesions from animals in a zoologic collection: IV. Endocrine glands. *J Zoo Anim Med* 17:24–28, 1986.

90. McMillan FD, Barr B, Feldman EC: Functional pancreatic islet cell tumor in a cat. *JAAHA* 21:741–746, 1985.

91. O'Brien TD, Norton F, Turner TM, et al: Pancreatic endocrine tumor in a cat: Clinical, pathological, and immunohistochemical evaluation. *JAAHA* 26:453–457, 1990.

92. Priester WA: Pancreatic islet cell tumors in domestic animals. Data from 11 colleges of veterinary medicine in the United States and Canada. *J Natl Cancer Inst* 53:227–229, 1974.

93. Myers NCIII, Andrews GA, Chard-Bergstrom C: Chromogranin A plasma concentration and expression in pancreatic islet cell tumors of dogs and cats. *Am J Vet Res* 58:615–620, 1997.

94. Nielsen SW: Neoplastic diseases, in Catcott EJ (ed): *Feline Medicine and Surgery*. Santa Barbara, CA, American Veterinary Publications, 1964, pp 156–176.

95. Carpenter JL, Andrews LK, Holzworth J: Tumors and tumor-like lesions, in Holzworth J (ed): *Diseases of the Cat. Medicine and Surgery*. Philadelphia, WB Saunders, 1987, pp 407–596.

96. Middleton DJ, Watson ADJ: Duodenal ulceration associated with gastrin-secreting pancreatic tumor in a cat. *JAVMA* 183:461–462, 1983.

97. van der Gaag I, van den Ingh TSGAM, Lamers CBHW, et al: Zollinger-Ellison syndrome in a cat. *Vet Q* 10:151–155, 1988.

98. Blunden AS, Wheeler SJ, Davies JV: Hyperparathyroidism in the cat of probable primary origin. *J Small Anim Pract* 27:791–798, 1986.

99. den Hertog E, Goossens MMC, van der Linden-Sipman JS, et al: Primary hyperparathyroidism in two cats. *Vet Q* 19:81–84, 1997.

100. Kallet AJ, Richter KP, Feldman EC, et al: Primary hyperparathyroidism in cats: Seven cases (1984–1989). *JAVMA* 199:1767–1771, 1991.

101. Marquez GA, Klausner JS, Osborne CA: Calcium oxalate urolithiasis in a cat with a functional parathyroid adenocarcinoma. *JAVMA* 206:817–819, 1995.

102. Sueda MT, Stefanacci JD: Ultrasound evaluation of the parathyroid glands in two hypercalcemic cats. *Vet Radiol Ultrasound* 41:448–451, 2000.

103. Doster AR, Armstrong DL, Bargar TW: Seminoma and parathyroid adenoma in a snow leopard *(Panthera unica)*. *J Comp Pathol* 100:475–480, 1989.

104. Zaki FA, Liu S–K: Pituitary chromophobe adenoma in a cat. *Vet Pathol* 10:232–237, 1973.

105. Zaki F, Harris J, Budzilovich G: Cystic pituicytoma of the neurohypophysis in a Siamese cat. *J Comp Pathol* 85:467–471, 1975.

106. Davidson MG, Nasisse MP, Breitschwerdt EB, et al: Acute blindness associated with intracranial tumors in dogs and cats: Eight cases (1984–1989). *JAVMA* 199:755–758, 1991.

107. Peterson ME, Taylor RS, Greco DS, et al: Acromegaly in 14 cats. *J Vet Intern Med* 4:192–201, 1990.

108. Goossens MMC, Feldman EC, Nelson RW, et al: Cobalt 60 irradiation of pituitary gland tumors in three cats with acromegaly. *JAVMA* 213:374–376, 1998.

109. Eigenmann JE, Wortman JA, Haskins ME: Elevated growth hormone levels and diabetes mellitus in a cat with acromegalic features. *JAAHA* 20:747–752, 1984.

110. Abrams-Ogg ACG, Holmberg DL, Stewart WA, et al: Acromegaly in a cat: Diagnosis by magnetic resonance imaging and treatment by cryohypophysectomy. *Can Vet J* 34:682–685, 1993.

111. Meij B, Voorhout G, van den Ingh TSGAM, et al: Transsphenoidal hypophy-

112. Zaki FA, Hurvitz AI: Spontaneous neoplasms of the central nervous system of the cat. *J Small Anim Pract* 17:773–782, 1976.

113. Middleton DJ, Culvenor JA, Vasak E, et al: Growth hormone-producing pituitary adenoma, elevated serum somatomedin C concentrations and diabetes mellitus in a cat. *Can Vet J* 26:169–171, 1985.

114. Heinrichs M, Baumgärtner W, Krug-Manntz S: Immunocytochemical demonstration of growth hormone in an acidophilic adenoma of the adenohypophysis in a cat. *Vet Pathol* 26:179–180, 1989.

115. Morrison SA, Randolf J, Lothrop CD: Hypersomatotropism and insulin-resistant diabetes mellitus in a cat. *JAVMA* 194:91–94, 1989.

116. Lichtensteiger CA, Wortman JA, Eigenmann JE: Functional pituitary acidophil adenoma in a cat with diabetes mellitus and acromegalic features. *Vet Pathol* 23:518–521, 1986.

117. Elliott DA, Feldman EC, Koblik PD, et al: Prevalence of pituitary tumors among diabetic cats with insulin resistance. *JAVMA* 216:1765–1768, 2000.

118. Furuzawa Y, Une Y, Nomura Y: Pituitary dependent hyperadrenocorticism in a cat. *J Vet Med Sci* 54:1201–1203, 1992.

119. Schwedes CS: Mitotane (o,p'-DDD) treatment in a cat with hyperadrenocorticism. *J Small Anim Pract* 38:520–524, 1997.

120. Zerbe CA, Nachreiner RF, Dunstan RW, et al: Hyperadrenocorticism in a cat. *JAVMA* 190:559–563, 1987.

121. Kipperman BS, Nelson RW, Griffey SM, et al: Diabetes mellitus and exocrine pancreatic neoplasia in two cats with hyperadrenocortism. *JAAHA* 28:415–418, 1992.

122. Peterson ME, Steele P: Pituitary-dependent hyperadrenocorticism in a cat. *JAVMA* 189:680–683, 1986.

123. Immink WFGA, van Toor AJ, Vos JS, et al: Hyperadrenocorticism in four cats. *Vet Q* 14:81–85, 1992.

124. Usher DG: Hyperadrenocorticism in a cat. *Can Vet J* 32:326, 1991.

125. Gembardt C, Loppnow H: Zur pathogenese des spontanen diabetes mellitus der katze. II. Mitteilung: Azidophile adenome des hypophysenvorderlappens und diabetes mellitus in zwei fällen. *Berl Münch Teirärztl Wschr* 89:336–340, 1976.

126. Duesberg CA, Nelson RW, Feldman EC, et al: Adrenalectomy for treatment of hyperadrenocorticism in cats: 10 cases (1988–1992). *JAVMA* 207:1066–1070, 1995.

127. Nelson RW, Feldman EC, Smith MC: Hyperadrenocorticism in cats: Seven cases (1978–1987). *JAVMA* 193:245–250, 1988.

128. Watson PJ, Herrtage ME: Hyperadrenocorticism in six cats. *J Small Anim Pract* 39:175–184, 1998.

129. Goossens MMC, Meyer HP, Voorhout G, et al: Urinary excretion of glucocorticoids in the diagnosis of hyperadrenocorticism in cats. *Dom Anim Endocrin* 12:355–362, 1995.

130. Valentine RW: Feline hyperadrenocorticism: A rare case. *Feline Pract* 24:6–11, 1996.

131. Meijer JC, Lubberink AAME, Gruys E: Cushing's syndrome due to adrenocortical adenoma in a cat. *Tijdschr Diergeneesk* 103:1048–1051, 1978.

132. Jones CA, Refsal KR, Lerner RW: Adrenocortical adenocarcinoma in a cat. *JAAHA* 9:137–143, 1992.

133. Fox JG, Beatty JO: A case report of complicated diabetes mellitus in a cat. *JAAHA* 11:129–134, 1975.

134. Daley CA, Zerbe CA, Schick RO, et al: Use of metyrapone to treat pituitary-dependent hyperadrenocorticism in a cat with large cutaneous wounds. *JAVMA* 202:956–960, 1993.

135. Johnston SD, Mather EC: Feline plasma cortisol (hydrocortisone) measured by radioimmunoassay. *Am J Vet Res* 40:190–192, 1979.

136. Peterson ME, Kintzer PP, Foodman MS, et al: Adrenal function in the cat: Comparison of the effects of cosyntropin (synthetic ACTH) and corticotropin gel stimulation. *Res Vet Sci* 37:331–333, 1984.

137. Sparkes AH, Adams DT, Douthwaite JA, et al: Assessment of adrenal function in cats: Responses to intravenous synthetic ACTH. *J Small Anim Pract* 31:2–5, 1984.

138. Zimmer C, Hörauf A, Reusch C: Ultrasonographic examination of the adrenal gland and evaluation of the hypophyseal-adrenal axis in 20 cats. *J Small Anim Pract* 41:156–160, 2000.

139. Peterson ME, Kemppainen RJ: Comparison of intravenous and intramuscular routes of administering cosyntropin for corticotropin stimulation testing in cats. *Am J Vet Res* 53:1392–1395, 1992.

140. Peterson ME, Kemppainen RJ: Dose-response relation between plasma concentrations of corticotropin and cortisol after administration of incremental

sectomy for treatment of pituitary-dependent hyperadrenocorticism in 7 cats. *Vet Surg* 30:72–86, 2001.

MANAGEMENT OF SPECIFIC DISEASES

doses of cosyntropin for corticotropin stimulation testing in cats. *Am J Vet Res* 54:300–304, 1993.

141. Smith MC, Feldman EC: Plasma endogenous ACTH concentrations and plasma cortisol responses to synthetic ACTH and dexamethasone sodium phosphate in healthy cats. *Am J Vet Res* 48:1719–1724, 1987.

142. Zerbe CA, Refsal KR, Peterson ME, et al: Effect of nonadrenal illness on adrenal function in the cat. *Am J Vet Res* 48:451–454, 1987.

143. Medleau L, Cowan LA, Cornelius LM: Adrenal function testing in the cat: The effect of low dose intravenous dexamethasone administration. *Res Vet Sci* 42:260–261, 1987.

144. Peterson ME, Graves TK: Effects of low dosages of intravenous dexamethasone on serum cortisol concentrations in the normal cat. *Res Vet Sci* 44:38–40, 1988.

145. Myers NC, Bruyette DS: Feline adrenocortical diseases: Part I–Hyperadrenocorticism. *Semin Vet Med Surg Small Anim* 9:137–143, 1994.

146. Howell MJ, Pickering CM: Calcium deposits in the adrenal glands of dogs and cats. *J Comp Pathol* 74:280–285, 1964.

147. Ross MA, Gainer JH, Innes JRM: Dystrophic calcification in the adrenal glands of monkeys, cats and dogs. *AMA Arch Pathol* 60:655–661, 1955.

148. Cartee RE, Bodner STF, Gray BW: Ultrasound examination of the feline adrenal gland. *J Diagn Med Sonog* 9:327–330, 1993.

149. Boord M, Griffin C: Progesterone secreting adrenal mass in a cat with clinical signs of hyperadrenocorticism. *JAVMA* 214:666–669, 1999.

150. Willard MD, Nachreiner RF, Howard VC, et al: Effect of long-term administration of ketoconazole in cats. *Am J Vet Res* 47:2510–2513, 1986.

151. Duesberg C, Peterson ME: Adrenal disorders in cats. *Vet Clin North Am Small Anim Pract* 27:321–347, 1997.

152. van Sluijs FJ, Sjollema BE: Adrenalectomy in 36 dogs and 2 cats with hyperadrenocorticism. *Tijdschr Diergeneesk* 117:29S, 1992.

153. Ahn A: Hyperaldosteronism in cats. *Semin Vet Med Surg Small Anim* 9:153–157, 1994.

154. Eger CE, Robinson WF, Huxtable CRR: Primary aldosteronism (Conn's syndrome) in a cat; a case report and review of comparative aspects. *J Small Anim Pract* 24:293–307, 1983.

155. Flood SM, Randolph JF, Gelzer ARM, et al: Primary hyperaldosteronism in two cats. *JAAHA* 35:411–416, 1999.

156. MacKay AD, Holt PE, Sparkes AH: Successful surgical treatment of a cat with primary aldosteronism. *J Feline Med Surg* 1:117–122, 1999.

157. Yu S, Morris JG: Plasma aldosterone concentration of cats. *Vet J* 155:63–68, 1998.

158. Patnaik AK, Erlandson RA, Lieberman PH, et al: Extra-adrenal pheochromocytoma (paraganglioma) in a cat. *JAVMA* 197:104–106, 1990.

159. Chun R, Jakovljevic S, Morrison WB, et al: Apocrine gland adenocarcinoma and pheochromocytoma in a cat. *JAAHA* 33:33–36, 1997.

160. Holzworth J, Coffin DL: Pancreatic insufficiency and diabetes mellitus in a cat. *Cornell Vet* 43:502–512, 1953.

161. Henry CL, Brewer WG, Montgomery RD, et al: Clinical vignette: Adrenal pheochromocytoma. *J Vet Intern Med* 7:199–201, 1993.

162. Maher ER: Pheochromocytoma in the dog and cat: Diagnosis and management. *Semin Vet Med Surg Small Anim* 9:158–166, 1994.

163. Port CD, Maschgan ER, Pond J, et al: Multiple neoplasia in a jaguar *(Panthera onca)*. *J Comp Pathol* 91:115–122, 1981.

164. Hruban Z, Carter WE, Meehan T, et al: Retroperitoneal paraganglioma in a tiger *(Panthera tigris)*. *J Zoo Anim Med* 19:231–234, 1988.

165. Rossmeisl JH, Scott-Moncrieff JCR, Siems J, et al: Hyperadrenocorticism and hyperprogesteronemia in a cat with an adrenocortical adenocarcinoma. *JAAHA* 36:512–517, 2000.

166. Becker TJ, Perry RL, Watson GL: Regression of hypertrophic osteopathy in a cat after surgical excision of an adrenocortical carcinoma. *JAAHA* 35:499–505, 1999.

167. Biller DS, Bradley GA, Partington BP: Renal medullary rim sign: Ultrasonographic evidence of renal disease. *Vet Radiol Ultrasound* 33:286–290, 1992.

TUMORS OF THE REPRODUCTIVE TRACT

Antony S. Moore and Gregory K. Ogilvie

45

MALE REPRODUCTIVE TRACT TUMORS

CLINICAL BRIEFING

Common Presentation	Testicular and prostatic tumors are very rare. Prostatic adenocarcinoma may cause hematuria and dysuria.
Staging and Diagnosis	MDB, abdominal radiographs, ultrasonography, and urine culture and sensitivity testing.
Treatment	
Initial	Surgery may be curative for early tumors.
Adjunctive	Chemotherapy with doxorubicin or carboplatin potentially useful for metastatic tumors (unproven).
Supportive	Analgesia as needed.

▶ TESTICULAR TUMORS

There are very few reports of testicular tumors in cats. In a large European survey of testicular tumors in domestic mammals, none were reported in cats.[1] According to a North American source, only two testicular tumors in cats were described in detail over a 35 year period[2]; both occurred in DSH cats. One cat was a bilateral cryptorchid. Both cats had bilateral Sertoli cell tumors, but neither had signs of feminization. Metastases to the liver and a concurrent mast cell tumor of the spleen were noted in one cat; the second had a seminoma in one testicle in addition to the Sertoli cell tumor.[3] The same paper cites a testicular teratoma reported in 1938, a testicular "cancer" in 1937, and a metastasizing testicular carcinoma in 1916.[3] A 13-year-old cat with an embryonal carcinoma of the testis was mentioned in another survey.[4]

The paucity of reports of testicular tumors in DSH cats has been ascribed to the common practice of castration. The greater number of testicular tumors seen in captive wild Felidae would seem to support this assumption.

Staging for cats with testicular tumors should include an MDB and abdominal ultrasonography. An excisional biopsy should be performed for diagnosis and is essentially the treatment of choice when followed by appropriate supportive care.

NONDOMESTIC FELIDAE

Sertoli cell tumors have been reported in two clouded leopards *(Neofelis nebulosa nebulosa)*[5,6] and two jungle cats *(Felis chaus)*.[6,7]

Emaciation was the primary problem in one 23-year-old jungle cat that had concurrent gastric adenocarcinoma, thyroid adenocarcinoma, and renal adenoma. No treatment was attempted. The testicular tumor was less than 3 cm in diameter, unilateral, and probably incidental.[7] In an 11-year-old Bengal circus tiger *(Panthera tigris)*,[8] intermittent seizures and loss of dominance within a group of tigers led to the finding of a 10 × 8 × 6 cm testicular mass. Unilateral castration was performed, and the cat was once again the dominant male 2 months later.[8]

Seminoma has been described in two snow leopards *(Panthera unicia)*.[6,9] Treatment was not attempted in an emaciated 20-year-old.[6] Hemicastration was performed in a 12-year-old with fertility problems; 3 months later, the cat again had no viable sperm and a second seminoma was present in the other testicle. No metastases were found in this cat.[9]

▶ PROSTATIC TUMORS

Incidence, Signalment, and Etiology

Prostatic adenocarcinoma is a rare tumor in cats. Six cases have been reported in DSH and DLH cats ranging in age from 11 to 22 years.[2,10–12] A benign tumor, a fibroadenoma, was reported, but no details were provided.[13] At least two of the cats with carcinomas were castrated.[11]

Clinical Presentation and History

All cats were presented for lower urinary tract signs, including hematuria; four were also dysuric and obstructed.[2,11] Constipation was a problem in one other cat.[12]

Staging and Diagnosis

In addition to an MDB, abdominal ultrasonography and urine culture and sensitivity testing should be performed.

A mass at the pelvic brim was palpated on rectal examination in two cats,[2] while radiographs disclosed a 2 cm mass that was confirmed on rectal palpation in another cat.[10] Ultrasonography showed an ovoid mass measuring 1.7×1.8 cm caudal to the urinary bladder and an enlarged iliac lymph node. Ultrasound-guided fine-needle aspiration was able to obtain a diagnostic sample.[11] Despite lymphatic and blood vessel invasion, no tumor showed evidence of metastasis at the time of diagnosis.

Treatment

Due to the limited number of case reports, it is difficult to suggest an ideal treatment regimen for prostatic tumors. Surgical intervention followed by subsequent chemotherapy is probably warranted, but treatment should be determined on an individual basis. One cat was treated by prostatectomy alone and lived 3 months before it was euthanized due to local metastasis that occluded the ureter and caused hydronephrosis.[12] Another cat was treated by prostatectomy and adjuvant chemotherapy using doxorubicin and cyclophosphamide.[10] The tumor recurred locally 10 months after surgery, and no further treatment was attempted. Supportive care, including postoperative analgesia, should be provided as part of the treatment regimen. Nutritional support may also be necessary after surgical resection.

FEMALE REPRODUCTIVE TRACT TUMORS

▶ OVARIAN TUMORS

CLINICAL BRIEFING

Common Presentation	Granulosa cell tumors and dysgerminomas are most common. Mostly unilateral, but both tumor types can be bilateral. Hormonal activity can lead to estrous behavior and/or aggression. Large tumors may occur and cause signs related to size.
Staging and Diagnosis	MDB and abdominal ultrasonography. Peritoneal cavity metastases are most common. Abdominocentesis and fluid cytology are indicated.
Treatment Initial	Ovariectomy may be palliative but is rarely curative.
Adjunctive	Carboplatin chemotherapy potentially useful (unproven).
Supportive	Analgesia and antiinflammatories, particularly with peritoneal metastases.

Ovarian tumors are not commonly diagnosed in the cat. Of 56 ovarian tumors reported in the literature, there were 26 granulosa cell tumors, 11 dysgerminomas, 6 interstitial cell tumors, 6 carcinomas, 5 teratomas, 2 sex cord tumors, and a cystadenoma.

GRANULOSA CELL TUMORS

Incidence, Signalment, and Etiology

Except for one pseudo-hermaphrodite male, all 26 reported cats with granulosa cell tumors were females.[14] Affected cats ranged in age from 6 months to 20 years (median, 7 years), and six cats (23%) were 3 years old or younger. There were 17 DSHs, 1 DLH, 3 Siamese, and 1 Persian.[2,3,14-19] Most tumors were unilateral, although bilateral tumors have been reported.[19] Two tumors have also occurred in an ovarian remnant, one at 23 months and one at 8 years after ovariectomy.[2]

Clinical Presentation and History

Granulosa cell tumors appear to be hormonally active in some cats. Five cats were presented because of continual estrous signs[2,14,19] that had been occurring for up to 23 months. A further five cats had prolonged estrus or abnormal or irregular estrous cycles[2,14,15,17] that were associated with aggressive behavior changes[2] or hair thinning.[19] Large tumors may cause abdominal distension that is noticed by the owner.[15,19] Masses from 8 to 10 cm in diameter have been reported[16,18,19] and may be associated with less specific signs of vomiting, anorexia, and lethargy. Tumor rupture and intraabdominal bleeding occurred in one cat.[14] A microscopic granulosa cell tumor was an apparently incidental finding in one cat with a uterine squamous cell carcinoma.[39]

Staging and Diagnosis

Staging of cats with a suspected granulosa cell tumor includes an MDB, abdominal ultrasonography, abdominocen-

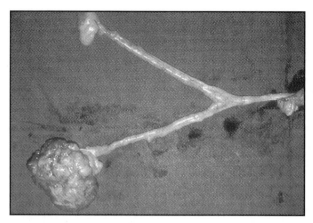

Figure 45-1: *An ovarian granulosa cell tumor in a cat. Surgical removal is the treatment of choice, although metastases are common. (Courtesy of W. Dernell)*

tesis, and fluid cytology.

Abdominal swelling may be due to the tumor mass, although peritoneal metastases resulting in peritoneal effusion may cause similar clinical signs. Metastasis, mainly within the abdominal cavity, occurs frequently, although lung metastases were seen in four cats.[14,15,18,19]

Metastases to the abdominal wall, omentum, and mesentery in six cats also involved one or more abdominal organs, including the spleen, liver, and kidneys. The hormonal activity of granulosa cell tumors was evident by secondary uterine effects in three cats that had a cystic endometrium.[19] One cat had an atrophic contralateral ovary,[18] and one had concurrent mammary adenocarcinoma.[19]

Treatment

Surgical resection is the treatment of choice, and exploratory laparotomy will allow the surgeon to examine the abdomen for the presence of metastases (Figure 45-1). Surgical removal of the tumor by ovariectomy provided palliation for 5 months in one cat,[2] 7 months in a second cat,[17] and 10 months in a third cat[16]; metastases were found at these times, and the cats were euthanized. Apparent cure was attained in two cats that had tumorous ovarian remnants removed, although follow-up times were not stated.[2]

While chemotherapy is largely unexplored in this disease, experience in other species and limited application in two cats[a] would suggest that intravenous or intracavitary chemotherapy with carboplatin may prove therapeutic. Supportive care, including analgesia, antiinflammatories, nutritional support, and antiemetics, should be provided as needed.

DYSGERMINOMAS

Incidence, Signalment, and Etiology

Dysgerminomas are rare. Of the 11 reported dysgerminomas in cats, 9 were in DSHs and 2 occurred in Siamese.

[a]Ogilvie GK: Personal observations.

All cats were female, although one had an ovotestis.[14] Affected cats ranged in age from 1 to 17 years, but 10 animals were 7 years old or younger.[14,20–22] Tumors were bilateral in three cats.[14,22]

Clinical Presentation and History

Dysgerminomas are supposedly hormonally inactive, yet two cats (both Siamese) were presented for continuous estrous[14] or masculine behavior.[20] Tumors ranged in size from 1 × 2 cm in diameter to 1 kg in weight.[19,20] The largest two tumors were histologically mixed with teratoma and did not appear to have metastasized. Bilateral dysgerminomas were found at routine ovariohysterectomy in a 1-year-old cat.[22]

MDB = minimum database; includes CBC, biochemical profile, urinalysis, FeLV/FIV serology, T_4 testing, and thoracic radiographs (three views).

Staging and Diagnosis

Although information about the metastatic potential of this tumor is limited, metastasis to the omentum was reported in three cats.[14,21] Staging should therefore include an MDB and analysis of any abdominal fluid. Abdominal ultrasonography is the preferred imaging modality.

Treatment

Ovariohysterectomy was performed in two cats. Omental metastases were also removed at the time of surgery in one cat,[21] which was euthanized 3 months later with metastases to lung, liver, adrenal gland, kidney, peritoneum, and pleura. A young cat in which the tumor was an incidental finding at ovariohysterectomy was still alive with no evidence of disease 2 years later.[22]

INTERSTITIAL CELL TUMORS

These rare tumors have been reported in five DSH cats, the youngest of which was 2 months of age.[14] A further cat reported to have an interstitial cell tumor was thought to have a nonfunctional pleomorphic sarcoma based on histopathologic review.[2]

Surgical removal is the treatment of choice after the cat has been evaluated for metastatic disease as outlined for other ovarian tumors.

TERATOMAS

Incidence, Signalment, and Etiology

These tumors are also rare and occur mostly in younger

cats (age range, 7 months to 3 years).[2,14,19,20,23] However, teratoma mixed with dysgerminoma was seen in two 6-year-old cats.[19,20] Of cats for which breed was cited, three were DSHs and one was a Persian.

KEY POINT

Ovarian granulosa cell tumors and carcinomas appear to be highly malignant, while teratomas may be less likely to metastasize.

Clinical Presentation and History

Abdominal distension due to a 1.1 kg tumor caused both decreased activity and appetite in one cat.[23] Similar sized tumors were seen in a 3-year-old Persian[14] and two cats with mixed teratoma and dysgerminoma.[19,20] Sudden death due to rupture and hemorrhage from the teratoma was seen in two cats, and the tumor was only 1.5 cm in diameter in one animal.[20] The other cat had delivered a litter of kittens 3 weeks previously.[19]

Staging and Diagnosis

No metastases have been reported for these tumors, although one large tumor invaded the abdominal wall.[19] Staging should include an MDB and abdominal radiographs. Abdominal ultrasonography should be performed prior to laparotomy as it may help prepare the surgeon for a potentially difficult resection.

Treatment

In the one cat treated by ovariohysterectomy, there was no evidence of tumor 1 year after surgery.[23]

ADENOCARCINOMA

The majority of female ovarian adenocarcinomas have been reported without clinical details[13,24] or were cited by other investigators.[19] A 5-year-old cat with hair loss and abdominal swelling due to ascites was found on necropsy to have bilateral ovarian adenocarcinoma with peritoneal metastasis as well as spread to liver and lungs.[19] An 11-year-old Siamese with nonspecific gastrointestinal signs was found to have a hemoabdomen when surgery was performed to remove a 5 cm ovarian adenocarcinoma and multiple small omental metastases. The cat died suddenly 10 days later. This cat had not had an estrous cycle since it was 3 years of age.[25]

CYSTADENOMA

Bilateral cystadenomas were seen in a 10-year-old DSH.[14]

SEX CORD TUMORS

Incidence, Signalment, and Etiology

These tumors are very rare and have been described in three DSH cats (6, 6, and 9 years of age).[19,26,27] One cat was multiparous.[27]

Clinical Presentation and History

In the two cats for which information was available, virilization and aggressive behavior were evidence of the hormonal effects of the tumor. In addition, prolonged estrus was seen in one of the cats and a purulosanguinous vaginal discharge occurred in the other.[19,27] Endometrial hyperplasia was circumstantial evidence of a hormonal effect in a third cat.

Staging and Diagnosis

Tumors in two cats were between 6 and 8 cm in diameter; no cats had evidence of metastasis. Large tumors such as these should be evident on abdominal palpation. Staging should include an MDB, abdominal imaging, and analysis (including cytology) of any abdominal fluid.

Treatment

Ovariohysterectomy was performed in all three cats. There was no follow-up in one case,[26] and in another there was regression of clinical signs with no evidence of disease 3 years later.[19] In the third cat, aggressive behavior resolved within 3 days of surgery and "never came back."[27] The prognosis for cats with ovarian sex cord tumors may be cautiously optimistic following surgery.

NONDOMESTIC FELIDAE

A 13-year-old snow leopard *(Panthera unicia)* had abdominal distension due to a large right ovarian dysgerminoma. Unilateral ovariectomy was performed, but follow-up information was not provided.[28] A survey of reproductive disorders in zoo animals found both an ovarian cystadenoma and a granulosa cell tumor in two black leopards *(Panthera pardus).*[29,30] A 17-year-old lioness *(Panthera leo)* was found to have multiple leiomyomas in the uterus and both ovaries.[19]

A 17-year-old jaguar *(Panthera onca)* with a history of poor breedability died with a distended abdomen. On necropsy, bilateral ovarian cystadenocarcinomas were found to have metastasized to the lungs, liver, and peritoneum.[31] Interestingly, jaguars may be predisposed to development of ovarian cystadenocarcinomas. In a survey of 66 wild Felidae, 12 were jaguars and 9 (75%) of these had ovarian papillary cystadenocarcinoma. The affected jaguars ranged in age from 12 to 24 years (average, 17 years). Only 5 of the 9 cats had received progestin contraceptives.[32] No other cat in this survey of 66 animals had an ovarian cystadenocarcinoma.

▶ UTERINE TUMORS

C L I N I C A L B R I E F I N G	
Common Presentation	Benign adenomas, fibromas, and leiomyomas occur. Adenoma can progress to adenocarcinoma. Carcinomas may result in signs of pyometra. Leiomyomas may be associated with cystic ovaries.
Staging and Diagnosis	MDB and abdominal ultrasonography. Metastases are common and widespread for carcinomas and leiomyosarcomas.
Treatment Initial	Ovariohysterectomy is curative for benign tumors but only palliative for malignant tumors.
Adjunctive	Chemotherapy unproven; consider carboplatin or doxorubicin.
Supportive	Analgesia or antiinflammatories as needed.

ADENOMYOSIS

Adenomyosis is described as proliferation of ectopic endometrium within the myometrium that causes enlargement of the uterus. Six cases have been reported without detail.[33] Clinical signs reported in three cats (a 7-year-old Burmese and two 9-year-old Siamese) included pseudopregnancy,[34] abdominal distention and vulvar discharge,[2] and vomiting.[35] Surgical removal by hysterectomy is likely to be curative.[2]

ADENOMAS OR ENDOMETRIAL POLYPS

Incidence, Signalment, and Etiology

Adenomas or endometrial polyps are a rare and likely underreported disease condition. Three early reports are cited with little detail.[2] More clinical details were provided in a series of 14 cats[36] ranging in age from 4[2] to 15[36] years. There were 8 DSHs, 1 Siamese, and 1 Persian; breed information was not provided for the other cats.[36]

Clinical Presentation and History

Ten cats had endometrial hyperplasia, which was concurrent with pyometra in two cats. Adenomas ranged in size from 0.5 cm in diameter to 5 × 7 cm. There was no evidence of malignant transformation,[16] although a 16-year-old cat with metastatic uterine adenocarcinoma also had five endometrial polyps.[2]

Staging and Diagnosis

Collection of an MDB and abdominal ultrasonography are recommended.

Treatment

Surgery is probably necessary for definitive diagnosis; although not reported, hysterectomy is likely to be curative.

Routine analgesia is recommended for postoperative discomfort, and nutritional support may be required.

MALIGNANT EPITHELIAL TUMORS

Malignant epithelial tumors of the uterus are rare in cats. Adenocarcinomas have been reported in 12 cats, carcinosarcomas in 2 cats,[37,38] and squamous cell carcinoma in 1 cat.[39] These tumors are grouped here as "carcinomas" as there is no apparent clinical difference in biologic behavior.

Incidence, Signalment, and Etiology

No details were available for 1 cat.[40] Of 12 other cats, 10 were DSHs, 1 was Siamese, and 1 was Persian. Ages of affected cats ranged from 5 to 16 years, with 10 cats being 11 years of age or older.[2,33,37–39,41–43] A local depressed immune reaction during fetal growth may lead to tumor growth in some cats. Circumstantial evidence for this comes from nonclinical data in which growth of uterine adenocarcinoma followed experimental inoculation of tumor cells in 3 pregnant cats.[44] Of the clinical cases, however, an 11-year-old Persian was nulliparous[33] and an 11-year-old DSH had been spayed at the age of 5 years.[39]

Clinical Presentation and History

Malignant epithelial tumors often cause nonspecific illness and clinical signs relating to abdominal discomfort. Vaginal discharge that was purulent,[39] serous,[33] or hemorrhagic[37] was a feature in five cats.[2,45] This discharge had continued for 3 months in two cats[33,37] and for 1 year in another.[38] Less specific signs of lethargy and anorexia were also common. Two cats were constipated due to pelvic obstruction,[39,43] and another had diarrhea.[2] Carcinoma metastases to the brain and eyes caused ataxia and blindness in one cat that had experienced dystocia 2 months previously.[45] Two cats died acutely.[39,41]

Staging and Diagnosis

Staging should include an MDB, abdominal ultrasonography, and analysis (including cytology) of any abdominal fluid. A mass was palpable in the abdomen in 3 cats,[37,39,43] and the uterine horns were greatly enlarged in three other cats.[2,33,38] Metastases to the peritoneum caused carcinomatosis and ascites in 1 cat.[2] Abdominal ultrasonography should be used to distinguish uterine enlargement or a mass from other organomegaly. Metastases or vascular invasion were reported in all cats for which clinical details or necropsy findings were provided, and metastases were widespread in most cats. Vascular invasion of tumor cells without gross evidence of metastases was seen in 2 cats.[2,38] In 10 other cats, metastases were commonly found on the peritoneum (6 cats), lungs (5 cats), and in the abdominal lymph nodes (4 cats). Other sites of metastasis seen in 2 or fewer cats included kidney, liver, ovary, pleura, brain, eyes, and adrenal and peripheral lymph nodes.

Treatment

Ovariohysterectomy was attempted in two cats. A stump recurrence of the tumor (6 weeks after surgery in one cat[37] and 12 weeks after surgery in the other[39]) was accompanied by widespread metastases that had not been evident at the time of surgery.

KEY POINT

Uterine carcinomas are highly malignant.

BENIGN MESENCHYMAL TUMORS

These benign tumors are often removed as clinically silent entities at the time of routine ovariohysterectomy and are therefore probably underreported. Fibromas have been reported in an 8-year-old Siamese[38] and two DSH cats (10 and 12 years old).[4,46] Three other cases are cited.[2] One cat was anorectic, weak, and vomiting. On physical examination, a painful, palpable 10 cm uterine mass was removed by ovariohysterectomy.[46]

Leiomyomas have been reported in eight cats, and six more were cited without clinical details.[2,47] The eight cats ranged in age from 3 to 15 years (average, 9 years). Tumors were multiple in four cats, with up to five tumors in one 3-year-old. Leiomyomas extended to involve the vagina in a 15-year old cat. Tumors usually involved the body of the uterus and ranged in size from 3 mm to 8 cm in diameter. Five cats with uterine leiomyomas also had ovarian cysts, and three cats had concurrent endometrial hyperplasia. Two cervix-obstructing leiomyomas were found on laparotomy in a cat with dystocia.[47] Treatment was not reported for any cat, but surgical resection by hysterectomy is the logical approach.

A uterine hemangioma was diagnosed in an 8-year-old DSH cat that had a vaginal discharge and abdominal distension for 6 months prior to becoming depressed and anorectic. On laparotomy, an 11 cm diameter uterine mass was associated with uterine torsion. The outcome of treatment was not reported.[48]

KEY POINT

Benign mesenchymal uterine tumors may be associated with cystic changes in the ovaries.

LEIOMYOSARCOMA

Leiomyosarcomas are distinguished from leiomyomas on histopathology by their high mitotic index.[2] Four cats between 10 and 17 years of age were reported to have uterine leiomyosarcomas.[2,42] Details were not available for one case; two others showed anorexia and weight loss associated with pyometra and a 9 to 10 cm uterine mass. These two cats also had metastases to peritoneal surfaces, sternal lymph node, and lungs. A 2 cm mass was found on routine ovariohysterectomy in the fourth cat.

Surgical removal by ovariohysterectomy is recommended. Chemotherapy using doxorubicin or carboplatin as described in Chapter 51 may be a logical adjunctive treatment due to the potential for intraabdominal metastases. Supportive care involves postoperative analgesia, nutritional support when indicated, and antiemetic administration if chemotherapy is attempted. The efficacy of therapy for this tumor has not been reported.

NONDOMESTIC FELIDAE

Adenocarcinoma of the uterus has been reported in a lioness *(Panthera leo)*[49] and a 13-year-old Bengal tigress *(Panthera tigris)*.[50] Although it seems unlikely to have been an inciting cause, the tigress had been treated with melengestrol acetate more than 52 months previously. The tumor in this cat consisted of multiple nodules up to 4 cm in diameter with infiltration of the ovary and perirenal fat as well as metastasis to the sublumbar lymph nodes.

Progestin contraception may have been an inciting cause of a uterine adenocarcinoma in a 12-year-old jaguar *(Panthera onca)*.[51] This cat had received weekly megestrol acetate for years prior to developing diabetes mellitus and carcinomatosis due to widespread intraabdominal metastases from the uterine tumor.

In another study of 19 uterine cancers in wild Felidae, four species—tigers *(Panthera tigris)*, jaguars *(Panthera onca)*, leopards *(Panthera pardus)*, and lions *(Panthera leo)*—were affected.[52] Fifteen of these cats had endometrial carcinomas, 3 had leiomyosarcoma, and 1 had both. Affected cats ranged in age from 9 to 24 years with the exception of one 5-year-old tiger. Melengestrol acetate (17 cats) and megestrol acetate (1 cat) had been used for contraception in 18 of these cats with uterine carcinoma.

A 20-year-old jaguar (Panthera onca) with nonspecific signs of anorexia and lethargy had a small (<1 cm) uterine leiomyosarcoma that had metastasized to regional lymph nodes and the liver.[53] This cat also had a metastatic mammary carcinoma.

A lioness with leiomyomas of the uterus and ovaries has been reported.[19] In addition, a 14-year-old clouded leopard (Neofelis nebulosa) was found to have a leiomyofibrosarcoma of the uterus that had metastasized to the lung.[54] A leopard (Panthera pardus) was found to have a uterine leiomyoma.[29]

▶ VAGINAL TUMORS

The majority of reported vaginal tumors are benign. Two fibromas[4,13] and a myxoma[24] were reported. A 12-year-old cat and a 15-year-old cat were reported to have leiomyofibroma, and one of these cats also had leiomyomas of the uterus.[2]

Two DSHs (8 and 14 years of age) were presented for constipation (chronic in one cat).[55] Neither cat was treated; necropsy revealed a solitary leiomyoma in each cat (8 cm in one and 4 cm in the other). The latter cat also had a mammary adenocarcinoma in its axilla.

A leiomyosarcoma that was occluding the uterine and vaginal lumen was found in a 12-year-old pregnant cat. No treatment was reported.[2]

An invasive granular cell tumor of the vulva, presumably a type of soft tissue sarcoma, was described in one cat.[56]

Surgical removal is the treatment of choice for vaginal tumors, and a vulvovaginectomy may be required in some cats. Evaluation by abdominal ultrasonography for any local extension is suggested prior to surgery. Analgesia and nutritional support are recommended postoperatively.

NONDOMESTIC FELIDAE

A 13-year-old multiparous Bengal tigress (Panthera tigris) had difficulty urinating and defecating. At ovariohysterectomy, an 11 cm myxoma was found to be attached to the dorsal vaginal wall. There was no evidence of disease 8 months after surgical resection of the mass.[57]

REFERENCES

1. Reifinger M: Statistiche untersuchungen zum vorkommen von hodentumoren bei haussäugetieren. J Vet Med 35:63–72, 1988.
2. Carpenter JL, Andrews LK, Holzworth J: Tumors and tumor-like lesions, in Holzworth J (ed): Diseases of the Cat. Medicine and Surgery. Philadelphia, WB Saunders, pp 407–596, 1987.
3. Meier H: Sertoli-cell tumor in the cat. Report of two cases. North Am Vet 37:979–981, 1956.
4. Joshua JO: Reproductive system, in: The Clinical Aspects of Some Diseases of Cats. London, William Heinemann Medical Books Ltd, 1965, pp 119–140.
5. Effron M, Griner L, Benirschke K: Nature and rate of neoplasia found in captive wild mammals, birds and reptiles at necropsy. J Natl Cancer Inst 59:185–198, 1977.
6. Doster AR, Armstrong DL, Bargar TW: Seminoma and parathyroid adenoma in a snow leopard (Panthera unica). J Comp Pathol 100:475–480, 1989.
7. Sagartz JW, Garner FM, Sauer RM: Multiple neoplasia in a captive jungle cat (Felis chaus)—Thyroid adenocarcinoma, gastric adenocarcinoma, renal adenoma, and Sertoli cell tumor. J Wildl Dis 8:375–380, 1972.
8. Michalska Z, Gucwinski A, Kocula et al: Sertoli cell tumour in Bengal tiger (Panthera tigris tigris). Akademie-Verlag, Erkrankungen der Zootiere Verhandlungsbericht des XIX Internationalen Symposiums uber die Erkrankungen der Zootiere 18:305–307, 1977.
9. Karesh WB, Kunz LL: Bilateral testicular seminoma in a snow leopard. JAVMA 189:1201, 1986.
10. Hubbard BS, Vulgamoot JC, Liska WD: Prostatic adenocarcinoma in a cat. JAVMA 197:1493–1494, 1990.
11. Bigliardi E, Parmigiani E, Morini G: Neoplasia prostatica. Summa 16:79–80, 1999.
12. Tommasini M, Assin R, Lombardo S: Ureteral transposition in the colon of a cat affected by prostatic carcinoma [abstract 28]. Vet Surg 23:217, 1994.
13. Cotchin E: Neoplasia; in Wilkinson GT (ed): Diseases of the Cat and Their Management. Melbourne, Blackwell Scientific Publications, 1983.
14. Gelberg HB, McEntee K: Feline ovarian neoplasms. Vet Pathol 22:572–576, 1985.
15. Aliakbrai S, Ivoghli B: Granulosa cell tumor in a cat. JAVMA 174:1306–1308, 1979.
16. Azuma Y, Matsuo Y, Chen B-Y: Granulosa cell tumor in a cat with unilateral renal agenesis. J Jpn Vet Med Assoc 45:324–327, 1992.
17. Arbjerg J: Extra-ovarian granulosa cell tumor in a cat. Feline Pract 10:26–32, 1980.
18. Baker E: Malignant granulosa cell tumor in a cat. JAVMA 129:322–324, 1956.
19. Norris HJ, Garner FM, Taylor HB: Pathology of feline ovarian neoplasms. J Pathol 97:138–143, 1969.
20. Dehner LP, Norris HJ, Garner FM, Taylor HB: Comparative pathology of ovarian neoplasms. III. Germ cell tumours of canine, bovine, feline, rodent and human species. J Comp Pathol 8:299–310, 1970.
21. Gruys E, van Duk JE, Elsinghorst AM, van der Gaag I: Four canine ovarian teratomas and a nonovarian feline teratoma. Vet Pathol 13:455–459, 1976.
22. Andrews EJ, Stookey JL, Helland DR, Slaughter LJ: A histopathological study of canine and feline ovarian dysgerminomas. Can J Comp Med 38:85–89, 1974.
23. Basaraba RJ, Kraft SL, Andrews GA, et al: An ovarian teratoma in a cat. Vet Pathol 35:141–144, 1998.
24. Nielsen SW: Neoplastic diseases, in Catcott EJ (ed): Feline Medicine and Surgery. Santa Barbara, CA, American Veterinary Publications, 1964, pp 156–176.
25. Röcken H: Ovarialtumor und ovaraplasie bei einer katze. Tierärztl Prax 11:245–247, 1983.
26. Hofmann W, Arbiter D, Scheele D: Sex cord stromal tumor of the cat: So-called androblastoma with Sertoli-Leydig cell pattern. Vet Pathol 17:508–513, 1980.
27. Röcken H: Ein fibrothekom als faktor für einen verhaltensschaden bei einer katze. Der Praktische Tierarzt 4:344–346, 1984.
28. Karesh WB, Russell R: Ovarian dysgerminoma in a snow leopard (Panthera unica). J Zoo Anim Med 19:223–225, 1988.
29. Schmidt RE, Hubbard GB, Fletcher KC: Systematic survey of lesion from animals in a zoologic collection: V. Reproductive system and mammary gland. J Zoo Anim Med 17:28–33, 1986.
30. Hubbard GB, Schmidt RE, Fletcher KC: Neoplasia in zoo animals. J Zoo Anim Med 14:33–40, 1983.
31. Bossart GD, Hubbell G: Ovarian papillary cystadenocarcinoma in a jaguar (Panthera onca). J Zoo Anim Med 14:73–76, 1983.
32. Munson L: A high prevalence of ovarian papillary cystadenocarcinomas in jaguars (Panthera onca). Vet Pathol 31:604, 1994.
33. Cotchin E: Spontaneous uterine cancer in animals. Br J Cancer 18:209–227, 1964.
34. Gelberg HB, McEntee K: Pathology of the canine and feline uterine tube. Vet Pathol 23:770–775, 1986.
35. Pack FD: Feline uterine adenomyosis. Feline Pract 10:45–47, 1986.
36. Gelberg HB, McEntee K: Hyperplastic endometrial polyps in the dog and cat. Vet Pathol 21:570–573, 1984.
37. Evans JG, Grant DI: A mixed mesodermal tumour in the uterus of a cat. J Comp Pathol 87:635–638, 1977.
38. Papparella S, Roperto F: Spontaneous uterine tumors in three cats. Vet Pathol 21:257–258, 1984.

39. Meier H: Carcinoma of the uterus in the cat: Two cases. *Cornell Vet* 46:188–200, 1956.

40. Puttannaiah GB, Seshadri SJ, Mohiyudeen S: A rare case of adenocarcinoma of uterus in a cat. *Curr Res Univ Agric Sci (Bangalore)* 4:156–158, 1975.

41. Belter LF, Crawford EM, Bates HR: Endometrial adenocarcinoma in a cat. *Pathol Vet* 5:429–431, 1968.

42. Berkin S, Tekeli Ö, Ünsüren H: Bir kedide uterusun mezensimal-mix tümörü. *A Ü Vet Fak Derg* 29:219–226, 1982.

43. Preiser H: Endometrial adenocarcinoma in a cat. *Pathol Vet* 1:485–490, 1964.

44. Minke JMHM, Hensen EJ, Misdorp W: Uterine carcinomas in mother cats after intrafetal inoculation of allogeneic tumor cells (K248 C and P). *Vet Immunol Immunopathol* 46:361–366, 1995.

45. O'Rouke MD, Geib LW: Endometrial adenocarcinoma in a cat. *Cornell Vet* 60:598–604, 1970.

46. Sorribas CE: Submucous uterine fibroma in a cat. *Mod Vet Pract* 68:493, 1987.

47. Nava GA, Sbernardour U: Distocia materna nella gatta da leiomioma del corpo dell'utero. *Clin Vet Rassegna Polizia Sanitaria Higiene* 90:521–525, 1967.

48. Fukui K, Matsuda H: Uterine haemangioma in a cat. *Vet Rec* 113:375, 1983.

49. Lombard LS, Witte EJ: Frequency and types of tumors in mammals and birds of the Philadelphia Zoological Garden. *Cancer Res* 19:127–141, 1959.

50. Linnehan RM, Edwards JL: Endometrial adenocarcinoma in a bengal tiger *(Panthera tigris bengalensis)* implanted with melengestrol acetate. *J Zoo Anim Med* 22:130–134, 1991.

51. Kollias GV, Calderwood-Mays MB, Short BG: Diabetes mellitus and abdominal adenocarcinoma in a jaguar receiving megestrol acetate. *JAVMA* 185:1383–1386, 1984.

52. Munson L, Stokes JE, Harrenstein LA: Uterine cancer in zoo felids on progestin contraceptives. *Vet Pathol* 32:578, 1995.

53. Frazier KS, Hines II ME, Ruiz C, et al: Immunohistochemical differentiation of multiple metastatic neoplasia in a jaguar *(Panthera onca)*. *J Zoo Wildl Med* 25:286–293, 1994.

54. Winter H, Göltenboth R: Metastasierendes leiomyofibrosarkom bei einem nebelparder *(Felis nebulosa griff)*. *Kleintierpraxis* 24:199–201, 1979.

55. Wolke RE: Vaginal leiomyoma as a cause of chronic constipation in the cat. *JAVMA* 143:1103–1105, 1963.

56. Patnaik AK: Histologic and immunohistochemical studies of granular cell tumors in seven dogs, three cats, one horse, and one bird. *Vet Pathol* 30:176–185, 1993.

57. Kollias GV, Bellah JR, Calderwood-Mays M, et al: Vaginal myxoma causing urethral and colonic obstruction in a tiger. *JAVMA* 187:1261–1262, 1985.

MAMMARY TUMORS

Antony S. Moore and Gregory K. Ogilvie

46

► FELINE MAMMARY FIBROADENOMATOSIS

C L I N I C A L B R I E F I N G	
Common Presentation	Usually young intact females, sometimes pregnant. Occasionally affects female and male cats treated with progestins. Multiple glands in young cats are typically very swollen and painful. Older cats may have a single affected gland.
Staging and Diagnosis	Signalment or history of progestin administration is suggestive of the condition. Perform coagulation profile in addition to MDB before attempting surgery. Regression may occur following spay or progestin withdrawal but may take months.
Treatment	
Initial	Cease exogenous progestins. Consider spay.
Adjunctive	Surgery only if solitary gland affected. Ulceration, hemorrhage, postoperative sepsis, and thromboembolism are potential sequelae.
Supportive	Antiinflammatories and analgesia are necessary, particularly if multiple glands are affected. Appetite stimulants and nutritional support may be necessary.

Incidence, Signalment, and Etiology

Feline mammary fibroadenomatosis describes a massive hypertrophy of the mammary epithelium, myoepithelium, and fibroblasts.[1,2] Other terms for this benign condition include pericanalicular fibroadenoma, total fibroadenomatous change, benign mammary hypertrophy, mammary adenomatosis, fibroglandular hypertrophy, fibroepithelial hyperplasia, and fibroadenomatous hypertrophy. Unlike mammary carcinoma, which is rare in males, this condition is seen in both males and females, particularly those receiving progestins such as megestrol acetate[3,4] or medroxyprogesterone acetate.[4] One study suggested that up to 40% of mammary tumors were fibroadenomatous,[5] although this figure appears higher than that reported by most other investigators.

Feline mammary fibroadenomatosis is generally a disease of young cats. In four studies totaling 77 cats, 48 were less than 18 months of age (range, 10 weeks to 10 years).[3,4,6,7] All young affected cats were intact females. All were pregnant in one study,[3] while pregnancy was less common in other studies.[4,6,8,9]

Three of 19 young affected cats were Siamese in one study.[4] This is of interest considering that Siamese are predisposed to developing mammary carcinoma. In a second study of 30 cats, 7 were tricolor (also known as calico or tortoiseshell) and there were no Siamese. This large number of tricolors was three times the expected incidence, reflecting the increased risk for this breed to develop mammary carcinoma.[6]

Of the 77 cats mentioned above, 29 were 2 years of age or older and 12 of these 29 (5 castrated males, 5 spayed females, and 2 intact females) had received prior progestin therapy. There were no Siamese in this older group, and the only affected purebred was a Persian.[4]

It is generally believed that there is a strong link between the role of progestins and this disease. Regression after cessation of hormonal therapy, ovariohysterectomy,[3,7] or abortion when pregnant[4] provides strong evidence for the role of progestins in the development of this disease. The cumulative dosage of megestrol acetate given to affected cats in one study was between 300 and 600 mg over 1 to 5 years.[3] Hypertrophy may occur soon after progestin therapy is started. One cat developed mammary masses within 7 weeks of starting oral progestins.[10]

In a separate study of 39 cats treated with oral progestins, 6 developed some sort of mammary pathology including 3 cats with fibroadenomatous hyperplasia.[11] It is interesting to note that despite the widespread use of progestins for contraception in nondomestic Felidae, fibroadenomatous hyperplasia has not been reported in these species.

Clinical Presentation and History

Although younger cats usually have multiple affected glands, older cats often have hypertrophy of only one or two mammary glands, most often the inguinal glands. Swelling of affected glands often occurs rapidly,[8] and an individual gland may weigh up to 500 g.[6] Such massive swelling may cause pain and discomfort[12] as well as mechanically interfere with walking (Figure 46-1). Glands are edematous and discolored and may be difficult to clinically distinguish from mastitis or rapidly progressing neoplasia.

MDB = minimum database; includes CBC, biochemical profile, urinalysis, FeLV/FIV serology, T_4 testing, and thoracic radiographs (three views).

Staging and Diagnosis

The signalment of the affected cat, particularly if the history includes progestin administration, should raise the index of suspicion for this condition. Because this is a nonneoplastic condition, staging beyond an MDB is probably unnecessary. If surgery is contemplated, a coagulation profile should be obtained because coagulopathies have been reported in affected cats. Hypertrophy is rarely encapsulated and often extends between multiple glands.[8] Histologically, the mitotic rate approaches that of mammary carcinomas.[13]

Treatment

Regression of mammary hypertrophy has been seen following cessation of progestin therapy, abortion, ovariohysterectomy, and occasionally spontaneously.[14] Regression may take up to 5 months to complete.[3,6]

KEY POINT

Cats with fibroadenomatosis are usually young intact females with large, fast-growing mammary gland swellings that may cause pain and discoloration of the overlying skin and an abnormal gait.

Surgical resection of a gland is feasible only in cats with solitary or few affected glands. Mastectomy coupled with withdrawal of progestins and/or ovariohysterectomy provides good long-term control. However, care should be taken in selection of cases for surgery as complications (ulceration, hemorrhage, and postoperative sepsis) may be common, particularly in cats with a large volume of inflamed mammary tissue.[6] In one study, 3 of 27 cats treated by mastectomy died and 2 of these 3 developed pulmonary thromboembolism.[6] Mastectomy is best reserved for cats with solitary lesions, and multiple lesions should probably be allowed to regress. The efficacy of antiinflammatory agents in this condition has not been reported, but their use may be helpful in some cats. Complete nursing care, including analgesics, appetite stimulants, nutritional support, and fluids, is considered essential due to the painful nature of the disease.

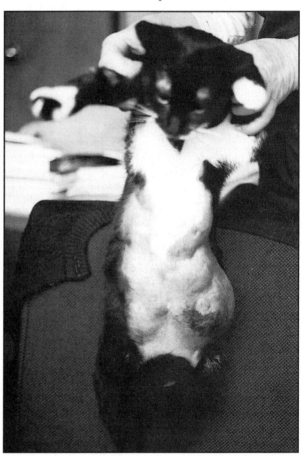

Figure 46-1: *Mammary fibroadenomatosis is usually seen in young female cats or cats treated with progestins. The swelling is often massive and subject to trauma, which can cause discomfort.*

▶ BENIGN MAMMARY TUMORS

CLINICAL BRIEFING

Because benign mammary tumors are rare, any solitary mammary tumor in a cat should be staged as if it were a malignant tumor before proceeding with surgical excision. If surgical excision is complete and the lesion is benign, no further treatment is necessary. However, the owner should be encouraged to palpate the mammary chain for new nodules every 2 to 4 weeks. Veterinary examinations should be scheduled every 6 months to check for recurrence or new, potentially malignant, tumors.

Incidence, Signalment, and Etiology

The majority of mammary tumors detected clinically in domestic cats are malignant. In four large series totaling 439 cats with mammary tumors, only 36 had benign tumors, emphasizing the importance of approaching all mammary tumors as if they were malignant.[6,15-17] Tumors were mostly adenomas, although intraductal papilloma was described in one cat[15] and one cat had a benign mixed mammary tumor in addition to an adenoma.[6]

Estrogen and progesterone receptors were present in greater numbers in benign lesions than in malignant lesions, although this finding may have been influenced by the use of iatrogenic progestin treatment in 12 of 14 cats assayed.[18] Both estrogen and progestin receptors were found in 9 of 13 adenomas assayed, while 2 of 13 had progestin receptors only.[18]

The signalment for cats with benign tumors is similar to that of cats with malignant mammary tumors. Most are DSHs[66] and tend to be older (median age, 6 years).[18] Young cats (less than 1 year of age) are occasionally reported.[15,18] Of 32 cats for which such information was available, 15 were spayed females and none were male.[6,15,18]

Staging and Diagnosis

See discussion for malignant mammary tumors.[6,18]

Treatment

Surgical excision of a mammary adenoma should be curative, although a cat will occasionally have a benign and a malignant tumor concurrently,[17] implying that risk factors for the development of a malignant tumor may be shared in some cats with mammary adenoma. Owners should be counseled to palpate their cats carefully for the presence of any new masses in the mammary chain following excision of an adenoma.

Analgesics and surgical wound care are essential. Nutritional support should be considered if anorexia or weight loss are associated with the disease or therapeutic intervention.

▶ MALIGNANT MAMMARY TUMORS

CLINICAL BRIEFING

Common Presentation	Usually adenocarcinoma or solid carcinoma. Mostly seen in older (median age, 11 years) spayed and intact females. Spayed cats are about half as likely to develop mammary tumors. Siamese are predisposed. Exogenous progestins may increase risk. Ulceration is common; tumors are often multiple and found in two or more glands.
Staging and Diagnosis	MDB and palpation and biopsy of inguinal and/or axillary lymph nodes. Thoracic radiographs are important because pulmonary metastases are most common. Abdominal ultrasonography to look for hepatic, splenic, or renal metastases and involvement of intraabdominal lymph nodes.

Prognostic Factors	
Breed	DSHs have longer survival.
Age	Younger cats have longer survival.
Tumor volume	Cats with tumors that are ≤3 cm^3 have longer survival.
Metastasis	Worse survival.
Well-differentiated tumors (low mitotic rate; little cellular or nuclear pleomorphism)	Longer survival.
Low AgNOR counts	Longer survival.
Histologically complete resection	Longer survival.

Treatment	
Initial	Surgery unlikely to be curative due to high rate of lymphatic invasion but may be palliative. Wide margins are important; mastectomy, not lumpectomy, should be performed. Full chain mastectomy if multiple glands affected or if regional lymph node involved.
Adjunctive	Chemotherapy using doxorubicin improves survival, particularly if there is lymphatic invasion. Drugs such as carboplatin, cyclophosphamide, and paclitaxel may have efficacy. Radiation therapy unproven but may improve local control.
Supportive	Analgesia, nutritional support, and nursing care may be necessary after surgery, particularly full chain mastectomy. Appetite stimulants may be needed if doxorubicin is administered.

MANAGEMENT OF SPECIFIC DISEASES

Incidence, Signalment, and Etiology

Mammary epithelial tumors are the most common type of feline mammary tumor, with adenocarcinomas and solid carcinomas predominating. Mixed mammary tumors are rare, accounting for only 4 of 227 tumors in one case series.[6] Mammary sarcomas are extremely rare[19–21] and appear to be slow to metastasize.[22]

Mammary carcinomas are seen in older cats (median age, 10 to 12 years). Cats as young as 2 years old may be affected,[6,23] although it is rare for cats younger than 5 years of age to have mammary carcinoma.[6] Mammary carcinoma may be seen in cats over the age of 20 years.[6,21,23,24] According to one study, the relative risk for a female cat developing mammary carcinoma increases steadily with age, especially in intact cats.[17]

KEY POINT

Older cats may have worse survival rates after surgical resection of a mammary carcinoma.

The effect of neutering on development of mammary carcinoma is less clear in cats than in dogs, although there is some evidence to suggest that neutering may prevent mammary tumor development. In one study, the relative risk for a spayed female developing mammary carcinoma was approximately half that of an intact cat.[17] Of 671 cats in seven studies,[6,15,17,18,24–26] only 6 male cats were affected,[6,17,18,26] 358 (34%) of the females were intact, and 307 were spayed. In one of these studies, the average age of spaying was 6 years of age but ranged from 6 months to over 16 years; only 11 of 85 cats (13%) were spayed in their first year of life.[24] In another study, early spaying did not completely eliminate the risk of developing a mammary carcinoma; 17% of spayed cats were less than 1 year of age at the time of ovariohysterectomy.[11] The time from spaying to first detection of carcinoma varied from 17 to 144 months (median, 38 months) in a group of 52 cats.[17] Earlier studies that reported a preponderance of affected intact female cats may have reflected neutering practices at the time rather than a true increased risk.[16] Parity does not seem to affect the incidence of mammary carcinoma; 35 of 64 (55%) spayed cats had had a litter, while 52 of 83 (63%) intact cats had also given birth.[24]

Male cats with mammary carcinoma have often been treated with progestins. Although quite rare, spontaneous mammary carcinoma is occasionally reported in males.[27]

While DSH and DLH cats are most commonly reported with mammary carcinoma, tricoloreds are the only DSH cats that have been shown to be at increased risk for developing the disease. Tricolor cats comprised 12% of the cats with mammary carcinoma in a study of 227 cats, while they account for only 7% of the general population.[6]

Even more striking is the increased incidence of mammary carcinoma in the Siamese breed seen in American,[6,15,17,25,28,29] Japanese,[26] and European studies.[24] Of 735 cats for which breed was reported, there were 190 (26%) Siamese, 15 Persian, and 1 each Angora, Abyssinian, Burmese, and Russian Blue. Siamese accounted for 51 of 227 (22%) affected cats in one study but comprised only 5% of the general population.[6] In another study, Siamese were found to have twice the risk for developing mammary carcinoma, although the risk seemed to plateau at 9 years of age instead of increasing with age as it did in DSH cats.[17]

Reports from the 1970s found that viral particles were associated with mammary carcinomas in cats. Both type A and type C particles were described.[29–31] Transmission experiments reported over a period of 7 years failed to demonstrate an increased risk for mammary tumor development.[30,32,33] A viral etiology for mammary carcinoma is unlikely.

While the role of exogenous progestins in promoting mammary carcinoma development has been well described for nondomestic Felidae, it is less clearly defined for domestic breeds. Cats receiving depot injections of medroxyprogesterone acetate for contraception, dermatologic conditions, or behavioral modification may be at increased risk for developing carcinoma. Three of 5 cats developed mammary carcinoma after 4 to 5 years of progestin treatment.[34] In another study, 6 of 39 cats treated with oral progestins developed mammary pathology and 2 of these had carcinoma.[11] Conversely, only 1 of 132 cats with mammary carcinoma in another study had received medroxyprogesterone acetate. Treatment in that cat was extended (9 years).[17]

Although earlier studies were unable to detect estrogen receptors in feline mammary carcinomas,[32,35] they were able to demonstrate progesterone receptors.[36] A recent study showed both estrogen and progesterone receptors to be present in mammary carcinomas, although in lower numbers and fewer tumors compared with benign tumors.[18] More than half of the cats with carcinoma in that study had received some progestin treatment, which may have complicated the receptor status of the tumors. As for all treatments, the potential risks of using progestins in cats should be weighed against the benefits. If it is possible to avoid the use of progestins, the risk of later development of mammary carcinoma is probably decreased.

Signalment factors shown to be prognostic for survival after surgical resection of mammary carcinoma include breed (DSH cats had longer survival times in one study)[37] and age (older cats having worse survival rates).[24] These findings have not been reported in other studies.[23]

Clinical Presentation and History

Mammary carcinomas in cats may remain undetected by owners until they become quite large or ulcerative, even if a previous mass was detected. Thus mammary carcinoma is often advanced by the time a veterinarian is consulted. In one study from the 1950s, the time from owner detection to treatment ranged from 2 weeks to 4 months,[16] while another study from the 1980s found that the median time from owner detection to treatment was 5 months, although the delay ranged up to 72 months.[24] Clearly cat owners need to be educated regarding early detection and treatment of these tumors. In contrast, veterinarians seem aware of the serious nature of mammary tumors in cats. Of 199 cats presented to veterinarians with a mammary tumor, all were treated surgically within 1 week.[24]

Tumor volume varies widely; a median of 3 cm³ was seen in one study, but tumor size ranged up to 13 cm³.[24] Nearly half of the tumors were ulcerated at the time of presentation.[24,38,39]

Mammary carcinoma is solitary in approximately half of the cats reported in U.S. studies (201 of 393 cats[6,11,15]), but 85% of cats (202 of 237) in a European study had a solitary tumor.[24] Multiple gland involvement may mean that only two or three glands are involved. However, in some cats the entire mammary chain is affected either unilaterally or bilaterally,[15,40] possibly as the result of lymphatic spread rather than multiple synchronous primary tumors (Figure 46-2).

Cats have only one abdominal mammary gland on each side (dogs have three), and the posterior thoracic gland is situated more caudally than in the dog. However, there is more frequent anastomosis between the thoracic and abdominal lymph drainage in cats,[41] although there does not appear to be lymphatic anastomosis across the midline.[16]

Tumors are more likely to occur in the third and fourth mammary glands, with approximately the same numbers occurring in the left or right glands[6,24] (Figure 46-3).

KEY POINT

Cats with large mammary tumors (>3 cm in diameter) have a poor prognosis for long-term survival after surgery alone.

On palpation, the regional lymph nodes (axillary or inguinal) may not be enlarged; only 6% of cats in one study had regional lymphadenopathy at their first veterinary intervention.[24] It should be noted that normal-sized lymph

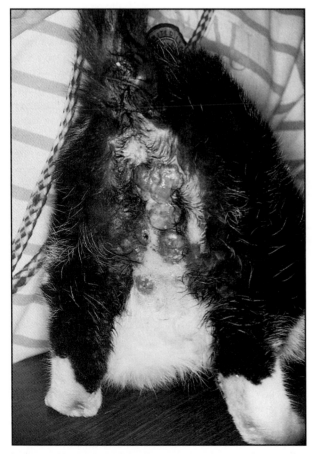

Figure 46-2: Multiple ulcerated mammary carcinomas in the inguinal region of a cat.

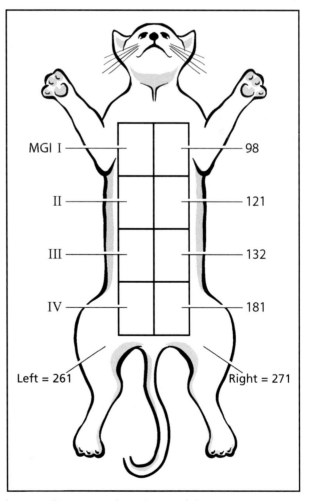

Figure 46-3: Diagram showing locations of solitary mammary tumors found in cats.[6,24] (Illustration by Beth Mellor; MGl = mammary gland)

MANAGEMENT OF SPECIFIC DISEASES

nodes may still contain tumor cells; in the same study, 27% of cats had histologic evidence of mammary carcinoma metastases to the lymph nodes.

Most cats are presented due to the detection of a mass or ulcerated area. However, widespread metastases may cause significant morbidity related to anorexia, dyspnea, and cough due to pulmonary or pleural metastases or even neurologic symptoms due to cerebral metastases.[38] Bone[39] and eye[42] metastases are rare reasons for presentation in a cat with mammary carcinoma.

The only clinical factor shown to be an independent predictor of survival for cats after surgery for mammary carcinoma is tumor diameter, with a worse prognosis for larger tumors.[24] In other studies, cats with small tumors had both longer remission after surgery and longer survival times[26,28,37] (Figure 46-4 and Tables 46-1 and 46-2). This re-

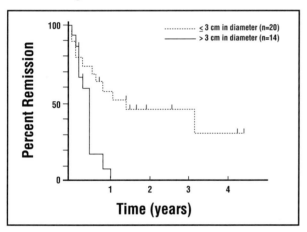

Figure 46-4: *Cats with tumors 3 cm or less in diameter have a much greater chance of tumor control by surgery alone than do cats with larger tumors. (From Ito T, Kadosawa M, Mochizuki M, et al: Prognosis of malignant mammary tumors in 53 cats.* J Vet Med Sci *58:723–726, 1996; with permission)*

TABLE 46-1[28]
Tumor Size Related to Survival after Surgery

Tumor Size (cm³)	No. of Cats	Median Survival (years)
1–8	54	>3
9–27	19	2
>28	8	0.5

TABLE 46-2[26]
Tumor Size Related to Survival after Surgery

Tumor Size (cm³)	No. of Cats	Median Survival (months)	% Alive at 2 Years
≤3	28	9	49.1
>3	25	5	0

iterates the need for early detection and action by both caregivers and veterinarians alike.

Staging and Diagnosis

Feline mammary carcinoma is an invasive and often rapidly metastatic tumor. A standard staging protocol involves at least an MDB; careful visual and digital assessments of the extent of the primary and metastatic tumors are also essential. Invasive tumors may extend to involve venules in the surrounding tissue and adjacent mammary glands and the dermis, causing ulceration.

More than one quarter of affected cats have evidence of regional lymph node metastasis at the time of first diagnosis.[24] The axillary or inguinal lymph nodes are most frequently involved, although the sternal lymph node may be enlarged in some cats. Necropsy revealed evidence of metastases in 120 of 129 cats that had undergone surgery to treat mammary carcinoma. The axillary or inguinal lymph node was affected in more than 80% of cats, while the sternal node was involved in 30% of cats. The majority of cats with sternal lymph node involvement also had pleural or pulmonary metastases.[43,44]

Pulmonary metastases occur more frequently than regional lymph node metastases.[15,17,20,21,43,44] In one study, 29 of 43 cats with mammary carcinoma had radiographic evidence of pulmonary metastases.[26] Involvement of the pleural surfaces is also common[6] and usually occurs with concurrent pulmonary metastases.[43,44] Pulmonary metastases usually appear as a miliary pattern on thoracic radiographs and may obliterate normal lung.[45] Pulmonary metastases appear to occur with equal frequency in cats with carcinomas affecting the caudal glands as in those with tumors of the cranial glands.[43]

KEY POINT

Lymph node metastasis is a poor prognostic sign.

Metastasis to other organs or systems is less common, although nearly 25% of cats had hepatic metastases in one study.[43] Metastases to the spleen, kidney, adrenal gland, peritoneal surfaces, and heart have been reported (Figure 46-5).[6,15,16,38–40] Bone metastases have been reported in a small number of cats. Cats with appendicular metastases were lame,[39,46] while two cats with rib and thoracic vertebral metastases were asymptomatic.[46] The radiographic appearance of these metastases is primarily lytic with little evidence of periosteal reaction (Figure 46-6).[46] The bone marrow was infiltrated in one cat with mammary carcinoma,[6] and CNS metastases caused neurologic signs in another cat.[38]

Prognostically, the finding of lymph node metastasis at diagnosis was highly associated with poor survival following

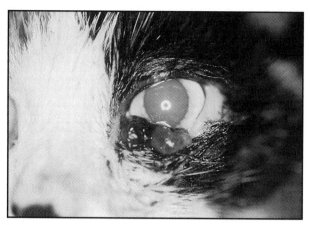

Figure 46-5: *Metastases to lung and regional lymph nodes are most common, but other sites, such as seen in this cat with a periocular metastasis, are occasionally involved.*

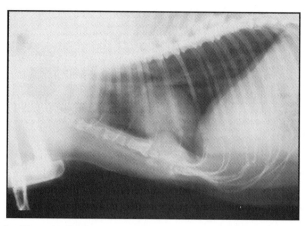

Figure 46-6: *Pulmonary metastases and a metastasis to the sternum were seen in this cat 8 months after surgery for a mammary adenocarcinoma. (Courtesy of K.M. Rassnick)*

surgery (Figure 46-7). The finding of distant metastases was likewise a poor prognostic factor.[24] Staging of cats according to World Health Organization (WHO) criteria takes into account the size of the tumor as well as the presence of lymph node or distant metastases. WHO staging in one study also found the presence of metastases to be a poor prognostic sign for survival after surgery[26] (Figures 46-7 and 46-8 and Table 46-3).

Multiple histologic criteria have been examined in feline mammary carcinoma, and some histologic factors have recently been examined for prognostic significance following surgical excision of a mammary carcinoma. The histologic types of carcinoma were catalogued in one study as tubular adenocarcinoma (35%), papillary adenocarcinoma (8%),

and solid carcinoma (14%). However, another 32% of tumors were classified as a mixture of two or more of these histologic types.[24] Another study found that the histologic type of tumor was not prognostic for survival,[47] although proliferating cell nuclear antigen (PCNA) staining (a measure of proliferative rate) increased from papillary cystic carcinomas to tubular adenocarcinomas to solid carcinomas.[13] Rarely, an anaplastic carcinoma will contain giant cells,[48] and there may be associated myofibroblast proliferation.[49] The clinical relevance of the histologic subtype and these rare variants would seem to be of little consequence to the veterinary clinician.

Other studies have looked at grading systems for mammary tumors regardless of the histologic subtype. These sys-

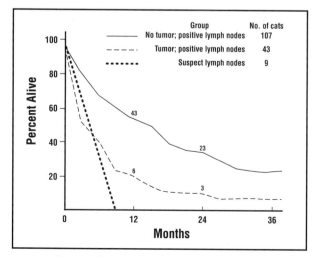

Figure 46-7: *Metastasis to the regional lymph nodes was correlated with decreased survival after surgery in this study. In addition, cats with lymphatic vessel invasion on histopathology were more likely to have lymph node metastasis. (From Weijer K, Hart AAM: Prognostic factors in feline mammary carcinoma. J Natl Cancer Inst 70:709-716, 1983; by permission of Oxford University Press)*

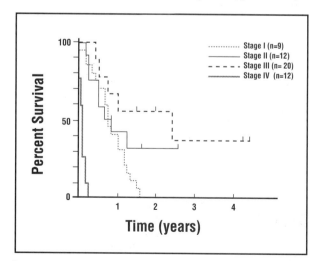

Figure 46-8: *Cats with small tumors and no evidence of metastases (Stage I) had a median survival of 29 months; median survival time for cats with Stage II disease was 12.5 months; Stage III, 9 months; and Stage IV, 1 month. (From Ito T, Kadosawa T, Mochizuki M, et al: Prognosis of malignant mammary tumor in 53 cats. J Vet Med Sci 58:723–726, 1996; with permission)*

TABLE 46-3
WHO Staging Related to Survival After Surgery

WHO Stage	Median Survival (months)	Description
I	29	T < 1 cm, no N
II	12.5	T < 1 cm and N OR T = 1–3 cm ± N
III	9	T > 3 cm OR T < 3 cm + fixed N
IV	1	Any T or N with M

M = distant metastases; N = lymph node metastases; T = tumor

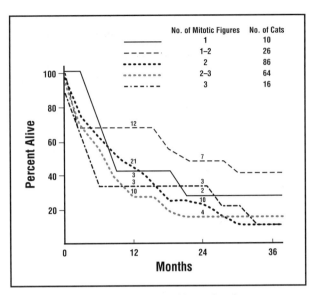

Figure 46-9: *Histologic measurement of the number of mitoses was strongly associated with survival in this study. (From Weijer K, Hart AAM: Prognostic factors in feline mammary carcinoma.* J Natl Cancer Inst *70:709–716, 1983; by permission of Oxford University Press)*

tems rely on subjective appraisal of nuclear variation, mitotic figures, differentiation of epithelial elements, invasion of lymphatics or surrounding stroma, lymphoid cellular reaction, and ductular development.[15,23,50] Only one system was applied prognostically, classifying tumors as well, moderately, or poorly differentiated.[23] There appeared to be prognostic value to this system (Table 46-4).

The majority (60%) of tumors were moderately differentiated, and within that subset there appeared to be a prognostic advantage if myoepithelial differentiation was seen in the tumor.[23]

KEY POINT

Histologic grading (mitotic count, cellular pleomorphism) is prognostic for survival in cats with mammary carcinoma.

In another study, the presence of necrosis within the tumor and an increasing number of mitotic figures were associated with shorter survival times (Figures 46-9 and 46-10).[24]

In an effort to reduce the subjectivity inherent in such grading systems, one study digitally scanned representative nuclei from mammary carcinomas and studied the nuclear profile and nuclear form. This study found that nuclear area, anisokaryosis, and nuclear shape were not prognostic for survival, although the presence of nuclear polymor-

phism was associated with poor survival.[47]

Immunohistochemical staining of feline mammary carcinomas for the intermediate filaments vimentin and various cytokeratins has shown that these stains may be used to subclassify mammary tumors.[51,52] The percentage of cells expressing vimentin varied from 25%[51] to 75%,[52] and vimentin expression was felt to reflect tumor reversion to more primitive cell types. Vimentin expression is associated with poor prognosis in human breast cancer patients, but the outcome of disease in cats and its association with vimentin expression was not studied here.

The number of silver staining regions (AgNORs) within the nuclei of cancer cells correlates with the number of cells in S phase (i.e., cellular proliferation). Despite early studies implying the contrary,[53] increasing AgNOR counts have been correlated with poor prognosis in cats with mammary carcinoma.[54] While there was no relationship between AgNOR numbers and histologic type, increasing counts correlated with poor survival. It appears that AgNOR counts of less than 5.9 correlated with a higher 1 year survival rate (78%) than counts greater than 5.9 (22%; Table 46-5).

TABLE 46-4
Histologic Grade Related to Survival after Surgery[23]

Grade	No. of Cats	% of Total	% Alive 12 Months after Surgery
Well differentiated	7	12.7	100
Moderately differentiated	33	60	54.5
Poorly differentiated	15	27.3	0

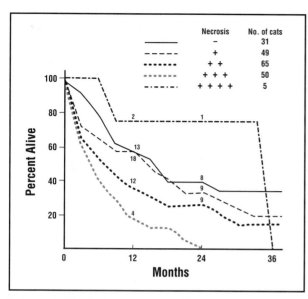

	Necrosis	No. of cats
	–	31
	+	49
	+ +	65
	+ + +	50
	+ + + +	5

Figure 46-10: *Histologic measurement of the amount of necrosis was strongly associated with survival in this study. (From Weijer K, Hart AAM: Prognostic factors in feline mammary carcinoma.* J Natl Cancer Inst *70:709–716, 1983; by permission of Oxford University Press)*

TABLE 46-5
AgNOR Count and Relation to Survival after Surgery[54]

AgNOR Count	No. of Cats	Percent (No.) Alive at 1 Year
<4.2	10	80% (8)
4.2–5.1	10	70% (7)
5.2–6.7	10	90% (9)
6.8–8.1	11	18% (2)
>8.1	10	10% (1)

MDB = minimum database; includes CBC, biochemical profile, urinalysis, FeLV/FIV serology, T_4 testing, and thoracic radiographs (three views).

In summary, the clinician should take histologic findings of mitotic count, nuclear and cellular pleomorphism, and tubule formation into account when looking for prognostic factors. These criteria combined with staging information gained from thoracic radiographs, and abdominal ultrasonography, the presence or absence of lymph node metastases, and tumor size should allow the veterinarian to assess the prognosis for an individual cat with mammary carcinoma. If AgNOR staining becomes widely available, additional prognostic information may be obtained.

Treatment

Feline mammary carcinomas are invasive, and the high rate of lymphatic involvement mandates aggressive treatment. The entire affected mammary chain should be removed with wide surgical margins, although the efficacy of this treatment is less clear than would be desired. Because of metastatic spread, surgical excision alone is unlikely to result in a cure; however, the extent of surgery appears to play a role in reducing local recurrence and survival times.[16] In addition, the histologic completeness of resection appears to correlate with survival.[24]

Two studies that looked at the effect of conservative surgery (removing only the affected gland and adjacent tissue) compared with radical surgery (unilateral or bilateral mastectomy) found no difference in survival between the two groups.[26,28] In one of these two studies, the 2 year survival rates were similar— 33.3% and 17.3% for radical and conservatively treated groups, respectively—but there was a marked difference in recurrence rates (0% and 43.4%, re-

spectively). This difference was not statistically significant.[26] The other study found that the radical surgery was associated with longer remission (Figures 46-11 and 46-12).[28] The definition of radical surgery was defined by the surgeon in both of these studies, although it appears that histopathology may be a more accurate method to define the completeness of surgery.[24] In a study of 153 cats treated surgically, 137 were thought by the surgeon to have been treated radically and 16 conservatively. On histologic review, only 103 of 137 were defined as having "radical" margins, while 21 of 137 and 3 of 16 were felt to have narrow margins. Resection was incomplete in the remaining cats. The histologic completeness of resection correlated with survival.[24]

It should be remembered that cats with small lesions or tumors that have not invaded the basement membrane (i.e., cancer in situ) may be cured by surgery. Definitive surgery should not be delayed for incisional or needle biopsies if the owner is agreeable to surgery.

The overall median remission for 34 cats treated surgically was 6 months, and fewer than one third of the cats were free of recurrence 2 years after surgery. Median survival for these cats was 1 year.[26] In another study, 45% of cats were alive 1 year after surgery.[23] The cause of death is most commonly attributed to recurrence or metastases.

In another study, cats with WHO stage II (27 cats) or III (9 cats) mammary carcinoma that were treated by radical full chain mastectomy had no recurrence a median of 10.4 months after surgery; median survival time was 21.3 months.[55] The addition of immunotherapy did not improve survival (discussed below). Overall, tumor control was significantly longer in cats with stage II tumors than those with stage III tumors (13.3 months vs. 2.9 months, respec-

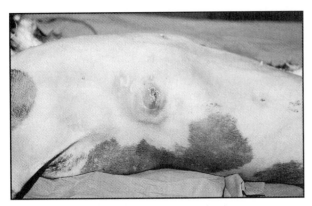

Figure 46-11: A large ulcerated mammary tumor should be removed with the widest possible margins, and regional lymph nodes should be biopsied at the time of surgery.

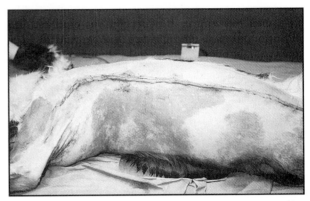

Figure 46-12: The cat shown in Figure 46-11 was treated via full chain mastectomy because other tumor nodules were palpated.

tively). At the end of the study, fewer than half of the cats with stage II tumors had died, while half the cats with stage III tumors were dead 4.2 months after surgery.[55]

KEY POINT

Aggressive, radical mastectomy is warranted for feline mammary carcinoma. The surgeon should submit the entire specimen for histologic review to ensure that complete margins have been obtained.

Chemotherapy

Due to the high metastatic potential of mammary carcinoma, chemotherapy would appear to be the most likely treatment modality to improve survival as an adjuvant to surgery. At present, doxorubicin appears to be the agent of choice. However, few studies have reported the use of chemotherapy.

Twenty-six cats received five doses of doxorubicin (1 mg/kg IV every 3 weeks) following surgery for mammary carcinoma. Whether the tumor was being resected for the first time or was recurrent did not influence survival unless the tumor could not be completely resected. Survival time after surgery was shorter in cats with incompletely excised tumors. The overall median survival was 25 to 41 weeks.[56] Cats with stage II disease that had not been previously treated with surgery had the longest survival times (median, 73 weeks). These cats in particular seem to benefit from doxorubicin chemotherapy.

In another study, 14 cats with measurable tumors received doxorubicin (30 mg/m² IV every 2 weeks) for five treatments following biopsy. Nine cats had a partial response, and 2 cats had some reduction in tumor size.[57] The cats lived 10 to 61 weeks (median, 31 weeks), but cats that responded did not necessarily live any longer than those that did not. Anorexia was the most common toxicity, occurring in 6 of

the 14 cats; vomiting and alopecia were also noted.[57]

Doxorubicin (30 mg/m² IV every 3 weeks) was combined with cyclophosphamide (100 mg/m² daily for 4 days) to treat 14 cats with inoperable or metastatic mammary carcinomas. Three cats with lung metastases had a complete response to treatment for 26 to 49 weeks, and 2 cats had shorter partial responses (one for 7 and the other for 21 weeks).[25] Twelve cats were anorectic; for some of these cats, the dose of doxorubicin was reduced to 20 mg/m² every 5 weeks.

Doxorubicin appears to be the drug of choice in treating mammary carcinoma. A dose of 1 mg/kg IV given every 3 weeks for five total treatments results in a beneficial effect; the major toxic side effect is anorectia. Concurrent appetite stimulants may be necessary with doxorubicin treatment.

Other chemotherapeutics such as carboplatin have not been evaluated but may have efficacy in treatment of mammary carcinoma. Paclitaxel has shown anecdotal efficacy against mammary carcinoma.[a] Vincristine and methotrexate appear to be ineffective in preventing metastatic spread of feline mammary carcinoma.[11,26] Cyclophosphamide as a single agent had no effect on survival when used as an adjuvant to surgery in 10 cats.[26]

Radiation Therapy

Radiation therapy has not been extensively used in the treatment of mammary carcinoma, but it may be effective in preventing local recurrence. Anecdotally, it may result in regression of inoperable recurrent local disease; however, due to the risk of radiation damage to underlying tissue (lung, kidneys) only shallow penetrating low energy radiation, such as an electron beam from a linear accelerator, can be safely utilized (Figure 46-13).

Immunotherapy

Immunotherapy has not been shown to diminish recurrence rate or improve survival time in cats with mammary

---

[a]AS, Ogilvie GK: Personal observations.

carcinomas. Postsurgical immunotherapy with *Corynebacterium parvum*,[58] a cocktail of *Streptococcus pyogenes* and *Serratia marcescens*,[11] or levamisole (5 mg/kg PO three times/week)[37] did not significantly improve outcomes compared with surgery alone. Postsurgical administration of liposome-encapsulated muramyl-tripeptide-phosphatidyl ethanolamine (L-MTP-PE) has been shown to improve survival for dogs with various tumors through targeted macrophage activation, but there was no improvement in time to tumor recurrence or survival times in cats with mammary carcinoma treated using adjuvant L-MTP-PE.[55]

Supportive Care

Analgesia is essential during and after surgical removal of any mammary tumor. Antiemetics can be helpful at reducing the adverse effects of chemotherapy, and supplemental feeding methods and appetite stimulants must be considered in all patients to facilitate healing and prevent weight loss during therapy. In addition, treatment of underlying secondary problems such as renal or heart disease is important.

NONDOMESTIC FELIDAE

Incidence, Signalment, and Etiology

Mammary carcinomas have been described in numerous species in captivity. Carcinomas appear to be most common in tigers *(Panthera tigris)*[59,60] but are also common in jaguars *(Panthera onca)*.[60,61] Other species recorded less frequently include lions *(Panthera leo)*,[46,60,62] cougars *(Felis concolor)*, leopards *(Panthera pardus)*, and jungle cats *(Felis chaus)*.[63] Only one benign tumor type, multiple cystic mammary adenomas, has been reported in a snow leopard *(Unica uncia)*[60]

Affected cats were older; 17 tigers ranged in age from 8.5 to 20 years (median, 12.5 years), while 7 jaguars had a median age of 15.7 years. No nondomestic cat under the age of 10 years has been reported with mammary carcinomas.[60]

According to a survey in which 31 nondomestic Felidae with mammary tumors were compared with a database of unaffected cats, tumors were more frequent in cats that were exposed to melengestrol acetate. Silicone implants containing melengestrol acetate are widely used for contraception in captive Felidae. Interestingly, the occurrence of tumors was not associated with the duration of exposure or with higher cumulative dosages.[60] It was suggested that an unidentified carcinogenesis threshold may exist for mammary carcinoma. Melengestrol acetate implants were more commonly used in jaguars and lions than other species. The duration of implant use in affected cats ranged from a median of 6 years for tigers to a median of 9 years for jaguars, with some individuals being exposed for up to 12.5 years.[60]

KEY POINT

The use of melengestrol implants increases the risk of mammary carcinogenesis in Felidae.

Clinical Presentation and History

As would be expected, mammary carcinoma is usually advanced when discovered in nondomestic Felidae. Most cats are examined for signs relating to metastases. Lameness due to bone metastases and neurologic signs due to skull and vertebral metastases have been seen in two lions,[46,62] and pleural effusion due to pulmonary and pleural metastases caused dyspnea in a tiger.[59]

In a larger group of 31 cats, nonspecific signs of anorexia and lethargy were most common, with vomiting, weight loss, diarrhea, and abdominal distension less commonly seen.[60] The primary tumor was ulcerated in nearly 30% of affected cats; respiratory difficulty due to thoracic metastasis and lymphatic obstruction due to nodal metastases were less common.

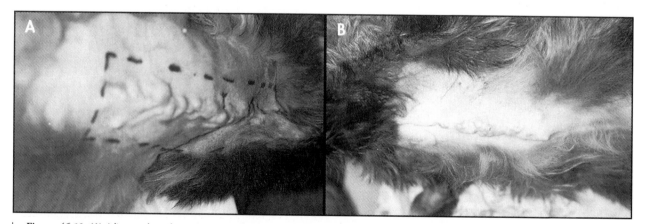

Figures 46-13: *(**A**) Adjuvant chemotherapy is warranted in a cat with mammary carcinoma and lymphatic vessel invasion to try to prevent distant metastases. In some cats, multiple local recurrence along the suture line shown may contribute to morbidity. (**B**) Radiation therapy may significantly reduce the tumor size and associated inflammation. This is the same cat as shown in **A** after radiation therapy.*

Staging and Diagnosis

As stated, metastases are widespread at the time of diagnosis, presumably due to the late recognition of this tumor by caregivers. Metastases, seen in 28 of 31 cats, affected (in order of decreasing frequency) lymph nodes, lungs, liver, adrenal gland, spleen, peritoneum, heart, ovary, and uterus. Metastases to kidney, bone, intestine, eyelid, and vagina were rare.[60]

Radiographically, metastases to bones appear primarily osteolytic without obvious periosteal reaction.[46] Thoracic radiographs showed metastases in 60% of cats in another study.[60] Abdominal radiographs were not very sensitive in disclosing metastases to abdominal organs. Interestingly, 7 of 25 affected cats for which serum chemistry was available showed evidence of hypercalcemia.[60]

Treatment

Most nondomestic cats with mammary carcinoma have not been treated due to the presence of metastases. A snow leopard with multiple mammary adenomas was treated, presumably successfully, by surgery.[64]

It is difficult to guess as to the rapidity of tumor progression in affected cats. A 12-year-old Siberian tiger with multiple mammary nodules and possible lung metastases lived 16 months before pleural effusion and progressive metastases necessitated euthanasia.[59]

Prevention of mammary carcinoma may be a more realistic goal. Avoidance of progestins in all captive Felidae, particularly in jaguars and tigers, may reduce the incidence dramatically. Ovariohysterectomy may be a better alternative for contraception in these cats.

Analgesics are essential due to the painful nature of the disease. Prednisone did not palliate neurologic signs due to bone metastases in a lioness.[62]

REFERENCES

1. Nimmo JS, Plummer JM: Ultrastructural studies of fibro-adenomatous hyperplasia of mammary glands of 2 cats. *J Comp Pathol* 91:41–50, 1981.
2. Hayden DW, Johnson KH, Ghobrial HK: Ultrastructure of feline mammary hypertrophy. *Vet Pathol* 20:254–264, 1983.
3. Hinton M, Gaskell CJ: Non-neoplastic mammary hypertrophy in the cat associated either with pregnancy or with oral progesterone therapy. *Vet Rec* 100:277–280, 1977.
4. Hayden DW, Johnston SD, Kiang DT, et al: Feline mammary hypertrophy/fibroadenoma complex: Clinical and hormonal aspects. *Am J Vet Res* 42:1699–1701, 1981.
5. Bostock DE: Canine and feline mammary neoplasms. *Br Vet J* 142:506–515, 1986.
6. Carpenter JL, Andrews LK, Holzworth J: Tumors and tumor-like lesions, in Holzworth J (ed): *Diseases of the Cat. Medicine and Surgery.* Philadelphia, WB Saunders, 1987, pp 407–596.
7. Bloom F, Allen HL: Feline mammary hypertrophy. *Vet Pathol* 11:561, 1974.
8. Allen HL: Feline mammary hypertrophy. *Vet Pathol* 10:501–508, 1973.
9. Graham TC, Wilson J: Mammary adenoma associated with pregnancy in the cat. *Vet Med Small Anim Clin* 67:82–84, 1972.
10. Seiler RJ, Kelly WR, Menrath VH, Barbero RD: Total fibroadenomatous change of the mammary glands of two spayed cats. *Feline Pract* 9:25–29, 1979.
11. Hayes AA, Mooney S: Feline mammary tumors. *Vet Clin North Am Small Anim Pract* 15:513–520, 1985.
12. Norris PJ, Blunden A: Fibro-adenoma of the mammary glands in a kitten. *Vet Rec* 104:233, 1979.
13. Preziosi R, Sarli G, Benazzi C, Marcato PS: Detection of proliferating cell nuclear antigen (PCNA) in canine and feline mammary tumors. *J Comp Pathol* 113:301–313, 1995.
14. Mandel M: Benign mammary hypertrophy. *Vet Med Small Anim Clin* 70:846–847, 1975.
15. Hayden DW, Nielsen SW: Feline mammary tumours. *J Small Anim Pract* 12:687–697, 1971.
16. Nielsen SW: The malignancy of mammary tumors in cats. *North Am Vet* 33:245–252, 1952.
17. Hayes Jr HM, Milne KL, Mandell CP: Epidemiological features of feline mammary carcinoma. *Vet Rec* 108:476–479, 1981.
18. Rutteman GR, Blankenstein MA, Minke J, Misdorp W: Steroid receptors in mammary tumours of the cat. *Acta Endocrinologica* 125:32–37, 1991.
19. Hayden DW, Ghobrial HK, Johnson KH, Buoen LC: Feline mammary sarcoma composed of cells resembling myofibroblasts. *Vet Pathol* 23:118–124, 1986.
20. Überreiter VO: Die tumoren der mamma bei hund und katze. *Wien Tierärztl Mschr* 8:481–503, 1968.
21. Überreiter VO: Die tumoren der mamma bei hund und katze. *Wien Tierärztl Mschr* 415–442, 1968.
22. Hampe JF, Misdorp W: Tumours and dysplasias of the mammary gland. *Bull WHO* 50:111–133, 1974.
23. Castagnaro M, Casalone C, Bozzetta E, et al: Tumour grading and the one-year post-surgical prognosis in feline mammary carcinomas. *J Comp Pathol* 119:263–275, 1998.
24. Weijer K, Hart AAM: Prognostic factors in feline mammary carcinoma. *J Natl Cancer Inst* 70:709–716, 1983.
25. Jeglum KA, deGuzman E, Young KM: Chemotherapy of advanced mammary adenocarcinoma in 14 cats. *JAVMA* 187:157–160, 1985.
26. Ito T, Kadosawa T, Mochizuki M, et al: Prognosis of malignant mammary tumor in 53 cats. *J Vet Med Sci* 58:723–726, 1996.
27. Thiéry PG: Épithélioma de la mamelle chez un chat castré. *Recueil Méd Vét* 122:258–261, 1946.
28. MacEwen EG, Hayes AA, Harvey HJ, et al: Prognostic factors for feline mammary tumors. *JAVMA* 185:201–204, 1984.
29. Feldman DG, Gross L: Electron microscopic study of spontaneous mammary carcinomas in cats and dogs: Virus-like particles in cat mammary carcinomas. *Cancer Res* 31:1261–1267, 1971.
30. Weijer K, Calafat J, Daams JH, et al: Feline malignant mammary tumors. II. Immunologic and electron microscopic investigations into a possible viral etiology. *J Natl Cancer Instit* 52:673–679, 1974.
31. Calafat J, Weijer K, Daams H: Feline malignant mammary tumors. III. Presence of particles and intracisternal A-particles and their relationship with feline leukemia virus antigens and D-114 virus antigens. *Int J Cancer* 20:759–767, 1977.
32. Weijer K: Feline mammary tumours and dysplasias. Conclusions based on personal studies and some suggestions for future research. *Vet Q* 2:69–74, 1980.
33. Misdorp W, Weijer K: Animal model: Feline mammary carcinoma. *Am J Pathol* 98:573–576, 1980.
34. Hernandez FJ, Chertack M, Gage PA: Feline mammary carcinoma and progestogens. *Feline Pract* 5:45–48, 1975.
35. Hamilton JM, Else RW, Forshaw P: Oestrogen receptors in feline mammary carcinomas. *Vet Rec* 99:477–479, 1976.
36. Elling H, Ungemach FR: Progesterone receptors in feline mammary cancer cytosol. *J Cancer Res Oncol* 100:325–327, 1981.
37. MacEwen EG, Hayes AA, Mooney S, et al: Evaluation of effect of levamisole on feline mammary cancer. *J Biol Resp Modif* 5:541–546, 1984.
38. Atasever A, Kul O: Metastase eines mammakarzinoms im zentralnervensystem bei einer katze. *Dtsch Tierärztk Wschr* 103:472–474, 1996.
39. Waters DJ, Honeckman A, Cooley DM, DeNicola D: Skeletal metastasis in feline mammary carcinoma: Case report and literature review. *JAAHA* 34:103–108, 1998.
40. Field EH: A contribution of the study of malignant growths in the lower animals. *JAMA* 23:982–985, 1894.
41. Silver IA: Symposium on mammary neoplasia in the dog and cat—I. The anatomy of the mammary gland of the dog and cat. *J Small Anim Pract* 7:689–696, 1966.
42. Wilcock BP, Peiffer Jr RJ, Davidson MG: The causes of glaucoma in cats. *Vet Pathol* 27:35–40, 1990.
43. Weijer K, Head KW, Misdorp W, Hampe JF: Feline malignant mammary tu-

mors. I. Morphology and biology: Some comparisons with human and canine mammary carcinomas. *J Natl Cancer Inst* 49:1697–1704, 1972.

44. Weijer K, Hampe JF, Misdorp W: Mammary carcinoma in the cat. A model in comparative cancer research. *Arch Chirurgicum Neerlandicum* 25:413–425, 1973.

45. Katsurada F, Okino T: Uber krebs bei katzen. *Jap J Cancer Res* 32:343–348, 1938.

46. Kas NP, van der Heul RO, Misdorp W: Metastatic bone neoplasms in dogs, cats and a lion (with some comparative remarks on the situation in man). *Zbl Vet Med (A)* 17:909–919, 1970.

47. De Vico G, Maiolino P: Prognostic value of nuclear morphometry in feline mammary carcinomas. *J Comp Pathol* 114:99–105, 1997.

48. Della Salda L, Sarli G, Benazzi C, Marcato PS: Giant cells in anaplastic mammary carcinoma of the dog and cat. *J Comp Pathol* 109:345–360, 1993.

49. Tateyama S, Shibata I, Yamaguchi R, et al: Participation of myofibroblasts in feline mammary carcinoma. *Jpn J Vet Sci* 50:1048–1054, 1988.

50. Scanziani E, Mandelli G: Contributo allo studio della classificazione dei tumori mammari felini—Histologic classification of feline mammary tumors. *Alti-della Societa, Italiana-della Scienze Veterinarie* 39:552–554, 1986.

51. Ivanyi D, Minke JMHM, Hageman C, et al: Cytokeratins as markers of initial stages of squamous metaplasia in feline mammary carcinomas. *Am J Vet Res* 54: 1095–1102, 1993.

52. de las Mulas JM, del los Monteros AE, Bautista MJ, et al: Immunohistochemical distribution pattern of intermediate filament proteins and muscle actin in feline and human mammary carcinomas. *J Comp Pathol* 111:365–381, 1994.

53. De Vico G, Maiolino P, Restucci B: Silver-stained nucleolar (Ag-NOR) cluster size in feline mammary carcinomas: Lack of correlation with histological appearance, mitotic activity, tumour stage, and degree of nuclear atypia. *J Comp Pathol* 113:69–73, 1995.

54. Castagnaro M, Casalone C, Ru G, et al: Argyrophilic nucleolar organiser regions (AgNORs) count as indicator of post-surgical prognosis in feline mammary carcinomas. *Res Vet Sci* 64:97–100, 1998.

55. Fox LE, MacEwen EG, Kurzman ID, et al: L-MTP-PE treatment of feline mammary adenocarcinoma. *Proc 14th Annu Conf Vet Cancer Soc*:107–108, 1994.

56. Mauldin GE, Mooney SC, Patnaik AK, Mauldin GN: Adjuvant doxorubicin for feline mammary adenocarcinoma. *Proc 14th Annu Conf Vet Cancer Soc*:41, 1994.

57. Stolwijk JAM, Minke JMHM, Rutteman GR, et al: Feline mammary carcinomas as a model for human breast cancer. II. Comparison of in vivo and in vitro Adriamycin sensitivity. *Anticancer Res* 9:1045–1048, 1989.

58. Misdorp W: Incomplete surgery, local immunostimulation, and recurrence of some tumour types in dogs and cats. *Vet Q* 9:279–286, 1987.

59. Hruban Z, Carter WE, Meehan T, et al: Complex mammary carcinoma in a tiger *(Panthera tigris)*. *J Zoo Anim Med* 19:226–230, 1988.

60. Harrenstien LA, Munson L, Seal US: Mammary cancer in captive wild felids and risk factors for its development: A retrospective study of the clinical behavior of 31 cases. *J Zoo Wildl Med* 27:468–476, 1996.

61. Frazier KS, Hines II ME, Ruiz C, et al: Immunohistochemical differentiation of multiple metastatic neoplasia in a jaguar *(Panthera onca)*. *J Zoo Wildl Med* 25:286–293, 1994.

62. Gillette EL, Acland HM, Klein L: Ductular mammary carcinoma in a lioness. *JAVMA* 173:1099–1102, 1978.

63. Munson L, Stokes JE, Harrenstein LA: Uterine cancer in zoo felids on progestin contraceptives. *Vet Pathol* 32:578, 1995.

64. Chandra S, Laughlin DC: Virus-like particles in cystic mammary adenoma of a snow leopard. *Cancer Res* 35:3069–3074, 1975.

MANAGEMENT OF SPECIFIC DISEASES

TUMORS OF THE RESPIRATORY TRACT

47

Antony S. Moore and Gregory K. Ogilvie

NASOPHARYNGEAL POLYPS

CLINICAL BRIEFING

Common Presentation	Usually young cats (<2 years of age). Cough, gagging after eating, nasal signs, or otic discharge; often mild but progressive. Peripheral vestibular disease may be present.
Staging and Diagnosis	MDB and skull radiographs, including bullae; CT scan of bullae if radiographs are equivocal. Endoscopy of nasopharynx and otic examination with biopsy.
Treatment Initial	Surgical excision may require bulla osteotomy and separate aural surgery for complete resection. Recurrence after complete removal is rare.
Supportive	Preoperative antiinflammatories do not seem to help. Postoperative analgesia as needed.

Incidence, Signalment, and Etiology

Polyps of the nasopharynx are thought to arise in either the eustachian tube or the tympanic bullae.[1] While polyps are often inflamed when they occur in the nasopharynx, those within the middle ear are often quiescent. It is possible that trauma in the nasopharynx creates secondary inflammation.[2]

KEY POINT

Not all cats with nasopharyngeal polyps are young.

The majority of affected cats are less than 2 years of age (26 of 31 cats in one survey were less than 1 year old).[3] Cats as old as 15 years have been described,[4] and some cats have mild signs for years prior to diagnosis.[5]

Of cats for which breed information was provided, 18 were DSHs. Three Himalayan cats less than a year old, including two littermates, have been described.[2,6] In addition, a Siamese, a Persian, and an Abyssinian were reported.[1,4,5] Of cats for which the information was available, 13 were male (7 castrated) and 9 were female (6 spayed).

Clinical Presentation and History

Nasal signs such as discharge, sneezing, snuffling, and stertor are commonly noted, may have been present from birth or soon afterwards, and often have been occurring for many months.[2,7] Signs may be mild enough to be tolerated by an owner for 1 to 2 years prior to presentation.[1,5] Cough-

ing is occasionally noted in a cat with nasopharyngeal polyps.[2] Cats may be dysphagic or have episodes of choking or gagging, particularly when eating.[1,3,6,8] Large polyps may cause ventral deviation of the soft palate.

Otorrhea is common and has been reported in some older cats.[3-5] The otic discharge is most often purulent but may be ceruminous or even hemorrhagic.[4]

Signs of peripheral neurologic disease are less common, although a head tilt was seen in 4 of the 12 cats in one series. Circling as well as dysequilibrium that may be accompanied by nystagmus has been reported.[4,5,7,9]

KEY POINT

Skull radiographs, and CT scan if available, should be performed to assess the tympanic bullae in cats with suspected nasopharyngeal polyps.

Staging and Diagnosis

Staging includes at least an MDB, thorough otic examination, endoscopy and biopsy of the nasopharynx, skull radiographs, and/or CT scan. Skull radiographs may sometimes disclose a soft tissue density in the nasopharynx, and thus it is important to obtain open-mouth radiographs to outline both of the tympanic bullae. Bullae may have thickened margins or be filled with a soft tissue density. The bullae were involved either by polyp extension or accumulation of debris in 37 of 56 reported cases.[1-6] Bulla involvement has implications for treatment. CT will outline the bullae with more detail if radiographs are equivocal. Bilateral polyps have occasionally been reported.[2,5]

Treatment

It has been strongly recommended that bulla osteotomy be performed if there are signs of tympanic bulla involvement.[3,7,10] When the bullae are opened, drainage should be established and samples collected for bacteriologic culture and sensitivity testing. Although a persistent Horner's syndrome has been described in some cats following bulla osteotomy,[5,11] it is mostly a transient complication. In a series of 25 cats undergoing bulla osteotomy for treatment of nasopharyngeal polyps, 24 developed Horner's syndrome, which resolved within 1 month of surgery in 21 cats.[3] In that same study, a cranial nerve palsy occurred in 1 of 31 cats and 1 cat died.[3] In another report, 7 cats with inflammatory polyps treated with bulla osteotomy were free of disease an average of 17 months after surgery (range, 5 to 36 months without recurrence).[7] Two of these cats required a separate aural surgery. Transient Horner's syndrome resolved by 4 weeks postoperatively in all cats (Figure 47-1).

KEY POINT

Bulla osteotomy should be performed if there is evidence of bulla involvement.

On occasion, it may be necessary to split the soft palate to gain access to a nasopharyngeal polyp,[6] and a lateral ear resection may be required when polyps involve the otic canal.[4] Often the polyps may be removed by gentle traction as they arise on a long pedicle. Although corticosteroids have been used preoperatively in some cats, presumably to reduce inflammation,[1] there does not seem to be any advantage to this approach. Postoperative analgesia, however, is warranted as supportive care for these cats.

MDB = minimum database; includes CBC, biochemical profile, urinalysis, FeLV/FIV serology, T_4 testing, and thoracic radiographs (three views).

Of the treated cats reported, the vast majority had complete resolution of signs. Recurrence seems to be rare even when the polyp is removed by traction. Regrowth following surgery was noted in only 6 of 31 cats in one series.[3] Traction to rupture the pedicle was successful in preventing recurrence for follow-up periods of 4 months to 3 years[1,2,4,5] and was considered "uniformly successful" in another study.[8] Recurrences may develop as soon as 5 weeks[2] or as long as 14 months[4] after surgery. One cat had a recurrence 9 months after surgery, and polyps were removed four times in the after 20 months. There was no recurrence for 20 months following the last surgery.[5] Repeated surgeries may be warranted in selected cases. Additional information on treating otic polyps may be found in Chapter 41.

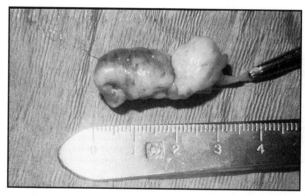

Figure 47-1: A pedunculated nasopharyngeal polyp removed by traction from a young cat. Many cats have bulla involvement, and bulla osteotomy is required for surgical success. (Courtesy of S.M. Cotter)

NASAL TUMORS

Tumors of the nasal planum, particularly squamous cell carcinoma (SCC), are often included in early surveys of "nasal" tumors. This section describes only intranasal tumors. SCC of the nasal planum is discussed in Chapter 50.

CLINICAL BRIEFING

Common Presentation	Carcinomas are most common; sarcomas and benign tumors are rare. Usually affect older cats. Nasal discharge and epistaxis are less common than facial deformity, snuffling, and sneezing. Seizures are rare.
Staging and Diagnosis	MDB, nasal radiographs, CT scan, and palpation of lymph nodes. Suction biopsy using catheter, rhinoscopy, or curettage may not be successful. Rhinotomy may be necessary to obtain diagnosis. Metastasis is rare.

(continued)

Treatment	
Initial	Surgery alone unlikely to be curative; best results obtained with radiation, either alone or postoperatively.
Adjunctive	Chemotherapy probably not needed, but carboplatin likely to be most effective.
Supportive	Appetite stimulants and warmed food will help because of affected cats' poor ability to smell food. Topical eye care following radiation therapy.

BENIGN NASAL TUMORS

Adenomas have been described in four cats ranging in age from 11 to 15 years.[12,13] Two were DSHs (one male and one female), and one was a male Siamese. No further clinical details were available.

Fibroma and fibropapilloma were mentioned in one survey.[13] A hemangioma, first noticed as a nasal deformity 2 years prior to surgery, occurred in a 10-year-old spayed female Siamese. The tumor was removed surgically after epistaxis occurred.[14] A chondroma in a 3-year-old male cat with a 1 year history of nasal signs recurred 3 months after surgical removal.[15] Another 3-year-old Siamese with chondroma was not treated and was lost to follow-up.[16] Benign tumors, particularly papillomas and fibromas, may be difficult to distinguish from inflammatory nasal polyps. If there are many blood vessels, nasal polyps may appear to be hemangiomas.[14] A nasal polyp in a 1-year-old spayed female Russian blue was removed by rhinotomy and had not recurred 12 months later. The author also cited 44 cases of nasal polyps that occurred in Italy.[17]

NASAL CARCINOMAS

This discussion of nasal carcinomas includes all cats with a diagnosis of adenocarcinoma (28 cats), undifferentiated carcinoma (27 cats), and SCC (7 cats). Although nasal SCC has been reported to have a more "sunburst" appearance on radiographs,[14,16,18] there is insufficient data available to distinguish clinically between subtypes.

Incidence, Signalment, and Etiology

Of the 62 cats reported with carcinoma of the nasal cavity, no signalment details were provided for 16[13,19] and a further 26 were discussed in studies that combined data from cats with carcinomas and those with mesenchymal tumors.[14,20]

Ages of the remaining cats ranged from 6 months[15] to 14 years[12,15,16,18,21,22] (median age, 10.5 years). Only 7 cats were 6 years of age or younger. There were 10 females and 16 males. In other surveys, the male:female ratio for all nasal tumors was 2:1,[13] 0.8:1,[14] and 0.9:1.[20] Breeds were not consistently noted, but 28 domestic cats, 8 Siamese, and 1 Persian were reported.[12,14,16,18,21,22] In two other surveys that grouped all histologic types of nasal tumors, 7 of 46 cats were Siamese and 2 were Persian.[15,20] It is interesting to speculate that the longer nasal passages of the Oriental breeds may predispose these cats to nasal tumor malignancies in a manner similar to "long-nosed" dogs.

Clinical Presentation and History

Nasal discharge is less common in cats than in dogs, and epistaxis occurs in only one third of cats. Discharge is often unilateral.[19,20] Sneezing, snuffling, snorting, and dyspnea are more common and may occur with or without nasal discharge. These signs are often worse when the cat is grooming, eating, or sleeping. Ocular discharge due to blockage of the nasolacrimal duct is common,[16] while seizures may indicate extension of the tumor into the brain. Facial deformity and exophthalmos or enophthalmos due to orbital invasion may be present in up to 70% of cases (Figures 47-2 and 47-3).[20] Signs relating to nasal carcinoma had been present for 4 weeks to 8 months in one report[14] and 1.5 weeks to 4.5 years in another[15] (median, 6 months).

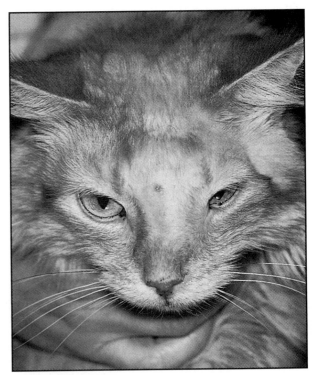

Figure 47-2: *Facial deformity in a cat with recurrent nasal carcinoma after being treated with radiation. This cat subsequently responded to carboplatin chemotherapy.*

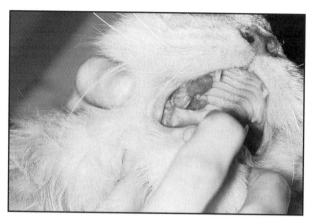

Figure 47-3: Nasal adenocarcinoma may occasionally erode the palate, causing signs and clinical appearance of an oral tumor.

Staging and Diagnosis

In addition to an MDB, staging for nasal carcinoma should include evaluation of lymph nodes and nasal radiographs and CT scan followed by a nasal biopsy. Nasal radiographs, which should include lateral, frontal, and open mouth views (Figure 47-4), will usually demonstrate a nasal opacity or erosion of turbinates, which may occur without an obvious mass lesion.[15,16] Radiographic changes such as deviation of the nasal septum or facial mass and nasal turbinate destruction were the most common findings in two studies[19,20]; however, the same changes can be seen in some cats with rhinitis or cryptococcosis. Neoplasia is more likely in cats with unilateral radiographic lesions showing lysis of lateral bone, nasal turbinate destruction, or tooth loss.[19]

KEY POINT

Epistaxis is less common in cats with nasal carcinoma than it is in dogs.

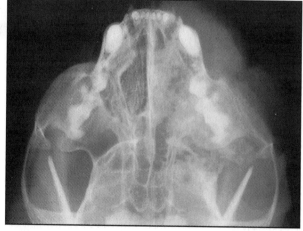

Figure 47-4: An open-mouth radiograph will best demonstrate turbinate destruction and a soft tissue mass. A left nasal tumor with sinus involvement was seen in this elderly cat. (Courtesy of S.M. Cotter)

Closed nasal biopsy using a suction technique may be productive, but no method has 100% diagnostic accuracy without rhinotomy. Most surgeons avoid rhinotomy in cats. One paper described a high success rate for brush cytology as a diagnostic tool in cats with chronic nasal disease[12]; a small cylindrical brush is introduced into the nasal cavity under endoscopic guidance. After "brushing" the lesion, the sample is smeared on glass slides for cytologic evaluation. Nine of 85 samples were nondiagnostic due to a poor sample. Of the 53 samples for which case follow-up was available, the diagnosis of a malignancy was not made in 6 of 17 cats with cancer, and 1 cat that actually had an adenocarcinoma was diagnosed cytologically as having an adenoma.[12] This technique shows promise and has the advantage of being noninvasive.

CT is necessary to accurately delineate the margins of the tumor, particularly if radiation therapy is to be used to treat the tumor (Figure 47-5).

Metastases are uncommon. Two cats with nasal tumors had metastases to the retropharyngeal lymph nodes and lungs, and a carcinoma eroded the cribriform plate to invade the brain in three other cats.[14,15] Nasal SCC metastasized to the submandibular lymph nodes in one cat,[18] although it may actually have had an oral tumor. An undifferentiated nasal carcinoma metastasized to lymph nodes in a cat that had had nasal signs for 17 months prior to diagnosis,[15] illustrating the need for thoracic radiographs and a thorough lymph node examination.

Treatment

One cat that received no treatment lived 4 months before euthanasia, but most cats that were not treated died considerably sooner.[15] Surgery alone (rhinotomy and debulking) was the treatment for five cats with nasal carcinomas. Two cats died in the postoperative period. Tumor recurrence was noted 1 week after surgery in one of the three re-

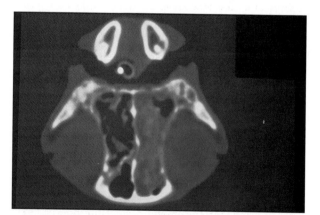

Figure 47-5: A CT scan will allow more accurate delineation of the extent of a nasal tumor and enable accurate planning for radiation therapy. This left-sided nasal carcinoma in a 15-year-old cat is clearly extending into the sinuses.

maining cats, 4 weeks after surgery in the second, and 12 weeks after surgery in the third. Survival times for the first two cats were 3 and 6 weeks, respectively, and the third was lost to follow-up.[15]

Radiation therapy markedly improved the prognosis for most cats. Surgical debulking of the tumor followed by orthovoltage radiation (25–50 Gy) was used to treat six cats with nasal carcinoma.[21] One was still alive 26 months after treatment, and another died without evidence of tumor 40 months after treatment. No recurrence was seen in four cats. Two cats died without evidence of recurrence 5 months after therapy, but one had renal failure and the other had renal lymphoma. Recurrence was noted in one cat 62 months after treatment and in a second at 21 months after treatment; the latter cat was retreated and had another 6 month remission.

Surgery and cobalt-60 irradiation (40–42 Gy) was used to treat three cats. One cat was euthanized due to local tumor extension 3 weeks after treatment; another had tumor recurrence 10 months after treatment, was treated a second time, and had a second recurrence 5 months later. Surgery for the second recurrence was performed at 13 months after the initial treatment; two more surgeries for recurrences were performed at 15 and 21 months after the initial treatment. A fifth recurrence (24 months after the first treatment) was not treated.[15]

KEY POINT

Radiation therapy is very effective for the treatment of feline nasal carcinoma.

Two cats were treated with megavoltage radiation but no surgery; one received 35 Gy and the second 40 Gy. One cat died 2 months later of renal failure while the other cat had no evidence of disease 41 months after treatment.[22] Another cat with a nasal SCC that was treated in the same manner developed local recurrence 2 months after radiation.[16]

Of 10 cats treated with either Cobalt-60 or orthovoltage radiation (44–48 Gy), all of those with nasal carcinoma had either local recurrence of tumor growth or distant metastases (one to mandibular lymph node and one to lungs) within 11 months of starting treatment.[20] Acute side effects of radiation, including moist desquamation and ocular damage, were much less likely to occur in cats compared with dogs with nasal tumors.[20] It may therefore be possible to increase the dose of radiation used in cats and improve these control and survival statistics (Figure 47-6).

Mitoxantrone caused a partial remission for 48 days in a cat with nasal carcinoma,[23] and carboplatin induced complete response for 6 months in one cat and 17 months in a second; both had failed to respond to radiation therapy.[24] Treatment with cyclophosphamide or vincristine in two cats did not cause any remission of tumors that recurred after radiation.[20] Carboplatin, alone or as an adjunct to radiation therapy, appears to be the most likely candidate for chemotherapeutic treatment of feline nasal carcinoma.

Supportive care is critical in the treatment of these cats and should include appropriate analgesia and nutritional support. Warming the food and administering appetite stimulants are warranted due to affected cats' reduced ability to smell. If radiation therapy is used, topical eye care will be necessary during the period of acute reaction. An enteral feeding tube should be considered if therapy is likely to be prolonged.

NASAL SARCOMAS

Intranasal sarcomas have been reported as undifferentiated (8 cats), fibrosarcoma (10 cats), chondrosarcoma (2 cats), osteosarcoma (4 cats), and hemangiosarcoma (4 cats).[13,14,19,20,22,25–27] Details regarding these cases are absent or included with epithelial tumors in three reports[13,19,20] and are available only for 2 cats with chondrosarcoma and 2 with osteosarcoma.[25,26] A 13-year-old spayed female Siamese was treated for nasal chondrosarcoma with a linear accelerator (40 Gy). The tumor recurred 6 months later.[22] A 6-year-old female DSH with a 2 year history of sneezing and diagnosed as having chondrosarcoma was treated surgically, but recurrence was noted 6 months later.[14] Surgical removal of a polypoid osteosarcoma twice over a 14 week period was insufficient to control the tumor in a 6-year-old male.[26] Six cats with either fibrosarcoma or undifferentiated sarcoma were treated with radiation therapy. Their survival times were not distinguished from cats with carcinoma treated the same way, although there were some long-term survivors.[20] One of these cats developed pulmonary metastases; in another, a recurrent tumor invaded the cribriform plate to involve the brain. Median survival for all cats was less than 10 months.

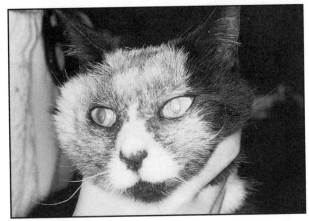

Figure 47-6: *Hair color change in the radiation field of 10-year-old cat treated for bilateral nasal carcinoma. Acute side effects of radiation are less common in cats than in dogs treated for nasal carcinoma.*

As with carcinomas, the higher apparent tolerance of cats than dogs for the acute side effects of radiation may allow larger doses to be delivered and therefore it may be possible to achieve better control of nasal sarcoma. An 11-year-old Siamese treated with radiation for nasal osteosarcoma had a 2 year remission[25] (see Chapter 37).

OLFACTORY NEUROBLASTOMA

CLINICAL BRIEFING	
Common Presentation	Nasal signs accompanied by CNS signs are most common and result from extension through the cribriform plate. Probably FeLV related.
Staging and Diagnosis	As for other nasal tumors (including FeLV serology). CNS signs mandate CT scan. Highly metastatic.
Treatment Initial	Radiation therapy most likely to be successful but unlikely to be curative because of the high metastatic rate.
Adjunctive	Chemotherapy probably warranted, but high rate of FeLV makes prognosis poor. Doxorubicin or carboplatin unproven.
Supportive	Antiinflammatory agents for CNS signs, but corticosteroids may worsen FeLV viremia. Appetite stimulants as needed. Prognosis very poor.

Incidence, Signalment, and Etiology

There are seven reports of these tumors in six cats (one cat was reported twice.)[15,28] Other terms used for this tumor in the veterinary literature include sympathicoblastoma and esthesioneuroblastoma.

One cat was diagnosed with a sympathicoblastoma,[13] but no clinical details were provided. The other tumors occurred in three DSHs and two Siamese (one bluepoint). Ages ranged from 5 to 15 years, and four cats were female (three spayed). The male was castrated.[28,29] All tested cats have been concurrently infected with FeLV, and it is suggested that this tumor is an FeLV-induced neoplasm. An unreported 8-year-old FeLV-positive male cat that was included in a report of a cluster household[30] was later diagnosed with esthesioneuroblastoma.[a]

Clinical Presentation and History

Signs referable to the respiratory system, such as sneezing, dyspnea, unilateral nasal discharge, wheezing, and cough, were present in four of the five cats described above.[28,29] One of these cats developed protrusion of the eye and deformity over the sinus and was euthanized.[28] The other three cats with nasal signs, plus one other cat, had signs referable to the CNS, including circling, ataxia, hindlimb paresis, compulsive pacing, bilateral amaurosis, behavior changes, and coma. The tumor invaded through the cribriform plate to the brain in all five cats.

Staging and Diagnosis

Nasal and CNS signs should prompt critical evaluation of the cribriform plate by radiographs or CT. Additional staging should be similar to that for other nasal tumors: an MDB (including FeLV serology), evaluation of lymph nodes, and biopsy of the mass. Cervical lymph node metastases were seen in two of five cats.[28,29] Testing for FeLV was not performed in two cats[28]; of the other three, one was FeLV antigenemic and one had FeLV in the CSF. Furthermore, FeLV DNA was extracted from the tumor of all three cats and from a metastasis to the mandibular lymph node in one.[29] FeLV could not be demonstrated in normal brain tissue of any of these three animals. This unusual tumor is therefore very likely to be a FeLV-induced neoplasm.

Treatment

No treatment has been described. Radiation therapy may be a possibility, but the rapid progress, high metastatic rate, and presence of concurrent FeLV infection make the prognosis poor. Chemotherapy using doxorubicin or carboplatin, which is unproven in treatment of this disease, may also be attempted.

While antiinflammatories may be used in an attempt to palliate CNS signs, immunosuppression due to corticosteroid treatment may actually worsen FeLV viremia and speed the course of the disease. Appetite stimulants and other nutritional support are often required in cats with olfactory neuroblastoma.

> **KEY POINT**
>
> *Olfactory neuroblastoma is commonly associated with FeLV infection.*

[a]Cotter SM: Personal communication.

NASAL LYMPHOMA

CLINICAL BRIEFING	
Common Presentation	Similar to other nasal tumors, particularly nasal discharge. Usually affects older, FeLV-negative cats but also seen in FeLV-positive cats.
Staging and Diagnosis	MDB, abdominal ultrasonography, bone marrow aspiration. CT scan prior to radiation therapy. FeLV-positive cats more likely to have systemic disease and poor prognosis. Diagnosis is as for other nasal tumors.
Treatment Initial	Radiation therapy or chemotherapy alone or in combination equally effective for nasal disease, but chemotherapy needed for cats with systemic disease. Long survivals possible in FeLV-negative cats.
Supportive	Appetite stimulants and analgesics as needed. Food may be warmed to improve aroma. Topical eye care following radiation therapy.

Incidence, Signalment, and Etiology

In a survey investigating the causes of nasopharyngeal disease in cats, lymphoma, seen in 26 of 53 (49%) cats, was the most common diagnosis.[31]

Sixty-eight cases of nasal lymphoma have been reported in the literature, although no clinical details were provided for 8.[13,19] The ages of the other 60 cats (23 females and 34 males) ranged from 2 to 19 years (median, 8 years). There were 34 DSHs, 11 DLHs, 2 Persians, 7 Siamese, 3 Burmese, 1 Maine Coon, and 1 Tonkinese.[12,15,21,22,32–34] Nine of 35 cats tested for FeLV were seropositive,[22,34,35] but not all of the other cats were tested.

Clinical Presentation and History

Signs on presentation are indistinguishable from those exhibited by cats with other nasal tumors. In order of decreasing frequency, reported signs include nasal discharge, dyspnea, epistaxis, stertor, facial deformity, anorexia, epiphora, exophthalmos, and sneezing.[34] Signs had been present for 6 to 8 weeks in 2 cats[15,32] and for 3 days to 82 weeks (median, 8 weeks) in a large study of 43 cats.[34]

MDB = minimum database; includes CBC, biochemical profile, urinalysis, FeLV/FIV serology, T_4 testing, and thoracic radiographs (three views).

Staging and Diagnosis

Brush cytology correctly identified nasal lymphoma in five of six cats; one cat with lymphoma was thought to have rhinitis, and one cat with lymphocytic-plasmacytic rhinitis

was identified as having lymphoma.[12] Rhinotomy may still be needed to obtain a diagnosis in some cats, as discussed in the section on nasal carcinomas.

Cats with nasal lymphoma should be staged as outlined in Chapter 36, which includes an MDB, abdominal radiographs and/or ultrasonography as appropriate, nasal CT or MRI, and bone marrow aspiration. In a series of 145 cats with lymphoma, 14 had nasal lymphoma. Only 1 of those 14 cats had a T cell tumor, and no cat was FeLV positive.[36]

KEY POINT

A cat with nasal lymphoma should be clinically staged for systemic disease using radiography, ultrasonography, and bone marrow aspiration in addition to the MDB. A CT scan or MRI should be used to image intranasal lesions.

In four case reports, the disease was multicentric, involving the kidneys and lymph nodes,[15] the kidney, lymph nodes, and spleen,[32] the spleen and lymph nodes,[35] and the larynx and trachea.[33] In a large study, only 3 of 46 cats with nasal lymphoma had evidence of systemic disease at initial presentation. Cats that were FeLV positive had a higher risk of developing systemic disease during and after treatment (4 of 7 cats) than did those that were FeLV negative (2 of 27 cats).[34]

Treatment

The tumor recurred in 4 weeks in a cat treated only with surgical curettage and rhinotomy,[32] and another cat hemorrhaged to death during surgery.[34] Radiation has a role in controlling nasal lymphoma and may be curative in cats without systemic involvement.

A cat that received 45 Gy of orthovoltage radiation following biopsy showed local recurrence 6 months later. Another cat treated with rhinotomy and the same radiation protocol died of unrelated causes with no evidence of tumor 19 months later; a second cat that underwent rhinotomy and received the same radiation protocol plus vincristine, cyclophosphamide, and methotrexate chemotherapy died 67 months later; this cat likewise had no evidence of tumor when it died.[21]

Six cats treated with a linear accelerator (8 Gy in two animals, one of which was FeLV antigenemic; 40–44 Gy in the other four) and no chemotherapy had no evidence of disease 12 to 69 months after treatment.[22,37]

Radiation (18 fractions to a total dose of 54 Gy in 4 cats and 3 fractions to a total dose of 30 Gy in 6 cats) was used concurrently with multiagent chemotherapy to treat nasal lymphoma in 10 cats. Three cats in the first group and 4 in the second had a complete response that was ongoing 4 to 55 months later. The 3 cats that failed to respond died within 3 months.[38] Fifteen cats that failed to respond to chemotherapy were treated with radiation therapy; 9 cats responded, but 13 died of systemic disease in less than 3 months. Two cats were alive and in remission, 1 at 8 months and 1 at 38 months after treatment.[38] Coarsely fractionated radiation therapy may have the same efficacy as conventional fractionation in the treatment of feline nasal lymphoma.

In a study comparing radiation versus chemotherapy versus a combination of the two, immunoblastic histologic phenotype and FeLV antigenemia were associated with poor survival, but the treatment modality did not influence outcome.[34] Survival times were not statistically different whether a cat received radiation, chemotherapy, or a combination thereof. In this study, 5 of 6 cats had a complete clinical response to radiation therapy alone and 6 of 8 cats responded to combined therapy. The median survival did not vary significantly between these two groups (593 days versus 178 days, respectively).[34] Ten of 19 cats treated with chemotherapy only had a complete response, and their overall survival was 151 days.

KEY POINT

FeLV antigenemia is a poor prognostic sign for cats with nasal lymphoma.

As for all cats with nasal tumors, supportive care, particularly nutritional support, is critical for a successful outcome. Inability to smell food may greatly decrease a cat's willingness to eat, making appetite stimulants and warming of food necessary. Antiemetics may also be appropriate if chemotherapy is used, and topical eye care is necessary during the period of acute reaction following radiation therapy to the head. Appropriate analgesia should also be administered as needed to ensure the patient's comfort. An enteral feeding tube should be considered if therapy is likely to be prolonged.

LARYNGEAL TUMORS

A laryngeal adenoma that caused almost complete obstruction of the airway was described in a series of cats with respiratory diseases,[39] and granulomatous disease that mimicked neoplasia but was responsive to corticosteroids was reported in three cats.[40] All other reported laryngeal tumors in cats have been malignant.

CLINICAL BRIEFING

Common Presentation	Lymphoma, SCC, and adenocarcinoma all have similar signs of dyspnea progressing to respiratory distress. Dysphonia may precede acute signs.
Staging and Diagnosis	MDB, laryngeal ultrasonography or endoscopy, lymph node evaluation, and biopsy of the tumor. Lymphoma staging should include bone marrow aspiration and abdominal ultrasonography. All tumor types are usually associated with systemic disease or metastases.
Treatment	
Initial	Surgery unlikely to be palliative or curative. Radiation therapy unproven but probably best for local control.
Adjunctive	Chemotherapy for lymphoma (see Chapter 36) and carcinomas; doxorubicin and carboplatin unproven but may be effective in slowing metastases if not already present.
Supportive	Analgesics as needed. Gastrostomy tube if definitive treatment attempted. Tracheostomy may be necessary if acute dyspnea is present and may need to be in place long term if definitive treatment is attempted.

LARYNGEAL LYMPHOMA

Incidence, Signalment, and Etiology

Of the 11 cats reported, no case details were provided for 1.[41] Ages of affected cats ranged from 2 to 17 years (median, 10 years). Eight were DSHs, 1 was Burmese, and 1 was a DLH.[33,42] Nine cats were male (6 castrated), and 1 was a spayed female. FeLV testing was not performed on these cats.

Clinical Presentation and History

Dyspnea, the most common sign, was present for 6 weeks to 4 months prior to presentation. Dyspnea progressed to acute respiratory distress in two cats, and a third cat became cyanotic. Other respiratory signs such as cough, gagging, and stertor were seen in some cats. Aphonia and voice changes occurred in two cats. Horner's syndrome was seen in one cat, and nasal discharge occurred in a cat that had nasal involvement.

Staging and Diagnosis

Lymphoma should always be considered a systemic disease; of eight cats in one series, two had nasal and tracheal involvement as well as retropharyngeal and cervical lymph node involvement.[33] One cat in another study had intestinal and lymph node involvement.[43] Necropsy information was not available for all cats. It would be wise to perform complete staging procedures (as outlined in Chapter 36) for any cat with laryngeal lymphoma.

Ultrasonography was shown to be an excellent imaging technique for laryngeal tumors in cats, and ultrasound-guided biopsy resulted in fewer complications than biopsy via the oropharynx.[44] Five cats had masses that protruded into the laryngeal lumen,[33] while three cats had diffuse laryngeal thickening.[33,42]

Treatment

No treatment was reported for cats with laryngeal lymphoma. Radiation for control or palliation of the local disease and chemotherapy for systemic lymphoma (as outlined in Chapter 36) would be the most likely to succeed.

A tracheostomy may be necessary prior to definitive treatment if the cat is in acute respiratory distress. Nutritional support—including appetite stimulants, placement of an enteral feeding tube, and antiemetic therapy—and analgesia to minimize discomfort associated with this disease and its treatment are often necessary.

SQUAMOUS CELL CARCINOMA (SCC)

Incidence, Signalment, and Etiology

The median age of six cats with laryngeal SCC was 14 years (range, 5 to 18 years). There were four DSHs, one DLH, and one Burmese.[14,33,42,45,46] A seventh cat that probably had a laryngeal SCC was also reported.[47]

Clinical Presentation and History

A cat that was dyspneic and coughing for 6 years was presumed to have asthma. This cat became acutely cyanotic before presentation. A second cat that had been dyspneic for 1 year and coughing and inappetent for 3 months presented with acute stridor. Severe dyspnea and hypersalivation were the presenting signs in another cat.[47] Signs of aphonia for 1 month and respiratory distress, coughing, and gagging for 2 months preceded acute stridor in two other cats.[45,46] One cat gagged if it attempted to purr.[45]

Staging and Diagnosis

SCC appeared as an annular constriction that was invasive deep into laryngeal tissues and the surrounding pharynx in most cats.[14,42,46] In one cat, multiple 2 mm to 1 cm masses were found in the lumen of the larynx and trachea and extended to the tracheal bifurcation and major bronchi.[33] Radiographs, which disclosed a mass occluding the laryngeal lumen and thickening of the epiglottis in two cats,[45,46] may also appear normal. Visualization of the larynx directly using a laryngoscope or endoscope is recommended. Metastases to the regional lymph nodes were seen in one cat,[47] but no metastases were reported in the others. Complete staging, including an MDB, laryngeal ultrasonography or endoscopy, evaluation of lymph nodes, and biopsy of the tumor, is recommended.

Ultrasound-guided biopsy may be less invasive than the intraluminal route to confirm a diagnosis of laryngeal neoplasia.[44]

Treatment

One cat that was not treated was euthanized due to dysphagia within 3 weeks of diagnosis.[45] A local excision was attempted in one cat, but the animal died due to respiratory distress 2 days after surgery. Neoplastic cells were found invading deep into the wall of the larynx.[46] Anecdotally, the size of the mass reduced markedly in a 12-year-old castrated male DSH treated with 48 Gy (using a linear accelerator) and concurrent carboplatin chemotherapy,[b] but the tumor soon recurred. Because of the invasive nature of this tumor, radiation therapy appears the most likely to be successful. Oral SCC is resistant to radiation whereas cutaneous SCC is very sensitive to the effects of radiation therapy. Radiation therapy, in combination with chemotherapy, may provide the best control of this disease. Supportive care, as described for lymphoma of the larynx, is important if treatment is to be attempted. A tracheostomy may be necessary prior to definitive treatment.

---

[b]Moore AS: Personal observation.

LARYNGEAL ADENOCARCINOMA

Incidence, Signalment, and Etiology

Three cats with this tumor have been reported. Two were DSHs (a 10-year-old castrated male and a 15-year-old female) and the other was a 13-year-old castrated Manx.[33,48,49]

Clinical Presentation and History

Recent onset of dysphonia, dyspnea, cough, and respiratory distress was seen in these cats.[33,48,49]

Staging and Diagnosis

Complete staging, including the MDB, laryngeal ultrasonography or endoscopy, evaluation of lymph nodes, and biopsy of the tumor, is recommended. While no metastases were seen in one cat,[33] both of the other two cats had metastases to the cervical lymph nodes. One cat had additional metastases to the lungs, spleen, and adrenal glands.[48]

Treatment

Laryngeal resection was attempted in the Manx. The cat died acutely 4 days after surgery due to a tracheal occlusion even though tracheostomy and pharyngostomy tubes were placed. Despite the wide resection, tumor cells had invaded into surrounding musculature, and there were metastases to regional lymph nodes.[49]

Radiation therapy may be a potential method of palliation, although there are no reports of its use. Carcinomas of some sites are very sensitive to the effects of radiation therapy. Radiation therapy in combination with chemotherapy may provide the best control of this disease. Again, appropriate supportive care as described for laryngeal lymphoma is critical for the success of treatment and is necessary to minimize discomfort.

Nondomestic Felidae

A 14-year-old male lion (*Panthera leo*) had shown progressive exercise intolerance and dyspnea over several months and aphonia for the 2 months preceding presentation. Bronchoscopy revealed a pedunculated laryngeal neurofibroma (Schwannoma). The tumor was surgically excised and treated with 40 Gy of cobalt-60 radiation therapy. The lion was able to vocalize in 5 days and was free of disease 9 months later.[50]

TRACHEAL TUMORS

CLINICAL BRIEFING

Common Presentation	Lymphoma and carcinomas cause similar signs of dyspnea, which can be severe. Carcinomas are usually intrathoracic; lymphoma may be anywhere.
Staging and Diagnosis	MDB, bronchoscopy, and biopsy. Metastatic rate for carcinomas is uncertain. Lymphoma staging, including bone marrow aspiration and abdominal ultrasonography.
Treatment Initial	Local excision may be palliative; segmental tracheal resection may give long-term control for carcinomas. Lymphoma is best treated with chemotherapy (see Chapter 36).
Adjunctive	Postoperative chemotherapy may be warranted for carcinomas. Carboplatin or doxorubicin unproven but most likely to be effective.
Supportive	Appetite stimulants; consider gastrostomy tube if definitive treatment is planned. Analgesics as needed.

Tumors of the trachea are uncommon. Four of 11 cats described in the literature were Siamese.[51-54] The other cats were DSHs (5 cats), DLH (1 cat), or Persian-cross (1 cat). Eight cats had epithelial tumors, and 3 cats had lymphoma. In addition, a 6-year-old cat with an adenoma at the tracheal bifurcation that was causing regurgitation and dyspnea was reported.[55]

CARCINOMAS

Incidence, Signalment, and Etiology

The age range of the eight affected cats was 2 to 12 years (median age, 9.5 years). For those with available information, there were four males (two castrated) and two spayed females. Four cats had adenocarcinoma, two had SCC, and two had other carcinomas.

Clinical Presentation and History

With the exception of one young cat[56] that had a few days' history of dyspnea, cats with tracheal carcinoma had a 6 week to 6 month history of signs referable to the respiratory tract.[51,52,57,58] These signs encompassed severe dyspnea that included open-mouth breathing[58] or even cyanosis.[58]

Cough, gagging, and stridor were also described. One cat had recently been anorectic,[51] but this finding was not described in other cats.

Two cats had carcinoma at the tracheal bifurcation.[42,57] Tumors in the other cats occurred anywhere from the thoracic inlet[52,53,58] to the intrathoracic trachea.[42,51,56] Seven cats had a single tracheal mass, and one cat had two masses at the thoracic inlet.[58] Masses were sometimes large (2 cm in one cat),[51] and in one cat a single mass had extended along the length of the trachea.[52]

Staging and Diagnosis

Staging should involve the MDB, bronchoscopy, and biopsy. Thoracic radiographs were able to demonstrate a tracheal mass in three cats,[51,53,57] and one cat had a fractured rib, presumably from the effort of coughing.[57] Bronchoscopy was successfully used to visualize masses located anywhere from the thoracic inlet to the tracheal bifurcation in two cats. If bronchoscopy is being considered for diagnosis or treatment, it is important that the veterinarian is trained in endoscopic technique before attempting the procedure. Bronchoscopy was used to remove the mass from one cat, but a second cat died during the procedure.[56]

No metastases were seen on thoracic radiographs from cats with tracheal carcinoma,[51] even after prolonged remission.[57] There were likewise no metastases on necropsy in at least two cats.[56,58]

Treatment

Thoracotomy and tracheostomy were performed in three cats. One cat had an extensive infiltrative tumor and was euthanized.[52] Tracheal resection was performed in the other two; to obtain surgical margins around the tumor, a 2.5[51] or 3[53] cm length of trachea needed to be resected. There was no follow-up beyond surgical recovery in one cat,[51] but the other had no evidence of disease 1 year after surgery.

An 8 × 5 × 3 mm tracheal mass was inadvertently suctioned from the tracheal bifurcation during bronchoscopy in one cat. The signs were relieved and the cat was normal until the tumor recurred 11 months later. Repeated suction removed the regrowth, and the cat was asymptomatic for a further 6 months, at which time recurrence led to euthanasia.[57]

At least one cat had no response to corticosteroids.[52]

Chemotherapy may be warranted postoperatively. Based on their efficacy for the treatment of other carcinomas, carboplatin or doxorubicin may be the best options for adjunctive treatment.

Appetite stimulants, enteral feeding tube placement, antiemetic administration, and analgesia may be necessary to optimize supportive care for and treatment of cats with this disease.

LYMPHOMA

Incidence, Signalment, and Etiology

Three Siamese (7-year-old male,[54] 9-year-old male,[53] and 13-year-old female[59]) and an 11-year-old DSH male[52] have been reported with this disease. One cat was FeLV positive,[54] two were FeLV and FIV negative,[53,59] and the fourth was not tested.

Clinical Presentation and History

Signs similar to those seen with tracheal carcinoma have been described, with dyspnea occurring most frequently. Onset of signs was more acute in this group of cats than in cats with tracheal carcinoma.

Staging and Diagnosis

Staging as described in Chapter 36, including an FeLV antigen test as part of the MDB, should be performed as systemic disease may also be present.[52] Radiographs may not reveal a mass; however, a mass was seen in either the cervical trachea[54] or at the thoracic inlet[52,53] (Figure 47-7) in all three cats in which bronchoscopy was used. Ribs 7 through 13 were unilaterally fractured in one cat, presumably as a result of coughing.[54] The tumor was a B cell neoplasm in one cat[59] and of uncertain derivation in the others.

Treatment

Three cats were treated. In one cat, 3 cm of trachea was resected and the tumor regrew within 10 days. A second resection was not possible, and the cat was euthanized.[53] A second cat in which 1.8 cm of trachea was resected died 4 months later with renal and gastrointestinal lymphoma,[52] but there was no local tumor regrowth. The third cat, which was FeLV positive, had four tracheal rings removed surgically and was treated with vincristine, cyclophosphamide, and prednisone. There was no evidence of disease 8 months later.[54]

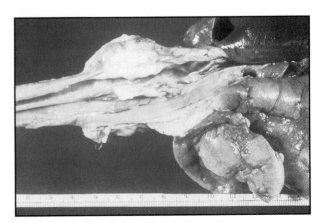

Figure 47-7: *Tracheal lymphoma at the thoracic inlet caused dyspnea and inappetence in a 15-year-old cat.*

Radiation may have a role in the control of tracheal lymphoma and may be curative in cats without systemic involvement. The treatment of choice would be radiation (or surgery) to control local tracheal disease and adjuvant chemotherapy as described in Chapter 36.

LUNG TUMORS

CLINICAL BRIEFING

Common Presentation	Most are carcinomas; sarcomas and benign tumors are very rare. Mostly affects older cats; signs are nonspecific. Respiratory signs, which are often chronic, are seen in only 50% of cats. Vomiting, lameness due to musculoskeletal metastases, and ataxia may be seen.
Staging and Diagnosis	MDB, thoracocentesis, and cytology; ultrasound-, fluoroscopic-, or CT-guided biopsy. Bronchoscopy with cytologic brushing. Careful musculoskeletal examination and abdominal ultrasonography.
Treatment Initial	Lung lobectomy for solitary tumors.
Adjunctive	Postoperative chemotherapy with doxorubicin and carboplatin may be palliative for metastatic disease (unproven).
Supportive	Antiinflammatories and analgesics for musculoskeletal metastases. Appetite stimulants as needed.

Incidence, Signalment, and Etiology

There are over 300 reports of lung tumors in cats. At least partial signalment data is available for 257 of these cats.

The most common tumors of the lung are of epithelial derivation; only three sarcomas have been described.[60,61] In addition, most tumors are malignant, with adenoma[60,61] and adenomatosis[62] described in only three cats. Most tumors derive from the bronchi and bronchial glands and are subdivided as adenocarcinoma and adenosquamous carcinoma; tumors from alveoli are similarly divided. SCC is less common, and some carcinomas are classified as anaplastic. To the veterinary clinician, there appears to be very little need to distinguish between these lung tumor types, as all are aggressive tumors that are often diagnosed late in the course of disease. Ages of cats with lung tumors ranged from 2 to 20 years, with very few cats under the age of 5 being reported.[14,60,63–65] The average age in all reported series of cats is 12 years.[14,60,61,63,66] There may be a female gender predilection; 93 cats were male and 134 were female, and most were castrated or spayed. Most affected cats were DSHs (165 cats) or DLHs (14 cats). Twelve cats were Siamese, 9 were Persian, 2 were Himalayan, 2 were Russian Blue (Maltese), and 1 was a Scottish Fold. Seven cats were purebred crosses.[60]

Clinical Presentation and History

Nonspecific signs of malaise, such as weight loss, lethargy, and anorexia, were the most common signs at presentation in three series encompassing 103 cats.[60,63,66] Signs had been present for an average of 2 to 5 weeks and up to 36 weeks in one study.[60] Other signs, such as diarrhea, polydipsia, polyuria, and fever, were less common.[60,63] Signs referable to the respiratory system occurred in one third to more than half the cats in some studies,[60,63,67] although many cats do not show respiratory signs and instead are presented for problems caused by metastases.[60,68] Dyspnea and tachypnea, the most commonly observed respiratory signs in cats with pulmonary carcinomas, had been present for days to 4 months prior to presentation.[60] Some cats had had signs for longer than 1 to 2 years.[14,63,65] Another sign referable to the respiratory system, coughing that is more often nonproductive than productive (27% versus 12% of cats, respectively), may also be present for months.[60,61] Wheezing has been reported,[60,66] but hemoptysis is rare.[60,66] Other occasionally reported respiratory signs include cyanosis and panting with exertion.[14]

Vomiting has been reported in approximately 20% of affected cats in case series and case reports. In some cats this sign is associated with tumor infiltration and constriction of the esophagus that could interfere with motility. Lameness has been commonly reported although, the large number of case reports associating lameness with pulmonary neoplasia may reflect the interesting natural history of the disease rather than true prevalence. Lameness was present in only 5% to 25% of cats in case series. Lameness may be present for up to 3 months prior to presentation (average, about 4 weeks). Metastases to the digits causing swelling, permanent exsheathment of multiple nails, paronychia, or cellulitis with loose claws (Figure 47-8) is the cause of lameness in some cats,[64,70,72-76] while metastases to muscles may cause lameness in others.[69,77,78] A cat that has multiple digital adenocarcinomas may be thought to have a primary malignancy of the sweat glands. It is equally or even more likely to have metastases from a primary lung tumor.[79] In a series of 19 cats with metastases from pulmonary carcinoma to the nail bed, 6 cats had multiple digits involved and the tumor sometimes invaded the interarticular space, causing lysis of the second and third phalanxes.[68] In a series of 64 cats with digital carcinomas, 56 had metastases from a pulmonary tumor and only 8 had a primary nailbed SCC. Primary adenocarcinoma of the digits was not observed.[80]

Hypertrophic osteopathy associated with pulmonary carcinoma was a reported cause of lameness in three cats.[6,77,78] The periosteal new bone production affected the long bones of all three and included the humeri in two cats (Figure 47-9); the lower limbs were less affected in one cat.[81] The primary lung lesion in all three of these cats was a large solitary carcinoma.

KEY POINT

A cat with multiple digital tumors should be evaluated for the presence of a primary lung tumor.

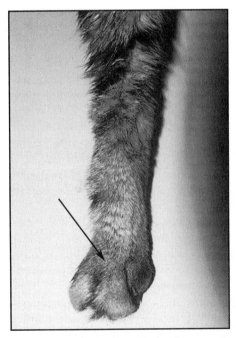

Figure 47-8: Lameness caused by digital metastasis (arrow) from a pulmonary tumor may be the presenting complaint in a cat without any respiratory signs.

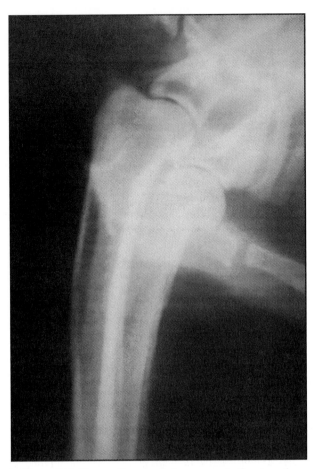

Figure 47-9: Hypertrophic osteopathy is a rare sequela of a primary lung tumor and often affects the proximal (rather than distal) extremities, as occurred this 15-year-old cat with a pulmonary tumor.

Ataxia of recent onset was reported in 21% of cats with lung tumors.[60] Paresis, paralysis, anisocoria, and uveitis have also been reported and are due to metastases to either the muscle[78,82] or the eyes.[63,76,82,83] Paraneoplastic polyneuropathy was suspected in one cat with paraparesis,[78] and hypercalcemia was found in a cat with metastatic SCC that was probably of pulmonary origin.[84]

Staging and Diagnosis

Although thoracic radiographs should be part of the MDB for any cat with suspected cancer, they are particularly critical to search for a primary lung tumor in cats with such respiratory signs as dyspnea, tachypnea, and cough. The presence of a primary lung tumor should likewise be considered for cats with chronic vomiting, musculoskeletal carcinoma, or multiple paronychia.

Thoracic radiographs may show a solitary well-circumscribed mass (Figure 47-10), solitary lobar consolidation (Figure 47-11), multiple well-circumscribed masses, or possibly a diffuse bronchointerstitial pattern of involvement that can mimic the appearance of feline asthma.[63] The cau-

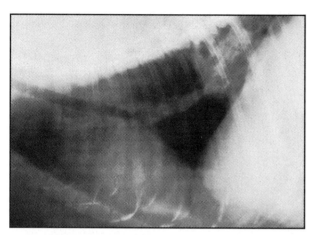

Figure 47-10: A solitary pulmonary mass may be an incidental finding. This radiograph is from an elderly Tonkinese presented for vomiting but that did not have respiratory signs. The diagnosis was pulmonary adenocarcinoma. (Courtesy of K.M. Rassnick)

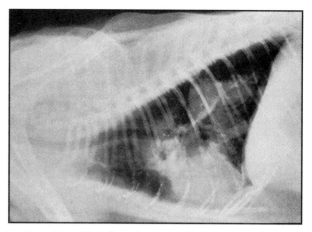

Figure 47-11: The radiographic appearance of a lung tumor may vary. The tumor appears as a consolidated lung lobe in this cat.

dal lung lobes are more likely than the cranial lobes to be affected when a solitary tumor is present, but diffuse lung involvement is common, occurring in about 25% of cases.[60,63] Tumor mineralization is rare.[64] Metastases to the tracheobronchial lymph nodes may not always be radiographically apparent in cats.[61] Pleural effusion may obscure a mass or hinder radiographic interpretation (Figures 47-12 and 47-13). Pleural effusion is seen in up to one third of cats[60,66] and may be severe.[14,60,61,63,66,70] In a series of 82 cats with pleural effusion of all causes, pulmonary carcinoma was confirmed to be the cause in 5 cats.[85] Cytologic examination of the effusion may be diagnostic for carcinoma; 12 of 13 samples obtained by thoracocentesis in one series of cats were diagnostic for pulmonary carcinoma.[60] This procedure had a lower positive yield in other series (3 of 16 cats).[61,72,85]

Preoperative diagnosis may also be obtained by ultrasound-guided fine-needle aspiration or by blind aspiration. These techniques were successful in 20 of 25 cats in one se-

ries.[60] Fluoroscopic-guided aspiration nearly always obtained diagnostic samples in another study,[86] and guidance of aspiration or biopsy using CT may be the most accurate for small or less peripheral lesions.[87] Endoscopic bronchiolar brushing was used to obtain diagnostic samples in 5 of 7 cats,[60] but transtracheal wash was nondiagnostic in 1 cat despite diffuse involvement of lungs.[14]

Systemic metastases from primary lung tumors are very common and may be the reason for presentation in a cat without respiratory signs. Lameness due to metastases preceded signs of dyspnea and cough by 3 weeks to 3 months in some cats[70,75] and up to 11 months in another cat.[88]

In a survey of the literature, intrathoracic metastases were slightly more common than extrathoracic. Intrathoracic metastases were found in regional lymph nodes, pleura, and mediastinum. However, metastases to the kidney, skeletal muscles, and heart occurred almost as frequently. Bone metastases to digits, appendicular skeleton, and axial skeleton (including vertebrae) were also common. Less common metastatic sites included the gastrointestinal tract, spleen,

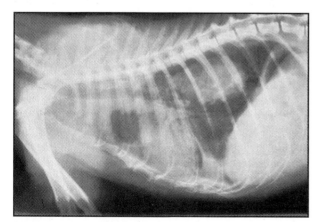

Figures 47-12: Pleural effusion due to pleural metastases from a large caudodorsally located carcinoma may obscure radiographic detail.

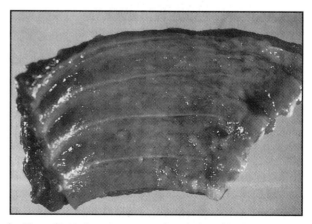

Figure 47-13: A necropsy specimen showing plaque-like pleural metastases from a primary lung tumor.

liver, and skin, while brain, eye, adrenal gland, and urinary bladder metastases were reported in more than one cat. Metastases to the thyroid gland, salivary gland, and pancreas were each reported once.

Due to the frequency of metastases, abdominal ultrasound and a careful musculoskeletal examination should be performed in addition to the MDB, thoracocentesis and fluid cytology, and biopsy when staging cats with this disease.

Treatment

Treatment was reported in six cats for which lameness was the presenting sign. Amputation of affected digits (one cat)[73] or the forelimb (one cat)[88] was performed in the absence of respiratory signs. Both cats were dead of the pulmonary disease and other metastases within 2 months. Corticosteroids were used in one of these cats for 9 months before surgery to relieve the musculoskeletal pain[88] and improved the lameness in two other cats.[64,65] In another series of 19 cats with lameness due to digital metastases, surgical excision of the affected digits did little to prolong the median survival time of 2 months.[68] Other sites of metastases and continued lameness were common reasons for euthanasia of the cats in that series.

MDB = minimum database; includes CBC, biochemical profile, urinalysis, FeLV/FIV serology, T$_4$ testing, and thoracic radiographs (three views).

Removal of a pulmonary tumor from a cat with hypertrophic osteopathy (HO) did not resolve the HO; 8 weeks later, new pulmonary masses and renal and skeletal metastases led to euthanasia.[89] No treatment was prescribed for another cat with HO, and the cat was euthanized due to poor mobility an astonishing 17 months later.[81]

Stapling equipment provides a rapid and safe method of removing pulmonary tumors in cats (Figure 47-14).[90]

Primary lung tumors were surgically removed from 21 cats in one study.[91] A solitary lobe was removed from 19 cats, while both the left cranial and caudal lobes were removed from 2 cats; surgical margins were considered adequate. Tracheobronchial lymph node or pleural metastases were seen at surgery in 4 of these cats. Eighteen cats died due to metastatic disease between 2 weeks and 51 months

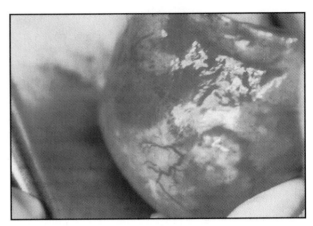

Figure 47-14: *A lung lobectomy may provide long-term palliation and possibly cure if the lesion is small and localized. Tumors such as these could be removed by stapling equipment.*

after surgery (median survival, approximately 4 months). Three cats were lost to follow-up 4 to 13 months after surgery. Nine cats with poorly differentiated tumors had a median survival of 2.5 months, which was significantly shorter than for the 12 cats with moderately differentiated tumors (13 months).

Chemotherapy has not been reported for cats with lung tumors, although two cats that received unspecified drugs died within 1 week of treatment.[85] A cat with metastatic SCC of the lung was given doxorubicin and cyclophosphamide; 3 weeks later, tumors were 25% smaller and hypercalcemia had normalized. This minor response lasted 111 days, at which time the cat died of renal disease.[92]

Although there are no published data, doxorubicin and possibly carboplatin may improve postsurgical survival in cats undergoing lung lobectomy for pulmonary carcinomas.

Supportive care, including antiinflammatory drugs and analgesia for musculoskeletal metastases, is required to minimize discomfort associated with this disease. Appetite stimulants, nutritional support, and antiemetic therapy may also be necessary, particularly postoperatively and after chemotherapy administration.

Nondomestic Felidae

Pulmonary adenocarcinoma was diagnosed in a male snow leopard *(Panthera unicia)*,[93] a cheetah *(Acinonyx jubatus jubatus)*,[94] and an 18-year-old female cougar *(Felis concolor)*.[95] The cougar was found to have concurrent bile duct carcinoma and bilateral thyroid adenocarcinomas that may have contributed to its sudden death.

A pulmonary adenoma was reported in a Siberian tiger *(Panthera tigris)*.[93] A 15-year-old golden cat *(Felis temmincki)* had signs of respiratory distress, anorexia, and uremia before death. A multifocal pulmonary SCC had also metastasized to its kidneys.[96]

REFERENCES

1. Bedford PGC, Coulson A, Sharp NJH, Longstaffe JA: Nasopharyngeal polyps in the cat. *Vet Rec* 109:551–553, 1981.

2. Stanton ME, Wheaton LG, Render JA, Blevins WE: Pharyngeal polyps in two feline siblings. *JAVMA* 186:1311–1313, 1985.

3. Kapatkin A, Matthiesen DT, Noone K, et al: Results of surgical treatment for nasopharyngeal inflammatory polyps in 31 cats. *Vet Surg* 18:59, 1989.

4. Harvey CE, Goldschmidt MH: Inflammatory polypoid growths in the ear canal of cats. *J Small Anim Pract* 19:669–677, 1978.

5. Lane JG, Orr CM, Lucke VM, Gruffydd-Jones TJ: Nasopharyngeal polyps arising in the middle ear of the cat. *J Small Anim Pract* 22:511–522, 1981.

6. Elkins AD: Resolving respiratory distress created by a nasopharyngeal polyp. *Vet Med* 82:1234–1235, 1987.

7. Trevor PB, Martin RA: Tympanic bulla osteotomy for treatment of middle-ear disease in cats: 19 cases (1984–1991). *JAVMA* 202:123–128, 1993.

8. Baker G: Nasopharyngeal polyps in cats. *Vet Rec* 111:43, 1982.

9. Pearson GR, Hart CA: A case of otitis in a domestic cat. *J Small Anim Pract* 21:333–338, 1980.

10. Ader PL, Boothe HW: Ventral bulla osteotomy in the cat. *JAAHA* 15:757–762, 1979.

11. Williams JM, White RAS: Total ear canal ablation combined with lateral bulla osteotomy in the cat. *J Small Anim Pract* 33:225–227, 1992.

12. Caniatti M, Roccabianca P, Ghisleni G, et al: Evaluation of brush cytology in the diagnosis of chronic intranasal disease in cats. *J Small Anim Pract* 39:73–77, 1998.

13. Madewell BR, Priester WA, Gillette EL, Snyder SP: Neoplasms of the nasal passages and paranasal sinuses in domesticated animals as reported by 13 veterinary colleges. *Am J Vet Res* 37:851–856, 1976.

14. Carpenter JL, Andrews LK, Holzworth J: Tumors and tumor-like lesions, in Holzworth J (ed): *Diseases of the Cat. Medicine and Surgery.* Philadelphia, WB Saunders, 1987, pp 407–596.

15. Cox NR, Brawner WR, Powers RD, Wright JC: Tumors of the nose and paranasal sinuses in cats: 32 cases with comparison to a national database (1977 through 1987). *JAAHA* 27:339–347, 1991.

16. Gilger BC, McLaughlin SA, Whitley RD, Wright JC: Orbital neoplasms in cats: 21 cases (1974–1990). *JAVMA* 201:1083–1086, 1992.

17. Galloway PE, Kyles A, Henderson JP: Nasal polyps in a cat. *J Small Anim Pract* 38:78–80, 1997.

18. Peiffer Jr RL, Spencer C, Popp JA: Nasal squamous cell carcinoma with periocular extension and metastasis in a cat. *Feline Pract* 8:43–46, 1978.

19. O'Brien MG, Withrow SJ, Straw RC, et al: Total and partial orbitectomy for the treatment of periorbital tumors in 24 dogs and 6 cats: A retrospective study. *Vet Surg* 25:471–479, 1996.

20. Theon AP, Peaston AE, Madewell BR, Dungworth DL: Irradiation of nonlymphoproliferative neoplasms of the nasal cavity and paranasal sinuses in 16 cats. *JAVMA* 204:78–83, 1994.

21. Evans SM, Hendrick M: Radiotherapy of feline nasal tumors. *Vet Radiol* 30:128–132, 1989.

22. Straw RC, Withrow SJ, Gillette EL, McChesney AE: Use of radiotherapy for the treatment of intranasal tumors in cats: Six cases (1980–1985). *JAVMA* 189:927–929, 1986.

23. Ogilvie GK, Moore AS, Obradovich JE, et al: Toxicoses and efficacy associated with the administration of mitoxantrone to cats with malignant tumors. *JAVMA* 202:1839–1844, 1993.

24. Wood CA, Moore AS, Frimberger AE, et al: Phase I evaluation of carboplatin in tumor bearing cats. *Proc Vet Cancer Soc 16th Annu Conf*:39–40, 1996.

25. Lord PF, Kapp DS, Schwartz A, Morrow DT: Osteogenic sarcoma of the nasal cavity in a cat: Postoperative control with high dose-per-fraction radiation therapy and metronidazole. *Vet Radiol* 23:23–26, 1982.

26. Gehring VH, Schröder U: Nasenpolypen bei einer 6 jährigen katze. *Berl Münch Teirärztl Wschr* 74:54, 1961.

27. Scavelli TD, Patnaik AK, Mehlaff CJ, Hayes AA: Hemangiosarcoma in the cat: Retrospective evaluation of 31 surgical cases. *JAVMA* 187:817–819, 1985.

28. Cox NR, Power RD: Olfactory neuroblastomas in two cats. *Vet Pathol* 26:341–343, 1989.

29. Schrenzel MD, Higgins RJ, Hinrichs SH, et al: Type C retroviral expression in spontaneous feline olfactory neuroblastomas. *Acta Neuropathol* 80:547–553, 1990.

30. Cotter SM, Essex M, Hardy Jr WD: Serological studies of normal and leukemic cats in a multiple-case leukemia cluster. *Cancer Res* 34:1061–1069, 1974.

31. Allen HS, Broussard J, Noone K: Nasopharyngeal diseases in cats: A retrospective study of 53 cases (1991–1998). *JAAHA* 35:457–461, 1999.

32. Legendre AM, Carrig CB, Howard DR, Dade AW: Nasal tumor in a cat. *JAVMA* 167:481–483, 1975.

33. Saik JE, Toll SL, Diters RW, Goldschmidt MH: Canine and feline laryngeal neoplasia: A 10 year survey. *JAAHA* 22:359–365, 1986.

34. Klein MK, Powers BE, Johnson CS, et al: Feline nasal lymphoma: A retrospective analysis, submitted 1999.

35. Van Der Riet FdStJ, McCully RM, Keen GA, Forder AA: Lymphosarcoma in a cat. *J South Afr Vet Assoc* 54:57–59, 1983.

36. Vail DM, Moore AS, Ogilvie GK, Volk LM: Feline lymphoma (145 cases): Proliferation indices, cluster of differentiation 3 immunoreactivity, and their association with prognosis in 90 cats. *J Vet Intern Med* 12:349–354, 1998.

37. Elmslie RE, Ogilvie GK, Gillette EL, McChesney-Gillette S: Radiotherapy with and without chemotherapy for localized lymphoma in 10 cats. *Vet Radiol* 32:277–280, 1991.

38. North SM, Meleo K, Mooney S, Mauldin GN: Radiation therapy in the treatment of nasal lymphoma in cats. *Proc 14th Annu Conf Vet Cancer Soc*:21, 1994.

39. Gibbs C: Radiographic examination of the pharynx, larynx and soft-tissue structures of the neck in dogs and cats. *Vet Annu* 26:227–241, 1986.

40. Tasker S, Foster DJ, Corcoran BM, et al: Obstructive inflammatory laryngeal diseases in three cats. *J Feline Med Surg* 1:53–59, 1999.

41. Harvey CE, O'Brien JA: Surgical treatments of miscellaneous laryngeal conditions in dogs and cats. *JAAHA* 18:557–562, 1982.

42. Carlisle CH, Biery DN, Thrall DE: Tracheal and laryngeal tumors in the dog and cat: Literature review and 13 additional patients. *Vet Radiol* 32:229–235, 1991.

43. Patterson DF, Meier H: Surgical intervention in intestinal lymphosarcoma in two cats. *JAVMA* 127:495–498, 1955.

44. Rudorf H, Brown P: Ultrasonography of laryngeal masses in six cats and one dog. *Vet Radiol Ultrasound* 39:430–434, 1998.

45. O'Handley P, Stickle R: What is your diagnosis? *JAVMA* 191:1492–1493, 1987.

46. Wheeldon EB, Amis TC: Laryngeal carcinoma in a cat. *JAVMA* 186:80–81, 1985.

47. Collet MP: Cancer primitif du larynx chez une chatte. *Bull Soc Sci Vet Lyon* 38:219–226, 1935.

48. Lieberman LL: Feline adenocarcinoma of the larynx with metastasis to the adrenal gland. *JAVMA* 125:153–154, 1954.

49. Vasseur PB, Patnaik AK: Laryngeal adenocarcinoma in a cat. *JAAHA* 17:639–641, 1981.

50. Paul-Murphy J, Lloyd K, Turrel JM, et al: Management of a Schwannoma in the larynx of a lion. *JAVMA* 189:1202–1203, 1986.

51. Cain GR, Manley P: Tracheal adenocarcinoma in a cat. *JAVMA* 182:614–616, 1983.

52. Beaumont PR: Intratracheal neoplasia in two cats. *J Small Anim Pract* 23:29–35, 1982.

53. Zimmermann U, Müller F, Pfleghaar S: Zwei fälle von histogenetisch unterschiedlichen trachealtumoren bei katzen. *Kleintierpraxis* 37:409–412, 1992.

54. Schneider PR, Smith CW, Feller DL: Histiocytic lymphosarcoma of the trachea in a cat. *JAAHA* 15:485–487, 1979.

55. Glock R: Primary pulmonary adenomas of the feline. *Iowa State Vet* 23:155–156, 1961.

56. Veith LA: Squamous cell carcinoma of the trachea in a cat. *Feline Pract* 4:30–32, 1974.

57. Neer TM, Zeman D: Tracheal adenocarcinoma in a cat and review of the literature. *JAAHA* 23:377–380, 1987.

58. Lobetti RG, Williams MC: Anaplastic tracheal squamous cell carcinoma in a cat. *Tydskr S Afr Vet Ver* 63:132–133, 1992.

59. Kim DY, Kim JR, Taylor HW, Lee YS: Primary extranodal lymphosarcoma of the trachea in a cat. *J Vet Med Sci* 58:703–706, 1996.

60. Hahn KA, McEntee MF: Primary lung tumors in cats: 86 cases (1979–1994). *JAVMA* 211:1257–1260, 1997.

61. Barr F, Gruffydd-Jones TJ, Brown PJ, Gibbs C: Primary lung tumours in the cat. *J Small Anim Pract* 28:1115–1125, 1987.

62. Moulton JE, von Tscharner C, Schneider R: Classification of lung carcinomas in the dog and cat. *Vet Pathol* 18:513–528, 1981.

63. Koblik PD: Radiographic appearance of primary lung tumors in cats. *Vet Radiol* 27:66–73, 1986.

64. Brown PJ, Hoare CM, Rochlitz I: Multiple squamous cell carcinoma of the digits in two cats. *J Small Anim Pract* 26:323–328, 1985.

65. Carr SH: Secondary hypertrophic pulmonary osteoarthropathy in a cat. *Feline Pract* 1:25–26, 1971.

66. Mehlhaff CJ, Mooney S: Primary pulmonary neoplasia in the dog and cat. *Vet Clin North Am Small Anim Pract* 15:1061–1068, 1985.

67. Carpenter RH, Hansen JF: Diffuse pulmonary bronchiolo-alveolar adenocarcinoma in a cat. *Calif Vet* 4:11–14, 1982.

68. Gottfried SD, Popovitch CA, Goldschmidt MH, Schelling C: Metastatic digital carcinoma in the cat: A retrospective study of 36 cats (1992–1998). *JAAHA* 36:501–509, 2000.

69. Jerram RM, Guyer CL, Braniecki A, et al: Endogenous lipid (cholesterol) pneumonia associated with bronchogenic carcinoma in a cat. *JAAHA* 34:275–280, 1998.

70. Moore AS, Middleton DJ: Pulmonary adenocarcinoma in three cats with non-respiratory signs only. *J Small Anim Pract* 23:501–509, 1982.

71. Teunissen VGHB, Stokhof AA: Tumoren in der Brusthöhle. *Kleintierpraxis* 26: 501–506, 1981.

72. Loser C, Lawrenz B, Werner H-G, et al: Primäre lungentumore mit metastasierung in die phalangen bei der katze. *Jahrgang* 43:425–442, 1998.

73. Pollack M, Martin RA, Diters RW: Metastatic squamous cell carcinoma in multiple digits of a cat: Case report. *JAAHA* 20:835–839, 1984.

74. Scott-Moncrieff JC, Elliott GS, Radovsky A, Blevins WE: Pulmonary squamous cell carcinoma with multiple digital metastases in a cat. *J Small Anim Pract* 30:696–699, 1989.

75. May C, Newsholme SJ: Metastasis of feline pulmonary carcinoma presenting as multiple digital swelling. *J Small Anim Pract* 30:302–310, 1989.

76. Jacobs TM, Tomlinson MJ: The lung-digit syndrome in a cat. *Feline Pract* 25: 31–36, 1997.

77. Schmitz JA, Bailey DE, Bailey RB: Bronchogenic carcinoma in a cat presenting as rear leg lameness. *Feline Pract* 8:18–22, 1978.

78. Chauvet AE, Shelton GD: Neuromuscular weakness as a primary clinical sign associated with metastatic neoplasia in two cats. *Feline Pract* 25:6–9, 1997.

79. Meschter CL: Disseminated sweat gland adenocarcinoma with acronecrosis in a cat. *Cornell Vet* 81:195–203, 1991.

80. van der Linde-Sipman JS, van den Ingh TSGAM: Primary and metastatic carcinomas in the digits of cats. *Vet Q* 22:141–145, 2000.

81. Roberg J: Hypertrophic pulmonary osteoarthropathy. *Feline Pract* 7:18–22, 1977.

82. Hamilton HB, Severin GA, Nold J: Pulmonary squamous cell carcinoma with intraocular metastasis in a cat. *JAVMA* 185:307–309, 1984.

83. Gionfriddo JR, Fix AS, Niyo Y, et al: Ocular manifestations of a metastatic pulmonary adenocarcinoma in a cat. *JAVMA* 197:372–374, 1990.

84. Dorn AS, Harris SG, Olmstead ML: Squamous cell carcinoma of the urinary bladder in a cat. *Feline Pract* 8:14–17, 1978.

85. Davies C, Forrester SD: Pleural effusion in cats: 82 cases (1987–1995). *J Small Anim Pract* 37:217–224, 1996.

86. McMillan MC, Kleine LJ, Carpenter JL: Fluoroscopically guided percutaneous fine-needle aspiration biopsy of thoracic lesions in dogs and cats. *Vet Radiol* 29:194–197, 1988.

87. Tidwell AS, Johnson KL: Computed tomography-guided percutaneous biopsy in the dog and cat: Description of technique and preliminary evaluation in 14 patients. *Vet Radiol Ultrasound* 35:445–446, 1994.

88. Gustafsson P, Wolfe D: Bone-metastasizing lung carcinoma in a cat. *Cornell Vet* 58:425–430, 1968.

89. Gram WD, Wheaton LG, Snyder PW, et al: Feline hypertrophic osteopathy associated with pulmonary carcinoma. *JAAHA* 26:425–428, 1990.

90. LaRue SM, Withrow SJ, Wykes PM: Lung resection using surgical staples in dogs and cats. *Vet Surg* 16:238–240, 1987.

91. Hahn KA, McEntee MF: Prognosis factors for survival in cats after removal of a primary lung tumor: 21 cases (1979–1994). *Vet Surg* 27:307–311, 1998.

92. Klausner JS, Bell FW, Hayden DW, et al: Hypercalcemia in two cats with squamous cell carcinomas. *JAVMA* 196:103–105, 1990.

93. Effron M, Griner L, Benirschke K: Nature and rate of neoplasia found in captive wild mammals, birds and reptiles at necropsy. *J Natl Cancer Inst* 59:185–198, 1977.

94. Munson L, Nesbit JW, Meltzer DGA, et al: Diseases in captive cheetahs (*Acinonyx jubatus jubatus*) in South Africa: A 20-year retrospective survey. *J Zoo Wildl Med* 30:342–347, 1999.

95. Kennedy GA, Strafuss AC: Multiple neoplasia in an aged cougar. *J Zoo Anim Med* 7:24–26, 1976.

96. Rao AT, Acharjyo LN: Squamous cell carcinoma in the lungs of a golden cat (*Felis temmincki*). *J Zoo Anim Med* 16:6–8, 1985.

CARDIOVASCULAR TUMORS

Anthony S. Moore and Gregory K. Ogilvie

48

Tumors of the cardiovascular system are rare in cats. While primary cardiac hemangiosarcoma is common in dogs, it has not been described in cats. Hemangiosarcoma from the mesentery and spleen has been reported to metastasize to the heart in cats.[1–3] Further discussion of hemangiosarcoma is found in Chapter 43.

In a series of 66 cats with pericardial disease, 12 cats had a neoplasm.[4] Lymphoma was the most common neoplasia found and caused effusion in 5 of 6 cats. Metastatic tumors causing pericardial disease included mammary carcinoma (3 cats), melanoma (1 cat), tonsillar adenocarcinoma (1 cat), and pulmonary carcinoma (1 cat). Metastasis to sites other than the heart was noted in all of these cats, and some had pleural effusion or ascites in addition to pericardial effusion.

A fibrosarcoma of the left atrial wall caused pericardial and pleural effusion and had metastasized to lung and liver in a 9-year-old DLH.[5] In another report, a myxoma that was well encapsulated arose from the endocardial free wall of the right atrium, almost obliterating that space, and caused sudden death in a 6-year-old DSH.[6] A rhabdomyosarcoma of the right ventricular wall that also involved pericardium but did not metastasize caused pleural and pericardial edema and dyspnea in a 7-year-old DSH. Despite the local pericardial metastases, pericardial fluid analysis was not diagnostically helpful in this cat.[7] None of the three cats with mesenchymal tumors were treated.

Other tumors reported to metastasize to the heart or pericardium include salivary carcinoma, pulmonary carcinoma, and melanoma.[8]

CHEMODECTOMA[a]

CLINICAL BRIEFING	
Common Presentation	Palpable neck mass in patients with carotid body tumor. Pericardial or pleural effusions causing dyspnea are seen with heart base tumors.
Staging and Diagnosis	MDB, cardiac ultrasonography, and biopsy (definitive diagnosis probably requires surgery). Cytology of any effusion unlikely to be diagnostic. Metastasis may be common for aortic body tumors.
Treatment Initial	Surgery may be curative for carotid body tumors; likely to be only palliative for cardiac tamponade (pericardectomy) in cats with aortic body tumors.
Adjunctive	Radiation therapy for cervical tumors; not possible for thoracic tumors. Chemotherapy unproven.
Supportive	Palliative thoracocentesis or pericardiocentesis prior to palliative pericardectomy. Analgesia postoperatively.

CAROTID BODY TUMORS

Only three of these tumors have been described,[9–11] and another[12] was probably an aortic body tumor and is discussed below. Cats ranged in age from 9 to 15 years.

All three cats had a 2 to 3 cm mass in the neck. One cat had signs of excessive salivation and inappetence and recovered from surgical resection with only ptosis of the ipsilateral eyelid.[9] Unfortunately, no further follow-up information was available. One cat had a locally invasive tumor, but no other clinical details were provided.[10]

AORTIC BODY TUMORS

Incidence, Signalment, and Etiology

Nine aortic body tumors have been reported in cats, including one "carotid body" tumor[12] and a "metastatic intestinal carcinoid" for which no primary tumor was identified.[13] Signalment was available for eight cats; ages ranged from 7 to 16 years (median, 9 years). Seven were DSHs, and one was

---

[a]Chemodectoma is a term that encompasses both aortic and carotid body tumors.

Siamese.[12-19] Signalment was not reported for one cat.[8]

Three cats were dyspneic due to pleural effusion[14,16,19] (concurrent with pulmonary edema in one cat[19]), and a fourth was dyspneic due to widespread pulmonary metastases.[12] One cat had a mild cough.[15] Other nonspecific signs such as inappetence, weight loss, and vomiting were also reported by owners. One cat that was diagnosed on necropsy had died a week after surgery for pyometra.[17]

Staging and Diagnosis

Radiographs were obtained in most cats and showed a heart base mass with dorsal tracheal elevation. Two cats had pulmonary metastases,[12,18] and three more had pleural effusion that obscured the cardiac silhouette.[14,16] The mass can be very large (e.g., 1.5 times the size of the heart in one cat).[19] Cardiac ultrasonography disclosed a heart base mass between the aorta and left pulmonary artery and the base of the heart. Multiple masses were seen in one cat,[13] and the mass extended to invade and surround the atria in others.[8,14,15] Masses ranged in size from 2 to 6 cm.

Pericardial effusion was seen in three cats[13,16,17] and was sufficient to cause tamponade in one of these three animals.[13] Cytology of any effusion is unlikely to be diagnostic but is recommended in addition to an MDB as part of a complete staging scheme.

Ultrasound-guided fine-needle aspiration was performed in two cats[15,16]; in both cases a neuroendocrine tumor was diagnosed cytologically, with chemodectoma or thyroid carcinoma as the main possibilities. A technetium scan in one cat ruled out an active thyroid neoplasm.[15] Definitive diagnosis will most likely require a thoracotomy, although CT-guided biopsy may be possible in some cats.[20,21] Tumor emboli were common in the cats that were necropsied. Emboli and metastases were found in the pericardium, epicardium, myocardium, and pulmonary arteries in three cats.[8,17,18] Metastasis to lungs, mediastinal lymph nodes, and liver was seen in four cats.[8,13,17,18] Metastasis to the sternal lymph node was not radiographically apparent in one cat but was seen on necropsy.[19]

The tumor was highly infiltrative in some cats, invading pericardium and atrial wall[8,17] or the intercostal muscles.[18] There was evidence of tracheal invasion in one treated cat, but this did not occur until nearly 2 years after initial diagnosis[14]; metastases were not seen in this patient or another that died 13 months after diagnosis.[15]

It appears that there is some variation as to the metastatic behavior of these tumors. Thoracic radiographs should be examined for pulmonary metastases and cardiac ultrasonography used to evaluate cardiac and vascular structures and identify cardiac tamponade resulting from pericardial effusion.

Treatment

Intermittent thoracentesis was used to control chylothorax in one cat for 4 months prior to pericardectomy.[14] This cat became asymptomatic for 19 months after pericardectomy but then died of renal failure due to metastatic renal carcinoma. The aortic body tumor was considered unresectable in this cat[14] as well as two others that underwent thoracotomy.[15,16] One cat was euthanized 48 hours after surgery,[16] while the other cat was found dead 13 months after surgery.[15] A worsening cough was the only sign of the trachea invasion and bronchial occlusion identified on necropsy.

> **KEY POINT**
>
> *Pericardial tamponade may be caused by a heart base chemodectoma or a pericardial lymphoma.*

This tumor appears to be slow growing in some cats. Surgical excision is usually impossible and unlikely to be curative or even palliative. Symptomatic and supportive treatment may result in long survival. Palliation may be provided via thoracocentesis or pericardiocentesis; ideally, a pericardectomy should be performed to relieve cardiac tamponade. Analgesia is essential in managing discomfort in these cats. Neither radiation therapy nor chemotherapy is likely to be practical for these tumors.

CARDIAC LYMPHOMA

CLINICAL BRIEFING

Common Presentation	Syncope due to pericardial effusion or dysrhythmias. May be solitary but is often part of systemic disease.
Staging and Diagnosis	MDB, cardiac ultrasonography, ECG, abdominal ultrasonography, and bone marrow aspiration. Cytology of pericardial or pleural effusion (often not diagnostic). Other systemic lymphoma often present.

Treatment	
Initial	Chemotherapy (as described in Chapter 36) is favored due to presence of systemic disease.
Supportive	Pericardiocentesis or thoracocentesis for symptoms. Appetite stimulants and analgesia as needed.

Incidence, Signalment, and Etiology

The heart is commonly involved by infiltration in patients with widespread multicentric lymphoma; however, such infiltration is rarely of clinical significance. There are few reports of cardiac disease due to lymphoma. In a series of 66 cats with pericardial disease, 6 cats had cardiac lymphoma.[4] All but 1 of the 9 reported cats with cardiac lymphoma were 10 years of age or older.[4,22-24] At least 2 cats were positive for FeLV[22,23]; this information was not available for others.

Clinical Presentation and History

Extensive infiltration of the heart by lymphoma may result in clinical cardiac disease (Figure 48-1). Syncope of only a few days duration was seen in two cats.[22,23] A third cat had paroxysmal atrial tachycardia.[24] Of six cats with pericardial disease, five had pericardial effusion (2–6 ml) and three of these also had pleural effusion; one of these three also had ascites.[4] All had multicentric lymphoma, as did at least one other cat.[22]

Staging and Diagnosis

The cause of collapse was cardiac tamponade due to pericardial effusion in one cat,[22] a large compressive heart base mass in another,[23] and an infiltrative cardiomyopathy in a third.[24]

Pericardiocentesis was performed in two cats. It was not diagnostic for lymphoma as it showed only a modified transudate without neoplastic cells.[4,22] Thoracic radiographs

showed cardiomegaly in two cats; the condition was better elucidated by cardiac ultrasonography.[4,22,23] Most cats had multicentric disease, although one appeared to have a solitary, primary cardiac lymphoma.[23]

Due to the high incidence of multicentric disease, complete staging as outlined in Chapter 36 should be performed for all cats diagnosed with or suspected of having lymphoma. Staging should include an MDB, cardiac and abdominal ultrasonography, electrocardiography, and bone marrow aspiration. Cytology of any pericardial or pleural effusion should also be performed but often will not be diagnostic.

MDB = minimum database; includes CBC, biochemical profile, urinalysis, FeLV/FIV serology, T_4 testing, and thoracic radiographs (three views).

Treatment

Treatment with prednisone had no effect on a large solitary heart base lymphoma in one cat.[23] Chemotherapy with vincristine, cyclophosphamide, and prednisone improved cardiac function but did not result in a complete remission in a cat that was euthanized due to progressive disease 4 weeks after diagnosis.[22] More aggressive chemotherapy may have better results; see Chapter 36 for details.

Pericardiocentesis or thoracocentesis may palliate symptoms of effusions. Nutritional support may be necessary, and appropriate analgesia should be administered to minimize discomfort.

REFERENCES

1. Scavelli TD, Patnaik AK, Mehlaff CJ, et al: Hemangiosarcoma in the cat: Retrospective evaluation of 31 surgical cases. *JAVMA* 187:817–819, 1985.
2. Patnaik AK, Liu S-K: Angiosarcoma in cats. *J Small Anim Pract* 18:191–198, 1977.
3. Kraje AC, Mears EA, Hahn KA, et al: Unusual metastatic behavior and clinicopathologic findings in 8 cats with cutaneous or visceral hemangiosarcoma (1981–1997). *JAVMA* 214:670–672, 1999.
4. Rush JE, Keene BW, Fox PR: Pericardial disease in the cat: A retrospective evaluation of 66 cases. *JAAHA* 26:39–46, 1990.
5. Ryan CP, Walder EJ: Feline fibrosarcoma of the heart. *Calif Vet* 8:12–14, 1980.
6. Campbell MD, Gelberg HB: Endocardial ossifying myxoma of the right atrium in a cat. *Vet Pathol* 37:460–462, 2000.
7. Venco L, Kramer L, Sola LB, et al: Primary cardiac rhabdomyosarcoma in a cat. *JAAHA* 37:159–163, 2001.

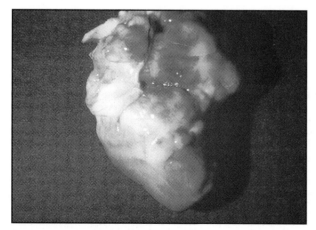

Figure 48-1: Extensive infiltration of cardiac muscle by lymphoma in a 2.5-year-old cat with multicentric disease.

MANAGEMENT OF SPECIFIC DISEASES

8. Tilley LP, Bond B, Patnaik AK, et al: Cardiovascular tumors in the cat. *JAAHA* 17:1009–1021, 1981.

9. Carpenter JL, Andrews LK, Holzworth J: Tumors and tumor-like lesions, in Holzworth J (ed): *Diseases of the Cat. Medicine and Surgery.* Philadelphia, WB Saunders, 1987, pp 407–596.

10. Yates WDG, Lester SJ, Mills JHL: Chemoreceptor tumors diagnosed at the Western College of Veterinary Medicine 1967–1979. *Can Vet J* 21:124–129, 1980.

11. Nielsen SW: Neoplastic diseases, in Catcott EJ (ed): *Feline Medicine and Surgery.* Santa Barbara, CA, American Veterinary Publications, 1964, pp 156–176.

12. Collins DR: Thoracic tumor in a cat. *Vet Med Small Anim Clin* 59:459, 1964.

13. Lusk Jr RH, Ettinger SJ, Barr EA: Ultrasound diagnosis of a feline heart tumor. *Calif Vet* 41:9–10, 1987.

14. Fossum TW, Forrester SD, Swenson CL, et al: Chylothorax in cats: 37 cases (1969–1989). *JAVMA* 198:672–678, 1991.

15. Tillson DM, Fingland RB, Andrews GA: Chemodectoma in a cat. *JAAHA* 30:586–590, 1994.

16. Paola JP, Hammer AS, Smeak DD, et al: Aortic body tumor causing pleural effusion in a cat. *JAAHA* 30:281–285, 1994.

17. Buergelt CD, Das KM: Aortic body tumor in a cat, a case report. *Pathol Vet* 5:84–90, 1968.

18. George C, Steinberg H: An aortic body carcinoma with multifocal thoracic metastases in a cat. *J Comp Pathol* 101:467–469, 1989.

19. Willis R, Williams AE, Schwarz T, et al: Aortic body chemodectoma causing pulmonary oedema in a cat. *J Small Anim Pract* 42:20–23, 2001.

20. Tidwell AS, Johnson KL: Computed tomography-guided percutaneous biopsy: Criteria for accurate needle tip identification. *Vet Radiol Ultrasound* 35:440–444, 1994.

21. Tidwell AS, Johnson KL: Computed tomography-guided percutaneous biopsy in the dog and cat: Description of technique and preliminary evaluation in 14 patients. *Vet Radiol Ultrasound* 35:445–446, 1994.

22. Brummer DG, Moise NS: Infiltrative cardiomyopathy responsive to combination chemotherapy in a cat with lymphoma. *JAVMA* 195:1116–1119, 1989.

23. Meurs KM, Miller MW, Mackie JR, et al: Syncope associated with cardiac lymphoma in a cat. *JAAHA* 30:583–585, 1994.

24. Machida N, Yamaga Y, Kagota K, et al: Paroxysmal atrial tachycardia in a cat. *J Jpn Vet Med Assoc* 44:1030–1033, 1991.

THYMOMA, MESOTHELIOMA, AND HISTIOCYTOSIS

49

Anthony S. Moore and Gregory K. Ogilvie

▶ THYMOMA

<table>
<tr><td colspan="2" align="center">C L I N I C A L   B R I E F I N G</td></tr>
<tr><td>Common Presentation</td><td>Dyspnea, often acute but sometimes chronic, is the most common sign. Secondary immune diseases such as myasthenia gravis, polymyositis, and dermatitis may be seen. Usually occurs in older FeLV-negative cats.</td></tr>
<tr><td>Staging and Diagnosis</td><td>MDB; thoracocentesis if fluid is present. Ultrasonography and guided needle biopsy. Serum AChRAb prior to surgery (Note: cats may be asymptomatic). Serum creatinine kinase and electromyography if myositis suspected. Cross-match for blood transfusion prior to surgery. Metastasis is very rare.</td></tr>
<tr><td>Treatment
Initial
Adjunctive

Supportive</td><td>
Surgical resection is usually curative, but have blood transfusion available.
Usually not required. For invasive tumors, may try prednisone, COP (cyclophosphamide, vincristine, and prednisone), doxorubicin, or carboplatin (unproven). Radiation for tumors extending into neck area; thoracic irradiation unwise due to surrounding lung.
Stabilize patients with myasthenia gravis using pyridostigmine and prednisone prior to surgery. Antifungals or antibiotics for secondary skin infections. Thoracocentesis may be necessary. Analgesia and nutritional support as needed.</td></tr>
</table>

Incidence, Signalment, and Etiology

Thymoma is an epithelial malignancy of the thymus. Mature lymphocytes are able to proliferate on the malignant stroma and may outnumber the epithelial component. Despite the high proportion of lymphocytes in thymoma, these cells are mature and not themselves malignant. All cats with thymoma tested for FeLV have been negative.[1-6]

Of the 64 cats with thymoma reported in the literature, 42 were DSHs, 8 were DLHs, 11 were Siamese, 1 was Persian, and 2 were Abyssinian.[4,7-9]

Of cats for which complete signalment was available, 36 were male (31 castrated) and 26 were female (21 spayed). The median age of affected cats was between 9 and 10 years[1,5,10] (range, 18 months[11] to 11 years[1]).

Clinical Presentation and History

A thymoma will occasionally be an incidental radiographic finding,[10] but most cats show signs referable to the thoracic cavity or to a paraneoplastic condition associated with the thymoma.

Dyspnea is the most common clinical sign and may be present for days or up to 1 year prior to veterinary advice being sought.[1,2,5,7,11-15] One study described clinical signs as occurring for up to 3 years prior to diagnosis.[10] Occasionally, respiratory distress is acute, resulting in cyanosis or even sudden death.[16-20] Care should be taken during physical examination as pleural effusion may cause cats with thymoma to become rapidly decompensated. As is the case for cats with mediastinal lymphoma, thoracocentesis should be attempted in cats with absent ventral bronchovesicular sounds or an incompressible anterior thorax prior to subjecting them to stressful procedures that could result in death (e.g., radiographs).[11,13]

Other respiratory signs such as cough can be chronic, occurring for weeks to months prior to presentation.[3,10,13,15,19,21] Nasal discharge and choking are less commonly reported.[6,13] One cat experienced pain when lifted under the sternum.[2]

Vomiting or regurgitation, possibly as a result of esophageal compression, has been reported infrequently in case reports[7,22] but occurred in 4 of 12 cats in a case series.[10] Other nonspecific signs of inappetence and anorexia have been reported in up to 50% of cats with thymoma.[1,10,19,21]

Cats with thymoma may be immunocompromised, possibly due to interference with T lymphocyte function by the tumor. One 13-year-old cat with thymoma was originally presented for septic polyarthritis.[18] In a series of cats with thymoma, one cat was further compromised by a fungal pyogranulomatous pleuritis that resulted in postsurgical death.[10] A cat with an exfoliative dermatitis exacerbated by *Malassezia pachydermatis* yeast infection had resolution of all signs following surgery for thymoma.[6] Another cat had a *Microsporum canis* infection superimposed on dermatitis.[23]

Paraneoplastic conditions reported in cats with thymoma include a nonpruritic dermatis, polymyositis, and myasthenia gravis. These conditions can occur alone or in combination.

Thymoma in association with a nonpruritic, seborrheic alopecia that involved the ventral neck, abdomen, thorax, medial limbs, and paws was seen in four cats. Two of these cats also had a coat color change from orange to white.[23,24] Histologically, all cats had a cutaneous lymphoid cellular infiltrate. All four cats were orange, as was another cat with generalized moist dermatitis reported in a case series of cats with thymoma.[1] The same condition has also been reported in a black DSH[25] and four other cats for which coat color was not reported.[1,5,6,9]

In one cat, generalized dermatitis occurred in conjunction with dysphagia and generalized muscular weakness,[25] and another cat with dermatitis also had intermittent hindlimb ataxia that progressed to become severe.[6] This latter cat had a moderate (fourfold) increase in creatine kinase, suggesting polymyositis. Polymyositis has likewise been described in three cats with thymoma but no dermatitis. Lymphoid and monocytic infiltration of muscle was a microscopic feature of all three cats, and in two cats the myositis also affected the myocardium.[1] Ataxia was reported as the reason for presentation in a 15-year-old Persian.[7]

Myasthenia gravis is another cause of ataxia and weakness in cats with thymoma. Affected cats may show dysphonia,[4,10] megaesophagus, and regurgitation as well as weakness that may be so severe as to cause ventroflexion of the neck and inability to stand.[14] These signs can progress very rapidly.

Myasthenia gravis can be confirmed indirectly by administering edriphonium chloride (0.25–0.5 mg/cat); cats with myasthenia gravis should show immediate improvement in strength.[14,26] Direct confirmation is obtained by demonstration of anti-cholinesterase receptor antibodies (AChRAb) in the cat's serum.[4,10] It is possible that some of the cats previously described as having polymyositis may actually have

had unconfirmed myasthenia gravis; the two conditions may also be concurrent.[4] AChRAb may not be present in cats without clinical signs,[3] but their presence can predict postsurgical occurrence of myasthenia gravis.[10] Thymoma is not the only cause of myasthenia gravis; in a series of 105 cats with myasthenia gravis, only 27 (26%) had a mediastinal thymoma.[27]

A case of hypertrophic osteopathy was described in an 18-month-old cat with a 6 month history of dyspnea; a thymoma was found on necropsy.[11] Interestingly, the periosteal reaction involved the more proximal long bones but spared the carpi, tarsi, and distal limbs.

Staging and Diagnosis

The major diagnostic differential in cats with thymoma is lymphoma. As a general rule, cats with thymoma are older and FeLV negative; however, a biopsy is required for cats, particularly young ones, to confirm the diagnosis.

Radiographically, the anterior mediastinum may be completely obliterated by a large tumor,[7] but the mass may be closer to the cardiac shadow than to the rostral anterior mediastinal limits in cats with smaller tumors (Figure 49-1). On ultrasound the mass is usually cystic with variably sized, multiple cysts (Figure 49-2) or occasionally one very large cyst.[3]

It may be necessary to perform thoracocentesis prior to any diagnostic tests, particularly in cats that appear unstable, and the fluid obtained should be examined. This fluid will usually contain small lymphocytes rather than lymphoblasts that would be exfoliated from lymphoma.[12,15,16,21] Mast cells, eosinophils, and malignant epithelial cells found in conjunction with mature lymphocytes should increase suspicion of thymoma. Erythrophagocytosis has also been reported.[10]

Definitive diagnosis is made by fine-needle aspiration or biopsy. Ultrasound guidance is helpful, particularly for very cystic tumors. Aspiration cytology may show a predominance of small lymphocytes mixed with epithelial cells and mast cells. Occasionally, a fine-needle aspirate will be misdiagnosed as lymphoma,[25] resulting in inappropriate treatment.[6] Biopsy is definitive, and in samples that have a very high proportion of lymphocytes, immunohistochemical staining for cytokeratin intermediate filaments will discriminate rare malignant epithelial cell clusters that would be missed on cytology or routine histopathologic staining.[7,28,29]

If thymoma is diagnosed or suspected and surgery contemplated, a serum AChRAb level should be obtained as clinical signs of myasthenia may not always be obvious prior to surgery.[10] A serum AChRAb titer above 0.30 nmol/L is diagnostic for myasthenia gravis,[27,30] although cats with

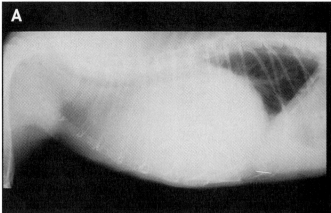

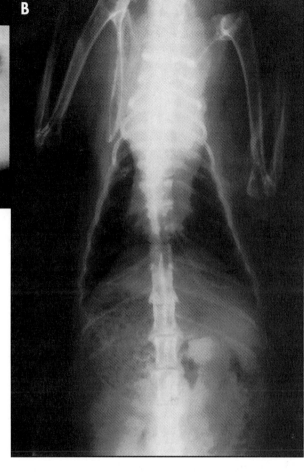

*Figure 49-1: The anterior mediastinal mass seen in these thoracic radiographs (lateral [**A**] and ventrodorsal [**B**] views) was diagnosed as a thymoma. Distinguishing between lymphoma and thymoma may be difficult on radiographs, and biopsy is required.*

titers below 10 nmol/L may not show muscular weakness at diagnosis. Early diagnosis will allow appropriate treatment prior to surgery and will improve the chances for an uncomplicated outcome.[4,10,14]

For cats in which a myositis is suspected, serum creatine kinase should be measured and electromyography considered.[4,6] Tests for FeLV and FIV have been uniformly negative in all tested cats but should be included as part of the MDB because a positive result may increase suspicion for lymphoma.

Metastasis is very rare. Two cats with thymoma that had areas of squamous cell carcinoma within cysts developed vascular invasion or metastases to the parietal pleura and intrathoracic lymph nodes.[12] These findings are similar to those in a cat with thymic squamous cell carcinoma (not thymoma) arising within the thymus that metastasized to lungs and sternal lymph nodes.[31] Another cat with a pri-

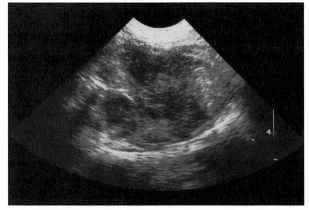

Figure 49-2: The cystic structure of thymoma is clearly demonstrated in this ultrasonograph. Ultrasonographic guidance will help ensure that a representative biopsy is obtained. (Courtesy of D. Penninck)

marily epithelial thymoma had pulmonary and renal metastases.[19] Pulmonary metastases were described in one other cat.[22] Multiple thymomas without obvious metastases were reported in one cat.[1] Second malignancies are uncommon: One cat had a thyroid carcinoma,[7] and one had a biliary cystadenoma.[20]

Treatment

Surgical resection of thymoma is usually successful and often curative (Figure 49-3). A median sternotomy is required to gain access to a large mediastinal mass in most cats.[10]

In a series of 12 cats treated with surgery alone,[10] the thymoma was well encapsulated in 5 cats and was adhered to the pericardium, parietal pleura, or cranial vena cava in 7. Despite the fact that the tumor was incompletely excised visually in 3 cats, the outcome for most patients was excellent. One cat died due to postoperative hemorrhage, and 3 cats required a blood transfusion but survived. A second cat died due to fungal pleuritis, presumably secondary to immunosuppression. Of the 10 surviving cats, 1 had unilateral laryngeal paralysis that resolved over 32 months. Myasthenia gravis occurred in 2 cats postoperatively (see below). Four

MANAGEMENT OF SPECIFIC DISEASES

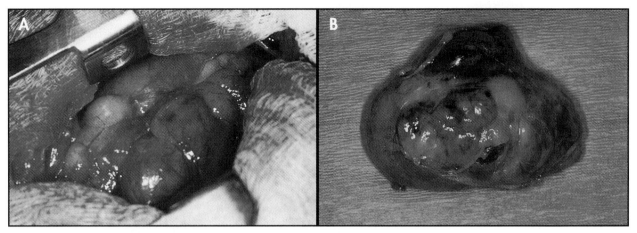

Figure 49-3: *At surgery (**A**), this thymoma appeared large and invasive; however, it was encapsulated (**B**), and complete excision was achieved. Careful attention to hemostasis is important for this surgical procedure. (Courtesy of J. Berg)*

cats died of other causes without evidence of thymoma; deaths occurred at 18, 32, 45, and 62 months after surgery. The median follow-up period for the 6 remaining cats that survived surgery was 21 months (range, 6–36 months).

<hr>

KEY POINT

Surgical excision of thymoma is usually curative.

<hr>

Similar good success was seen in other cats following surgery[6] and implied in other reports, although long-term follow-up information was not available.[14,18]

Surgery has been unsuccessful in only a small number of cats. In one cat, tumor regrowth around the vena cava and carotid artery and through the sternotomy site occurred 2 years after surgery.[8] Another cat had extension of the thymoma from the anterior mediastinum, through the thoracic inlet, and to the level of the thyroid gland. Two surgeries were performed to remove it, but thymoma recurred in the thorax 8 months later. A third surgery was performed, and the cat was treated with cyclophosphamide and cytosine arabinoside. It was disease-free 8 weeks later.[2] The surgeon should be aware that cervical extension of an intrathoracic thymoma may occur in some cats. A third cat in which surgery was incomplete experienced tumor recurrence 70 days after surgery.[15] A cat with squamous cell carcinoma arising in thymoma cysts developed metastases 36

MDB = minimum database; includes CBC, biochemical profile, urinalysis, FeLV/FIV serology, T₄ testing, and thoracic radiographs (three views).

days after surgery.[12]

The role of chemotherapy in the management of feline thymoma is uncertain; however, chemotherapy should be considered, particularly for cats with invasive tumors. A cat that was treated with cyclophosphamide, vincristine, and prednisone (COP) had a slight improvement in demeanor but progressive ataxia. This cat improved dramatically following surgery.[6] Another cat treated with COP for suspected lymphoma had spectacular improvement in muscle strength and skin disease and was radiographically free of disease when chemotherapy was stopped after 5 months. The tumor rapidly regrew, and the cat was euthanized.[25] A cat treated with prednisone alone prior to surgery did not respond but was alive 1 year after tumor resection.[3]

A cat in which thymoma recurred 70 days after surgery was treated with COP and cytosine arabinoside following tumor recurrence and had a complete remission for longer than 11 months.[15] Another cat treated with surgery and bleomycin died due to other causes 18 months after treatment. The efficacy of bleomycin in this cat is obviously difficult to assess.[15] A cat with unresectable thymoma responded for 5 months to doxorubicin treatment.[a] Similarly, there is anecdotal information regarding carboplatin chemotherapy, but no results are available.

Radiation is currently being employed in dogs with unresectable thymomas. Three cats treated for unresectable thymoma with external beam radiation therapy have had survival times longer than 1 year.[b]

Supportive care is essential and should include nutritional support when necessary. Antiemetics and analgesics should be used as needed. The major role for supportive care is to improve quality of life for cats with unresectable tumors or to control paraneoplastic signs such as myasthenia gravis.

<hr>

[a]Moore AS: Personal observation.
[b]Ogilvie GK: Personal observation.

Palliation by drainage of cysts is not recommended when definitive surgery is possible. Drainage of a large cystic thymoma every 4 to 6 weeks for 4 months[3] and thoracocentesis to drain a chylothorax for 6 months[1] was sufficient to palliate two cats. In contrast, surgery to remove the tumor in one of these cats caused long-term remission.[3]

Myasthenia gravis in cats with thymoma is associated with circulating AChRAb. One cat discussed above[6] and another cat[4] had progressive weakness and ataxia despite receiving corticosteroids. The latter cat developed a megaesophagus and, after surgery, aspiration pneumonia.[4] This cat had a partial response to dexamethasone and a good response to neostigmine (0.125 mg SQ q8h). Long-term treatment with pyridostigmine (2.4 mg PO q12h) and prednisone (5 mg PO daily) resulted in resolution of the megaesophagus in 3 months. Interestingly, the clinical response did not correlate with serum AChRAb levels, which rose from 15.9 nmol/L at surgery to 18.3 nmol/L 8 weeks later (normal, <0.3 nmol/L).

Two other cats in which signs of myasthenia gravis became apparent following surgery were treated following a positive edrophonium test. Pyridostigmine and prednisone resulted in dramatic improvement for 9 months after surgery in one cat and 62 months in the other. Treatment was discontinued in the second cat after 24 months.[10]

Another cat was treated with neostigmine and dexamethasone for 1 month and then pyridostigmine rectally prior to surgery.[14] Treatment prior to surgery is probably warranted for a cat that has signs of myasthenia gravis but does not have obvious respiratory signs related to the thymoma. If respiratory signs are present, concurrent surgery and treatment for myasthenia gravis may be the most prudent course to follow.

THYMIC CYSTS

Incidence, Signalment, and Etiology

Four cats with thymic cysts (or thymic branchial cysts) have been reported. Signs were very similar to those described for cats with thymoma, and responses to treatment were likewise similar. It may not be clinically relevant to distinguish between the two.

All reported cases have been in DSHs; there were three females (two spayed) and one castrated male. These cats were 5, 8, 10, and 13 years of age.[18,26,32]

Clinical Presentation and History

Signs of myasthenia gravis were found in two cats, and one of these also had dyspnea.[18,26] A final histologic diagnosis was not pursued in one of these cats.[18]

A third cat was dyspneic.[18] The fourth cat had sublingual squamous cell carcinoma, and the anterior mediastinal mass was an incidental finding.[32]

Staging and Diagnosis

Staging should be performed as outlined for thymoma. Ultrasound-guided fine-needle aspiration was used to obtain a diagnosis in three cats. Small lymphocytes were noted in two cats,[18,26] and mast cells and epithelial cells were an additional finding in one.[18] Aspiration of fluid led to radiographic resolution of the mass in the third cat.[32] An edrophonium test was positive in two cats.[18,26]

Treatment

Surgery is probably the treatment of choice for these cysts, just as it is for thymoma; the beneficial effects, however, are unknown. Chemotherapy has also been used. For example, dyspnea and signs of myasthenia completely resolved in one cat treated with pyridostigmine, prednisone, and chlorambucil; the cat was weaned off medication and was free of disease 18 months after treatment was started. No final diagnosis was made.[18] Treatment with prednisone for 2 weeks prior to and 8 weeks after surgery resulted in a reduction in AChRAb levels to normal and resolution of clinical signs in a cat with a thymic cyst.[26] Interestingly, this cat's unaffected sibling had a positive AChRAb titer and its unaffected mother had an equivocal titer.

A third cat was treated with prednisone to decrease the size of the mediastinal mass. Follow-up treatment with vincristine and L-asparaginase did not shrink it further, and surgery to remove a thymic branchial cyst was performed. The cat had no evidence of disease 10 months later.[18]

▶ MESOTHELIOMA

C L I N I C A L   B R I E F I N G

Common Presentation	Ascites and/or pleural or pericardial effusion usually associated with severe acute signs. Occasionally chronic.
Staging and Diagnosis	MDB, cytology of effusion (but may not be distinguished from reactive mesothelial cells), ultrasonography. Biopsy often requires surgery. Perform coagulation profile prior to surgery.

(continued)

MANAGEMENT OF SPECIFIC DISEASES

Treatment	
Initial	No definitive treatment reported. Chemotherapy unproven.
Supportive	Fluid centesis may be palliative. Analgesia and nutritional support often necessary.

Incidence, Signalment, and Etiology

Mesothelioma is a rare cause of effusion in any of the body cavities in cats. There are eight reported cases in cats ranging from 1 to 17 years of age[33,34] (median age, 5 years). Three of the reported cats were Siamese,[35–37] and the rest were DSHs. There is no gender predilection. While asbestos has been linked to development of mesothelioma in humans and dogs, there have been too few cases in cats to explore this potential etiology.

Clinical Presentation and History

The clinical signs associated with mesothelioma in cats depend to some extent on the body cavity involved and hence the organ(s) most affected. The proliferation of malignant mesothelial cells results in considerable fluid accumulation, presumably due to reduced lymphatic drainage, and possible production of fluid secondary to inflammation induced by the tumor. The resulting ascites and/or pleural or pericardial effusion may prove life-threatening in cats with relatively small tumor burdens.

KEY POINT

Mesothelioma is a rare cause of body cavity effusion in cats.

Emaciation was a clinical finding in three cats,[33,37,38] and one cat was moribund.[36] Nonspecific signs of lethargy, anorexia, or intermittent vomiting predominated in other cats. These nonspecific signs were associated with dyspnea in two cats with mesothelioma of the pleural cavity.[33,36] Dyspnea due to abdominal fluid accumulation was also a sign in one of five cats with a clinically obvious abdominal effusion.[34,35,37–39] Abdominal swelling may be acute,[35] although recurrent ascites had been investigated over a 2 year period in one cat.[40] One cat had pericardial mesothelioma, which caused cardiac tamponade and clinical signs of coughing, anorexia, and lethargy.[41]

Staging and Diagnosis

Fluid is usually an exudate but may be a transudate (even in the same cat at different times).[40] Fluid analysis following thoracocentesis, abdominocentesis, or pericardiocentesis usually reveals basophilic mononuclear cells that can be interpreted as either reactive mesothelial cells or mesothelioma. It is very difficult to distinguish cytologically between these two possibilities, and the clinician may need to obtain a tissue biopsy to confirm a suspected diagnosis of mesothelioma.

Radiographs often prove of limited value due to fluid obscuring details of abdominal or thoracic cavities. There may be displacement of abdominal viscera if masses associated with the mesothelioma are large.[37] In the cat with pericardial mesothelioma, a large globular cardiac silhouette on radiographs led to a diagnosis of cardiac tamponade.[41]

KEY POINT

It is often impossible to distinguish cytologically between reactive and malignant mesothelial cells.

The presence of fluid makes ultrasonography the imaging modality of choice. Ultrasonography may reveal an abdominal mass or masses that can involve the mesentery, omentum, stomach wall, spleen, liver, or diaphragm, but usually only the peritoneal surface of these viscera is affected. Negative contrast imaging with pericardial injection of carbon dioxide as reported in one of the cases[41] would now be better performed using ultrasonography to disclose a pericardial mass or masses. Ultrasound-guided biopsy may be difficult or impossible due to the small size of the lesion(s), and the clinician may still need to perform an exploratory surgery to obtain a diagnosis; however, the potential for such a procedure to be therapeutic or even palliative is remote. Because nutritional support is so important, placement of an assisted feeding tube is often indicated at the time of biopsy.

Metastases were not seen in one cat treated symptomatically for more than 2 years.[40] In two cats with pleural and one cat with pericardial mesothelioma, there was no evidence of metastases on autopsy, despite multiple masses on visceral parietal surfaces.[33,36,41]

One cat had a solitary liver mass.[38] In another, the spleen, diaphragm, and diaphragmatic lung lobe were invaded.[35] The lungs and mediastinal lymph nodes were affected in two other cats.[34,37] In one of these two cats, a second report detailed spread of the tumor by lymphatic drainage from the abdomen via the cranial mesenteric and sternal and cranial mediastinal lymph nodes.[37,42]

One cat had concurrent systemic mast cell disease affecting the spleen, blood, and bone marrow. The authors suggested that a terminal disseminated intravascular coagulation (DIC) may have facilitated metastases,[34] although another cat with chronic DIC had no metastases from an abdominal mesothelioma.[40]

In addition to ultrasonography, cytology, and biopsy, a coagulation profile should be performed prior to any attempted surgical intervention in cats with suspected mesothelioma.

Treatment

No treatment was attempted in three cats. Prednisone was used in an attempt to palliate two additional cats. Slight improvement was noted for a week in one cat, but the animal was then euthanized at laparotomy.[38] Signs in the second cat (which may have been related to mast cell disease) improved for 5 months, at which time the animal became anorectic and died suddenly due to thromboembolic disease.[34] Pericardectomy in one cat led to its perioperative death.[41]

One cat with recurrent ascites was treated with ab-dominocentesis to remove 1 to 2 L of fluid three times over a 2 year period. Three exploratory laparotomies were performed, but after the third surgery, the frequency of abdominocentesis needed to be increased. The cat died due to thromboembolic disease.[40]

Intracavitary cisplatin has proven palliative for dogs with mesothelioma but should not be used in cats as it causes fatal pulmonary edema. Systemic doxorubicin or carboplatin chemotherapy has not been evaluated in the treatment of this disease, although chemotherapy would certainly be the treatment modality of choice. Intracavitary carboplatin is theoretically unlikely to be successful due to its poor tissue penetration, but anecdotal improvement for 3 to 6 months has been seen in three cats using this route of administration.[b] The prognosis for cats with mesothelioma remains grim.

Nondomestic Felidae

Pleural mesothelioma has been described in two female tigers (*Panthera tigris*; ages, 8 and 19.5 years). Clinical signs were not reported in one[43] and were nonspecific except for dyspnea and exercise intolerance in the other.[44]

On necropsy, the mesothelioma had metastasized to lungs, liver, and peritoneum in one tiger.[43] Metastases to the tracheobronchial and mediastinal lymph nodes were found in the other.[44] No treatment was described.

▶ MALIGNANT HISTIOCYTOSIS

CLINICAL BRIEFING	
Common Presentation	Very rare tumor; signs are nonspecific.
Staging and Diagnosis	MDB, bone marrow aspiration, and abdominal ultrasonography.
Treatment Initial	No successful treatment has been reported. Chemotherapy, as used for lymphoma, is most likely to be effective.
Supportive	Blood transfusions, antibiotics, and antiinflammatories may be palliative. Nutritional support should be provided as necessary.

Incidence, Signalment, and Etiology

Malignant histiocytosis has been described in only eight cats. All were adult DSHs (median age, 13 years; but seen in a cat as young as 1 year); six were from the United States,[45–48] one from Switzerland,[49] and one from France.[50] Five cats were FeLV and FIV negative[45–48,50]; the 1-year-old was FeLV positive,[48] and the other two were not tested.

Clinical Presentation and History

Nonspecific signs of listlessness, inappetence, and weight loss (Figure 49-4) were seen in all cats, and one cat was febrile.[45] On physical examination, four cats had prominent organomegaly and two of these had ascites. Two cats had pleural effusion. All but one of the cats were anemic. One cat showed neurologic signs.[48]

Staging and Diagnosis

The similarities of this disease to lymphoma mean that staging of cats with malignant histiocytosis should be similar to that performed in cats with lymphoma. This should include an MDB, bone marrow aspiration, and abdominal ultrasonography.

Radiographs showed an enlarged spleen and liver in three

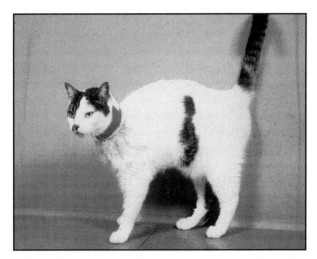

Figure 49-4: A cat with malignant histiocytosis showing weight loss. This cat also was anemic and lethargic. (Courtesy of L. Freeman)

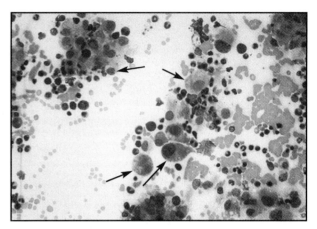

Figure 49-5: Bone marrow aspirate from the cat in Figure 49-4 showing dense histiocytic infiltration and erythrophagocytosis (arrows). (Courtesy of L. Freeman)

cats; two had pleural effusion, and one of these also had ascites. Ultrasonography confirmed organomegaly in three cats and disclosed pericardial effusion in one of those three.[45] Ultrasonography showed a mediastinal mass in one cat[46] that also had a nodule in the right caudal lung lobe. Thoracic radiographs in another revealed multiple cavitated masses.[48]

Anemia was marked (range, 9% to 20%). The anemia was regenerative in two cats[45,48] but was nonregenerative in four cats[48,50] despite a strong positive Coombs' reaction in one of them.[47] Anemia was not characterized in one cat.[49] Five cats were thrombocytopenic (platelet counts, 31,000 to 141,000/µl), and one of these was pancytopenic.

Serum bilirubin was elevated in five cats.[45,47,48] Four cats were hypoalbuminemic.[47,48]

Bone marrow aspiration was performed in four cats and showed erythrophagocytosis,[45–48] usually associated with a dense infiltration with histiocytes.[47] The percentage of histiocytes remained low in an anemic cat in which serial bone marrow aspirations were performed over a 5 week period.[50] Erythrophagocytosis by malignant histiocytes has also been demonstrated in other organs and is considered to be characteristic of histiocytosis (Figure 49-5).

Diagnosis was confirmed by demonstration of malignant histiocytes on bone marrow aspiration cytology alone or in conjunction with fine-needle aspiration cytology of spleen, liver, or lung. Further confirmation should be obtained by immunohistochemical staining with lysosyme[46,49] or by positive staining for the macrophage markers acid phosphatase, nonspecific esterase,[45,47] and α-1-antitrypsin.[48] A specific macrophage marker was also used in one cat.[46] Staining is often able to demonstrate clusters of histiocytic tumor cells that form nodules in the liver, lung, and spleen and infiltrate mesenteric lymph nodes. The lungs were involved in three cats and the brain in one cat.

Treatment

Two cats were not treated.[48,49] One cat received corticosteroids and cyclophosphamide as well as two blood transfusions over 9 days as treatment for presumed immune-mediated disease. There was no response, and the cat was euthanized due to worsening anemia and icterus.[45] Supportive treatment caused an initial improvement in three other cats, but they ultimately died 1 to 5 weeks later despite blood transfusions[48] or prednisone treatment.[50]

KEY POINT

Cats with histiocytosis should be clinically staged as if they had lymphoma.

Blood transfusions, prednisone, vincristine, and L-asparaginase were also ineffective in halting the progress of disease in another cat.[47] A final cat received an attenuated course of radiation therapy to its mediastinal mass before it deteriorated and was euthanized.[46]

Chemotherapy has limited efficacy in dogs with malignant histiocytosis; however, protocols used for treatment of lymphoma may be the best therapeutic approach for this rare tumor in cats. Blood transfusions, antibiotics, analgesics, and antiinflammatories may be palliative, and appropriate attention should be given to nutritional support.

REFERENCES

1. Carpenter JL, Holzworth J: Thymoma in 11 cats. *JAVMA* 181:240–251, 1982.
2. Martin RA, Evans EW, August JR, Franklin JE: Surgical treatment of a thymoma in a cat. *JAAHA* 22:347–354, 1986.
3. Galloway PEJ, Barr FJ, Holt PE, et al: Cystic thymoma in a cat with cholesterol-rich fluid and an unusual ultrasonographic appearance. *J Small Anim Pract* 38:220–224, 1997.
4. Scott-Moncrieff JC, Cook Jr JR, Lantz GC: Acquired myasthenia gravis in a cat with thymoma. *JAVMA* 196:1291–1293, 1990.
5. Day MJ: Review of thymic pathology in 30 cats and 36 dogs. *J Small Anim Pract* 38:393–403, 1997.

6. Forster-van Hufte MA, Curtis CF, White RN: Resolution of exfoliative dermatitis and *Malassezia pachydermatis* overgrowth in a cat after surgical thymoma resection. *J Small Anim Pract* 38:451–454, 1997.

7. Kirchhoff A, Walter JH: Thymome bei der katze: Makroskopische, histologische und immunohistochemische befunde. *Kleintierpraxis* 41:177–184,1996.

8. Carpenter JL, Andrews LK, Holzworth J: Tumors and tumor-like lesions, in Holzworth J (ed): *Diseases of the Cat. Medicine and Surgery.* Philadelphia, WB Saunders, 1987, pp 407–596.

9. Loveday RK: Thymoma in a Siamese cat. *J South Afr Vet Med Assoc* 30:33–34, 1959.

10. Gores BR, Berg J, Carpenter JL, Aronsohn MG: Surgical treatment of thymoma in cats: 12 cases (1987–1992). *JAVMA* 204:1782–1785, 1994.

11. Richards CD: Hypertrophic osteoarthropathy in a cat. *Feline Pract* 7:41–43, 1977.

12. Carpenter JL, Valentine BA: Brief communications and case reports. Squamous cell carcinoma arising in two feline thymomas. *Vet Pathol* 29:541–543, 1992.

13. Mettler F: Thymome bei hund und katze. *Schweiz Arch Tierheilk* 117:577–584, 1975.

14. van Oosterhout ICAM, Teske E, Vos JH, Koeman JP: Myasthenia gravis en een thymoom bij een kat. *Tijdschr Diergeneesk* 114:499–505, 1989.

15. Willard MD, Tvedten H, Walshaw R, Aronson E: Thymoma in a cat. *JAVMA* 176:451–453, 1980.

16. Kobayashi Y, Yoshida K, Sawashima K, et al: Thymoma in a cat. *J Jpn Vet Med Assoc* 46:582–584, 1993.

17. Dubielzig RR, DeLaney RG: A thymoma in a cat. *Vet Med Small Anim Clin* 75:1270–1272, 1980.

18. Malik R, Gabor L, Hunt GB, et al: Benign cranial mediastinal lesionas in three cats. *Aust Vet J* 75:183–187, 1997.

19. Middleton DJ, Ratcliffe RC, Xu FN: Thymoma with distant metastases in a cat. *Vet Pathol* 22:512–514, 1985.

20. Mackey L: Clear-cell thymoma and thymic hyperplasia in a cat. *J Comp Pathol* 85:367–371, 1975.

21. Gorman PD: What is your diagnosis? *JAVMA* 202:993–994, 1993.

22. Hauser B, Mettler F: Malignant thymoma in a cat. *J Comp Pathol* 94:311–313, 1984.

23. Scott DW, Yager JA, Johnston KM: Exfoliative dermatitis in association with thymoma in three cats. *Feline Pract* 23:8–13, 1995.

24. Godfrey DR: Dermatosis and associated systemic signs in a cat with thymoma and recently treated with an imidacloprid preparation. *J Small Anim Pract* 40:333–337, 1999.

25. Bonnard P, Dralez F: A propos d'un cas de thymome chez un chat. *Le Point Veterinaire* 23:1089–1094, 1992.

26. O'Dair HA, Holt PE, Pearson GR, Gruffydd-Jones TJ: Acquired immune-mediated myasthenia gravis in a cat associated with a cystic thymus. *J Small Anim Pract* 32:198–202, 1991.

27. Shelton GD, Ho M, Kass PH: Risk factors for acquired myasthenia gravis in cats: 105 cases (1986–1998). *JAVMA* 216:55–57, 2000.

28. Rae CA, Jacobs RM, Couto CG: A comparison between the cytological and histological characteristics in thirteen canine and feline thymomas. *Can Vet J* 30:497–500, 1989.

29. Vos JH, Stolwijk J, Ramaekers FCS, et al: The use of keratin antisera in the characterization of a feline thymoma. *J Comp Pathol* 102:71–77, 1990.

30. Ducoté JM, Dewey CW, Coates JR: Clinical forms of acquired myasthenia gravis in cats. *Compend Contin Educ Pract Vet* 21:440–447, 1999.

31. Anilkumar TV, Voigt RP, Quigley PJ, et al: Squamous cell carcinoma of the feline thymus with widespread apoptosis. *Res Vet Sci* 56:208–215, 1994.

32. Ellison GW, Garner MM, Ackerman N: Idiopathic mediastinal cyst in a cat. *Vet Radiol Ultrasound* 35:347–349, 1994.

33. Sugiyama M, Ohashi S, Mitani S, et al: A feline case of malignant mesothelioma in the pleura. *Bull Nippon Vet Zootech Coll* 26:3–8, 1977.

34. Kobayashi Y, Usuda H, Ochiai K, Itakura C: Malignant mesothelioma with metastases and mast cell leukaemia in a cat. *J Comp Pathol* 111:453–458, 1994.

35. Raflo CP, Nuernberger SP: Abdominal mesothelioma in a cat. *Vet Pathol* 15: 781–783, 1978.

36. Andrews EJ: Pleural mesothelioma in a cat. *J Comp Pathol* 83:259–263, 1973.

37. Akiyama K, Akiyama R, Suzuki Y: A case of feline peritoneal mesothelioma with psammoma bodies. *Jpn J Vet Sci* 44:975–979, 1982.

38. Umphlet RC, Bertoy RW: Abdominal mesothelioma in a cat. *Modern Vet Pract* 69:71–73, 1988.

39. Paola JP, Hammer AS, Smeak DD, Merryman JI: Aortic body tumor causing pleural effusion in a cat. *JAAHA* 30:281–285, 1994.

40. Schaer M, Meyer D: Benign peritoneal mesothelioma, hyperthyroidism, nonsuppurative hepatitis, and chronic disseminated intravascular coagulation in a cat: A case report. *JAAHA* 24:195–202, 1988.

41. Tilley LP, Owens JM, Wilkins RJ, Patnaik AK: Pericardial mesothelioma with effusion in a cat. *JAAHA* 11:60–65, 1975.

42. Suzuki Y, Sugimura M, Atoji Y, Akiyama K: Lymphatic metastasis in a case of feline peritoneal mesothelioma. *Jpn J Vet Sci* 47:511–516, 1985.

43. Rao AT, Acharjyo LN: Pleural mesothelioma in a tigress. *Indian J Vet Pathol* 18: 174–175, 1994.

44. Shin N-S, Kwon S-W, Kim D-Y, et al: Metastatic malignant mesothelioma in a tiger *(Panthera tigris)*. *J Zoo Wildl Med* 29:81–83, 1998.

45. Court EA, Earnest-Koons KA, Barr SC, Gould II WJ: Malignant histiocytosis in a cat. *JAVMA* 203:1300–1302, 1993.

46. Walton RM, Brown DE, Burkhard MJ, et al: Malignant histiocytosis in a domestic cat: Cytomorphologic and immunohistochemical features. *Vet Clin Pathol* 26:56–60, 1997.

47. Freeman L, Stevens J, Loughman C, Tompkins M: Clinical vignette: Malignant histiocytosis in a cat. *J Vet Intern Med* 9:171–173, 1995.

48. Kraje AC, Patton CS, Edwards DF: Malignant histiocytosis in 3 cats. *J Vet Intern Med* 15:252–256, 2001.

49. Gafner F, Bestetti GE: Feline maligne histiozytose und lysozymnachweis. *Schweiz Arch Tierheilk* 130:349–356, 1988.

50. Fritz D, Georges C, Hopfner CL: Malignant histiocytosis in a cat. *Feline Pract* 27:6–8, 1999.

MANAGEMENT OF SPECIFIC DISEASES

SKIN TUMORS

Antony S. Moore and Gregory K. Ogilvie

Cutaneous tumors are among the most visible to pet owners, and it is therefore understandable that skin tumors compose a large proportion of reported tumors in cats. The skin is also the first line of defense against a variety of environmental carcinogens.

There are some interesting differences in the pattern of skin tumor types found in different continents and countries. Countries that are closer to the equator, or perhaps those that have less ozone protection, have a higher incidence of actinically induced tumors such as squamous cell carcinoma (SCC; Table 50-1[1-6]). In addition, soft tissue sarcomas appear to be increasing in incidence, particularly in association with vaccination; this trend may not be universal because of variation in vaccination practices and may lead to further differences in skin tumor incidence around the world.

BENIGN SKIN TUMORS

The proportion of feline skin tumors that are benign varies by country. While basal cell tumors and mast cell tumors (MCTs) mostly have a benign course in cats, many other benign tumors seen in dogs (e.g., lipomas, papillomas, sebaceous/adnexal tumors) are rare in cats.

Excisional biopsy, as described in Section II, may often be curative. However, all excised tissue should be submitted for histopathologic examination as malignant skin tumors are common in cats.

CLINICAL BRIEFING	
Common Presentation	Hair matrix tumors are rare; Persian cats are predisposed. Papillomas are rare and tend to be viral induced. Plasmacytomas are rare. Lipomas may occur anywhere on the body; Siamese are predisposed.
Staging and Diagnosis	MDB. Cutaneous plasmacytoma may be associated with multiple myeloma, and thus complete staging with lymph node palpation, abdominal ultrasonography, urine and serum protein electrophoresis, and bone marrow aspiration is indicated.
Treatment	
Initial	Surgery has the potential to cure all tumors listed above.
Adjunctive	Chemotherapy with prednisone and melphalan if plasma cell tumor is associated with multiple myeloma.
Supportive	Analgesia after surgery. Antiemetics may be needed if chemotherapy is administered.

DILATED PORE OF WINER AND TRICHOEPITHELIOMA

Dilated pore of Winer is characterized by a cystic structure similar to an epidermal inclusion cyst or a trichoepithelioma, and it appears to be derived from the follicular sheath. Tumors may be initially raised and then "open-up" to leave a crater-like lesion but are neither pruritic nor painful. This benign tumor was described in 17 DSHs, 1 DLH, and 1 Siamese ranging in age from 1 to 14 years (median, 7 years); there was no apparent gender predilection. The lesion was on the head or neck in all but 4 of these 19 reported cats, and none had recurrence after surgical excision at periods ranging from 3 to 72 months (median, 8 months).[7-9]

Two trichoepitheliomas were diagnosed among 340 skin tumors; both occurred in DSH cats. One was 1 year old and the other was 10 years old. One tumor was on the chin.[1] A trichoepithelioma on the shoulder of an 11-year-old Siamese and a pilomatricoma on the shoulder of a 12-year-old Siamese were described in another report and appeared to be benign.[2] In a series of 32 trichoepitheliomas, the tail was affected in 8 cats and 1 cat had multiple tumors. Persian cats were more than five times more likely than other breeds to develop trichoepithelioma.[3] Pilomatricoma is a rare tumor in cats.[9]

TABLE 50-1
Worldwide Distribution of Feline Skin Tumors

Tumor Type	Percentage of Skin Tumors by Country						
	Southern United States[1]	Northern United States[2]	United States[3]	United Kingdom[4]	Germany[5]	Australia[6]	New Zealand[6]
Basal cell	26.1	21.8	14	14.8	11.4	13.2	20
MCT	21.1	20.0	12	7.7	5.6	5.4	4
Fibrosarcoma/Fibroma	17.9	16.4	16.5	28.1	43.9	14.5	8
SCC	15.2	4.5	9.6	17.4	7.2	49.1	54
Melanoma	0.8	2.3	0.3	2.7	2.7	0.4	0
Hemangioma	1.2	1.6	N/A	0.3	0.5	0.9	0

PILOLEIOMYOMA

A 12-year-old male Russian Blue had a rapidly growing nodular skin mass on its neck. The lesion was a low-grade muscle tumor with areas of osteoid metaplasia. The tumor was thought to arise from the arrector pili muscles. It was well circumscribed and completely excised.[10]

PAPILLOMA

A fibropapilloma in an 18-year-old female Siamese cat was mentioned in the literature,[1] but papilloma-virus associated tumors have been described in only three cats[11,12]: two purebred silver Persians and a Persian-cross (all castrated males; age range, 7 to 13 years). Two cats had received long-term corticosteroids or "hormonal" therapy for dermatologic and behavior problems,[11] and the other had severe peritonitis and pancreatitis.[12]

The lesions were described as multiple greasy, rough, and scaly plaques and were pigmented in two cats. The plaques ranged in size from 0.5 to 2.0 cm in diameter and affected the neck, shoulders, thorax, and forelegs of one cat for 2 years.[12] One cat was FeLV and FIV negative.[12] Papilloma virus was found in all three cats. Therapy was not described.

Fibropapillomas that were histologically similar to equine sarcoid were described in a 2-year-old Siamese-cross and a 13-year-old DSH.[13] The tumors were surgically removed from the lip and hind foot and did not recur. Viral analysis was not available.

CUTANEOUS PLASMACYTOMA

The majority of plasma cell tumors reported in cats are systemic in nature and are discussed in Chapter 37 under the heading Multiple Myeloma.

Few details were provided about the six cases of cutaneous plasmacytoma reported in the literature. A plasmacytoma was found on the back of a 13-year-old castrated male DSH,[14] and mucocutaneous plasmacytomas of the lip or gum were reported in a 10-year-old female DSH and an 8-year-old male

Persian.[15] A 0.5 cm plasma cell tumor developed suddenly below the right eye of a 3-year-old female Burmese.[16] The fifth cat, a 10-year-old castrated male DSH, had a tarsal cutaneous plasmacytoma with histologic evidence of associated amyloid. The tumor was metastatic to the popliteal and inguinal lymph nodes, and the cat had IgG globulinemia; globulins were also detected in the urine. The cat was treated with melphalan and prednisone, and the cutaneous mass reduced in size over the next month; nevertheless, the cat died due to pulmonary arterial thromboembolism 6 weeks after starting treatment. On necropsy, the retroperitoneal lymph nodes and spleen were infiltrated with metastatic plasma cells.[17] The sixth cat had multiple 3 mm cutaneous plasmacytomas, but there were no additional findings associated with myeloma other than a monoclonal globulin spike. However, 2 months later at necropsy, the bone marrow, liver, spleen, and kidneys were infiltrated with plasma cells.[2]

Solitary cutaneous plasmacytomas should be excised. Staging, including an MDB, excisional biopsy, evaluation of regional lymph nodes, bone marrow aspiration, urine and serum protein electrophoresis, and radiography and ultrasonography as described for multiple myeloma, should be performed. Adjunctive chemotherapy with prednisone and melphalan is recommended if the plasma cell tumor is associated with multiple myeloma.

Appropriate analgesia should be used in the postoperative period to minimize patient discomfort. Antiemetic therapy may be helpful in cats experiencing nausea associated with chemotherapy.

LIPOMA

Benign fatty tumors are variably reported in surveys of skin tumors. In surveys from the United Kingdom, Australia, and the United States totaling 685 cats,[1,6,18] only three lipomas were described; they were located on the dorsal trunk of a 12-year-old castrated male DSH[1] and 2 other cats.[6] In contrast, more than 5% of skin tumors in two pathology surveys from the Northeastern United States[2,3] and approximately 3% of 943 skin tumors diagnosed in Germany[5] and Switzerland[19] were lipomas. In one survey, 23 lipomas were seen, all in DSHs except for two Siamese and one Persian. The ages of cats ranged from 2 to 16 years (mean, 9.6 years). None of the cats were obese.[2] Tumors were solitary in most cats, although 7 (30%) had multiple tumors (5 cats had 2 tumors, 1 cat had 3, and 1 had many). Tumors were found only on the trunk or upper legs and were usually small, rarely reaching a size greater than 13 cm.[2] In another series of 179 cats with cuta-neous lipoma, 8 cats had multiple lipomas.[3] Lipomas oc-curred on the thorax and abdomen in 63 cats and on the limbs in 50 cats. Siamese were nearly three times more likely to develop lipoma than other breeds. Surgical removal of a lipoma should be curative, but the cat should be checked for multiple tumors prior to surgery.

Infiltrative lipoma, a tumor seen in dogs that is difficult to excise surgically, has only rarely been reported in cats. An infiltrative lipoma seen in one cat appeared to be cured by wide surgical excision.[20]

ADNEXAL TUMORS

BENIGN BASAL CELL TUMORS

CLINICAL BRIEFING	
Common Presentation	Benign tumors, usually as a solitary cystic or solid dermal mass on the head or body; commonly pigmented. Longhaired cats and Siamese may be predisposed.
Staging and Diagnosis	MDB and excisional biopsy.
Treatment Initial Adjunctive Supportive	 Surgery should be curative. None necessary. Analgesia after surgery.

MDB = minimum database; includes CBC, biochemical profile, urinalysis, FeLV/FIV serology, T_4 testing, and thoracic radiographs (three views).

Incidence, Signalment and Etiology

Basal cell tumors originate from basal cells of the epider-mis, hair follicles, sweat glands, or sebaceous glands. In three surveys,[1,2,18] basal cell tumors were the most common skin tumors in cats, accounting for 25% to 30% of cuta-neous tumors. In two other recent surveys, one from the United States[21] and one from Australia,[6] the incidence of basal cell tumors ranged from 10% to 13% of cutaneous tu-mors, while basal cell tumors accounted for 20% of cuta-neous tumors in a study from New Zealand.[6] The clinician should be aware that these are the most common melanocytic tumor in cats and that they are the most com-mon benign skin tumor despite the other terms (e.g., basal cell carcinoma, basosquamous carcinoma, basal cell epithe-lioma) sometimes used to describe this tumor. The terms *basal cell carcinoma* and *basosquamous carcinoma* are more correctly applied to invasive, less common malignant vari-ants[22] (see below). Some of these tumors were recently re-classified on the basis of their lineage as trichoblastoma.[9]

The median age of affected cats in all studies (842 cats) was 10 years (range, <1–20 years).[1–3,5,6,18,21]

Although an early study found a higher proportion of basal cell tumors in males,[18] five recent studies have not borne this out. In these studies, there were 392 males and 410 females affected[1–3,6,21]; furthermore, the distribution of neutered cats was almost equal in one of these studies.[21]

Breed information was provided for over 200 cats in two studies. There were 148 DSHs, 14 DLHs, 27 Siamese, 9 Per-sians, 5 Himalayans, and 3 Angoras reported.[1,21] In another study, 20 of 97 cats were Siamese, which was four times high-er than the hospital population.[2] In a series of 467 basal cell tumors from the United States, the majority of affected cats were DSHs, but there were also 71 DLHs, 31 Persians, and 27 Himalayans. These three breeds had an increased risk of developing basal cell tumors of 1.6, 3.3, and 2.1 times that of the general feline population, respectively.[3] In contrast, a Ger-man study found no predisposition in long-haired breeds.[5]

Clinical Presentation and History

Basal cell tumors are nearly always solitary, although a cat with multiple lesions affecting the rear legs and inguinal area has been described[23] and 0.2% to 1% of cats in three other surveys had multiple lesions affecting the face, abdomen, and flank.[2,3,6] While two studies found a predilection for the head and neck (180 of 466 affected cats), three other studies indicated that the dorsum and flank are more likely to be affected; in these five studies, of 694 cats in which the site was known, 232 tumors affected the trunk or back, 257 affected the head or neck, and 178 affected the limbs.[1,2,6,18,21] Basal cell tumor of the tail was seen in 1% to 3% of cats.[2,3] Tumors were usually small but ranged in size from less than 1 cm to 7 cm in diameter. In one study, fewer than 5% of basal cell tumors were larger than 2.5 cm in diameter.[21] They may occasionally be pedunculated.[2]

Tumors may remain static over a long period. In one study, tumors were present from weeks to 3 years (10 years in one cat) before owners sought veterinary advice.[18]

The appearance of basal cell tumors is variable. These tumors usually appear as well-demarcated, small, firm nodules that sharply elevate the overlying epidermis. Pigmentation seems to be more common in cystic tumors than in solid tumors (Figure 50-1), while solid tumors are more likely to be ulcerated.[1,21] Cystic tumors may consist of a single cyst but are often multilocular.

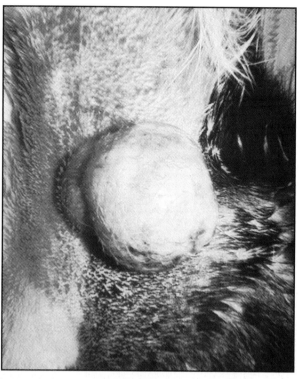

Figure 50-1: Solitary, pigmented basal cell tumor on the neck of a 13-year-old cat. These benign tumors are the most common pigmented skin tumor in cats. (Courtesy of G.H. Theilen)

> ## KEY POINT
>
> *The benign basal cell tumor is the most common melanocytic skin tumor in cats.*

Staging and Diagnosis

An MDB and excisional biopsy should be performed as staging for benign basal cell tumors. Local recurrence is rare after adequate surgical removal.

Treatment

Surgical excision appears to be curative in nearly all cats. In one study, the tumor recurred in 2 of 36 cats. In one of these cats, a recurrence 18 months after surgery was followed by a second recurrence 7 months later.[18] In two series of 188 cats, there were no recurrences after surgery and no metastases[21]; however, wide surgical margins should be obtained whenever possible. A cat with a basal cell tumor on the nasal planum was treated with a "nosectomy" and was free of disease 27 months later.[24]

Postoperative analgesia is indicated, particularly in more involved surgeries, such as removal of the nasal planum.

MALIGNANT BASAL CELL TUMORS

CLINICAL BRIEFING	
Common Presentation	Invasive, nonpigmented tumors usually located on the head and neck. Persian cats are predisposed.
Staging and Diagnosis	MDB and palpation and fine-needle aspiration of regional lymph nodes. Metastasis is rare.
Treatment	
Initial	Surgical excision.
Adjunctive	If excision is incomplete, consider radiation therapy. For metastatic tumors, consider doxorubicin and/or carboplatin. No adjunctive treatment proven to date.
Supportive	Analgesia after surgery.

Incidence, Signalment and Etiology

Basal cell tumors may show stromal invasion with a high mitotic index; 10 of 97 tumors had these characteristics in one study. All 10 were solid (not cystic) nonpigmented tumors.[2] Five of these tumors invaded vessels, and 1 had metastasized from the base of the ear to the prescapular lymph node. This is the only basal cell tumor reported to metastasize.[2] Another pathology survey differentiated basal cell carcinoma from basal cell tumors on the basis of deep dermal and subcutaneous invasion that incited a desmoplastic response (Figures 50-2 and 50-3).[3] While this survey documented 467 basal cell tumors, only 40 were classified as carcinoma.

Clinical Presentation and History

Carcinomas occurred on the head or neck in 19 of 40 cats, and Persians were four times more likely to develop this tumor.[3] Basal cell tumors appear capable of transforming into the more malignant variant.[3]

Staging and Diagnosis

Staging for malignant basal cell tumors should include an MDB, biopsy of the lesion, and palpation and fine-needle aspiration of regional lymph nodes.

Treatment

Malignant basal cell tumors are probably best treated as described for SCC. Surgical excision is the treatment of choice. Radiation following incomplete surgery is advisable, although no reports of treatment are published. Chemotherapy as described for SCC is probably the most practical adjunctive treatment. While there are no published reports of their efficacy, doxorubicin and carboplatin are the chemotherapeutic agents most likely to control metastasis. Appropriate analgesia should be administered postoperatively, and antiemetic therapy may be indicated if chemotherapy is used.

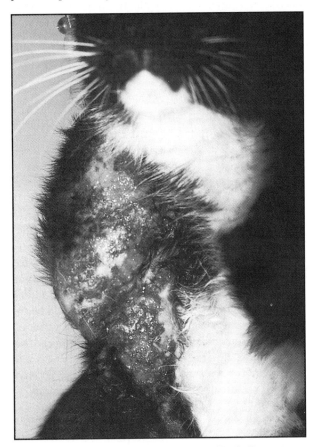

Figure 50-2: A less common malignant variant of basal cell tumor is seen in this cat with widespread intracutaneous invasion and metastasis. A deep desmoplastic response is evident. (Courtesy of K.M. Rassnick)

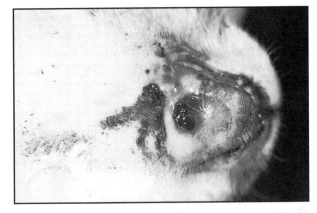

Figure 50-3: A malignant basal cell tumor on the chin of a 14-year-old Birman. This tumor was recurrent after radiation therapy.

TUMORS OF GLANDULAR TISSUE

▶ BENIGN GLANDULAR TUMORS

CLINICAL BRIEFING

Common Presentation	Both apocrine and sebaceous adenomas are usually solitary and located on the head or back. Both are rare, but apocrine is more common. Persians are predisposed to sebaceous adenomas. Tumors are often cystic (apocrine tumors).

Staging and Diagnosis	MDB and excisional biopsy.
Treatment Initial Adjunctive Supportive	 Surgical excision should be curative. None necessary. Analgesia after surgery.

APOCRINE GLAND ADENOMA

Other terms for these tumors include *papillary syringoadenoma* and *sweat gland cystadenoma*.

Incidence, Signalment, and Etiology

These tumors account for 1.6% to 5.4% of tumors in published surveys. There are 187 sebaceous adenomas reported in five surveys totaling 4,389 skin tumors.[1–3,6,18]

Signalment was available for 34 cats; except for 1 Siamese, all were DSHs.[1] Affected cats ranged in age from 7 to 27 years (average age in two surveys,[1,2] 12 years). Although there were more females than males in a survey that grouped benign and malignant apocrine skin tumors,[2] a larger survey of 142 cats with apocrine adenomas found no gender predilection.[3]

KEY POINT

Apocrine and sebaceous adenomas have a predilection for the head and dorsum.

Clinical Presentation and History

Apocrine gland adenomas have a predilection for the head, with nearly 60% of these tumors occurring at this site.[1–3,25] The back is the next most common reported site, while lesions of the neck, abdomen, perineum, and hind leg are rare. In one study,[3] fewer than 3% of 142 apocrine adenomas were multiple.

Apocrine adenomas are often fluctuant and may clinically appear to be cysts. Like basal cell tumors, they may appear darkly pigmented. Apocrine adenomas are rarely ulcerated,[25] despite having been present for months to years in some cats.

Treatment

Most apocrine gland adenomas are less than 1.5 cm in diameter, and surgical excision should be curative. Recurrence after surgery may respond to a more aggressive excision. One cat that had two recurrences in 6 months was free of tumor 3 years after a third surgery.[25] Analgesia is indicated postoperatively.

SEBACEOUS ADENOMA

Incidence, Signalment, and Etiology

Sebaceous gland hyperplasia may be difficult to differentiate from sebaceous adenoma in cats. Both are very rare. It is possible that hyperplastic lesions may progress to become an adenoma, but this is probably a rare event. One cat with multiple nodular sebaceous hyperplasia developed a single adenoma after 10 years.[2]

Sebaceous adenomas occur with equal frequency in male and female cats. In one survey, 5 of 54 cats were Persian and Persian cats were five times more likely than other breeds to develop these tumors.[3] In another survey, 3 of 15 cats with sebaceous adenoma were Siamese.[2]

Clinical Presentation and History

Sebaceous adenomas occur as a solitary sessile mass, usually located on the head or back. Multiple lesions occurred in only 1 of 48 cats.[3]

Treatment

Surgical excision should be curative. Analgesia should be used to minimize patient discomfort postoperatively.

▶ MALIGNANT GLANDULAR TUMORS

C L I N I C A L B R I E F I N G	
Common Presentation	Apocrine and sebaceous carcinomas are found on the head and limbs. Lesions are often ulcerated and invasive. Siamese are predisposed to develop apocrine carcinomas. Older female cats may be predisposed to sebaceous carcinomas.
Staging and Diagnosis	MDB; excisional biopsy, lymph node palpation, and abdominal ultrasonography if regional lymph nodes are abdominal. Metastasis possible but not widely reported. Digital apocrine carcinomas are most likely to be metastatic from a primary lung tumor. *(continued)*

Treatment	
Initial	Surgical excision may be curative.
Adjunctive	Radiation for incomplete excision. Chemotherapy with doxorubicin or carboplatin if metastatic.
Supportive	Analgesia after surgery. Antiemetics for chemotherapy-induced nausea.

APOCRINE GLAND ADENOCARCINOMA

Incidence, Signalment, and Etiology

Apocrine gland adenocarcinomas are less common than adenomas in all published surveys, accounting for about 2% to 3% of all feline skin tumors.[1-3,6,18] While apocrine adenomas are more likely to be found on the head, only about one third of apocrine adenocarcinomas occur in this location.[2,3] Apocrine adenocarcinomas are found on the legs in many cats.[1,3]

Like adenomas, apocrine adenocarcinomas occur with equal frequency in both males and females. Siamese appear to be at higher risk than other breeds for developing this tumor; 12 of 94 cats in two studies[2,3] were Siamese, making their risk of developing these tumors nearly three times greater than other breeds.

Clinical Presentation and History

Malignant apocrine gland tumors tend to be larger than adenomas, with an average size of 2.4 cm. They are also more often ulcerated than adenomas (Figure 50-4); more than half of the apocrine adenocarcinomas were ulcerated in one study.[2] When located on the ventral abdomen, they may resemble mammary tumors (Figure 50-5). Affected sites in one study included the pinnae, axilla, rump, thigh, thoracic wall, and perineum.[25]

Cats with a histologic diagnosis of apocrine adenocarcinoma of the digit may in fact have digital metastasis from a pulmonary carcinoma. In one study, 56 of 64 cats with digital tumors had metastases from a primary lung tumor. Primary digital SCC was diagnosed in 8 cats, and no cat had a primary digital adenocarcinoma[26] (see Chapter 47).

Staging and Diagnosis

Apocrine adenocarcinomas often have histologic evidence of stromal and lymphatic vessel invasion.[25] Careful palpation and fine-needle aspiration or biopsy of regional lymph nodes should be performed. Thoracic radiographs and abdominal ultrasonography will help identify enlarged distant lymph nodes as well as pulmonary metastases.

Treatment

Surgical excision should be wide and deep to completely remove this infiltrative tumor. Recurrence was not noted a year after excision of a small apocrine adenocarcinoma in one cat[27]; two cats did not have recurrence 5 months after surgical excision.[25] Radiation therapy may reduce the recurrence rate when excision is incomplete, but no published reports of efficacy exist. Chemotherapy for metastatic tumors has not been reported; doxorubicin and carboplatin may be effective. Analgesia should be considered postoperatively, and antiemetics may be needed if chemotherapy is administered.

SEBACEOUS ADENOCARCINOMA

Incidence, Signalment, and Etiology

These tumors occur in older cats (average age, 11.5

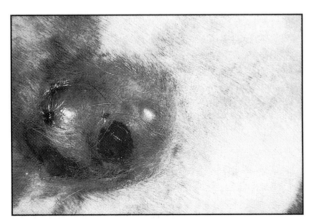

Figure 50-4: A solitary cystic and ulcerated apocrine adenocarcinoma on the right hip of an 11-year-old cat. Ulceration is more common in malignant glandular tumors than in the benign variants. (Courtesy of G.H. Theilen)

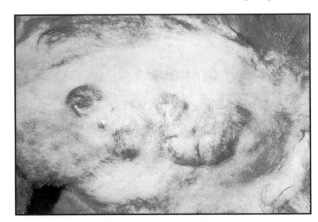

Figure 50-5: Invasive apocrine adenocarcinoma may clinically resemble mammary carcinoma. (Courtesy of A. Evans)

years). In two surveys totaling 30 cats with sebaceous adenocarcinoma, 21 (70%) were females and only 9 were spayed.[2,3]

Clinical Presentation and History

While about 40% of these malignant tumors occur on the head and neck, approximately 25% occur on the limbs or thorax. Like apocrine adenocarcinomas, malignant sebaceous tumors may be ulcerated.

Staging and Diagnosis

Too little information is available to make statements regarding metastasis for this tumor type, although one tumor was noted to invade lymphatic vessels.[2] No metastases were noted over a 1 year period in one cat and a 2 year period in a second cat. Staging should be performed as described for apocrine tumors.

Treatment

Surgical excision of an ulcerated sebaceous adenocarcinoma from the paw of an 18-year-old Siamese appears to have been successful as no recurrence or metastasis was present 1 year later. In contrast, three surgeries were performed over a 2 year period to remove a sebaceous adenocarcinoma from the tail base of a cat. This tumor had invaded lymphatic vessels.[2] This serves to emphasize the importance of obtaining wide surgical margins at the first surgery. As for apocrine adenocarcinomas, there are no published reports of the success of radiation and chemotherapy as adjunctive treatments for cats with sebaceous adenocarcinoma; however, radiation therapy may reduce the likelihood of recurrence after incomplete excision, and doxorubicin and/or carboplatin may be used in an attempt to control metastasis. Analgesia should be considered postoperatively, and antiemetics may be needed if chemotherapy is administered.

CUTANEOUS MELANOMA

CLINICAL BRIEFING

Common Presentation	Mostly affects older DSH cats; possibly more common in black and gray cats. Usually pigmented. Often found on the head (pinna and ear base), rarely multiple. Rapid growth and ulceration possible.
Staging and Diagnosis	MDB, evaluation of regional lymph nodes, and abdominal ultrasonography. Metastasis common and widespread. Histologic criteria, including mitotic index, not predictive of behavior.
Treatment Initial	Surgical excision unlikely to be curative, but it is possible.
Adjunctive	For incomplete excision, coarse fraction radiation therapy may reduce recurrence. Chemotherapy with carboplatin or doxorubicin unproven.
Supportive	Analgesia, appetite stimulants, and antiinflammatories if metastasis is present. Antiemetics if chemotherapy used.

Incidence, Signalment, and Etiology

DSH cats account for 164 of 176 reported cases of cutaneous melanoma; there were 5 DLHs and 6 Siamese included in these reports.[1,18,28–31] A white Manx is the only other purebred cat reported.[32] In one study, 35% of 64 cats were black or gray.

Cutaneous melanoma occurs most frequently in older cats (average age, 10–11 years[29–31]); however, cats as young as 2 years of age have been reported as having this tumor.[31,33] For 172 cats in which gender was stated, there was no strong predilection.[28–32] Signalment does not vary between cats with malignant or benign melanoma.[29,31]

Clinical Presentation and History

Cutaneous basal cell tumors are the most common dark pigmented skin tumor in cats (see previous section). Another lesion that could be mistaken for melanoma, particularly by owners, is "lentigo simplex." The occurrence of tiny black spots on the lips, gingiva, eyelids, and nasal plane in orange cats may be distinguished from melanoma by the signalment, slow rate of growth, and lack of a mass lesion. In a study of 11 cats 2 to 11 years of age, lentigo spots had been noticed to be present in 7 of the cats since they were less than a year old. In 5 cats followed for more than 2 years, no lesion transformed into a neoplasm.[34]

Approximately 80% of cutaneous melanoma in cats are black in color.[31] Apart from their color, melanomas of the skin have a variable appearance; they are nodular or papilloma-like in some cats and can be sessile, pedunculated, or crateriform. Ulceration is less commonly seen (Figure 50-6).

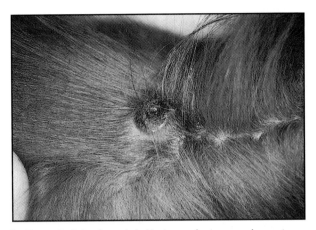

Figure 50-6: *An ulcerated, darkly pigmented cutaneous melanoma in a 12-year-old cat.*

No association has been found between clinical appearance (including ulceration) and prediction of malignant or benign behavior.[31] Cutaneous melanoma may be present for several years,[2] but rapid growth is often a feature noted by owners.[28] Rate of growth does not seem to correlate with biologic behavior.[31]

Cutaneous melanomas commonly occur on the head, in particular on the pinna and at the base of the ear[31]; 41 of 136 (30%) tumors occurred at these two sites.[2,3,28–30,33] Of the same 136 cats, tumors also occurred on the head and neck (including eyelids, lips ,and nares) in 39 cats, limbs (including three digital tumors) in 15 cats, trunk in 27 cats, and tail and perineum in 8 cats. Multiple tumors were seen in 5% of cats[28,31,32] and may signal metastatic spread of the tumor (Figure 50-7).[32]

Staging and Diagnosis

Any persistent or growing black tumor on the skin of a cat should be removed. While the biopsy result may confirm the diagnosis of melanoma, criteria to predict malig-

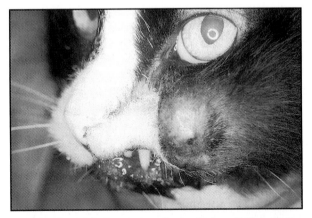

Figure 50-7: *Multiple cutaneous melanomas in the cat in Figure 50-6 were associated with widespread metastatic disease. No response was seen to doxorubicin or carboplatin chemotherapy.*

nant behavior are unclear. The conflicting findings reported below serve to emphasize the heterogeneous nature and variable behavior of this tumor.

Different classification schemes based on histologic criteria have been applied to cutaneous melanomas in cats. The predominant cell type in tumors may be classified as epithelioid, spindloid, round cell, or mixed. In addition, some recent studies have described signet ring or balloon-type cells as the predominant histologic type in melanomas that are often amelanotic.[30] In one study,[31] cutaneous melanomas of the epithelioid type were malignant in 80% of cases, spindloid tumors were malignant in only 29% of cases, and round cell tumors were malignant about half the time. In another study,[30] only 3 of 14 epithelioid (21%) and none of 4 spindloid tumors showed malignant behavior at the time of diagnosis. In this study, malignant behavior was seen in 1 of 7 mixed cell melanomas and 1 of 11 balloon cell melanomas, while 6 of 21 (29%) signet ring melanomas developed lymph node metastases or invaded lymphatics. Although the incidence of metastatic spread at the time of diagnosis was quite low (11 of 57 cats; 19%), local recurrence and regional lymph node metastasis were noted in 22 of 45 cats at follow-up 0.5 to 18 months after surgery.[30] An additional 15 cats died of unknown cause. The 18 month survival rate was therefore 18%. Prognosis for cats with melanoma appears to be poor regardless of the histologic type of the tumor.[30]

Other histologic criteria have been evaluated for their ability to predict biologic behavior. Tumors showing moderate to extensive nuclear atypia were likely to be malignant in 75% of cases, while those with little atypia were still likely to act malignantly about 40% of the time.[31]

KEY POINT

Histologic criteria are rarely prognostic in cats with cutaneous melanoma.

Mitotic index (number of mitoses/10 high power fields) was found to be somewhat predictive of biologic behavior (Table 50-2); however, 25% of the malignant tumors had a mitotic index of 0 and one third of cats with a high mitotic index had a benign tumor.[31] It is therefore hard to predict tumor behavior based on mitotic index in an individual cat.

Specific measurement of the cellular proliferation rate in melanoma by immunohistochemical detection of protein Ki67 was prognostic in a small study.[35] All cats that had a high proliferation index had a poor prognosis. This testing was performed on a small number of cats and is not widely available.

Inflammatory infiltration by lymphocytes and plasma cells was found to predict malignant behavior in one study[29] but not in another.[31] Similarly, necrosis and the presence of

TABLE 50-2
Mitotic Activity of Feline Cutaneous Melanomas[31]

Mitotic Index	Benign	Malignant
0	11	5
1	3	5
2–5	4	6
6–10	1	0
>10	2	4
Total	21	20

multinucleate giant cells were found to predict malignant behavior in one study[29] but not in two others.[30,31] Junctional activity (proliferation of cells along the dermal-epidermal junction) was found to predict benign behavior in one study[29] but was not addressed in two other studies.[30,31]

It is therefore prudent to say that all cutaneous melanomas in cats should be considered to have the potential to be malignant. Tumors with a high number of mitotic figures, marked nuclear atypia, and lymphoid infiltration may raise the level of concern, but even tumors that have all these features may still act benignly. The widespread nature of metastases (outlined below) should help direct the clinician toward staging procedures both prior to surgery and in the postoperative follow-up period.

Occasionally, a melanoma is too poorly differentiated to be accurately diagnosed on routine histopathology. Immunohistochemical staining for the S-100 protein is helpful in these cases.[35]

The regional lymph nodes are the most common metastatic sites for melanoma.[30] Other reported visceral sites of metastasis include, in order of decreasing frequency, lung, liver, kidney, spleen, pleura, heart, bone, pancreas, peritoneum, muscles, and meninges.[30] Metastases to other sites in the skin and to the stomach and mesentery have also been reported.[32]

Clinical staging prior to surgery should therefore include careful palpation and fine-needle aspiration of regional lymph nodes, ultrasonography, and a search for tumors in other external sites in addition to the MDB.

Treatment

Surgery has the potential to be curative in some cats with cutaneous melanoma. Eight of 45 cats with cutaneous melanoma were alive with no evidence of disease 3 to 60 months after surgery.[30] Similarly, 11 of the 15 cats (of 43 original cats) for which follow-up information was available were alive without recurrence of melanoma a median of 24 months (range, 6–66 months) after surgery.[29] This group of 11 cats included a 20-year-old cat that had a histologically malignant tumor of the pinna. Other cats have been found to have no evidence of disease 1 year after surgery.[28]

MDB = minimum database; includes CBC, biochemical profile, urinalysis, FeLV/FIV serology, T_4 testing, and thoracic radiographs (three views).

Recurrence is usually associated with metastases, although one cat had three surgeries for tumor recurrence and yet had no evidence of tumor recurrence or metastases 8 months after the third surgery.[28] Another cat had a recurrent tumor and a chain of infiltrated lymph nodes removed 7 months after the initial surgery but had no evidence of disease a further 19 months later.[33] Second surgeries may be warranted if staging does not reveal widespread metastases.

Radiation therapy given as coarse fractionation reduces local recurrence rate for dogs with melanoma and anecdotally may have similar efficacy in cats.[a] Metastasis is still possible after radiation therapy.

When metastases do occur, it is usually within 12 months of surgery.[28,30,33] There are few chemotherapeutic options for cats with metastatic melanoma. Some tumor regression was seen in one cat following carboplatin chemotherapy,[36] and doxorubicin may have some efficacy (unproven). The rarity of this tumor in cats means that any chemotherapeutic options for adjunctive treatment are based on anecdotal information.

Supportive care for cats with cutaneous melanoma should include postoperative analgesia, appetite stimulants and antiinflammatories if metastasis is noted, and antiemetics if chemotherapy is administered.

[a]Moore AS: Personal observation.

CUTANEOUS MAST CELL TUMORS

CLINICAL BRIEFING

Common Presentation	Affect cats of any age; Siamese are predisposed. Usually solitary but can be multiple. Often hairless and firm, up to 5 cm in diameter. Most common on head and neck. Need to differentiate from eosinophilic granuloma. Systemic involvement is rare.

(continued)

Staging and Diagnosis	MDB and excisional biopsy for solitary lesions. Histologic grading does not predict behavior. If multiple lesions are present, thoracic radiography, abdominal ultrasonography, buffy coat smear, and bone marrow aspiration should be performed to rule out systemic disease.
Treatment	
Initial	Surgical excision usually curative, but new lesions may arise. Spontaneous regression has been reported in Siamese cats with histiocytic tumors.
Adjunctive	Radiation therapy for incompletely excised tumors. Corticosteroids probably not effective. Other chemotherapy not reported; could try vinblastine or CCNU.
Supportive	Histamine or possibly serotonin antagonists for cutaneous reaction. Analgesia as needed.

Incidence, Signalment, and Etiology

MCTs are among the most common cutaneous tumors in cats in the United States, accounting for 12%[3] to 20%[1,2] of all skin neoplasms. These tumors are proportionally less common in Australia (4% to 5%) due to an increased number of sunlight-associated SCCs.[6] In an early U.K. survey, less than 2% of skin tumors were MCTs, but the reason for this low incidence is obscure.[18]

While the majority of affected cats are DSHs, Siamese are overrepresented. In six surveys totaling 732 cats with MCTs, there were 117 Siamese (16%).[1–3,37–39] In three of these surveys, Siamese cats were two[3] or three[1,2] times more likely to develop MCTs compared with the hospital population. Other purebreds reported are Persians,[1,40] Russian Blue (1 cat),[1] and Himalayan (1 cat).[39]

Siamese cats were also the youngest cats reported. A litter of 6-week-old kittens and an 8-week-old with same sire had histiocytic MCTs of the frontal and temporal areas of the head. The lesions regressed by the time all the kittens had reached 4 months of age.[41] In large surveys, the age of affected cats ranged to 21 years,[2] with an average age of 9 years in most surveys.[1–3] In a study comparing gender distribution with that of the general population, no predisposition was noted.[3]

Clinical Presentation and History

Cutaneous MCTs may be single, multiple, or diffuse (miliary). In two series encompassing 174 MCTs, 130 (75%) were solitary lesions that were hairless, firm, and between 2 and 5 cm in diameter (Figure 50-8).[2,38] Multiple lesions were seen in 12%[39] to 20%[2] of cats. About half of the cats with multiple tumors had a diffusely disseminated (miliary) distribution of tumors within the skin.[2] Diffuse miliary nodules may be a component of systemic MCT disease.[42–44] Cats that have been treated for systemic mast cell disease may relapse, even months later, with miliary[40,45,46] or solitary[40] cutaneous lesions. Further discussion of systemic mast cell disease is found in Chapter 42. Cats that have multiple tumors do not always develop systemic disease,[37] and cats with solitary tumors may later develop multiple cutaneous tumors

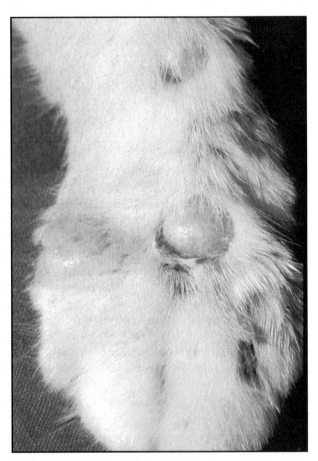

Figure 50-8: *Multiple raised alopecic MCTs on the paw of a cat. (Courtesy of B.R. Madewell)*

without evidence of systemic disease. These cats usually have 5 or fewer tumors[37,47] rather than the diffuse miliary distribution seen in cats with systemic disease. The exception to this rule may be Siamese cats, in which disseminated cutaneous tumors may spontaneously regress, even up to 2 years after diagnosis.[38]

Tumors are often noticed to have been present for

months[45,48,49] or years.[49] In one cat the tumor was present for 6.5 years prior to veterinary intervention.[2]

Tumors most commonly appear on the skin of the head and neck (Figure 50-9), with 227 of 444 tumors (51%) occurring here in two studies.[2,3] MCTs particularly affect the temples, pinnae (Figure 50-10), and periorbital regions.[2,40,48,49] Less frequently, MCTs are found on the feet and legs (18% to 20%) or trunk, abdomen, or flank (17%) and rarely in the perineum.[3,37,40] Solitary MCTs can appear plaque-like and may be misdiagnosed as eosinophilic granuloma based on their clinical appearance (Figures 50-11 and 50-12).[50] On the other hand, the clinician should be aware that mast cells are a common cell type in inflammatory lesions[51] and their presence on fine-needle aspiration or histopathology does not necessarily indicate a neoplastic process. In one study, 9 of 94 lesions previously diagnosed as MCTs on biopsy were reclassified as eosinophilic plaque.[38]

The release of vasoactive substances by the tumor causes the surrounding tissue to become pruritic and erythematous,[2] which may lead to self trauma and secondary ulceration.[37,40,42,45,49,52] Manipulation or fine-needle aspiration may cause erythema, hemorrhage, and/or edema around the site of an MCT,[27] and owners may report a tumor that appears to "grow" and shrink rapidly (Figure 50-13). Histamine has been implicated as the inciting substance, although serotonin appears to be a more important inflammatory mediator in feline mast cells.[53]

A bizarre, unique case report described malignant mast cells forming a continuous dermal band throughout the skin of a 1-year-old shorthaired cat.[54] Metastasis to regional lymph nodes had occurred, but there was no systemic involvement.

Staging and Diagnosis

Fine-needle aspiration will provide material for a cytologic diagnosis in most cats.[43] However, feline mast cells

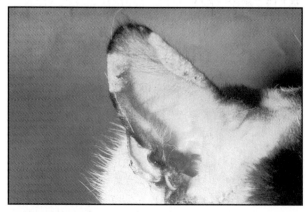

Figure 50-9: Solitary plaque-like erosive MCT on the head of a cat. (Courtesy of G.H. Theilen)

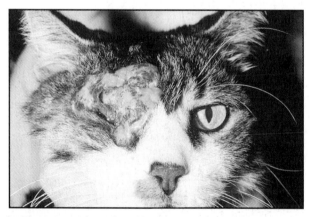

Figure 50-10: Plaque-like MCT on the pinna of a Siamese cat. Histiocytic MCTs in this breed may spontaneously regress. (Courtesy of B.R. Madewell)

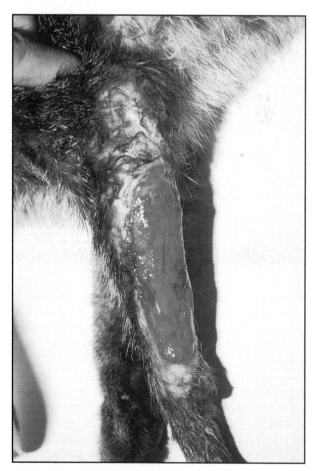

Figure 50-11: This ulcerated, plaque-like erosion on the skin of a cat's leg clinically resembles eosinophilic granuloma but was actually an MCT. The cat was treated palliatively by amputation. (Courtesy of G. Nesbitt)

MANAGEMENT OF SPECIFIC DISEASES

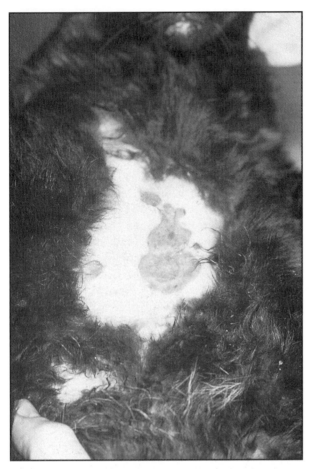

Figure 50-12: An ulcerated cutaneous lesion on the abdomen of a cat. Like the tumor seen in Figure 50-11, this lesion resembles an inflammatory eosinophilic granuloma. Biopsy should be performed on all lesions to ensure appropriate treatment. (Courtesy of G. Nesbitt)

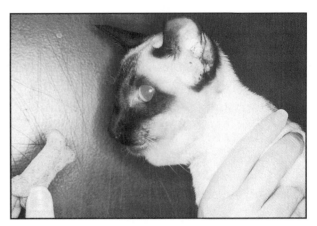

Figure 50-13: A 1-year-old Siamese with a cutaneous MCT of the ear base. After manipulation of the tumor, submandibular edema was considerable and the lesion was pruritic due to degranulation of mast cells.

may have very fine granules that are difficult to see; furthermore, they may not stain, even with toluidine blue, making an accurate cytologic diagnosis very difficult in some cases.[42] Thus biopsy is the preferred method to diagnose MCT. An MDB and excisional biopsy are recommended for staging a cat with a solitary MCT, whereas more extensive staging as described below should be performed when multiple or diffuse MCTs are present.

The behavior of cutaneous MCTs in dogs can be predicted by histologic grading; attempts to correlate biopsy findings with behavior have not been successful in cats.

In one study, 14 tumors were graded as dermal and well differentiated (Grade I), dermal to subcutaneous with moderate cellular pleomorphism (Grade II), and poorly differentiated (Grade III). Histologic grading did not correlate with recurrence or survival.[37] Eleven cats had no recurrence of the original tumor, although new tumors were found and treated surgically in five cats. The other three cats had static tumors for up to 5.5 years.

In another study, 9 of 10 tumors were classified as well differentiated and the tenth as moderately differentiated. Of those with well-differentiated tumors, 1 cat developed a second tumor a year after the first was removed and 2 cats developed multiple cutaneous lesions. One cat had intraabdominal disease.[47]

KEY POINT

Histologic grading does not predict the biologic behavior of cutaneous MCTs in cats.

This same grading system was used to classify MCTs from 32 cats, 4 of which had multiple tumors.[39] Eleven cats had Grade I tumors, 18 had Grade II tumors, and 3 had Grade III tumors. No cat died of MCT in over a year of follow-up, and grade of tumor did not correlate with tumor recurrence, which occurred in 5 cats (all within 1 year of surgery). Individual histopathologic criteria of mitotic rate, dermal infiltration, nuclear pleomorphism, and eosinophilic infiltration also failed to predict behavior.

A histiocytic form of MCT has been described.[38] Eighteen of 85 MCTs with a subcutaneous location and marked eosinophilic and lymphoid infiltrate were classified as histiocytic. Seventeen of the 18 cats were Siamese, and 14 were younger than 4 years of age. Nine cats had miliary tumors, and 5 had solitary lesions. Over a period of 2 years, 4 of 9 cats with miliary lesions developed multiple "crops" of tumor nodules with eventual complete spontaneous regression and remission. The other cats with histiocytic MCTs had a similar benign outcome to cats with nonhistiocytic solitary MCTs. Histiocytic MCTs occurred in 4 related Siamese kittens, and all regressed over 2 to 4 months.[41] All MCTs in Siamese cats are not histiocytic,[37] and the clinician should not rely on spontaneous remission as a mode of therapy.

Whether cats had solitary or multiple lesions did not predict future behavior in another report in which three of eight cats with solitary lesions and two of six cats with multiple lesions developed new cutaneous MCTs. All cats had five or fewer tumors.[37]

Histiocytic MCTs in Siamese cats may regress spontaneously.

It is often difficult to be certain whether a cutaneous MCT in a cat with systemic mast cell disease has spread to involve the viscera or whether the skin itself is a metastatic site. Cats with concurrent systemic disease[40,44–46] or that have cutaneous tumors long after treatment of systemic mast cell disease[55] are probably in the latter group. It appears that some MCTs may start as a cutaneous tumor and spread systemically,[38,42,43] although a short period between diagnosis of multiple cutaneous tumors and splenic tumors makes this a difficult "call."[42,43]

Accordingly, the clinician should clinically stage cats with multiple tumors or those with solitary tumors that are about to undergo extensive therapy. This staging procedure is covered more extensively in the section on MCTs in Chapter 42. In brief, a blood count and a buffy coat smear should be performed and a bone marrow aspirate obtained. Abdominal ultrasonography and thoracic radiography should be performed to rule out systemic disease. Concurrent mast cell disease has been found in the spleen, liver, and kidneys of cats with cutaneous lesions.[38,40,42–46] In one series, 15% of cats with cutaneous MCTs had evidence of systemic disease.[5] Regional lymph node metastasis has also been reported in up to 9% of affected cats,[5,40,42,49] and fine-needle aspiration of regional lymph nodes should be performed prior to surgery; however, such a metastatic pattern is less commonly seen than is spread to the spleen, liver, and bone marrow.[39]

Treatment

Surgery is the treatment of choice for cutaneous MCTs in cats. Many MCTs are only minimally invasive, but it is prudent to obtain wide margins if anatomically possible (Figure 50-14).

In one study of 30 cutaneous MCTs, surgical excision was histologically incomplete in 20, emphasizing the need for wide margins at surgery. However, only 2 of these 20 tumors recurred and did so within a year of surgery. Sixteen of the cats were followed for more than 3 years, and no cat died due to mast cell disease.[39] In another series of 14 cats, no tumor recurred locally but tumors arose at different cutaneous sites in 5 cats.[37] In a study that separated dermal and histiocytic MCTs, 42 cats with dermal tumors were treated via surgical excision; there was no tumor recurrence 1 year after surgery in 34 cats. Tumor recurred at the surgi-

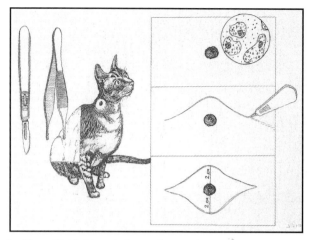

Figure 50-14: *Schematic showing the surgical approach to removing cutaneous MCT. Recurrence is rare after a complete excision. (From Elmslie RE, Ogilvie GK: Variables in behavior and management of mast cell tumors, in August JR (ed):* Consultants in Feline Internal Medicine, ed 2. *Philadelphia, WB Saunders, 1994, p 571; with permission)*

cal site (2 cats), and a new tumor developed at a distant cutaneous site (3 cats) or visceral site (3 cats) within a few months.[38] There was no recurrence after surgery in 5 cats with solitary histiocytic lesions.[38]

Four cats with 2 to 4 recurrent histiocytic MCTs had a second surgery and were then free of recurrence.[38] Tumor recurrence within 1 year was successfully treated with a second surgery in another cat.[47] Despite having metastasis to the regional lymph node, a third cat that had both a skin lesion and lymph node removed was free of disease 6 months later.[49]

In another series of 34 cats with follow-up after surgery, 14 cats (41%) had no recurrence over a period of 7 months to 6.5 years. Eight cats had recurrence locally or at a distant cutaneous site 3 weeks to 2 years (average, 7 months) after surgery, and two had metastases to the regional lymph node.[2] In 10 cats, tumors progressed to involve other organs or systems: One tumor affected the jejunum, one lesion involved the cranial mediastinum, two cats had mastocythemia, and six tumors involved the spleen.[2]

Radiation therapy appears to be effective for control of MCTs that cannot be completely excised; however, the efficacy of this modality remains anecdotal, and there are no published reports (Figures 50-15 and 50-16).

Corticosteroids do not seem to have a role in the adjunctive treatment of cutaneous MCTs in cats. Treatment with prednisone and cimetidine was not successful in reducing the number or size of cutaneous lesions in cats with systemic mast cell disease.[43] Triamcinolone ointment caused complete regression of a 2 mm MCT and a partial response in a 5 mm nodule, thereby enabling removal from the lateral canthus.[48] In contrast, triamcinolone applied topically or given parenterally had no effect on histiocytic MCTs in a litter of Siamese kittens. These lesions later regressed spontaneously.[41]

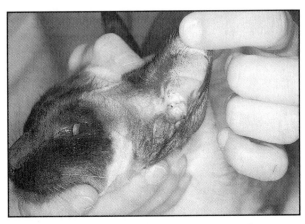

Figure 50-15: The same cat as shown in Figure 50-13; prednisone was administered for 1 year but failed to induce remission, so radiation therapy was instituted.

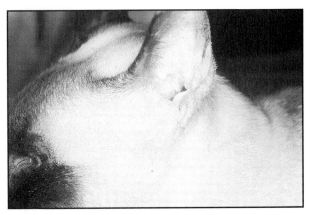

Figure 50-16: Four months after radiation therapy, regression of the MCT in the cat in Figure 50-15 is complete.

There are no published reports about the efficacy of chemotherapy as an adjunctive treatment for MCTs, but both vinblastine and CCNU are active agents against canine MCTs and may be logical agents to use.

MDB = minimum database; includes CBC, biochemical profile, urinalysis, FeLV/FIV serology, T_4 testing, and thoracic radiographs (three views).

Photodynamic therapy using Photofrin-I (a hematoporphyrin derivative that is no longer available) caused regression of a 3 mm MCT. However, the tumor recurred 5 months later and again 2 months after a second treatment.[56]

The pruritus associated with mast cell degranulation has been assumed to be due to histamine release, although the efficacy of antihistamines in relieving pruritus is inconsistent.[2,43] More recently, serotonin has been found to be the principle active amine following mast cell degranulation, and cyproheptadine causes specific blockade of the serotonin receptor in cats.[53] Cyproheptadine, rather than diphenhydramine, may be a good choice for pruritic cats with cutaneous MCTs.

SQUAMOUS CELL CARCINOMA

CLINICAL BRIEFING

Common Presentation	Sunlight (actinically) induced tumor in older cats. Cats that are lightly pigmented are predisposed. Black cats and Siamese have low risk. FIV-associated, possibly due to similar risk factors. Ulcerated lesions on head; early lesions look like a scratch.
Staging and Diagnosis	MDB. Metastasis is uncommon, but evaluate regional lymph nodes. Size of tumor predictive of outcome.
Treatment Initial	In situ lesions may regress with retinoid treatment (unpublished). Small (T_1 and T_2) lesions cured by most treatment options, including surgery, photodynamic therapy, cryotherapy, radiation therapy, and intralesional chemotherapy. Larger (T_3 and T_4) invasive tumors less responsive; surgery or radiation therapy gives best responses, possibly combine with intralesional chemotherapy.
Adjunctive	Chemotherapy rarely necessary due to low metastatic rate. Carboplatin, mitoxantrone, and doxorubicin may have efficacy (unproven).
Preventative	Keep cats with little skin pigment out of direct sunlight during midday. Use strategies to block ultraviolet light.
Adjunctive	Analgesia, appetite stimulants, antibiotics as needed, particularly in FIV-positive cats.

Incidence, Signalment, and Etiology

SCC is the most common skin tumor in cats from Australia and New Zealand, accounting for approximately 50% of all skin tumors.[6] This is probably due to the higher sunlight exposure in the southern hemisphere, as SCC is thought to be an actinically induced tumor. The incidence of SCC in the United States varies depending on the distance from the equator but, as in the United Kingdom, Germany, and Switzerland, does not exceed 20%.[1–3,5,18,19] In a Malaysian survey of neoplasms, the only tumor diagnosed in cats was SCC of the upper lip.[57]

DSHs predominated in a series of cats with cutaneous SCC. Breed information was available for 262 cats; there were 226 DSHs, 27 DLHs, 2 Persians, 2 Siamese, 3 Chinchillas, and 1 Manx.[1,22,24,58–60] Purebred cats were found to be significantly less likely to develop cutaneous SCC.[22] In particular, Siamese cats appear to be protected from developing this disease by virtue of their coat color.[61] Coat color, and specifically a lack of skin pigment and poor hair covering in areas of high sunlight exposure, have been recognized as risk factors for development of SCC in cats. This is particularly evident in the Mediterranean[62] and the Antipodes.[6] In two recent studies, cats that were white or partly white accounted for 73% (66 of 90)[63] and 95% (58 of 61)[60] of cats with SCC. In a large study of 106 cats, coat color in affected cats was compared with the general population, and white cats were found to have five times greater risk for developing SCC (Table 50-3).[22] In an earlier study, white cats were more than 13 times more likely to develop cutaneous (but not oral) SCC than all other cats combined,[61] and Siamese were at a lower risk. Sunlight may induce mutations in the tumor suppressor gene *p53*, allowing development of SCC.[64]

TABLE 50-3
Risk of Developing SCC Associated with Coat Color[22]

Coat Color	Odds Ratio	95% Confidence Interval
Orange (Ginger)	0.10	0.00–0.74
Black	0.11	0.00–0.80
Tabby	0.33	0.09–1.04
Gray	0.39	0.07–1.15
Orange and white	0.74	0.12–2.42
Tortoiseshell	1.0	Reference group
Black and white	1.18	0.47–3.06
Tabby and white	1.34	0.48–3.73
Silver	1.48	0.22–7.34
Grey and white	1.78	0.59–5.32
White	5.11	2.17–12.54

Older cats (median age, 12 years) are usually affected.[1,60] Cats as young as 1 year of age have been reported,[1,3,65] although this is uncommon. Actinic carcinogenesis would be expected to take a long time, and it is therefore not surprising that cats affected with SCC are an aging population. Most affected cats are neutered, and there does not appear to be a gender predilection.

FeLV has not been associated with SCC; FIV does appear to be associated with SCC, but it is uncertain if there is a direct causal relationship or whether the risk factors for FIV and actinic exposure (i.e., outside cats) are similar.[66] Ninety-five percent of cats in one study spent at least part of their time outdoors, presumably increasing their risk for both diseases.[60] FIV-positive cats account for 7% to 20% of cats with SCC in recent studies.[59,60,63]

Clinical Presentation and History

Cutaneous SCC is much more likely to affect the face than any other part of the body. In published studies totaling more than 600 cats, the overall incidence of cutaneous SCC varies but the proportion involving the face is between 80% and 90%[1,3,6,22] regardless of the geographic location. The nasal plane is the most common site of involvement, with the pinnae and eyelids the next most frequent sites. Cats with eyelid lesions usually have other lesions on the nasal plane or pinnae.[6,22] SCC is therefore a tumor that affects multiple facial cutaneous sites, which is again consistent with actinic induction. In one study, approximately 10% of cutaneous SCC affected the limbs[3]; the back, tail, and perineum are rarely affected.[1,3] SCC at these sites may not be associated with sunlight exposure. In one study, a Siamese cat had SCC of the genital skin and a Persian had a digital SCC. Multiple cutaneous SCC of other body sites has been termed *multicentric SCC in situ*, or *Bowen's disease*, and is described below.

Cutaneous SCC may often start as epidermal dysplasia following chronic sunlight exposure (Figure 50-17).[67] Dysplasia progresses to SCC in situ and will eventually form an invasive cutaneous tumor. When in the form of dysplasia or in situ carcinoma, the lesion may be easily overlooked by an owner. It often has the appearance of tenacious waxy debris that, when removed, reveals a reddened, sometimes slightly ulcerated area that does not bleed. A common reason for presentation is a "cat scratch" that will not heal. Crusting and ulceration may be severe in advanced cases, and destruction of normal tissue by the invading tumor is often

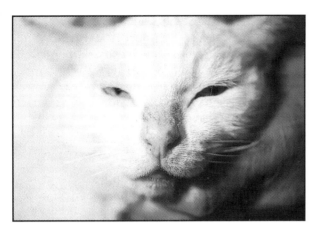

Figure 50-17: Epidermal dysplasia due to sunlight exposure on the nose of an 11-year-old white cat. (Courtesy of A. Evans)

marked (Figure 50-18).

Lesions may be present for months or even years prior to an owner seeking veterinary advice.[18] In one study, cutaneous SCC was present for an average of 18 months before treatment commenced.[22]

Staging and Diagnosis

Metastasis from cutaneous SCC of the face is uncommon and may occur only late in the course of disease. At the initiation of treatment, no cat (of 647 cats) has been reported to have metastases.[1,6,18,22,24,58–60,63,65,67–73]

In one study, metastasis to the parotid and pharyngeal lymph node occurred after treatment in only one cat with an SCC of the pinna.[18] In another study, 15 of 90 cats with SCC of the nasal plane were necropsied; 6 of these had metastases to the mandibular lymph node, and 1 cat had pulmonary metastases.[63] One other cat of 15 treated developed pulmonary metastases.[71] In another early study, cats that had poorly differentiated SCC of the eyelid, nares, pinna, lip, or shoulder had a poor outcome, with metastases (to

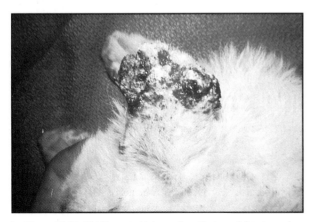

Figure 50-18: Thickly crusted lesion and cartilaginous deformity on the pinna of a 6-year-old white cat with SCC. (Courtesy of G.H. Theilen)

unspecified sites) occurring in 6 of 8 cats; only 1 cat developed metastases from a well-differentiated SCC 48 weeks after surgery.[58] This high rate of metastasis has not been recorded in other studies.

There does seem to be predictive prognostic value in staging the tumor size and depth of erosion[74] (Table 50-4 and Figure 50-19).

KEY POINT

The size of a cutaneous SCC is highly predictive for the likely success of any treatment modality.

This grading system also includes categories for lymph nodes (N) and distant metastasis (M) but, as stated above, no cat with cutaneous SCC has been reported to have metastases at the time of diagnosis. This should not discourage the clinician from carefully palpating regional lymph nodes. Fine-needle aspiration or biopsy is warranted if these nodes are enlarged. While thoracic radiographs are unlikely to disclose metastases, cats with SCC are generally an older population and thus radiographs should be included with blood work and a total serum T_4 level as part of the MDB. Cats should also be tested for FIV and FeLV. Although FIV-positive cats do not seem to be less likely to respond to treatment, they may experience a higher rate of treatment complications as outlined below.[63]

Treatment

Many different treatment modalities have been used to treat cutaneous SCC in cats, and depending on the stage of the tumor, most seem to be very effective. Selection of the appropriate treatment for any individual cat will depend not only on the stage of the tumor but also on the owner's willingness to accept side effects and cosmetic changes as well as the availability of such modalities as radiation or

TABLE 50-4
Tumor Staging System for Cutaneous SCC in Cats[74]

Stage	Size	Depth
T_{is}		Pre-invasive carcinoma (in situ)
T_1	<2 cm	Superficial
T_2	2–5 cm	Minimal invasion regardless of size
T_3	>5 cm	Invasion of subcutis regardless of size
T_4	Any size	Invasion of fascia, cartilage, muscle, or bone

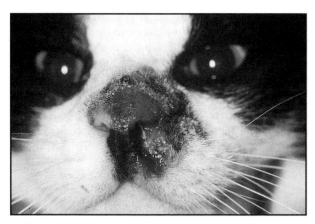

Figure 50-19: *A large, deeply invasive SCC in an FIV-positive cat. This tumor was staged as T_3 and response to radiation therapy was poor. Cats that are FIV positive are more likely to have complications from treatment with radiation.*

photodynamic therapy.

Precancerous actinic keratosis, or tumors that have not invaded beyond the basement membrane (T_{is}), may respond to retinoic acid derivatives/carotenoids. However, some of the available data are contradictory. Cats with solar dermatitis of the pinna were treated with a mixture of β-carotene and canthaxanthin (carotenoids), which are thought to reduce oxidative damage caused by solar radiation. Six cats that had erythema, increased pinna hyperesthesia, and hair loss but no ulceration had a good response within 2 to 4 weeks. Only two of four cats with cartilage deformity (curling) had a response, while cats with more advanced lesions did not respond to treatment.[75]

In contrast, seven cats with actinic epidermal dysplasia were treated with 13-*cis*-retinoic acid (Accutane®) for a median of 2 months. None showed improvement, and the lesion progressed to become SCC in three cats.[67] In the same study, an additional seven cats with SCC were treated with Accutane® but only one responded. This cat's lesion was reclassified as dysplasia after 162 days of treatment.

Etretinate (a newer retinoid that is no longer available) has been used at a dose of 10 mg/cat/day and anecdotally appears to result in regression of actinic keratoses and in situ lesions.[a] Doses of 20 mg/cat/day in two cats were associated with nonpruritic erythema and hair loss on the head, feet, ventral abdomen, and perineum that resolved on discontinuation of the drug.[a] Elevations in liver enzymes have been reported to occur in dogs receiving Etretinate. Etretinate is no longer marketed, but an analogous compound has been synthesized (acitretin; Soriatane®) and may be less toxic when used at the same dose as Etretinate. There are no reports of efficacy or toxicity for either agent in cats. If either is found to be useful, long-term treatment will probably be required in most cats.

Photodynamic therapy is an appropriate treatment for superficial lesions less than 1 cm in depth. In photodynam-

ic therapy, a drug that is capable of being activated by a certain wavelength of light is given systemically. After a variable period of time (dependent on the drug), drug levels in the tumor are higher than in surrounding normal tissue. The tumor and a normal tissue margin are irradiated with a laser of a specific wavelength to activate the drug, and the tumor tissue is damaged by oxygen free radical formation that is absent or minimal in surrounding normal tissue. The tumor size limitation is due to poor light penetration into tissue and blood below a depth of 1 cm.

The majority of photosensitizers are porphyrin derivatives. Eighteen cats with 19 SCC lesions were treated with a phthalocyanine dye.[68] The tumor in 9 of these cats was staged as T_{is} to T_2, and 7 of these 9 cats had a complete response after one treatment. In contrast, only 3 of 8 cats with a T_3 or T_4 lesion achieved a complete response. The 10 cats that responded had no evidence of recurrence 3 to 18 months after treatment. Complete response was achieved in one cat after a second treatment and in a second cat after a third treatment.

Side effects were mostly mild, with inappetence and sneezing due to scab formation at the treatment site predominating. Four cats that were allowed outside in daylight experienced generalized cutaneous sensitization. One owner euthanized the cat due to stertor caused by the nasal scab. More importantly, 1 of 18 cats[68] and 2 other cats in a separate report[76] developed acute hepatic necrosis and disseminated intravascular coagulation, presumably due to the photosensitizing drug. Only 1 of these 3 cats survived.

A novel photosensitizer (ethyl-Nile blue sulfur [EtNBS]) that rapidly clears after administration and therefore decreases the risk of generalized photosensitization was used to treat six cats.[59] Four cats with small lesions were free of tumor 9 to 38 months after treatment, while two cats with T_3 lesions did not respond. Toxicity was minimal in all cats. If photodynamic therapy is available, it may be a good treatment option for cats with T_{is}, T_1, or T_2 SCC lesions.

Topical 5-aminolevulinic acid cream was used to sensitize nasal planum (T_1) SCC in three cats prior to photodynamic therapy.[77] Complete resolution was obtained for 4 to 5 months.

Cryosurgery is another therapeutic option for cats with small superficial SCC. Liquid nitrogen was used to treat 163 SCC lesions on 102 cats. Tumor stage was not reported. A cryoprobe was used to monitor the temperature of the tissue, which was frozen to −25°C to −40°C twice with an intervening thaw cycle.[22] In this study, tumors of the pinnae and an area 3 to 5 mm below the lesion were cryosurgically amputated. Although this is a narrow margin and margins of at least 2 cm should routinely be obtained, the results of this study were impressive. Complete resolution was seen in all (50) pinna lesions and all (23) eyelid lesions treated in this manner. Nasal lesions did not have as good a response rate despite being frozen to –40°C. The authors conjectured that thawing might have been too rapid on the well-vascularized nares to sufficiently kill tumor cells. Complete resolution was seen in 73 of 90 (81%) nasal planum lesions; of these, 65 cats received only one treatment, 8 received two treatments (second treatment was administered a median of 18 months after the first), and two cats received a third treatment a median of 9 months after the second treatment. The median remission time for all 102 cats was 26.7 months (range, 1.2 to 122.9 months). Eighty-four percent of cats were tumor free 1 year after cryosurgery, and 58% were tumor free 7 years after treatment.[22] The 17 cats that failed to respond or in which the tumor recurred had a median remission of 6.6 months; 2 of these cats received multiple cryosurgical treatments. In another study, 11 cats with cutaneous SCC were treated with cryosurgery.[60] In this study, 8 of 11 tumors recurred a median of 6 months after treatment. Overall, these cats had a median remission duration of 8.5 months. Cryosurgery is probably most effective for T_{is}, T_1, and T_2 lesions.

Surgery was the only method of treatment for 13 cats with SCC in one study.[58] Tumors were located on the eyelid margins (4 cats), nasal plane (3 cats), ear tip (3 cats), lip (1 cat), flank (1 cat), and shoulder (1 cat). Surgical margins were histologically complete in all cats except for 1 with an eyelid tumor and 2 with tumors of the nasal plane. Follow-up times were not long, but survival times for the 3 cats with incomplete surgical margins ranged from 3 to 17 weeks. One cat with a pinna lesion was still alive 8 weeks after surgery and a second 66 weeks after surgery. Local recurrence and metastasis were the reason for death in the 8 remaining cats; median survival was 16 weeks.[58]

"Nosectomy" (removal of the nasal planum) was performed in eight cats with SCC of the nasal planum (Figure 50-20).[24] Three cats with deeply invasive (T_3 to T_4) lesions had tumor recurrence within 5 months of surgery, while five cats with less aggressive tumors were tumor free a median of 16 months after surgery. The authors stated that while most owners were initially apprehensive about the potential cosmetic result, all were satisfied with their cats' appearances.

In another study, surgical excision of the nasal plane (21 cats) or the pinna (18 cats) resulted in complete surgical margins in all but 7 cats. The tumor recurred in 2 of these cats in which surgical margins were incomplete.[60] The median disease-free interval for all 39 cats was 20 months, which was longer than for cryosurgery (8.5 months) in the same study.

Surgery of SCC lesions appears very successful for tumors in stages T_1 and T_2. Aggressive surgery is required to cure more advanced lesions (Figure 50-21).

Laser surgery was used to treat an SCC of the nasal plane in one cat.[78] The tumor recurred at intervals of 7 months, 4 months, and 3 months, but there was no recurrence 16 months after the fourth treatment. It is difficult to see any advantage of this approach over conventional surgery.

Radiation therapy is a generic term that covers a wide range of treatment strategies. The type of radiation used determines both the depth of radiation penetration and the total dose that can be safely delivered.

Radiation therapy with a strontium-90 handheld source delivers a very high dose of radiation that penetrates only 3 to 5 mm below the skin surface (Figure 50-22). Strontium-90 was used to treat small (T_{is} and T_1) lesions of the nasal plane in 25 cats.[72] One year after treatment, 22 cats (89%) were tumor free; the median progression-free survival time was 34 months.

Orthovoltage radiation delivers a moderate to high dose of radiation to a depth of 2 to 4 cm below the skin surface and has been used to treat more advanced tumors. Nine cats treated with orthovoltage had recurrence of tumor between 4 and 33 months after treatment (median, 7 months); only one cat had no evidence of tumor 72 months after treat-

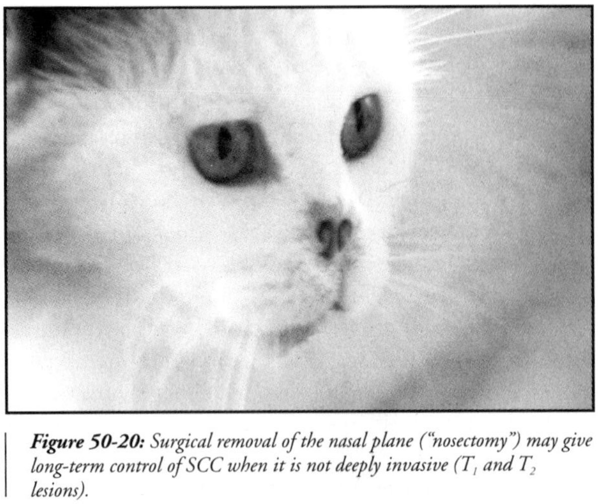

Figure 50-20: *Surgical removal of the nasal plane ("nosectomy") may give long-term control of SCC when it is not deeply invasive (T_1 and T_2 lesions).*

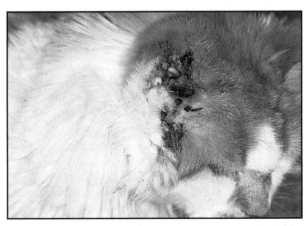

Figure 50-21: *It is important to obtain wide surgical margins with SCC of the pinna. This tumor recurred after multiple localized surgeries until it was inoperable at the ear base. Early pinnectomy may have been curative.*

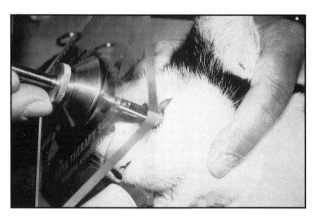

Figure 50-22: *A Strontium-90 radiation handheld probe can be used to treat shallow (T_1) lesions with a single application, as in this cat with an eyelid SCC. (Courtesy of A. Théon)*

TABLE 50-5
Progression-Free Survival (PFS) in 90 Cats with SCC Treated with Orthovoltage Radiation[63]

Stage	Average PFS (months)	1 Year Rate (%)	5 Year Rate (%)
T_1	53.2	84.9	56.0
T_2	27.8	66.8	10.6
T_3	18.8	45.5	—
T_4	15.3	50.5	—

ment.[71] In another study, 36 of 70 SCCs (in 62 cats) were advanced (T_3 or T_4), but this only marginally affected their response to orthovoltage treatment.[65] These cats were treated with a "coarse" fractionation protocol using 20 Gy given monthly until remission was achieved. Despite the fact that half the cats received more than 40 Gy (up to 230 Gy), no radiation toxicities were reported. While 32 of 33 cats with T_1 or T_2 tumors achieved complete clinical remission, 30 of 36 cats with more advanced lesions attained remission. Recurrence within 2 years of treatment was seen with 18 of 32 (56%) less advanced lesions and 14 of 30 (47%) more advanced tumors; 3 years after treatment, 9 of 32 (27%) and 7 of 30 (23%) cats, respectively, were free of tumor.

In the same study,[65] a further 26 cats received 30 Gy in three weekly fractions and 24 cats achieved a complete remission. In this group of cats, recurrence of tumor within 1 year was seen in 2 of 17 (12%) with T_1 or T_2 lesions and in 7 of 11 cats (64%) with advanced lesions.[65]

KEY POINT

Cats with SCC that are FIV positive are more likely than other cats to develop cutaneous toxicities following radiation therapy.

In a third study, 90 cats with SCC of the nasal plane received orthovoltage radiation (40 Gy in 10 fractions). Those cats with T_1 lesions had a mean progression-free survival of 53.2 months, which was significantly better than cats with T_3 or T_4 lesions (18.8 and 15.3 months, respectively; Table 50-5). Histologic grading did not predict recurrence or survival. However, as the percentage of proliferating cells within the tumor rose, the risk of recurrence increased.[63] Cats that were FIV positive were more likely to experience cutaneous side effects following radiation treatment. Ulceration was pronounced, particularly in cats with

tumors of the nasal plane.[63]

Nearly one third of the cats had more than one lesion, but this did not influence response or outcome for these cats.[63] Fifteen cats that relapsed 4 to 36 months after the first treatment were treated a second time. The median duration of their second remission was 25 months.

Megavoltage radiation using a cobalt-60 source was used to treat a total of 15 cats in two studies.[60,71] Megavoltage radiation allows deeper dose penetration, but this is not a significant advantage over orthovoltage radiation for treatment of a superficial skin tumor like SCC. Tumor recurred in 1 cat 3 months after treatment and in a second cat 31 months after treatment in one study.[71] Megavoltage radiation therapy was used only for invasive, advanced (T_3 and T_4) SCC in 11 cats.[60] The median disease-free interval was 12 months. High-energy radiation therapy using 72 MeV protons was considered somewhat effective in the treatment of 10 cats with SCC. Nine cats had a complete response to 40 Gy, but 4 cats had recurrence between 3.5 and 24 months after treatment.[73]

For high-stage (T_3 and T_4) SCC, radiation therapy administered prior to surgical excision may reduce the size of the tumor and improve response to treatment. Tumor control appeared to be good in two cats treated this way.[79]

The incidence of metastases from cutaneous SCC is low, and chemotherapy is rarely used. Two of the most effective drugs for the treatment of SCC in humans and dogs, cisplatin and 5-fluorouracil, cannot be used safely in cats; these drugs cause fatal acute pulmonary edema[80] and fatal neurotoxicity,[81-83] respectively. Despite this, a novel approach that mixed either cisplatin or 5-fluorouracil with bovine collagen matrix for injection into the tumor has been used safely to treat localized SCC in cats.[84] The collagen reduces absorption of the chemotherapy drug, apparently reducing systemic drug levels to a safe range. In this study, 118 lesions were treated at 1 to 2 week intervals, alternating to the other drug if only a partial (rather than complete) remission was seen. Although these cats were not "staged," tumor size influenced outcome. Complete response was seen in 75 cats (64%) in which the tumor volume averaged 0.06 cm³. The 23 cats

(19%) that had a partial response had an average tumor volume of 0.61 cm³. Ten cats did not respond. The duration of response was not reported.[84]

Carboplatin in purified sesame oil, administered into the tumor four times at 10 to 14 day intervals, caused a complete response in 10 of 15 cats.[70] The sesame oil acts similarly to bovine collagen matrix to reduce absorption of the chemotherapy drug, and hence plasma concentration over time is reduced when compared with an aqueous solution injected locally. The oil also reduced leakage from the injection site. Seven cats had tumor recurrence, and 4 of these recurrences were at the margin of the treated area, emphasizing the importance of infiltrating the drug widely around the tumor margins. Two cats were treated a second time and were still free of tumor, one at 15 months and the other at 24 months later. When adjusted for tumor stages, progression-free survival times were similar to those obtained with orthovoltage radiation therapy.[63]

It is possible that the combination of intratumor chemotherapy and radiation therapy may improve response rate and duration in cats with more advanced SCC.

Systemic chemotherapy for cats with SCC has been rarely reported. Mitoxantrone has not been reported to be of benefit.[60] Bleomycin was used to treat four cats with cutaneous SCC; one cat (the only one that received IV bleomycin) showed tumor response for 5 months.[69] No other reports of the efficacy of bleomycin are available.

Analgesia should be administered as needed for discomfort associated with treatment of SCC. Appetite stimulants, antiemetics, and antibiotics may also be indicated, depending on the type of therapy employed and the FIV status of the cat.

Prevention

Since SCC is usually an actinically induced cutaneous tumor, the owners of high-risk cats (i.e., white or partially white cats, particularly those with poor pigmentation of the nasal plane, eyelids, or pinnae) can take steps to reduce the risk of tumorigenesis.[85]

For indoor/outdoor cats, outside activity should be restricted to early morning and late afternoon, thereby avoiding the sun at its zenith. Cats that like to "sunbathe" in a favorite window can be protected from ultraviolet exposure by placing ultraviolet blocking film on the window.

Owners should be educated to recognize early precancerous changes in their cats' skin, and veterinarians should be prepared to undertake treatment before a lesion progresses to an advanced stage. These precautions are even more important in equatorial or tropical areas. Tattooing of lightly pigmented skin has not been shown to reduce the incidence of SCC.

MULTICENTRIC SCC IN SITU (BOWEN'S DISEASE)

CLINICAL BRIEFING

Common Presentation	Multiple in situ lesions can appear on any part of the body in older cats. Lack of pigment is not a predisposing cause. Usually small crusting nonpruritic plaques; multiple lesions may be seen.
Staging and Diagnosis	MDB. Metastases not reported with in situ lesions; if tumors are invasive, stage as for SCC. New lesions may arise.
Treatment Initial Adjunctive Supportive	Surgery or radiation therapy for small number of lesions. Retinoids have not been evaluated but may reduce risk of new lesions. Antiinflammatories and analgesics as needed.

Incidence, Signalment, and Etiology

This manifestation of SCC has been described only in the last 10 years, possibly because people are now looking for it or possibly because it is truly becoming more common. Only 32 cats (25 DSHs and 7 DLHs) have been reported to be affected.[86–88] Sunlight does not seem to be a factor in tumor development. Information regarding coat color was available for all cats, and only 9 had some white in addition to other colors such as black, gray, or brown. One cat was white.[88] In one study, 6 of 12 affected cats were solely indoor cats and 5 were mainly indoor cats.[86] It appears to be a disease of older cats; the median age in two studies was 11.5 to 12.5 years, and reported cats ranged in age from 5 to 20 years.[86–88] The majority of affected cats have been castrated males (13) or spayed females (18), with only 1 intact male reported.

An FeLV-related giant-cell dermatosis seen in cats is characterized by transformation of keratinocytes and was postulated to be a preneoplastic process.[89] However, this seems unlikely to be related to SCC in situ as none of 14 cats with

SCC in situ were FeLV positive and only 1 of 12 was FIV positive in one study.[88]

Papillomavirus has been identified in association with feline cutaneous SCC in situ, but a causal relationship has yet to be established.[90]

Clinical Presentation and History

Lesions are usually small (5 mm to 3 cm in diameter) and can be plaque-like or papillated, partially alopecic, and crusted. They are usually not pruritic, although they bleed easily if ulcerated. Some lesions are darkly pigmented, and such pigmentation often precedes ulceration.[88] One lesion had a cutaneous horn arising from the tumor.[91]

Lesions are often present for a long time before owners seek veterinary advice. For the 14 cats for which this information was available, 8 had had lesions for 1 to 2.5 years, 3 for more than 6 months, and the remaining 3 for 1 to 5 months.[86,87] Cats were often presented for a solitary lesion and developed further lesions within 2 to 12 months. Lesions were widely distributed, affecting the head, neck, thighs, shoulders, ventral abdomen, and paws.[86–88] Four cats had oral mucosal SCC lesions.[88]

Staging and Diagnosis

Despite the long clinical history in these cats, metastases have not been described, although multiple new cutaneous lesions may continue to appear and may coalesce. In two studies, three cats had solitary lesions, three had 2 lesions, one had 3 lesions, five had 4 lesions, three had 5 lesions, and two had 6 lesions. In another study, the number of lesions ranged from 2 to more than 30.[88] Most cats are FeLV negative, although one cat was concurrently infected with FeLV and had lymphoma and demodecosis.[87]

The histologic criteria for diagnosis include noninvasion of the basement membrane even in large lesions, cellular atypia, mitotic figures that are not in the basal layer, and disorder in maturation of the epidermis.[86] A biopsy should be performed in addition to an MDB in cats with crusting lesions that do not heal. If a diagnosis of Bowen's disease is obtained, the cat should be carefully examined for new lesions at 2 to 3 month intervals. Although metastases have not been reported, careful palpation of lymph nodes and

staging as for SCC should be performed. Lesions should be excised, rather than observed, as invasive SCC may develop from these low-grade lesions.[86]

> *MDB = minimum database; includes CBC, biochemical profile, urinalysis, FeLV/FIV serology, T_4 testing, and thoracic radiographs (three views).*

Treatment

No change in lesions was noted over a 2 month treatment period in three cats receiving topical isotretinoin.[86,87] Treatment with corticosteroids, progesterone, and alkylating agents was unsuccessful in controlling lesions in 5 cats.[88] Surgical excision is probably the treatment of choice for solitary lesions. Surgical excision was performed in 12 cats, and 11 had no evidence of tumor recurrence 4 to 20 months after surgery[86]; lesions recurred in the twelfth cat after 2 months. Although there was no local recurrence, 4 cats developed one to six lesions at new sites; these were also removed surgically. Surgical excision provided local tumor control in 4 cats in another study, but new lesions arose in other locations.[88] A cat that developed multiple SCCs in situ and was not treated died of an unrelated problem 8 months after initial diagnosis.[91]

In one cat, lesions on the face and trunk were treated with strontium-90 to a total dose of 150 Gy. The lesion on the trunk resolved, but the facial lesions did not change and the cat was euthanized. In another study, strontium-90 radiation therapy controlled eight treated lesions, although new lesions often occurred.[88]

Surgical excisions should be performed in a timely manner as lesions may progress to become more aggressive. Radiation therapy may be effective for local control of nonresectable lesions. Newer retinoids such as Soriatane® and chemotherapeutics as described for cutaneous SCC have not been evaluated in cats with multicentric SCC in situ. Antiinflammatory drugs and analgesia should be employed as necessary to minimize any discomfort associated with these skin lesions or their treatment.

SARCOMAS OF VESSELS

CUTANEOUS HEMANGIOSARCOMA AND HEMANGIOMA

C L I N I C A L   B R I E F I N G

Common Presentation	Affects older cats; may be more common in males. Cats with poorly pigmented skin may be predisposed. Possibly actinically induced. Sarcomas are often ulcerated or cause subcutaneous bleeding.

(continued)

Staging and Diagnosis	MDB and abdominal ultrasonography; evaluate regional lymph nodes. Lungs are the most common site for metastasis, but widespread metastasis is often seen.
Treatment	
Initial	Surgical excision needs to be wide.
Adjunctive	Incomplete excision may require radiation therapy (no published efficacy). Metastatic rate is high, so chemotherapy is warranted; doxorubicin, ifosfamide, and carboplatin are potentially effective drugs.
Supportive	Analgesia as needed; antiinflammatories may be palliative.

Incidence, Signalment, and Etiology

In two series of cats with hemangiosarcoma (*n* = 87), the skin was the most common site of occurrence (38 cats).[2,92] Hemangiosarcoma and hemangioma occurred in similar numbers in three surveys of skin tumors in cats.[5,18,93] Both hemangioma and hemangiosarcoma were more common in male cats in one survey; median age was 10 years in 7 cats with hemangioma (range, 7 to 15 years) and 12.5 years for 9 cats with hemangiosarcoma (range, 9 to 17 years). However, only a slight increase in gender incidence was noted in another study, in which 57.3% of 94 cats were male.[3]

The majority of reported cats have been DSHs,[1,2,92,93] but there has been no breed predisposition.[3] Interestingly, five of six cats for which coat color was known were white in one survey.[93] This, combined with an apparent predilection for the head and the histologic presence of associated elas-tosis, led the authors to propose that this tumor may be actinically induced in a manner similar to SCC. In contrast, a survey of skin tumors in cats from Australia found that fewer than 1% were hemangiomas, and hemangiosarcomas were not mentioned.[6] This same survey reported a very high incidence of cutaneous SCC.

Clinical Presentation and History

Ulceration and bleeding were features of hemangiosarcoma in the majority of cats in two surveys (Figures 50-23 and 50-24)[2,94] but were less common in others.[92,93] Subcutaneous bleeding (Figure 50-25) led to a rapid increase in tumor size in some cats[2] and may be the first sign noted by an owner. Ulceration may occur due to tumor invasion of the epidermis, self-trauma, or a combination of the two. Cutaneous hemangiosarcoma may occasionally invade underlying bone.[92]

Of 122 cats for which tumor location was stated, 32 tumors were found on the head. Common sites were the pinna (6), nares (2), lip (2), canthus, and face.[3,18,92-94] One of the cats had bilateral pinnae hemangiosarcoma.[93] Other locations included the limbs (38), abdomen (28), inguinal and perineal skin (10), back (5), neck (4), thorax (3), and tail (1). One cat had multiple tumors.[3] Similarly, in anoth-

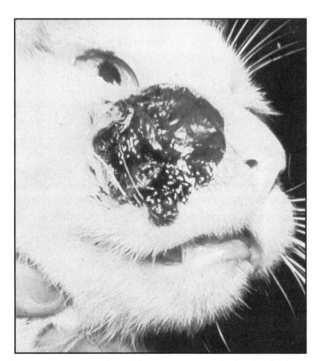

Figure 50-23: An ulcerated hemangiosarcoma on the face of a white cat. This tumor may be actinically induced, as is SCC. (Courtesy of B.R. Madewell)

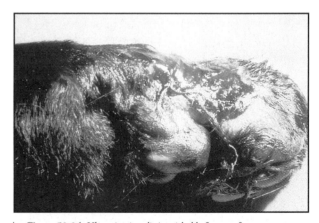

Figure 50-24: Ulceration is a distinguishable feature of hemangiosarcoma, as seen in this foot lesion in a 5-year-old cat. The metastatic rate from these tumors appears to be higher than for other soft tissue sarcomas. (Courtesy of A. Evans)

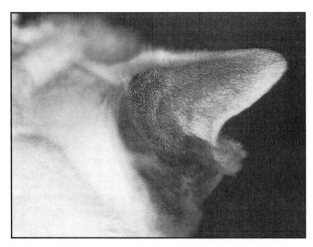

Figure 50-25: *Subcutaneous bruising and hemorrhage are obvious features of this hemangiosarcoma in a 6-year-old white cat.*

er survey, common locations were the head and axillary and inguinal regions, while tumors were less common on the flank and limbs.[2]

Hemangiomas were reported to occur in similar locations at similar incidences to hemangiosarcomas (Figure 50-26).[18,93]

Staging and Diagnosis

Although cutaneous hemangiosarcoma may be clinically suspected when a bleeding or bruising mass is observed, it may be difficult to distinguish among other more common soft tissue sarcomas histologically. Immunohistochemical staining for Factor VIII-related antigen appears to be helpful in determining the exact histogenesis of the tumor[93] and should be requested when the pathology report is equivocal. The true metastatic rate for cutaneous hemangiosarcoma has been difficult to determine, as local tumor regrowth occurs early and may precede development of macroscopic metastatic lesions; also, cats are often not necropsied. In

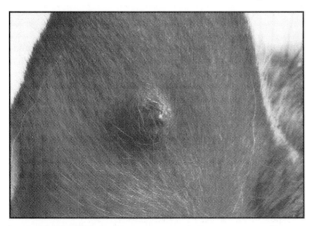

Figure 50-26: *The head is a common site for hemangioma as well as hemangiosarcoma. This benign lesion is not ulcerated and shows no bruising or bleeding. (Courtesy of A. Evans)*

two surveys, metastasis from cutaneous hemangiosarcoma was not observed.[92,93] In another study, metastasis to the lung was seen in 1 of 12 cats and multiple tumors involving the tail, mammary tissue, and gingiva occurred in another cat.[2] In a more recent study in which all cats were necropsied, metastases to lungs were seen in all 6 cats with cutaneous hemangiosarcoma. One of the 6 also had metastasis from a perineal tumor to the regional lymph node and spleen, and one had additional metastases to the kidney, eye, and heart.[94] In another survey, 2 of 5 cats had widespread distant metastases from a cutaneous hemangiosarcoma.[5] These studies imply a more aggressive behavior for hemangiosarcoma of the skin than has previously been recognized. Thoracic radiographs and abdominal ultrasonography should be performed in cats with cutaneous hemangiosarcoma in addition to a thorough physical examination including fine-needle aspiration of enlarged regional lymph nodes and collection of an MDB. Because tumors may be locally extensive, it is recommended that a CT scan or MRI be obtained prior to attempting surgical excision.

KEY POINT

Cutaneous hemangiosarcoma appears to have a higher metastatic potential than other soft tissue sarcomas.

Treatment

Surgery has been the primary treatment modality reported for cats with cutaneous hemangiosarcoma. In surveys documenting surgical treatment, recurrence was common but there was no information regarding completeness of excision. Recurrence was seen in 26 of 40 cats,[2,5,92–94] and metastasis was the cause of death in 8 of these cats.[5,94] Tumor recurrence was seen between 2 weeks and 12 months in all cats (average, 4 months) in two surveys.[2,92] Second surgeries were attempted in 4 cats. There was no evidence of recurrence in 2 of these cats,[92] while recurrences were detected 9 months later in 1 of the remaining cats and 12 months later in the second.[93] In one survey, median survival was 40 weeks, with 5 cats alive 18 to 112 weeks after surgery.[92]

Radiation therapy can reduce the local tumor recurrence rate for other soft tissue sarcomas, but the efficacy of this modality has not been reported for cutaneous hemangiosarcoma in cats (see Chapter 51).

Chemotherapy has been reported in only one cat. This cat received vincristine (0.4–0.5 mg/m² weekly) after resection of an inguinal mass[94] but developed pulmonary metastases and lived only 11 weeks. Chemotherapy is probably warranted due to the potential for metastasis. The chemotherapy agents doxorubicin, ifosfamide, and carboplatin have been shown to have efficacy against hemangiosarcoma in dogs, but the potential benefits of these drugs have not been explored in cats.

Surgical resection of cutaneous hemangioma should be curative.

Analgesia is indicated postoperatively in cats with cutaneous hemangiosarcoma and hemangioma. Antiinflammatories may be used palliatively.

CUTANEOUS LYMPHANGIOSARCOMA/LYMPHANGIOMA

CLINICAL BRIEFING

Common Presentation	Uncommon tumor; difficult to distinguish from hemangiosarcoma. Often occurs in subcutis of abdominal skin with fluid drainage.
Staging and Diagnosis	MDB, abdominal ultrasonography, and lymph node evaluation. Metastasis is common. Very locally invasive.
Treatment Initial	Surgery often not curative due to extensive subcutaneous invasion.
Adjunctive	Radiation therapy for incomplete excision possible but unproven. Chemotherapy as described for hemangiosarcoma probably valuable but untried.
Supportive	Analgesia and antiinflammatories may be palliative.

Incidence, Signalment, and Etiology

The distinction between the benign and malignant forms of this tumor may not be clinically relevant.

The skin is the most common reported site for lymphangiosarcoma in cats, but this tumor is rare. In a report of 7 cats with lymphangioma of the skin, 5 tumors were small and all 7 tumors occurred in the abdominal skin.[3] In another study, 4 of 12 lymphangiomas occurred in the skin.[95] In reports with clinical details, all 14 cats were DSHs[96-100] and the majority were male. The affected cats ranged in age from 6 to 15 years (median, 11 years).

Clinical Presentation and History

In reports with clinical details, the most commonly affected site was the subcutis of the caudal abdomen.[96-99] The lymphangiosarcoma appeared edematous and firm and showed evidence of self trauma and ulceration in 4 of 11 cats.[96-99] The overlying skin was moist and erythematous in these cats (Figure 50-27), and there was drainage of a clear fluid that had been intermittent for 8 months prior to presentation in one cat.[97]

One cat had lymphangiosarcoma in the subcutis of the neck,[96] and two other cats had a lymphangiosarcoma that started in the digit and extended to involve the thoracic wall.[99,100]

Staging and Diagnosis

Metastases have been noted soon after surgery to either the lungs[96] or spleen and liver.[96,97] Staging prior to treatment should include an MDB and abdominal ultrasonography. Local extension frequently makes this tumor inoperable,

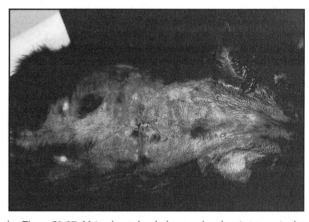

Figure 50-27: *Moist ulcerated and edematous lymphangiosarcoma in the abdominal skin of a cat, a common site for this rare tumor. (Courtesy of A. Evans)*

and it is recommended that a CT scan or MRI be obtained prior to attempting surgical excision.

Treatment

Extension of the tumor from the caudal abdominal skin to involve the muscles of the abdominal wall and thighs may render a lymphangiosarcoma inoperable.[98]

Survival times for 11 cats with caudal abdominal tumors that were treated surgically ranged from 3 days[96] to 9 months[97] (median, 2 months).[96,97,99] Local recurrence in conjunction with poor wound healing (2 cats), visceral metastases (2 cats), and invasion of the abdominal and thoracic walls leading to thoracic effusion (2 cats) were the causes of death in 6 cats; another cat with lymphangiosarcoma of the neck was euthanized because of local recurrence and poor wound healing 4 weeks after surgery.[96] Amputation of the affected limb did not prevent tumor recurrence in the thoracic wall in 2 cats with digital lymphangiosarcoma; tumor recurred 9 months after surgery in one cat and 10 months after surgery in the other. Neither cat had evidence of metastasis.[99,100]

Radiation therapy is a logical choice for adjunctive treatment of incompletely excised tumors, but there are no reports of this application. Chemotherapy, as discussed for hemangiosarcoma, may be valuable due to the high rate of metastasis but also remains unexplored. Analgesia and anti-inflammatories may be used postoperatively and as palliative therapy.

CUTANEOUS LYMPHOMA

CLINICAL BRIEFING

Common Presentation	Plaque-like pruritic and exfoliative lesions (often multiple) in older cats. May extend to involve deeper dermis. Affected cats usually FeLV negative.
Staging and Diagnosis	MDB, palpation and biopsy of regional lymph nodes even if not enlarged. Abdominal ultrasonography and bone marrow aspiration. Immunohistochemistry for T and B cell markers. Often associated with systemic lymphoma. Epidermotropic lymphoma is often of T cell derivation.
Treatment	
Initial	Surgery may be curative if lesion is solitary and there is no systemic spread.
Adjunctive	Best to assume disease is systemic and treat with multidrug chemotherapy (see Chapter 36). Radiation therapy for localized disease.
Supportive	Corticosteroids may be palliative, but do not use if chemotherapy contemplated. Radiation may be palliative for individual lesions. Analgesia for multiple or large lesions. Appetite stimulants as needed.

Incidence, Signalment, and Etiology

Lymphoma affecting the skin of cats can be divided into two distinct histopathologic types. The first is epidermotropic, while the other is not restricted to this site and may infiltrate more deeply. The epidermotropic variant is often termed *mycosis fungoides* and is usually assumed to be a T cell lymphoma. This form is less commonly seen in cats.

Cutaneous lymphoma affects older cats (average age in one study of 86 cats, 10.8 years[3]; median age in 29 individual cases reported, 12 years). However, cats younger than 1 year[3] and as old as 18 years[101] have been reported.

The majority of reported cats were DSHs, but three Siamese cats[101–103] and one Abyssinian[52] were also described. While 21 of the 29 individual cats reported have been male, a large survey found no increased incidence in male cats[3] despite a slightly higher incidence in castrated males.

Clinical Presentation and History

A plaque-like lesion is the most common clinical appearance in cats with cutaneous lymphoma.[3] These plaques are often erythematous[101,103–106] and have been described as "burnlike" in one cat where successive lesions appeared as others dried, sloughed, and scarred.[2] Occasionally these lesions are painful to the touch.[103] Less commonly, the lesion is nodular ranging from 1 mm[103] to 3 cm in diameter.[105–107]

Other cats will present with generalized erythroderma that resembles a fungal or bacterial infectious process but does not respond to topical or systemic antibiotics,[101,106,108,109] antihistamines,[106] or even prednisone.[106,110,111] The lesions may be hot to the touch.[106,108] Most lesions are pruritic, and pruritus can be severe, resulting in excoriation, induration, and ulceration of the affected skin.[101,105,106,108–110,112] There is often generalized scaliness or crusting due to epidermal exfoliation.[101,105,109,110,113] The variable clinical appearance of cutaneous lymphoma often complicates differentiation from other more common causes of dermatitis in cats (Figures 50-28 and 50-29).

While cutaneous lymphoma often starts as a solitary lesion (Figure 50-30), more lesions may appear as the disease progresses. In one study, 27% of lesions (22 of 82) were multiple in cats with cutaneous lymphoma.[3] One cat had 24 lesions.[114]

Cutaneous lymphoma does not have a predilection for any one site, with tumors of the head and neck, limbs, and trunk all occurring with approximately equal frequency. The tail is rarely affected[3] and may be the only area spared in cats

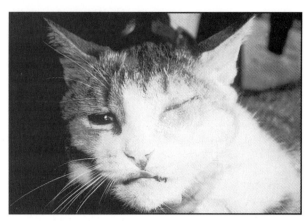

Figure 50-28: *Pruritic, crusting lesions on the face of a cat. Although this is cutaneous lymphoma, biopsy was required to differentiate it from other more common causes of dermatitis in cats. (Courtesy of A. Evans)*

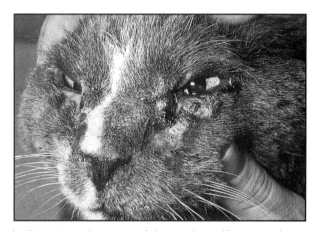

Figure 50-29: *Excoriation and ulceration due to self-trauma may be severe in cats with cutaneous lymphoma, as in this 12-year-old cat with multiple facial lesions. (Courtesy of A. Evans)*

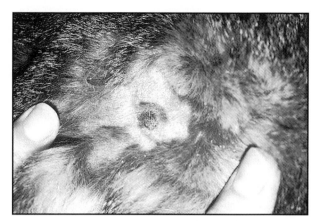

Figure 50-30: *A solitary cutaneous lymphoma lesion, such as in this cat, may precede multiple lesions and/or be associated with systemic lymphoma. Complete staging should be performed before treatment is attempted. (Courtesy of G. Nesbitt)*

three of five cats with cutaneous lymphoma were found on immunohistochemistry to have FeLV antigen associated with the tumor (one cat) or to have FeLV DNA amplified from tumor tissue by polymerase chain reaction (PCR)[116]; the latter was also found in another cat with cutaneous lymphoma.[112] All these cats had tested negative for FeLV on serology.

Staging and Diagnosis

Localized or generalized lymphadenopathy may be present in cats with cutaneous lymphoma. Enlargement seems to be an inflammatory reaction in some cats, while in others there is involvement with lymphoma.[101,105,109–112] A cat with normal-sized lymph nodes will occasionally be found to have lymphomatous infiltration.[101] Staging should include biopsy of the regional lymph node regardless of whether it is enlarged.

Radiographs rarely show evidence of systemic involvement, although infiltration of abdominal organs is often reported on necropsy.[2,102,110,114] Ultrasonography may be a better way to evaluate abdominal organs and should be performed in addition to radiography when staging cats with cutaneous lymphoma.

Bone marrow aspiration should be performed in addition to an MDB. Bone marrow infiltration by lymphoma has been reported in cats with cutaneous lymphoma.[101–103] There may also be abnormal circulating lymphocytes[101,107,109] or a lymphocytosis.[106,110] Although rare, cutaneous lymphoma may be seen concurrently with leukemia.[109] In such cases, the circulating malignant cells are termed *Sézary cells* and are characterized by large nuclei with highly convoluted nuclear membranes.

Biopsy is required for definitive diagnosis of cutaneous lymphoma. Histopathologic findings of epidermotrophism and accumulation of atypical pleomorphic lymphocytes in

with generalized involvement.[110] There is one report of cutaneous lymphoma affecting the gingival epithelium.[115]

The clinical history may be acute, with some cats having skin lesions for fewer than 4 weeks.[101] However, most cats have had a chronic history (up to years) before a diagnosis of cutaneous lymphoma is confirmed.[101,102,106,108,110,112]

KEY POINT

Cats with solitary cutaneous lymphoma often develop other lesions as the disease progresses.

Serum testing for FeLV and FIV has been negative in all tested cats[2,101,102,105–112,116] except for one FIV-positive animal.[114] However, uncharacterized C type virus particles have been associated with cutaneous lymphoma.[102] More recent evidence suggests that FeLV may have a role in at least some cutaneous lymphomas in cats. In a recent study,

Pautrier's microabscesses is pathognomonic for the variant of cutaneous lymphoma known as mycosis fungoides.[105,106,109–112] Mycosis fungoides is assumed to be a T cell variant of cutaneous lymphoma. This derivation was implied in earlier studies by the formation of "rosettes" with sheep red blood cells[105,107,111] or demonstration of increased blastogenesis to mitogen stimulation.[107] In recent studies, the T cell derivation has been more convincingly shown by immunohistochemical staining with the T cell antibody to CD-3.[106,112,113,116] Some cutaneous lymphomas have been shown to be of B cell derivation,[113] and one cat with cutaneous lymphoma developed hyperviscosity due to a monoclonal IgG, hypercalcemia, and pancytopenia.[103] Lymphoma derived from T cells is more difficult to treat in dogs, but this has not been confirmed in cats.[117]

KEY POINT

A cat with cutaneous lymphoma should be staged with biopsy of the lesion and the regional lymph node, radiography, ultrasonography, and a bone marrow aspiration in addition to an MDB.

Treatment

There have been few successful treatments reported for cats with cutaneous lymphoma.

Survival in untreated cats has varied widely. One cat lived 4 years with mycosis fungoides and was euthanized due to renal disease,[105] while two other cats were euthanized after being diagnosed with multiple cutaneous nodules.[101] Surgical excision of solitary lesions has been reported; however, recurrence developed in two cats within 4 weeks of surgery, prompting other treatments.[101] In one cat, amputation of the affected left hindlimb appeared successful, with no recurrence detected more than a year after surgery.[112] Even when surgery is successful in treating individual lesions, new lesions may arise within weeks.[114]

Neither oral nor topical prednisone appears to be successful in inducing remission,[101,106,112] although some reduction in pruritus may occur. One cat had no response despite 8 weeks of prednisone therapy at 5 mg/kg/day.[106] This cat responded dramatically to oral dexamethasone at a reducing dose from 0.2 mg/kg/day to 0.05 mg/kg/day and was clinically normal 12 months after treatment started.[106] Repeated skin biopsies in this cat showed improvement, but not complete remission, of the cutaneous lymphoma. Triamcinolone in combination with chlorambucil caused only stabilization of lesions in one cat for a period of 4.5 months.[101] Corticosteroids should not be used if chemotherapy is contemplated due to the risk of inducing chemotherapy resistance in the surviving tumor cells.

Chemotherapy with vincristine, cyclophosphamide, and prednisone caused a dramatic short-term improvement in lesions in two cats,[105,107] but new lesions appeared within 4 weeks in both cats. Cyclophosphamide in combination with the nonspecific immunomodulator levamisole caused stabilization of the lesions in another cat for 5 months.[101]

MDB = minimum database; includes CBC, biochemical profile, urinalysis, FeLV/FIV serology, T_4 testing, and thoracic radiographs (three views).

Fibronectin, believed to be an immunostimulator, was unsuccessful in causing remission of the lesion, although injection into the lesion did cause necrosis and sloughing.[111] Placental lysate may have slowed the progression of disease in another cat.[105] The specificity of cyclosporine for T lymphocytes led to its use in one cat with cutaneous lymphoma. Although the tumor lesion remained static, the dose of 15 mg/kg/day proved immunosuppressive and treatment was discontinued after 8 weeks due to secondary infection.[104]

Despite their utility in dogs with cutaneous lymphoma, the use of retinoic acid derivatives has not been widely reported in the treatment of feline cutaneous lymphoma. One report cited three cats treated with isotretinoin (Accutane®) at an oral dose of 1 mg/kg sid–bid.[110] A reduction in scaling and erythema but no objective reduction in the size of tumors was noted in all cats. Survival in these three cats ranged from 6 to 18 months. It is possible that newer drugs such as acitretin (Soriatane®; see section on treatment of SCC) may have efficacy against cutaneous lymphoma.

Radiation therapy (6 Gy using a cesium source) caused an objective response in the size of a preputial lesion in one cat.[105] Multiple lesions treated with Strontium-90 plesiotherapy regressed completely.[114] This modality may be appropriate for treatment of localized lesions, but the risk of toxicity to underlying organs and tissues prevents radiotherapy of multiple or generalized tumors. In addition, the high rate of noncutaneous, systemic lymphoma limits its usefulness. Palliative treatment of individual lesions with radiation is nonetheless an excellent option.

More aggressive chemotherapy with doxorubicin-based protocols (see Chapter 36) have not been reported for cutaneous lymphoma but should be investigated.

Appropriate analgesia should be administered as supportive care regardless of the treatment modality selected, and appetite stimulants may be necessary due to treatment-induced anorexia.

Nondomestic Felidae

Cutaneous tumors appear to be uncommon in nondomestic Felidae. Bowen's disease has been described in a snow leopard *(Panthera uncia)*, as have papilloma virus-induced cutaneous warts, which appeared as scaly plaques.[87,118] Papilloma virus has been associated with SCC in situ. A Bengal tiger *(Panthera tigris)* was found to have an adenoma of the merocrine gland in one survey of tumor types.[119] A 16-year-old Indian lion *(Panthera leo)* was found to have more than 20 cutaneous tumors ranging from 1 to 5 cm in diameter.[120] These hairless tumors were occasionally ulcerated and were found on biopsy to be poorly differentiated MCTs. There was no evidence of metastasis or systemic disease.

A 10-year-old male white tiger with a skin lesion that had been ulcerated for 8 months died in respiratory distress due to widespread metastatic melanoma. The elbow was believed to be the primary site.[121]

An abraded cutaneous hemangiosarcoma on the tail of a 6-year-old jaguar *(Panthera onca)* measured 5 cm in diameter.[122] Cryosurgery was unsuccessful in controlling this tumor, and the tail was amputated. Recurrence at the tail base and intrapelvic lymph nodes 4 months later led to euthanasia.

REFERENCES

1. Miller MA, Nelson SL, Turk JR, et al: Cutaneous neoplasia in 340 cats. *Vet Pathol* 28:389–395, 1991.
2. Carpenter JL, Andrews LK, Holzworth J: Tumors and tumor-like lesions, in Holzworth J (ed): *Diseases of the Cat. Medicine and Surgery*. Philadelphia, WB Saunders, 1987, pp 407–596.
3. Goldschmidt MH, Shofer FS: *Skin Tumors of the Dog and Cat*. New York, Pergamon Press, 1992.
4. Bostock DE: Neoplasms of the skin and subcutaneous tissues in dogs and cats. *Br Vet J* 142:1–19, 1986.
5. Stiglmair-Herb MTh: Hauttumoren bei katzeneine retrospektive studie. *Tierärztliche Umschau* 42:681–686, 1987.
6. Burrows AK, Lee EA, Shaw SE, et al: Skin neoplasms of cats in Perth. *Aust Vet Pract* 24:11–15, 1994.
7. Luther PB, Scott DW, Buerger RG: The dilated pore of Winer—An overlooked cutaneous lesion of cats. *J Comp Pathol* 101:375–379, 1989.
8. Scott DW, Flanders JA: Dilated pore of Winer in a cat. *Feline Pract* 14:33–36, 1984.
9. Abramo F, Pratesi F, Cantile C, et al: Survey of canine and feline follicular tumours and tumour-like lesions in central Italy. *J Small Anim Pract* 40:479–481, 1999.
10. Finnie JW, Leong ASY, Milios J: Multiple piloleiomyomas in a cat. *J Comp Pathol* 113:201–204, 1995.
11. Lozano-Alarcón F, Lewis II TP, Clark EG, et al: Persistent papillomavirus infection in a cat. *JAAHA* 32:392–396, 1996.
12. Carney HC, England JJ, Hodgin EC, et al: Papillomavirus infection of aged Persian cats. *J Vet Diagn Invest* 2:294–299, 1990.
13. Gumbrell RC, Rest JR, Bredelius K, et al: Dermal fibropapillomas in cats. *Vet Rec* 142:376, 1998.
14. Breuer W, Colbatzky F, Platz S, Hermanns W: Immunoglobulin-producing tumours in dogs and cats. *J Comp Pathol* 109:203–216, 1993.
15. Kyriazidou A, Brown PJ, Lucke VM: Immunohistochemical staining of neoplastic and inflammatory plasma cell lesions in feline tissues. *J Comp Pathol* 100:337–341, 1989.
16. Lucke VM: Primary cutaneous plasmacytomas in the dog and cat. *J Small Anim Pract* 28:49–55, 1987.
17. Carothers MA, Johnson GC, DiBartola SP, et al: Extramedullary plasmacytoma and immunoglobulin-associated amyloidosis in a cat. *JAVMA* 195:1593–1597, 1989.
18. Cotchin E: Skin tumours of cats. *Res Vet Sci* 2:353–361, 1961.
19. Jörger K: Hauttumoren bei katzen vorkommen und häufigkeit im untersuchungsgut (Biopsien 1984–1987) des institutes für veterinärpathologie Zürich. *Schweiz Arch Tierheilk* 130:559–569, 1988.
20. Esplin DG: Infiltrating lipoma in a cat. *Feline Pract* 14:24–25, 1984.
21. Diters RW, Walsh KM: Feline basal cell tumors: A review of 124 cases. *Vet Pathol* 21:51–56, 1984.
22. Clarke RE: Cryosurgical treatment of feline cutaneous squamous cell carcinoma. *Aust Vet Pract* 21:148, 1991.
23. Fehrer SL, Lin SH: Multicentric basal cell tumors in a cat. *JAVMA* 189:1469–1470, 1986.
24. Withrow SJ, Straw RC: Resection of the nasal planum in nine cats and five dogs. *JAAHA* 26:219–222, 1990.
25. Kalaher KM, Anderson WI, Scott DW: Neoplasms of the apocrine sweat glands in 44 dogs and 10 cats. *Vet Rec* 127:400–403, 1990.
26. van der Linde-Sipman JS, van den Ingh TSGAM: Primary and metastatic carcinomas in the digits of cats. *Vet Q* 22:141–145, 2000.
27. Macy DW: Darier's sign associated with a cutaneous mast cell tumour in a cat with multiple neoplasms. *J Small Anim Pract* 29:597–602, 1988.
28. Patnaik AK, Mooney S: Feline melanoma: A comparative study of ocular, oral, and dermal neoplasms. *Vet Pathol* 25:105–112, 1988.
29. Miller Jr WH, Scott DW, Anderson WI: Feline cutaneous melanocytic neoplasms: A retrospective analysis of 43 cases (1979–1991). *Vet Dermatol* 4:19–26, 1993.
30. van der Linde-Sipman JS, De Wit MML, van Garderen E, et al: Cutaneous malignant melanomas in 57 cats: Identification of (Amelanotic) signet-ring and balloon cell types and verification of their origin by immunohistochemistry, electron microscopy, and in situ hybridization. *Vet Pathol* 34:31–38, 1997.
31. Goldschmidt MH, Liu SMS, Shofer FS: Feline dermal melanoma: A retrospective study. *Vet Derm* 2:285–291, 1992.
32. Howard-Martin MO, Qualls Jr CW: Metastatic melanoma in a cat. *Feline Pract* 16:6–8, 1986.
33. Day MJ, Lucke VM: Melanocytic neoplasia in the cat. *J Small Anim Pract* 36:207–213, 1995.
34. Scott DW: Lentigo simplex in orange cats. *Comp Anim Pract* 23–25, 1987.
35. Roels S, Tilmant K, Ducatelle R: PCNA and Ki67 proliferation markers as criteria for prediction of clinical behaviour of melanocytic tumours in cats and dogs. *J Comp Pathol* 121:13–24, 1999.
36. Wood CA, Moore AS, Frimberger AE, et al: Phase I evaluation of carboplatin in tumor bearing cats. *Proc 16th Annu Conf Vet Cancer Soc*:39–40, 1996.
37. Buerger RG, Scott DW: Cutaneous mast cell neoplasia in cats: 14 cases (1975–1985). *JAVMA* 190:1440–1444, 1987.
38. Wilcock BP, Yager JA, Zink MC: The morphology and behavior of feline cutaneous mastocytomas. *Vet Pathol* 23:320–324, 1986.
39. Molander-McCrary H, Henry CJ, Potter K, et al: Cutaneous mast cell tumors in cats: 32 cases (1991–1994). *JAAHA* 34:281–284, 1998.
40. Head KW: Cutaneous mast-cell tumours in the dog, cat and ox. *Br J Dermatol* 70:389–408, 1957.
41. Chastain CB, Turk MA, O'Brien D: Benign cutaneous mastocytomas in two litters of Siamese kittens. *JAVMA* 193:959–960, 1988.
42. Crafts GA, Pulley LT: Generalized cutaneous mast cell tumor in a cat. *Feline Pract* 5:57–58, 1975.
43. Cohen SJ, Koch F: Cutaneous mastocytosis with metastases in a domestic cat. *Feline Pract* 10:41–43, 1980.
44. Goto N, Ozasa M, Takahashi R, et al: Pathological observations of feline mast cell tumor. *Jpn J Vet Sci* 36:483–494, 1974.
45. Bell A, Mason K, Mitchell G, Miller R: Visceral and cutaneous mast cell neoplasia in a cat. *Aust Vet Pract* 24:86–91, 1994.
46. Madewell BR, Gunn CR, Gribble DH: Mast cell phagocytosis of red blood cells in a cat. *Vet Pathol* 20:638–640, 1983.
47. Garner FM, Lingeman CH: Mast-cell neoplasms of the domestic cat. *Pathol Vet* 7:517–530, 1970.
48. Anderson WI: Efficacy of topical 5-fluorouracil and triamcinolone acetonide in feline cutaneous mast cell tumors. *Feline Pract* 15:34–35, 1985.
49. Meier H: Feline mastocytoma: Two cases. *Cornell Vet* 47:220–226, 1957.
50. Holzinger EA: Feline cutaneous mastocytomas. *Cornell Vet* 63:87–93, 1973.
51. Scott DW: Epidermal mast cells in the cat. *Vet Dermatol* 1:65–69, 1990.
52. Monlux WS: Mastocytoma in a feline—A case report. *Southwestern Vet* 6:153–154, 1953.

53. Padrid PA, Mitchell RW, Ndukwu IM, et al: Cyproheptadine-induced attenuation of type-I immediate-hypersensitivity reactions of airway smooth muscle from immune-sensitized cats. *Am J Vet Res* 56:109–115, 1995.

54. Brown CA, Chalmers SA: Diffuse cutaneous mastocytosis in a cat. *Vet Pathol*
27:366–369, 1990.

55. Barr MC, Butt MT, Anderson KL, et al: Spinal lymphosarcoma and disseminated mastocytoma associated with feline immunodeficiency virus infection
in a cat. *JAVMA* 202:1978–1980, 1993.

56. Cheli R, Addis F, Mortellaro CM, et al: Hematoporphyrin derivative pho-
tochemotherapy of spontaneous animal tumors: Clinical results with opti-
mized drug dose. *Cancer Lett* 23:61–66, 1984.

57. Seiler RJ, Punita I: Neoplasia of domestic mammals: Review of cases diagnosed at Universiti Pertanian Malaysia. *Kajian Veterinar* 11:80–84, 1979.

58. Bostock DE: The prognosis in cats bearing squamous cell carcinoma. *J Small
Anim Pract* 13:119–125, 1972.

59. Frimberger AE, Moore AS, Cincotta L, et al: Photodynamic therapy of naturally occurring tumors in animals using a novel benzophenothiazine photosensitizer. *Clin Cancer Res* 4:2207–2218, 1998.

60. Lana SE, Ogilvie GK, Withrow SJ, et al: Feline cutaneous squamous cell carcinoma of the nasal planum and pinnae: 61 cases. *JAAHA* 33:329–332, 1997.

61. Dorn CR, Taylor DON, Schneider R: Sunlight exposure and risk of developing cutaneous and oral squamous cell carcinomas in white cats. *J Natl Cancer
Inst* 46:1073–1078, 1971.

62. Ciampi L: Su deu casi di cancroide cutaneo nei gatti bianchi. *La Nuova Vet-
erinaria* 15:342–349, 1949.

63. Thèon AP, Madewell BR, Shearn VI, Moulton JE: Prognostic factors associated with radiotherapy of squamous cell carcinoma of the nasal plane in cats.
JAVMA 206:991–996, 1995.

64. Teifke JP, Löhr CV: Immunhistochemical detection of P53 overexpression in
paraffin wax-embedded squamous cell carcinomas of cattle, horses, cats and
dogs. *J Comp Pathol* 114:205–210, 1996.

65. Carlisle CH, Gould S: Response of squamous cell carcinoma of the nose of
the cat to treatment with X-rays. *Vet Radiol* 23:186–192, 1982.

66. Hutson CA, Rideout BA, Pedersen NC: Neoplasia associated with feline immunodeficiency virus infection in cats of Southern California. *JAVMA* 199:
1357–1362, 1991.

67. Evans EG, Madewell BR, Stannard AA: A trial of 13-cis-retinoic acid for treatment of squamous cell carcinoma and preneoplastic lesions of the head in cats.
Am J Vet Res 46:2553–2557, 1985.

68. Peaston AE, Leach MW, Higgins RJ: Photodynamic therapy for nasal and aural squamous cell carcinoma in cats. *JAVMA* 202:1261–1265, 1993.

69. Buhles WC, Theilen GH: Preliminary evaluation of bleomycin in feline and
canine squamous cell carcinoma. *Am J Vet Res* 34:289–291, 1973.

70. Thèon AP, Van Vechten MK, Madewell BR: Intratumoral administration of
carboplatin for treatment of squamous cell carcinomas of the nasal plane in
cats. *Am J Vet Res* 57:205–210, 1996.

71. Cox NR, Brawner WR, Powers RD, Wright JC: Tumors of the nose and
paranasal sinuses in cats: 32 cases with comparison to a national database
(1977 through 1987). *JAAHA* 27:339–347, 1991.

72. VanVechten MK, Thèon AP: Strontium-90 plesiotherapy for treatment of early squamous cell carcinomas of the nasal planum in 25 cats. *Proc 13th Annu
Conf Vet Cancer Soc*:107–108, 1993.

73. Kaser-Hotz B, Egger B, Ruslander D, et al: Radiation therapy of feline facial
squamous cell carcinoma with 72 MeV protons. *Proc 7th Europ Soc Vet Intern
Med*:113, 1997.

74. Owen LM: *TNM Classification of Tumors in Domestic Animals*. Geneva, World
Health Organization, 1980, pp 46–47.

75. Irving RA, Daz RS, Eales L: Porphyrin values and treatment of feline solar
dermatitis. *Am J Vet Res* 43:2067–2069, 1982.

76. Leach MW, Peaston AE: Adverse drug reaction attributable to aluminum
phthalocyanine tetrasulphonate administration in domestic cats. *Vet Pathol*
31: 283–287, 1994.

77. Stell AJ, Langmack K, Dobson JM: Treatment of superficial squamous cell
carcinoma of the nasal planum in cats using photodynamic therapy [abstract].
42nd BSAVA Congress, 1999.

78. Shelley BA, Bartels KE, Ely RW, Clark DM: Use of the neodymium:yttrium-
aluminum-garnet laser for treatment of squamous cell carcinoma of the nasal
planum in a cat. *JAVMA* 201:756–758, 1992.

79. Thèon AP, Peaston AE: Pre-operative irradiation of facial tumors in cats [ab-
stract 54]. *J Vet Intern Med* 6:122, 1992.

80. Knapp DW, Richardson RC, BeNicola DB, et al: Cisplatin toxicity in cats. *J
Vet Intern Med* 1:29–35, 1987.

81. Harvey HJ, MacEwen EG, Hayes AA: Neurotoxicosis associated with use of
5-fluorouracil in five dogs and one cat. *JAVMA* 171:277–278, 1977.

82. Henness AM, Theilen GH, Madewell BR, Crow SE: Neurotoxicosis associated with use of 5-fluorouracil. *JAVMA* 171:692, 1977.

83. Theilen GH: Adverse effect from use of 5-fluorouracil. *JAVMA* 191:276,
1987.

84. Orenberg EK, Luck EE, Brown DM, Kitchell BE: Implant delivery system:
Intralesinal delivery of chemotherapeutic agents for treatment of spontaneous
skin tumors in veterinary patients. *Clin Dermatol* 9:561–568, 1992.

85. Rogers KS: Feline cutaneous squamous cell carcinoma. *Feline Pract* 22:7–9,
1994.

86. Baer KE, Helton K: Multicentric squamous cell carcinoma in situ resembling
Bowen's disease in cats. *Vet Pathol* 30:535–543, 1993.

87. Miller Jr WH, Affolter V, Scott DW, Suter MM: Multicentric squamous cell
carcinomas *in situ* resembling Bowen's disease in five cats. *Vet Dermatol* 3:
177–182, 1992.

88. Turrel JM, Gross TL: Multicentric squamous cell carcinoma in situ (Bowen's
disease) of cats. *Proc 11th Annu Conf Vet Cancer Soc*:84, 1991.

89. Gross TL, Clark EG, Hargis AM, et al: Giant cell dermatosis in FeLV-positive
cats. *Vet Dermatol* 4:117–122, 1994.

90. LeClerc SM, Clark EG, Haines DM: Papillomavirus infection in association
with feline cutaneous squamous cell carcinoma in situ. *Proc Am Assoc Vet
Derm/Am Coll Vet Derm* 13:125–126, 1997.

91. Rees CA, Goldschmidt MH: Cutaneous horn and squamous cell carcinoma
in situ (Bowen's disease) in a cat. *JAAHA* 34:485–486, 1998.

92. Scavelli TD, Patnaik AK, Mehlaff CJ, Hayes AA: Hemangiosarcoma in the cat:
Retrospective evaluation of 31 surgical cases. *JAVMA* 187:817–819, 1985.

93. Miller MA, Ramos JA, Kreeger JM: Cutaneous vascular neoplasia in 15 cats:
Clinical, morphologic, and immunohistochemical studies. *Vet Pathol* 29:329–
336, 1992.

94. Kraje AC, Mears EA, Hahn KA, et al: Unusual metastatic behavior and clinicopathologic findings in 8 cats with cutaneous or visceral hemangiosarcoma
(1981–1997). *JAVMA* 214:670–672, 1999.

95. Lawler DF, Evans RH: Multiple hepatic cavernous lymphangiomas in an aged
male cat. *J Comp Pathol* 109:83–87, 1993.

96. Hinrichs U, Puhl S, Rutteman GR, et al: Lymphangiosarcomas in cats: A retrospective study of 12 cases. *Vet Pathol* 36:164–167, 1999.

97. Swayne DE, Mahaffey EA, Haynes SG: Lymphangiosarcoma and haemangiosarcoma in a cat. *J Comp Pathol* 100:91–96, 1989.

98. Patnaik AK, Liu S-K: Angiosarcoma in cats. *J Small Anim Pract* 18:191–198,
1977.

99. Walsh KM, Abbott DP: Lymphangiosarcoma in two cats. *J Comp Pathol* 94:
611–613, 1984.

100. Walton DK, Berg RJ: Cutaneous lymphangiosarcoma in a cat. *Feline Pract*
13:21–26, 1983.

101. Caciolo PL, Nesbitt GH, Patnaik AK, Hayes AA: Cutaneous lymphosarcoma
in the cat: A report of nine cases. *JAAHA* 20:491–496, 1984.

102. Dallman MJ, Noxon JO, Stogsdill P: Feline lymphosarcoma with cutaneous
and muscle lesions. *JAVMA* 181:166–168, 1982.

103. Dust A, Norris AM, Valli VEO: Cutaneous lymphosarcoma with IgG monoclonal gammopathy, serum hyperviscosity and hypercalcemia in a cat. *Can Vet
J* 23:235–239, 1982.

104. Rosenkrantz WS, Griffin CE, Barr RJ: Clinical evaluation of cyclosporine in
animal models with cutaneous immune-mediated disease and epitheliotropic
lymphoma. *JAAHA* 25:377–384, 1989.

105. Baker JL, Scott DW: Mycosis fungoides in two cats. *JAAHA* 25:97–101, 1989.

106. Kottkamp C, Walter JH, Löblich-Beardi B, Opitz M: Das kutane lym-
phosarkom der katze. *Kleintierpraxis* 41:357–366, 1996.

107. Legendre AM, Becker PU: Feline skin lymphoma: Characterization of tumor
and identification of tumor-stimulating serum factor(s). *Am J Vet Res* 40:1805–
1807, 1979.

108. Sent U, Pothmann M: A case of cutaneous lymphosarcoma associated with
mycosis fungoides in a cat. *Feline Pract* 24:6–9, 1996.

109. Schick RO, Murphy GF, Goldschmidt MH: Cutaneous lymphosarcoma and
leukemia in a cat. *JAVMA* 203:1155–1158, 1993.

110. Plant JD: Would you have diagnosed cutaneous epitheliotropic lymphoma in
these two cats? *Vet Med* 86:801–806, 1991.

111. Caciolo PL, Hayes AA, Patnaik AK, et al: A case of mycosis fungoides in a cat
and literature review. *JAAHA* 19:505–512, 1983.

112. Tobey JC, Houston DM, Breur GJ, et al: Cutaneous T-cell lymphoma in a
cat. *JAVMA* 204:606–609, 1994.

MANAGEMENT OF SPECIFIC DISEASES

113. Day MJ: Immunophenotypic characterization of cutaneous lymphoid neoplasia in the dog and cat. *J Comp Pathol* 112:79–96, 1995.

114. Foster SF, Charles JA, Swinney GR, Malik R: Multiple crusted cutaneous plaques in a cat. *Aust Vet J* 77:360, 1999.

115. Stebbins KE, Morse CE, Goldschmidt MH: Feline oral neoplasia: A ten year survey. *Vet Pathol* 26:121–128, 1989.

116. Jackson ML, Wood SL, Misra V, Haines DM: Immunohistochemical identification of B and T lymphocytes in formalin-fixed, paraffin-embedded feline lymphosarcomas: Relation to feline leukemia virus status, tumor site, and patient age. *Can J Vet Res* 60:199–204, 1996.

117. Vail DM, Moore AS, Ogilvie GK, Volk LM: Feline lymphoma (145 cases): Proliferation indices, cluster of differentiation 3 immunoreactivity, and their association with prognosis in 90 cats. *J Vet Intern Med* 12:349–354, 1998.

118. Sundberg JP, Van Ranst M, Montali R, et al: Feline papillomas and papillomaviruses. *Vet Pathol* 37:1–10, 2000.

119. Effron M, Griner L, Benirschke K: Nature and rate of neoplasia found in captive wild mammals, birds and reptiles at necropsy. *J Natl Cancer Inst* 59:185–198, 1977.

120. Stolte M, Welle M: Cutaneous mast cell tumours in a lion *(Pantherea leo)*: A light and transmission electron microscopical study. *J Comp Pathol* 113:291–294, 1995.

121. Rao AT, Acharjyo LN, Mohanty AK: Malignant melanoma in a white tiger. *Indian J Vet Pathol* 15:113–114, 1991.

122. Ladiges WC, Foster JW, Jones MH: Malignant hemangioendothelioma in a jaguar *(Panthera onca)*. *J Zoo Anim Med* 12:36–37, 1981.

SOF TISSUE SARCOMAS

51

Antony S. Moore and Gregory K. Ogilvie

CLINICAL BRIEFING	
Common Presentation	Firm dermal mass anywhere on the body; more common at injection sites. Ulceration may occur in large tumors. Injection site sarcomas usually occur in younger cats; increased risk with increased number of vaccinations at one site. FeSV may cause multiple tumors in young FeLV-positive cats. Fibrosarcoma, histiocytic sarcomas, and nerve-sheath sarcomas are most common.
Staging and Diagnosis	MDB; obtain history of previous injections. Abdominal ultrasonography. CT scan or MRI and biopsy prior to definitive treatment. Lymph node cytology if lymphadenopathy is present. Metastasis relatively uncommon but usually to lungs.
Treatment	
Initial	Wide and deep surgical excision if complete excision with 2 cm margins is possible. If not, consider pre- or postsurgical radiation therapy (treatment of choice).
Adjunctive	Radiation, particularly at high doses, after incomplete surgery improves local control. Metastatic rate is moderate but may be higher for injection site tumors. Doxorubicin and possibly carboplatin are active chemotherapeutic agents.
Supportive	Analgesia postoperatively. Consider gastrostomy or esophagostomy feeding tube if prolonged treatment considered. If radiation and chemotherapy are used, a vascular access port may be advantageous.

Incidence, Signalment, and Etiology

Soft tissue sarcomas are grouped together in this section because of apparent similarities in their biologic, and therefore clinical, behavior. Benign variants of these tumors are reported (e.g., fibroma, rhabdomyoma, etc.), but it is best to think of them as highly locally invasive, low-grade malignancies and to treat them in the same aggressive manner as tumors described as sarcomas.

Fibrosarcoma is the most common histologic diagnosis within this group of tumors. Histologic distinction may be difficult with other tumors. For example, confirmation of muscle origin (rhabdomyosarcoma) requires immunohistochemical staining for the intermediate filament desmin,[1,2] and histologic differentiation of neurofibrosarcoma from Schwannoma is possible only by using electron microscopy[3] or by identifying small bundles and palisades of cells called *Antoni type A pattern*.[4,5] Soft tissue sarcomas with a highly mucinous stroma are called *myxofibrosarcomas* or *myxosarcomas*.[6]

Two large studies totaling 712 cats are the source of epidemiologic data on soft tissue sarcomas.[6,7] One study of cats in the United States showed that DSH cats were nearly twice as likely as other breeds to develop fibrosarcomas.[6] In contrast, a German study showed no evidence of breed predispositions.[7]

The ages of affected cats ranged from 1 to 18 years, and there appears to be incidence peaks at 3 and 8 years of age.[7] Recent U.S. studies have shown an increased risk for young cats to develop injection site sarcomas (discussed below); however, the German study cited above[7] also showed a young age peak in cats diagnosed between 1970 and 1984, which is prior to changes in vaccination habits. Another explanation for the increased risk in young cats is the presence of feline sarcoma virus (FeSV; discussed below). These cats often have multiple tumors, as was the case in 10 of 174 cats (5.8%) in one of the two studies cited above[7] and 7 of 494 cats (1.4%) in the other.[6] Affected cats were between 3 and 7 years of age.[7] There was no obvious gender predilection in either study.

In one study, 58% of tumors affected the hindquarters and 39% affected the thorax.[7] More specific site distribution was provided for 494 cats[6]: 28 tumors (26%) were on the head and neck, 196 (40%) on the limbs, 52 (10.5%) on the back, 42 (8.5%) on the thorax, 56 (11%) on the abdomen, 12 (2%) on the tail, and 1 each (0.2%) on the perineum and scrotum.

Other specific site distributions have been noted. Four cats with rhabdomyoma of the pinna were described. Three of the cats were white, and all four cats had white pinnae.[8]

Myxosarcomas occurred most commonly on the limbs (16 of 23 tumors) in one study.[6]

MDB = minimum database; includes CBC, biochemical profile, urinalysis, FeLV/FIV serology, T₄ testing, and thoracic radiographs (three views).

There has been interest in chromosomal aberrations associated with soft tissue sarcoma, particularly those occurring at injection sites. A neurofibroma on the flank of a cat showed a trisomy of chromosome D2,[9] and a fibrosarcoma showed multiple copies of many chromosomes.[10] Other chromosomal aberrations have been noted.[11] Further information is included in the section on injection site sarcomas. Mutations in the tumor suppressor gene, *p53*, have also been identified in feline soft tissue sarcomas[12,13] but may not be specific to injection site sarcomas.[14,15]

KEY POINT

Soft tissue sarcomas that have a high mitotic rate are more likely to recur, and cats with these tumors often have short survival times.

Clinical Presentation and History

Soft tissue sarcomas are often dermal in origin, so the most common reason for presentation is a mass that the owner detected while grooming or petting the cat (Figure 51-1). Tumors can vary in size from 0.3 to 15 cm in diameter[7] and are typically not well demarcated. Ulceration is rare but may occur secondary to pressure necrosis of the skin overlying large tumors (Figure 51-2). Most tumors are firm, although some may be cystic or mucinous, which can

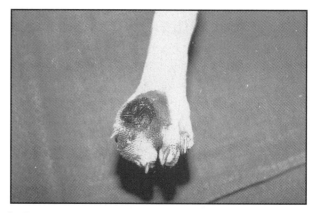

Figure 51-2: *Large tumors may cause pressure necrosis of overlying tissue and become ulcerated, as has happened to the nerve sheath tumor on the paw of this cat.*

make them feel soft.[7] Soft tissue sarcomas can be slow to enlarge, and owners may delay seeking veterinary advice for years after first detecting a mass. Tumors that infiltrate the underlying bone may cause lameness,[4,16–19] and those arising from the nerve sheath may cause weakness and pain.[20–22]

Staging and Diagnosis

Soft tissue sarcomas infiltrate far beyond the clinically palpable borders (Figures 51-3 and 51-4), and those affecting the nerve sheath may extend through bone to involve the spinal dura.[22,23] Therefore wide surgical excision is needed to ensure adequate tissue margins are obtained, and adjunctive radiation therapy is often necessary. A CT scan prior to surgery or radiation therapy will allow delineation of tumor margins and allow for all treatment options to be explored (Figures 51-5 and 51-6). MRI, if available, will also allow detailed examination of the tumor margins prior to treatment.

Metastasis appears to be uncommon, regardless of the subtype of soft tissue sarcoma. In one study, 8 of 84 cats

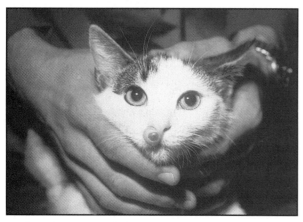

Figure 51-1: *A firm dermal mass occurring anywhere on the body may be a soft tissue sarcoma, as in this young cat with a facial fibrosarcoma.*

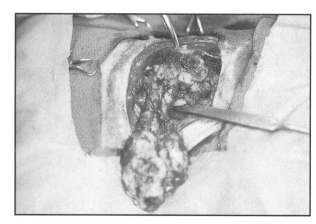

Figure 51-3: *Surgical exposure of an injection site sarcoma on the flank. Macroscopic tentacles of tissue invade deeper muscle and bone. Microscopic extensions also occur throughout the area, thereby compromising surgical excision.*

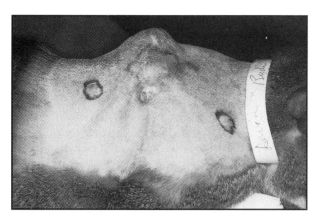

Figure 51-4: *A recurrent interscapular fibrosarcoma in an Abyssinian. The large central tumor has satellite tumors (ringed) more than 5 cm from the main mass, emphasizing the invasive nature of this tumor. Treatment with surgery or radiation is very difficult for extensive tumors like this.*

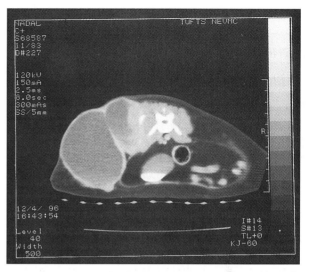

Figure 51-6: *A CT scan of the cat shown in Figure 51-5 reveals a multilobed tumor that extends to the lumbar vertebrae. A CT scan helps the surgeon or radiation therapist to plan treatment strategies.*

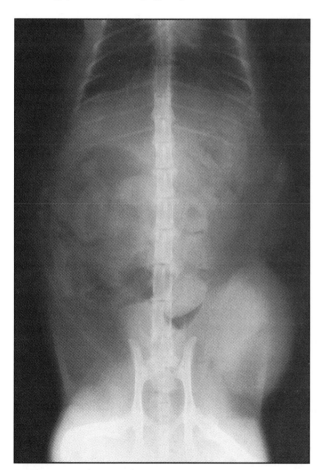

Figure 51-5: *This radiograph of a cat with a left paralumbar sarcoma reveals a soft tissue density but little detail.*

(10%) had confirmed metastases and another 12 had suspected but unconfirmed metastases (total = 26%).[7] In other studies, 32 of 158 cats (20.3%) had metastases.[19,24–27] Some investigators believe that the metastatic rate for injection site sarcomas may be higher than for sarcomas affect-

ing other sites. It is difficult to estimate the overall rate of metastasis because many older studies relied on surgical excision alone to control the tumor and most cats died as a result of local recurrence soon after surgery. Although metastases have been reported as soon as 5 weeks after surgery,[19,28] they are usually detected much later. Recent studies encompassing cats with injection site sarcomas[25,26] have included cats treated with radical surgical procedures and often adjunctive therapies such as radiation therapy. In these studies, local tumor control has improved, which may in turn increase the chances for occurrence, and therefore detection, of metastases.

Metastases have most often been described to the lung,[1,7,25,26,28] with occasional concurrent skin metastases.[26,28] Splenic metastases have been reported,[7] as has renal involvement.[1,7] Regional lymph node involvement appears to be uncommon, occurring in only 3 of 108 cats.[7,25,26,28] Thoracic radiographs do not usually disclose evidence of metastasis at the time of presentation[19,26] but should still be included as part of the MDB in staging procedures. Although lymph node involvement is uncommon, nodes should be palpated and fine-needle aspiration for cytologic evaluation performed if they are enlarged. Splenic metastases have been reported, albeit rarely, and thus abdominal ultrasonography is important for completeness of staging.

A preoperative biopsy is recommended to guide therapy. Radiation therapy prior to surgical excision may have advantages over postsurgical radiation (see the Treatment section). To reduce the size of the surgical scar that would need to be irradiated, an incisional or Tru-cut needle biopsy is preferred over an excisional biopsy. The degree of histologic differentiation and mitotic rate found on biopsy may be prognostic. In one study of 174 sarcomas, 91 (52%) were characterized as fibrosarcomas, 57 (33%) as pleomorphic sarcomas, 22 (13%) as spindle cell sarcomas, and 4 (2%) as undifferentiated.[7] Of 8 cats that developed confirmed metastases, 4 had pleomorphic tumors, 2 had fibrosarcomas, and 2 had spindle cell sarcomas.[7] The mitotic index can vary widely in feline soft tissue sarcoma.[29] In one study, the mitotic index of the tumor predicted recurrence and survival following surgery.[30] Nineteen cats with a mitotic index of 4 or less had a median survival of 128 weeks despite a 63% recurrence rate. In contrast, 16 cats with a mitotic index of 5 or greater survived a median of 16 weeks, and the recurrence rate was 75%.

Treatment

Surgery

Surgical excision has been the principal treatment modality for soft tissue sarcomas. Due to the extensive infiltration and invasion of surrounding normal tissue, it is necessary to resect a wide and deep (more than 2 cm) margin of normal tissue in all surgical planes around the palpable tumor (Figure 51-7). While this is often possible in larger species such as dogs and humans, it is rarely possible in cats, particularly following an initial unsuccessful attempt. Exceptions to this would be tumors on a distal limb or other extremity that can be amputated. For this reason the first attempt at surgical removal should be the definitive one, and wide surgical margins that include bone, muscle, and other structures should be obtained. For example, a cat with soft tissue sarcoma in the interscapular space would require resection that encompasses 2 cm or greater circumferential margins of normal tissue, including the dorsal process of the scapulae and dorsal spinous processes. The aim should be to remove the tissue "en bloc" without incising tumor tissue itself (Figure 51-8).

The surgeon should be aware that as soft tissue sarcomas grow, they compress a cuff of tumor cells to form a pseudocapsule, thereby giving the false impression that the sarcoma is encapsulated.

Because aggressive surgeries require specific surgical skills and adequate planning, the preferred approach is an incisional or Tru-cut needle biopsy prior to consulting with an experienced surgeon and/or radiation oncologist. As stated earlier, pretreatment staging should include a CT scan to more clearly define the tumor margins and areas of infiltration.

KEY POINT

A needle biopsy should be performed and a surgical oncologist and radiation therapist consulted before treatment of a soft tissue sarcoma is attempted.

In a study of 84 cats surgically treated for soft tissue sarcoma, 60 cats (70%) had tumor recurrence an average of 3.5 months later.[7] Tumors recurred as soon as 2.5 weeks and as long as 1.5 years after surgery. Only 34 of the 60 cats had a second surgery; the other 26 were euthanized. Of these 34 cats, 27 (80%) had a second recurrence and 12 of these were euthanized. Of the 84 cats originally treated, only 9

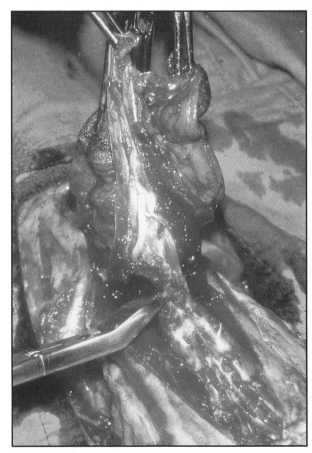

Figure 51-8: *Aggressive, deep excision of an interscapular fibrosarcoma should include the dorsal spinous and scapular processes as an "en bloc" resection.*

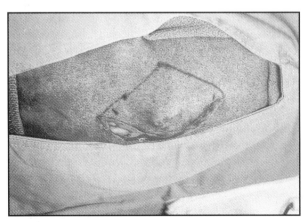

Figure 51-7: *Wide surgical excision of a sarcoma may still be unsuccessful because of the microscopic tentacles of tumor tissue.*

cats became disease free and only 4 of those were disease free longer than 18 months.[7] A similar recurrence rate of over 80% was seen in another study in which the median tumor-free period following surgical excision was 4 months.[31] Only 10% of 61 cats were tumor free a year after surgery in another study[28]; these cats had all been treated by wide excision or amputation.

Tumors that involve the limb often recur after an attempted local excision, but the likelihood of long-term control following amputation is high (Figure 51-9).[4,16,19,27,28,30] Similarly, tumors of the pinnae[8] or even nictitans[32] may be removed with complete surgical margins. For more extensive limb tumors that approach the pelvis, a hemipelvectomy may be required; if complete margins cannot be obtained, a rapid recurrence should be expected.[33] Procedures that are less aggressive than amputation, such as scapulectomy, may leave tumor cells and lead to recurrence.[18]

Aggressive surgical excisions in other areas may lead to long-term tumor control even after other methods have failed.[33] However, the first surgery should be considered definitive rather than relying on a second or third surgery for salvage. Wide resection on the chest wall or flank may require rib or body wall removal and the use of propylene mesh. Even with extensive surgery and reconstructive attempts, recurrences may still develop.[34]

Some prognostic factors following surgery were explored in one study of 35 cats.[25] Tumor location did not seem to affect whether a tumor recurred. However, cats that had a surgery with histologically complete margins had a median tumor-free survival of more than 16 months. Surgeries that had "dirty" margins led to tumor recurrence a median of 4 months after surgery, which is consistent with other studies cited above, and a median survival of only 9 months. In addition, cats that had not been treated with surgery prior to the definitive resection (i.e., this was their first surgery) had a median disease-free interval of longer than 16 months. In comparison,

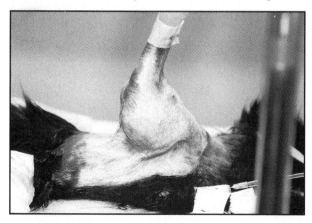

Figure 51-9: Soft tissue sarcomas of the distal limbs may be removed by amputation. Tumor infiltration still occurs, so complete forequarter or hindquarter amputation is preferred to ensure surgical margins are free of tumor cells.

cats that had undergone one or more attempts at excision prior to definitive surgery had a median disease-free interval of only 5 months and a median survival of 13 months.[25]

Radiation Therapy

Most early studies report very little efficacy for radiation therapy in reducing recurrence rates for soft tissue sarcoma. A combination of minimal surgical excision and low doses of radiation therapy probably contributed to the apparent ineffectiveness.[35–37] More recent studies suggest that the treatment of choice for this tumor type is aggressive surgery in combination with high doses of pre- or postoperative radiation therapy.

In two studies, cats were treated with brachytherapy using iridium-192 (^{192}Ir) implants after surgery. The dose in one study was 60 Gy[24] but was not provided in the other.[31] The recurrence rate in one study was 70% (11 of 16 cats), with a median survival of 8 months[24]; in the other group of cats, 50% of tumors recurred and the median disease-free interval was 12.5 months,[31] which was better than for cats in the same study treated with surgery alone (discussed previously).

Selection of cats with poor prognostic factors may have influenced outcome in another study in which ^{192}Ir brachytherapy or cobalt-60 teletherapy resulted in a median disease-free interval of only 4.5 months.[25] Information about radiation doses was not provided.

In a study of 31 cats treated with orthovoltage radiation to a dose of 51 to 60 Gy following incomplete surgical excision, the median tumor-free interval was 18 months and median survival was 22 months.[38] Acute toxicities were mild, but systemic toxicities led to the euthanasia of 6 cats, 2 due to pneumonitis and 4 due to renal failure. These toxicities occurred because of radiation of underlying structures when injection site sarcomas of the interscapular area or the flank were treated (Figure 51-10).

High-dose radiation therapy (57 Gy) was used to treat 25 cats with soft tissue sarcomas. An electron beam was used to deliver the radiation to most cats; this method delivers radiation to superficial tissues while sparing the underlying normal tissue, thereby avoiding toxicity. Median survival for all cats was 700 days.[39] In this small group of cats, the administration of doxorubicin chemotherapy was not associated with longer survival, but further studies are warranted as other anecdotal experience indicates that adjuvant chemotherapy may improve survival. Increasing numbers of surgeries prior to radiation were not associated with decreased survival.

Sarcoma recurrence after radiation may be due to improved tumor cell survival along the relatively hypoxic surgical scar. Hypoxia reduces the effectiveness of radiation therapy. One study investigated the efficacy of presurgical radiation therapy to an area surrounding the tumor followed by wide surgical excision.[26] The tumor recurred in 11 of 33

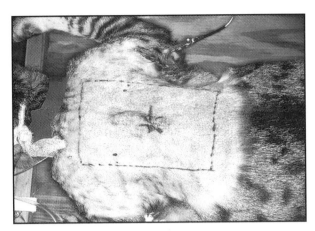

Figure 51-10: *Postoperative radiation should include 3 to 5 cm margins around the surgical scar. Even a small scar, as in this Ocicat, requires a radiation field that includes all lung fields. For this reason, preoperative radiation may be a preferred treatment, as it will reduce the area of normal tissue to be irradiated.*

cats, and 8 of 33 developed metastases (4 also experienced tumor recurrence). The tumor was more likely to recur quickly in cats in which surgical excision was incomplete after radiation therapy. Tumors recurred in the 5 cats with incomplete resection a median of 3.5 months after surgery, while those with complete resection were tumor free a median of 23 months after surgery.[26] Tumor volume at the time of radiation did not influence recurrence or survival, implying that even large tumors could be treated in this manner. Some cats developed transient pneumonitis, and wound dehiscence occurred and was repaired in 4 of 33 cats. It appears that radiation may act to "sterilize" the margins of a tumor, enabling a more effective surgical excision. A combination of radiation therapy and aggressive surgery may be the treatment of choice for feline soft tissue sarcomas.

KEY POINT

A combination of surgery and radiation therapy is probably the treatment of choice for soft tissue sarcomas.

Chemotherapy

There is very little information regarding chemotherapy in the treatment of soft tissue sarcomas in cats. The reportedly low metastatic rate has meant that chemotherapy is rarely used in an adjuvant setting. The higher metastatic rates now reported and the reduction in the rate of local recurrences following the use of surgery and radiation therapy indicate that chemotherapy may have an increasing role in the management of soft tissue sarcomas in cats.

Drugs that anecdotally appear to have no efficacy are vincristine, methotrexate, and cyclophosphamide.[19,27,35] Doxorubicin has been used with apparent success to treat cats

with local recurrence after surgery,[40] although other studies indicated no response to treatment.[35] Mitoxantrone did not influence tumor recurrence in a cat with soft tissue sarcoma.[33] The use of carboplatin chemotherapy did not seem to improve survival rates in another study,[25] although some oncologists believe that this drug is helpful. Similarly, studies are currently in progress to investigate the efficacy of ifosfamide,[a] a drug that is very effective against soft tissue sarcomas in humans.

In an investigation of a novel approach to treat recurrent sarcomas, IV bleomycin (0.5 mg/kg) was combined with electric stimulation of the sarcoma and immunotherapy.[41] Tumor regression was seen in only one cat, but survival appeared to be prolonged (5 months) compared with untreated cats (0.7 months).

In another study, either doxorubicin, mitoxantrone, or carboplatin was administered to seven cats in which sarcoma recurred after surgery and radiation.[26] The median survival for these cats was 3.5 months, and two cats were alive 10 to 22 months after treatment. Doxorubicin and carboplatin need to be further evaluated in the treatment of soft tissue sarcomas in cats, particularly as an adjuvant to surgery and radiation therapy.

Immunotherapy

Nonspecific immunomodulation using a mixed bacterial vaccine or levamisole had no obvious effect on recurrence rates or survival following surgical excision of soft tissue sarcomas.[19,27]

Acemannan is another nonspecific immunomodulator that has been evaluated in a small number of cats with fibrosarcoma. Cats were injected with 2 mg/kg intralesionally weekly for 6 weeks prior to surgery and megavoltage radiation therapy (60 Gy). The cats then received 1 mg/kg intraperitoneally weekly for 6 weeks and then monthly for 1 year. Of four cats so treated, one had tumor recurrence 8 months after surgery but the other three had no recurrence for 14 to 19 months after surgery.[42] The true contribution of acemannan to survival in these cats is difficult to evaluate.

Xenogeneic cells (Vero hIL-2) that secrete human recombinant interleukin-2 (hrIL-2) were infiltrated around the tumor at the time of surgical resection and implantation of ^{192}Ir seeds for brachyradiotherapy.[24] This infiltration was repeated 5 days later and another five times over the next 2 months. Of 16 cats treated by this protocol, two had local recurrence and three had metastases, with an overall median survival of 16 months. In comparison, 11 of 16 cats that did not receive Vero hIL-2 cells had tumor recurrence and a median survival of 8 months. Antibodies to the cells were detected after 5 days of treatment, and most cats had a local inflammatory reaction to injection. One cat developed anaphylaxis.[24]

---

[a]Rassnick K: Personal communication.

Immunotherapy may contribute to longer survival in cats treated with local therapies for fibrosarcoma. Further studies involving the use of specific immunomodulators are needed to define the role of immunotherapy.

Supportive Care

Supportive care is critical in the treatment of soft tissue sarcomas and should include appropriate analgesia, nutritional support (including placement of gastrostomy or esophagostomy tubes if prolonged treatment is considered), and antiemetic therapy if needed. The placement of a vascular access port will likely be helpful if radiation and/or chemotherapy is used because the multiple anesthesia and chemotherapy treatments result in poor peripheral vascular integrity.

INJECTION SITE (VACCINE ASSOCIATED) SARCOMAS

Incidence, Signalment, and Etiology

Soft tissue sarcomas that occur in the subcutis of the dorsal neck/interscapular area, flank/paralumbar area, dorsolateral thorax, and femoral musculature have been increasing in frequency (Table 51-1).[43] These sarcomas have been termed *injection site sarcomas* or *vaccine associated sarcomas* due to their anatomic location at common sites of SQ injection. One study showed an eightfold increase in the number of sarcomas diagnosed from 1988 to 1994 and a similar increase in the ratio of injection site to noninjection site sarcomas (Table 51-2).[44] In the 5 years from 1984 to 1988, injection site sarcomas outnumbered sarcomas at other sites only once, while between 1989 and 1992 they were the most common type.[44] This coincides with widespread rabies vaccination and availability of FeLV vaccines. In three large studies encompassing 773 cats with sarcomas, 489 tumors occurred at injection sites.[43–45]

Injection site sarcomas occur in younger cats more often than do sarcomas at noninjection sites, with a peak at 6 to 7 years of age (Figure 51-11).[43,44,46] The signalment of affected cats is otherwise similar whether the sarcoma is injection site related or not.[43]

These tumors are most commonly fibrosarcomas but may also be described as osteosarcoma, malignant fibrous histiocytoma (histiocytic sarcoma), giant cell tumor, myofibroblastic sarcoma, rhabdomyosarcoma, leiomyosarcoma, chondrosarcoma, undifferentiated sarcoma, neurofibrosarcoma/nerve sheath tumor, and liposarcoma. The majority of injection site sarcomas have been associated with vaccination, particularly rabies and FeLV vaccines.[44,45,47] Sarcomas have also been associated with feline panleukopenia, herpesvirus, and calicivirus vaccination[48,49] in countries where vaccination for rabies and FeLV are not common. Sarcomas appear to arise months to years after vaccination (Table 51-3).[44,47] Injection site sarcomas have also arisen at the site of antibiotic administration, SQ fluid administration,[44,49–51] long-acting corticosteroid injection,[48] or lufenuron injection (Program® 6 month injectable).[52]

There have been many estimates of the incidence of sarcomas that occur following vaccination. Most have been based on estimates of the number of cats truly vaccinated, and all rely on what could be incomplete or biased reporting of tumors.

TABLE 51-1
Sites of Soft Tissue Sarcomas in 170 Cats[43]

Location	Number (%)
Vaccination Sites	
Interscapular/scapular	30 (17.6)
Flank/paralumbar	27 (15.9)
Dorsolateral thorax	19 (11.2)
Dorsal area of back or neck	17 (10.0)
Femoral region	11 (6.5)
Nonvaccination Sites	
Head (including oral cavity)	31 (18.2)
Limbs (including scapula and inner thigh)	13 (7.6)
Bone	3 (1.8)
Tail	4 (2.4)
Other	10 (5.9)
Dubious Vaccination Site	
Ventrolateral neck	5 (2.9)
Total	**170 (100)**

TABLE 51-2
Sarcomas as a Ratio of Total Feline Pathology Accessions and Ratio of Injection Site (IS) to NonInjection Site (NIS) Sarcomas[43]

Parameter	1989	1990	1991	1992	1993	1994
Total cat accessions	1,855	1,244	1,314	1,215	1,184	1,129
Fibrosarcoma:total ratio	1.13	1.69	2.97	1.65	3.04	2.92
IS:NIS ratio	0.54	1.00	1.47	1.86	2.6	4.33

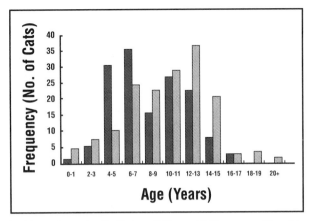

Figure 51-11: *Age distribution of 332 cats with fibrosarcoma. The solid bars are injection sites; shaded bars are noninjection sites. (From Kass PH, Barnes Jr WG, Spangler WL, et al: Epidemiologic evidence for a causal relation between vaccination and fibrosarcoma tumorigenesis in cats. JAVMA 203:396–405, 1993; with permission.)*

In California, one study estimated that 10 to 12 cats/100,000 would develop a sarcoma at a vaccination site.[44] A nationwide study involving 235 practitioners affiliated with the American Association of Feline Practitioners looked at the 1992 incidence of sarcomas in vaccinated cats.[53] This study found that 48% (158 of 329) were at vaccination sites and the incidence was 36 cats/100,000. Other estimates have ranged from 10/100,000 to 100/100,000.[54] One small study showed the risk of sarcoma formation to be 130/100,000 vaccinations.[48]

Injection site sarcomas are often associated with an inflammatory infiltrate, primarily macrophages, that are frequently reported to contain bluish "foreign material"[46,47] and may include giant cells.[46] In one study, aluminum was associated with this inflammation, leading to speculation that aluminum-containing adjuvants in vaccines may cause inflammatory changes that lead to carcinogenesis.[55] Trials with adjuvanted killed vaccines in 36 cats showed that 80%

to 100% of cats had a local inflammatory reaction following vaccination and that rabies vaccination created a larger inflammatory mass than did vaccination for FeLV.[50,54] Although reactions were most common with aluminum adjuvant vaccines, less common with non-aluminum adjuvant vaccines, and not seen with nonadjuvant vaccines, the size of the reaction was not related to the presence of aluminum. IM injection has been shown to cause the same reaction as SQ injection,[50] and sarcomas have occurred at IM injection sites,[48,56] although they appear to be less common at this location.[44]

One study showed an increasing risk of sarcoma formation with the use of killed vaccines.[48] The risk of sarcoma formation appears to be greatest following FeLV vaccination, with vaccinated cats being nearly three times more likely to develop a tumor than cats not receiving FeLV vaccine.[44] Rabies vaccination is less strongly associated with sarcoma formation, with vaccinated cats about twice as likely to develop a tumor.[44] Since adjuvants are used with killed vaccines and appear responsible for much of the inflammation, some investigators have suggested the preferential use of modified-live vaccination. However, some sarcomas have been associated with modified-live virus vaccination.[49]

The risk of sarcoma development increases with the number of vaccines given at a site (Figure 51-12). In one study, cats receiving three to four vaccinations in the interscapular region were nearly twice as likely to develop a sarcoma than if they received one vaccine at that site (Table 51-4).[44]

In one study of cats with sarcomas, vaccines received were cataloged according to their manufacturer. There were seven manufacturers of FVRCP vaccines, five manufacturers of FeLV vaccines, and eight manufacturers of rabies vaccines.[44] There was no association between manufacturers and tumor formation in this or other studies.[45]

It has been known that inflammation may cause sarcoma development in cats because ocular sarcomas at the site of

TABLE 51-3[44]
Details of 104 Cats with an Interscapular Sarcoma[a]

Vaccine Type	No. of Cats with Sarcoma That Received the Vaccine Within:				No. of Cats with Sarcoma That Did Not Receive This Vaccine at This Site
	2 Years	1 Year	6 Months	3 Months	
FVRCP	63	50	24	9	12
FeLV	47	41	20	7	32
Chlamydia	7	--	--	--	57
Rabies	33	22	15	4	48

[a]Becasue some cats received more than one vaccine type, numbers do not total 104.

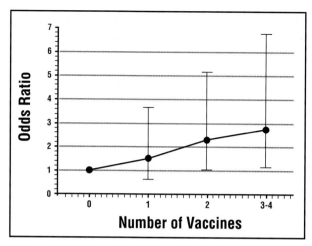

Figure 51-12: *The number of vaccines administered to the same injection site compared with the odds ratio of developing a soft tissue sarcoma within 1 year. (From Kass PH, Barnes Jr WG, Spangler WL, et al: Epidemiologic evidence for a causal relation between vaccination and fibrosarcoma tumorigenesis in cats.* JAVMA *203:396–405, 1993; with permission.)*

ocular trauma have been described[57,58] (see Chapter 40). Fibrosarcomas have also been induced by trauma in cats infected with FeSV.[59] FeSV requires FeLV as a "helper" virus in order to proliferate, so if FeSV were to be implicated in injection site sarcoma carcinogenesis, affected cats would be FeLV positive. Of 169 cats with sarcomas in one study, only 8 were FeLV positive and only 4 of these had injection site sarcomas.[44] In addition, of 36 cats tested for FIV, only 3 were antibody positive and only 1 of these had an injection site sarcoma. In a second study, all tested cats were FeLV and FIV negative.[45] Immunohistochemical staining of 130 injection site sarcomas showed no evidence of FeLV *gp70*, and polymerase chain reaction showed no evidence of FeLV in 100 injection site sarcomas.[60] It seems unlikely that FeSV is involved in injection site sarcoma development.

The development of sarcomas does seem to be related to the presence of oncogenes and mutations in tumor suppressor genes. Approximately 75% of injection sarcomas were found to contain *p53* and *c-kit* oncogene.[61] Approximately one third of tumors contained both mutated *p53* and *mdm-2*, and these tumors were histologically more anaplastic, perhaps explaining the aggressive biologic be-

TABLE 51-4[44]
Sarcoma in the Interscapular Region

No. of Vaccinations	Risk	Odds Ratio
0 (control)	1.0	
1	1.49	0.61–3.64
2	2.27	1.02–5.15
3 or 4	2.75	1.12–6.74

havior of some injection site sarcomas.

The current thinking is that individual cats may respond to inflammatory changes in a manner that predisposes to sarcoma formation. This is supported by the discovery of cats that have developed sarcomas at more than one injection site and the finding of injection site sarcomas in related cats.[50] Current studies to investigate the cytogenetics of injection site sarcomas may provide more information. Up-to-date information regarding research can be obtained from the Vaccine Associated Fibrosarcoma Task Force (http://www.avma.org/vafstf/default.asp).

MDB = minimum database; includes CBC, biochemical profile, urinalysis, FeLV/FIV serology, T_4 testing, and thoracic radiographs (three views).

Clinical Presentation and History

The occurrence of a mass at a site commonly used for SQ or IM injections should alert the clinician to the possibility of an injection site sarcoma. In particular, biopsy samples should be collected from a vaccination reaction that persists or starts to increase in size. In one study, most reactions following rabies or FeLV vaccination had resolved within 2 to 3 months[5]; some oncologists believe that a biopsy sample should be obtained when a vaccine reaction persists longer than 1 month.

Injection site sarcomas are more likely to appear in the subcutis, while noninjection site tumors occur more frequently in the dermis.[43] Injection site sarcomas are usually larger than sarcomas at other sites. In one study, 26 of 54 (48%) injection site tumors had a diameter of 4 cm or more and only one tumor was less than 1 cm in diameter.[45] In contrast, 16 of 63 (25%) sarcomas at other sites were at least 4 cm in diameter and 10 were less than 1 cm. It is possible that this reflects the inability of an owner to detect tumors at injection sites and emphasizes the need for owner education to improve early detection of tumors.

Staging and Diagnosis

Fine-needle aspiration of an injection site sarcoma may reveal a spindle cell sarcoma or mesenchymal tumor. The exact histologic diagnosis matters less than the classification as a soft tissue sarcoma. Most oncologists recommend an initial needle or incisional biopsy rather than an attempt at excisional biopsy. This is because an aggressive first surgery or presurgical radiation therapy will provide a better outcome than will treating a recurrence.

Injection site sarcomas often contain necrotic areas, probably secondary to vascular thrombosis and abscessation.[43] These tumors are more likely than noninjection site tumors to show lymphocytic and macrophage inflammation, often progressing to granulation tissue.[43,46] These inflammatory macrophages often contain phagocytosed bluish material,[47] which may be vaccine adjuvant.

Histologically, injection site sarcomas are locally invasive, have more mitotic figures, and appear more pleomorphic (less differentiated, more anaplastic) than noninjection site tumors.[43,47] Indeed, only injection site sarcomas showed production of osteoid, chondroid, or myxomatous tissue in one study.[43] The intercellular matrix was more variable in these tumors. Malignant fibrous histiocytoma (histiocytic sarcoma) was a diagnosis made only at injection sites in two studies[43,45] and appears to be associated with vascular invasion more commonly than other types of sarcomas.[43]

There may be increased risk of metastasis from injection site sarcomas. In one study, staging procedures prior to initial treatment revealed no evidence of metastasis in any cat.[45] However, following diagnosis and treatment, three cats developed pulmonary metastases and a fourth developed skeletal metastases from injection site sarcomas; only one cat developed pulmonary metastases from a noninjection site sarcoma.

Seven individual case reports have documented metastases from injection site sarcomas. Five cats had interscapular tumors,[48,62-65] three of which metastasized within 4 months of the first surgical excision. The other two cats had a tumor of the flank or hip.[54,55] The most common metastatic site was the lungs (five cats), followed by the liver (three), mediastinum (two), spleen (two), kidney (two), and eye, pancreas, and intestines (one each). Interestingly, abdominal metatases were all that were detected in two cats.[64,67]

In addition to needle biopsy of the tumor, staging for cats with suspected injection site sarcoma should include an MDB, thorough history of previous vaccinations and injections, and abdominal ultrasound. A CT scan or MRI should also be performed to allow delineation of the tumor margins for appropriate surgical planning. Regional lymph nodes should be palpated and aspirated if enlarged.

Treatment

Treatment options are the same as outlined for other soft tissue sarcomas. There is some concern that delaying surgery may increase the likelihood of metastasis.[67]

FELINE SARCOMA VIRUS ASSOCIATED SARCOMAS

Incidence, Signalment, and Etiology

FeSV was first isolated from multiple SQ fibrosarcomas in a 2-year-old female DSH.[68] FeSV is a recombinant virus formed when proviral DNA from the FeLV virus is combined with a cellular oncogene from the infected cat. FeSV also requires FeLV to provide certain genes in order to replicate.[59] This means that only cats infected with FeLV have the capacity to generate FeSV.

Because of the dependence on FeLV, the immunologic reactions to FeSV are essentially the same as for FeLV. Feline oncornavirus-associated cell membrane antigen (FOCMA) antibodies appear to protect against the formation of sarcomas and may cause tumor regression[69,70]; disappearance of FOCMA in experimentally infected cats leads to rapid recurrence and widespread metastasis of sarcomas.[69] FeSV has many different "strains." Seven strains have been isolated from cats between the ages of 14 months and 5 years with multiple tumors,[59,68,71] and two strains were isolated from solitary tumors in 7-year-old cats. The majority of cats with FeSV that were tested for FeLV have been FeLV positive (Table 51-5).

Clinical Presentation and History

Cats that have multiple soft tissue sarcomas should be considered potentially infected with FeSV/FeLV, particularly if the cat is younger than 5 years of age. Multiple tumors are sometimes seen in FeLV-negative cats[59] and as an injection site phenomenon.[50]

Staging and Diagnosis

Cats with multiple soft tissue sarcomas should be tested for FeLV by ELISA and/or IFA or by PCR if available. FeSV has been isolated from cats with solitary tumors, and these tumors may have a higher metastatic rate than sarcomas in cats without FeSV. Of six FeSV-positive cats with multiple tumors, three had metastases.[59] An FeLV-positive 10-month-old cat with multiple rapidly metastasizing sarcomas to regional lymph nodes and lungs probably had an FeSV-related tumor.[17] Cats with metastatic sarcomas should be tested for FeSV/FeLV. Some investigators believe that FeSV is a significant public risk as it has the experimental potential to infect non-Felidae.[72] Cats that have sarcoma and FeLV should

TABLE 51-5
FeLV Status of Cats with Sarcomas[59]

Age of Affected Cats	FeLV-Positive Cats	FeLV-Negative Cats
Cats with Solitary Tumors		
≤5 years	0	4
>5 years	0	34
Cats with Multiple Tumors		
≤5 years	19	0
>5 years	1	3

therefore be treated with this possibility in mind.

Staging should include an MDB, needle biopsy of the tumor(s), abdominal ultrasonography, and lymph node cytology if lymphadenopathy exists. If treatment is to be undertaken, a CT scan or MRI should be performed to examine the margins of the tumor(s).

Treatment

Some investigators believe that cats with FeSV-induced fibrosarcomas should be euthanized due to the public health risk of transspecies infection. Certainly treatment as outlined in the preceding sections would be difficult in an FeLV-positive cat due to potential for secondary problems. There have been no studies to show that these tumors are more or less likely to respond to treatment than non-FeSV-related sarcomas. Appropriate supportive care, including adequate analgesia and nutritional support, should be provided with any treatment undertaken.

NONDOMESTIC FELIDAE

Very few soft tissue sarcomas have been reported in non-domestic Felidae. A Bengal tiger (Panthera tigris tigris) was recorded as having a liposarcoma of an undisclosed site.[73] Another Bengal tiger had a leiomyosarcoma of the hind leg that was removed by amputation. Three years later, the cat was euthanized due to lethargy, anorexia, and the radiographic finding of pulmonary metastases.[74] Metastases affected the muscular fascia throughout the body as well as lungs, intraabdominal fat, urethra, pancreas, liver, gastric mucosa, and brain.

An 18-year-old female lion (Panthera leo) with a history of ascites and anorexia was found on necropsy to have multiple intraabdominal rhabdomyosarcomas.[75]

REFERENCES

1. de las Mulas JM, de los Monteros AE, Carrasco L, et al: Immunohistochemical distribution pattern of intermediate filament proteins in 50 feline neoplasms. Vet Pathol 32:692–701, 1995.

2. Moore AS, Madewell BR, Lund JK: Immunohistochemical evaluation of intermediate filament expression in canine and feline neoplasms. Am J Vet Res 50:88–92, 1989.

3. Jones SA, Strafuss AC: Scanning electron microscopy of nerve sheath neoplasms. Am J Vet Res 39:1069–1072, 1978.

4. Jones BR, Alley MR, Johnstone AC, et al: Nerve sheath tumours in the dog and cat. N Z Vet J 43:190–196, 1995.

5. Silva ALA, Serakides R: Schwannoma tipo Antoni A em gato. Arq Bras Med Vet Zootec 47:257–259, 1995.

6. Goldschmidt MH, Shofer FS: Skin Tumors of the Dog and Cat. New York, Pergamon Press, 1992.

7. Stiglmair-Herb VM, Ortmann U: Die fibrosarkome der katze unter besonderer berücksichtigung ihrer dignität. Kleintierpraxis 32:75–80, 1986.

8. Roth L: Rhabdomyoma of the ear pinna in four cats. J Comp Pathol 103:237–240, 1990.

9. Kalat M, Mayr B, Schleger W, et al: Trisomy D2 in a feline neurofibroma. Res Vet Sci 48:256, 1990.

10. Kalat M, Mayr B, Schleger W, et al: Chromosomal hyperdiploidy in a feline sarcoma. Res Vet Sci 51:227–228, 1991.

11. Mayr B, Wegscheider H, Reifinger M, Jugl T: Cytogenetic alterations in four feline soft-tissue tumours. Vet Res Comm 22:21–29, 1998.

12. Mayr B, Schaffner G, Kurzbauer R, et al: Mutations in tumour suppressor gene p53 in two feline fibrosarcomas. Br Vet J 151:707–713, 1995.

13. Mayr B, Reifinger M, Alton K, Schaffner G: Novel p53 tumour suppressor mutations in cases of spindle cell sarcoma, pleomorphic sarcoma and fibrosarcoma in cats. Vet Res Comm 22:249–255, 1998.

14. Kanjilal S, Banerji N, Fifer A, et al: p53 tumor suppressor gene alterations in vaccine-associated feline sarcoma. Proc 9th Annu Conf Vet Cancer Soc:48, 1999.

15. Hershey AE, Dubielzieg RR, Helfand SC: Overexpression of p53 in feline vaccine-assocated sarcomas. Proc 9th Annu Conf Vet Cancer Soc:32, 1999.

16. Cook JL, Turk JR, Tomlinson JL, et al: Fibrosarcoma in the distal radius and carpus of a four-year-old Persian. JAAHA 34:31–33, 1998.

17. Harasen GLG: Multicentric fibrosarcoma in a cat and a review of the literature. Can Vet J 25:207–210, 1984.

18. Trout NJ, Pavletic MM, Kraus KH: Partial scapulectomy for management of sarcomas in three dogs and two cats. JAVMA 207:585–587, 1995.

19. Brown NO, Patnaik AK, Mooney SC, et al: Soft tissue sarcomas in the cat. JAVMA 173:744–779, 1978.

20. Moon ML, Saunders GK, Martin RA: Vertebral osteosclerosis in a cat secondary to rhabdomyosarcoma. Vet Radiol 31:39–41, 1990.

21. Ruben JMS: Neurofibrosarcoma in a 19-year-old cat. Vet Rec 113:135, 1983.

22. Levy MS, Mauldin G, Kapatkin AS, Patnaik AK: Nonlymphoid vertebral canal tumors in cats: 11 cases (1987–1995). JAVMA 210:663–664, 1997.

23. Watrous BJ, Lipscomb TP, Heidel JR, Normal LM: Malignant peripheral nerve sheath tumor in a cat. Vet Radiol Ultrasound 40:638–640, 1999.

24. Quintin-Colonna F, Devauchelle P, Fradelizi D, et al: Gene therapy of spontaneous canine melanoma and feline fibrosarcoma by intratumoral administration of histoincompatible cells expressing human interleukin-2. Gene Therap 3:1104–1112, 1996.

25. Davidson EB, Gregory CR, Kass PH: Surgical excision of soft tissue fibrosarcomas in cats. Vet Surg 26:265–269, 1997.

26. Cronin K, Page RL, Spodnick G, et al: Radiation therapy and surgery for fibrosarcoma in 33 cats. Vet Radiol Ultrasound 39:51–56, 1998.

27. Brown NO, Hayes AA, Mooney S: Combined modality therapy in the treatment of solid tumors in cats. JAAHA 16:719–722, 1980.

28. Hershey AE, Sorenmo KU, Hendrick MJ, et al: Prognosis for presumed feline vaccine-associated sarcoma after excision: 61 cases (1986–1996). JAVMA 216:58–61, 2000.

29. Schwyn U, Crompton NEA, Blattman H, et al: Potential tumour doubling time: Determination of T$_{pot}$ for various canine and feline tumours. Vet Res Comm 22:233–247, 1998.

30. Bostock DE, Dye MT: Prognosis after surgical excision of fibrosarcomas in cats. JAVMA 175:727–728, 1979.

31. Devauchelle P: Interest and limits of brachytherapy (interstitial radiotherapy) as adjuvant treatment of feline soft-tissue sarcomas. Proc ESVIM 7:44, 1997.

32. Buyukmihci N: Fibrosarcoma of the nictitating membrane in a cat. JAVMA 167:934–935, 1975.

33. Straw RC, Withrow SJ, Powers BE: Partial or total hemipelvectomy in the management of sarcomas in nine dogs and two cats. Vet Surg 21:183–188, 1992.

34. Bowmann KLT, Birchard SJ, Bright RM: Complications associated with the implantation of polypropylene mesh in dogs and cats: A retrospective study of 21 cases (1984–1996). JAAHA 34:225–233, 1998.

35. Odenall JSJ, Cronje JDE, Bastanello SS: Chirurgiese en chemotherapeutiese behandeling van fibrosarcoma in n'Kat. J South Afr Vet Assoc 205–208, 1983.

36. Dommert R: Hemangiopericytoma in a cat. Southwestern Vet 14:149–150, 1961.

37. Hilmas DE, Gillette EL: Radiotherapy of spontaneous fibrous connective-tissue sarcomas in animals. J Natl Cancer Inst 56:365–368, 1976.

38. Bongiovanni S, Bengtson AE, Gliatto JM, et al: Prognostic indicators associated with adjuvant radiotherapy for cats with soft tissue sarcoma. Proc 19th Annu Conf Vet Cancer Soc:44, 1999.

39. Bregazzi VS, LaRue SM, McNiel E, et al: Treatment with a combination of doxorubicin, surgery, and radiation versus surgery and radiation alone for cats with vaccine-associated sarcomas: 25 cases (1995–2000). JAVMA 218:547–550, 2001.

40. Kleiter M, Leschnik M: Postoperative chemotherapie zur behandlung eines zweifach rezidivierten vakzine-assoziierten fibrosarkoms. Kleintierpraxis 43:295–302, 1998.

41. Mir LM, Devauchelle P, Quintin-Colonna F, et al: First clinical trial of cat soft-tissue sarcomas treatment by electrochemotherapy. Br J Cancer 76:1617–1622, 1997.

42. King GK, Yates KM, Greenlee PG, et al: The effect of acemannan immunostimulant in combination with surgery and radiation therapy on spontaneous

canine and feline fibrosarcomas. *JAAHA* 31:439–447, 1995.

43. Doddy FD, Glickman LT, Glickman NW, Janovitz EB: Feline fibrosarcomas at vaccination sites and non-vaccination sites. *J Comp Pathol* 114:165–174, 1996.

44. Kass PH, Barnes Jr WG, Spangler WL, et al: Epidemiologic evidence for a causal relation between vaccination and fibrosarcoma tumorigenesis in cats. *JAVMA* 203:396–405, 1993.

45. Hendrick MJ, Shofer FS, Goldschmidt MH, et al: Comparison of fibrosarcomas that developed at vaccination sites and at non-vaccination sites in cats: 239 cases (1991–1992). *JAVMA* 205:1425–1429, 1994.

46. Hendrick MJ, Brooks JJ: Postvaccinal sarcomas in the cat: Histology and immunohistochemistry. *Vet Pathol* 31:126–129, 1994.

47. Esplin DG, McGill LD, Meininger AC, Wilson SR: Postvaccination sarcomas in cats. *JAVMA* 202:1245–1247, 1993.

48. Lester S, Clemett T, Burt A: Vaccine site-associated sarcomas in cats: Clinical experience and a laboratory review (1982–1993). *JAAHA* 32:91–95, 1996.

49. Burton G, Mason KV: Do postvaccinal sarcomas occur in Australian cats? *Aust Vet J* 75:102–106, 1997.

50. Macy DW: Current understanding of vaccination site-associated sarcomas in the cat. *J Feline Med Surg* 1:15–21, 1999.

51. Gagnon A-C: Drug injection-associated fibrosarcoma in a cat. *Feline Pract* 28:18–21, 2000.

52. Esplin DG, Bigelow M, McGill LD, Wilson SR: Fibrosarcoma at the site of a lufenuron injection in a cat. *Vet Cancer Soc Newsl* 23:8–9, 1999.

53. Coyne MJ, Postorino Reeves NC, Rosen DK: Estimated prevalence of injection-site sarcomas in cats during 1992. *JAVMA* 210:249–251, 1997.

54. Macy DW, Hendrick MJ: The potential role of inflammation in the development of postvaccinal sarcomas in cats. *Vet Clin North Am Small Anim Pract* 26:103–109, 1996.

55. Hendrick M, Goldschmidt MH, Shofer F, et al: Postvaccinal sarcomas in the cat: Epidemiology and electron probe microanalytical identification of aluminum. *Cancer Res* 52:5391–5394, 1992.

56. Dubielzieg RR, Hawkins KL, Miller PE: Myofibroblastic sarcoma originating at the site of rabies vaccination in a cat. *J Vet Diagn Invest* 5:637–638, 1993.

57. Peiffer RL, Monticello T, Bouldin TW: Primary ocular sarcomas in the cat. *J Small Anim Pract* 29:105–116, 1988.

58. Dubielzig RR, Everitt J, Shadduck JA, Albert DM: Clinical and morphologic features of post-traumatic ocular sarcomas in cats. *Vet Pathol* 27:62–65, 1990.

59. Hardy Jr WD: The feline sarcoma viruses. *JAAHA* 17:981–997, 1981.

60. Ellis JA, Jackson ML, Bartsch RC, et al: Use of immunohistochemistry and polymerase chain reaction for detection of oncornaviruses in formalin-fixed, paraffin-embedded fibrosarcomas from cats. *JAVMA* 209:767–771, 1996.

61. Goad MEP, Lopez MK, Goad DL: Expression of tumor suppressor genes and oncogenes in feline injection-site associated sarcomas [abstract 129]. *J Vet Intern Med* 13:258, 1999.

62. Esplin DG, Campbell R: Widespread metastasis of a fibrosarcoma associated with a vaccination site in a cat. *Feline Pract* 23:13–16, 1995.

63. Rudmann DG, Van Alstine WG, Doddy F, et al: Pulmonary and mediastinal metastases of a vaccination-site sarcoma in a cat. *Vet Pathol* 33:466–469, 1996.

64. Sandler I, Teeger M, Best S: Metastatic vaccine associated fibrosarcoma in a 10-year-old cat. *Can Vet J* 38:374, 1997.

65. Briscoe C, Lipscomb T, McKinney LA: Pulmonary metastasis of a feline post-vaccinal fibrosarcoma. *Vet Pathol* 32:564, 1995.

66. Fulton LM, Bromberg NM, Goldschmidt MH: Soft tissue fibrosarcoma with intraocular metastasis in a cat. *Prog Vet Comp Ophthalmol* 1:129–132, 1991.

67. Esplin DG, Jaffe MH, McGill LD: Metastasizing liposarcoma associated with a vaccination site in a cat. *Feline Pract* 24:20–23, 1996.

68. Snyder SP, Theilen GH: Transmissible feline fibrosarcoma. *Nature* 221:1074–1075, 1969.

69. Aldrich CD, Pedersen NC: Persistent viremia after regression of primary virus-induced feline fibrosarcomas. *Am J Vet Res* 35:1383–1387, 1974.

70. Essex M, Klein G, Snyder SP, Harrold JB: Correlation between humoral antibody and regression of tumours induced by feline sarcoma virus. *Nature* 233:195–196, 1971.

71. Irgens K, Wyers M, Moraillon A, et al: Isolement d'un virus sarcomatogene felin a partir d'un firbrosarcome spontane du Chat: Etude de pouvoir sacomtagene in vivo. *C R Acad Sci Paris* 276:1783–1786, 1973.

72. Hardy WD Jr: Oncogenic viruses of cats: The feline leukemia and sarcoma viruses, in Holzworth J (ed): *Diseases of the Cat. Medicine and Surgery.* Philadelphia, WB Saunders, 1987, pp 246–268.

73. Effron M, Griner L, Benirschke K: Nature and rate of neoplasia found in captive wild mammals, birds and reptiles at necropsy. *J Natl Cancer Inst* 59:185–198, 1977.

74. Saunders G: Disseminated leiomyosarcoma in a Bengal tiger. *JAVMA* 185:1387–1388, 1984.

75. Starzynski W, Rokioki J: Abnormal findings from abdominal cavity of big felidae in Warsaw Zoo. *Erkrankungen der Zootiere,* 1974, pp 127–131.

ACEPROMAZINE (PromAce®)

Use:	Preanesthetic; sedative
How Supplied:	Injectable: 10 mg/ml in 50 ml vials
Dose:	0.025–0.05 mg/kg IV, SQ, or IM (use with butorphanol for painful procedures)

ACITRETIN (Soriatane®)

Use:	Antineoplastic agent; retinoic acid derivative
How Supplied:	Oral: 10 and 25 mg capsules
Dose:	10 mg/cat PO sid

ACTINOMYCIN D (Dactinomycin®)

Use:	Antineoplastic agent
How Supplied:	Injectable: 0.5 mg vials
Dose:	0.5–0.9 mg/m^2 IV slow infusion (over 20 min) q3wk

ALIMENTATION, ORAL (Osmolite HN®, Jevity®)

Use:	Nutritional supplement
How Supplied:	Oral liquid: 8 oz cans, 1.06 calories/ml
Dose:	Calculate animal's daily caloric requirement (DCR) Day 1: Give 0.25 DCR Day 2: Give 0.5 DCR Day 3 and beyond: Give total DCR divided into frequent feedings (four to seven meals/d) or by constant infusion

AMOXICILLIN
(Amoxi-Drop®, Amoxi-Tabs®, Amoxi-Inject®)

Use:	Broad-spectrum antibiotic
How Supplied:	Injectable: 250 mg/ml in 25 g vials Oral: 50, 100, 200, and 400 mg tablets; 50 mg/ml suspension in 15 ml bottles
Dose:	11 mg/kg (5 mg/lb) PO, SQ, or IM bid

AMOXICILLIN-CLAVULANIC ACID (Clavamox®)

Use:	Broad-spectrum antibiotic (effective against many penicillinase-producing pathogens)
How Supplied:	Oral: Fixed combination of 4 parts amoxicillin to 1 part clavulanic acid

(as the potassium salt); 62.5, 125, 250, and 375 mg tablets; 62.5 mg/ml suspension in 15 ml bottles

Dose:	13.75 mg/kg (6.25 mg/lb) PO bid

AMPICILLIN SODIUM

Use:	Broad-spectrum antibiotic
How Supplied:	Injectable: 1 g vials
Dose:	22 mg/kg (10 mg/lb) IM, IV, or SQ tid
Note:	Approximately 6% loss of potency/8 hr when mixed to 100 mg/ml and stored in a refrigerator

L-ASPARAGINASE (Elspar®)

Use:	Antineoplastic agent
How Supplied:	Injectable: 10,000 U/vials
Dose:	10,000 U/m^2 (or 400 U/kg) IM q7–21d

ASPIRIN (acetylsalicylic acid)

Use:	Analgesic, antipyretic, antiprostaglandin
How Supplied:	Oral: 80 and 325 mg tablets; 1 lb powder
Dose:	10 mg/kg (4.5 mg/lb) PO q48–72h prn for pain

ATROPINE

Use:	Anticholinergic, mydriatic, cycloplegia
How Supplied:	Injectable: 0.5 mg/ml in 100 ml vials 1% Ophthalmic ointment in 3.5 g tubes 1% Ophthalmic solution in 15 ml bottles
Dose:	0.04 mg/kg (0.02 mg/lb) IV, SQ, or IM

AZATHIOPRINE (Imuran®)

Use:	Immunosuppressive, antimetabolite
How Supplied:	Oral: 50 mg tablets
Dose:	0.3–1.0 mg/kg PO eod
Note:	Not recommended for use in cats by some authors because of potential for fatal toxicity and difficulty in accurate dosing

BLEOMYCIN (Blenoxane®)

Use:	Antineoplastic agent
How Supplied:	Injectable: 15 mg (15 U) vials (1 mg = 1 U)
Dose:	0.3–0.5 U/kg IM or SQ once weekly to an accumulated dose of 125–200 mg/m^2; IV push over at least 10 min

---

*Note: This section contains information on the most important and/or commonly discussed drugs in this book. Highly experimental agents or those with limited availability have not been included.

BUPIVACAINE (Marcaine®)

Use: Long-acting local anesthetic
How Supplied: 0.75% Injectable solution in 30 ml
                   single dose vials
Dose: 1–2 mg/4.5 kg for local blocks and/or
                   intrapleural infusion

BUPRENORPHINE (Buprenex®)

Use: Opioid agonist-antagonist
How Supplied: Injectable: 0.3 mg/ml in 1 ml ampules
Dose: 0.005–0.01 mg/kg IM, IV, or SQ
                   q4–12h
Note: Schedule V Controlled Substance

BUSULFAN (Myleran®)

Use: Antineoplastic agent
How Supplied: Oral: 2 mg tablets
Dose: 2 mg/m^2 PO sid

BUTORPHANOL (Torbugesic®, Torbutrol®)

Use: Central-acting analgesic, narcotic
                   agonist-antagonist
How Supplied: Injectable: 10 mg/ml in 50 ml vials
                   Oral: 5 mg tablets
Dose: Analgesia: 0.1–0.4 mg/kg IM, IV, or
                   SQ q1–4h
                   Somatic pain: 0.8 mg/kg IV q2h
                   Nausea and vomiting: 0.4 mg/kg IM q8h
Note: Butorphanol possesses antagonist
                   properties and will reverse the effects
                   of narcotics. Therefore do not give
                   butorphanol within 12 hours of any
                   pre- or intraoperative narcotics.
                   Schedule IV Controlled Substance

CALCIUM GLUCONATE/BOROGLUCONATE

Use: Hypocalcemia
How Supplied: 10% Injectable solution in 10 ml
                   ampules
                   23% solution in 500 ml vials
                   26% solution with Mg, P, and dextrose
                   in 500 ml vials (Norcalciphos™)
Dose: 1–1.5 ml/kg 10% solution IV (slowly
                   over 10–20 min)

CARBOPLATIN (Paraplatin®)

Use: Antineoplastic agent
How Supplied: Injectable: 50, 150, and 450 mg vials
Dose: 200–220 mg/m^2 IV q4wk
Note: Dilute with 5% dextrose in water to
                   10 mg/ml

CARPROFEN (Rimadyl®)

Use: Analgesic, antiinflammatory (Caution:
                   Not approved for use in cats in some
                   countries)
How Supplied: Oral: 25, 75, and 100 mg tablets
Dose: 4 mg/kg IV, IM, or SQ preoperatively,
                   reducing to 2 mg/kg PO q24h
                   postoperatively for up to 3 days.
Note: The use of carprofen for longer than
                   3 days is not recommended in the cat
                   due to toxicity (GI ulceration and
                   kidney damage).

CEFADROXIL (Cefa-Tabs®)

Use: First generation cephalosporin antibiotic
How Supplied: Oral: 50 and 100 mg tablets
Dose: 11–22 mg/kg (5–10 mg/lb) PO bid

CEFAZOLIN (Ancef®)

Use: First generation cephalosporin antibiotic
How Supplied: Injectable: 250 mg, 500 mg, and 1 g vials
Dose: 22 mg/kg (10 mg/lb) IV, IM, or SQ q8h
                   For surgical prophylaxis: give within 30
                   minutes of actual surgery and repeat
                   every 2.5 h

CEFOXITIN (Mefoxin®)

Use: Second generation cephalosporin antibiotic
How Supplied: Injectable: 1 g vials
Dose: 22 mg/kg (10 mg/lb) slow IV tid

CEPHALEXIN (Keflex®)

Use: First generation cephalosporin antibiotic
How Supplied: Oral: 25 mg/ml suspension in 100 ml
                   bottles; 250 and 500 mg capsules or
                   tablets
Dose: 11–22 mg/kg (5–10 mg/lb) PO tid

CHLORAMBUCIL (Leukeran®)

Use: Antineoplastic agent
How Supplied: Oral: 2 mg coated tablets
Dose: 6 mg/m^2 sid (or equivalent thereof in 1
                   week's time)

CHLORPHENIRAMINE
(Aller-Chlor®, Chlor-Trimeton®)

Use: Antihistamine
How Supplied: Oral: 4 mg tablets
Dose: 2–4 mg PO sid–bid

CHLORPROMAZINE (Thorazine®)

Use:	Tranquilizer, antiemetic
How Supplied:	Injectable: 25 mg/ml in 2 ml ampules
Dose:	0.5 mg/kg IM or SQ q6–8h

CIMETIDINE (Tagamet®)

Use:	H_2-receptor antagonist
How Supplied:	Oral: 100, 200, and 300 mg tablets
	Injectable: 150 mg/ml in 2 and 8 ml vials
Dose:	2.5 mg/kg (1.14 mg/lb) PO or slow IV push bid

CISAPRIDE (Propulsid®)

Use:	Cholinergic enhancer, GI emptying adjunct
How Supplied:	Oral: 10 mg tablets
Dose:	0.1–0.5 mg/kg PO given 30 min before meals up to tid

CISPLATIN (Cis-Diamminedichloroplatinum II)
(Platinol®)

Use:	Antineoplastic agent
How Supplied:	Injectable: 1 mg/ml in 10, 50, and 100 mg vials
Dose:	Intralesional use only
Note:	Not for IV use in cats—FATAL

CLINDAMYCIN (Antirobe®)

Use:	Antibiotic
How Supplied:	Oral: 25, 75, and 150 mg capsules; 25 mg/ml solution in 20 ml bottles
Dose:	12.5 mg/kg (5.7 mg/lb) PO bid for 28 d for toxoplasmosis

CYCLOPHOSPHAMIDE
(Cytoxan®, Endoxan®, Neosar®)

Use:	Antineoplastic agent
How Supplied:	Oral: 25 and 50 mg tablets
	Injectable: 100 mg, 200 mg, 500 mg, 1 g, and 2 g vials (reconstituted with 20 ml of D5W to make 10 mg/ml)
Dose:	250 mg/m² IV or PO q3wk for 4–8 treatments
	OR
	50 mg/m² PO or IV sid on days 3, 4, 5, and 6 following doxorubicin administration

CYPROHEPTADINE (Periactin®)

Use:	Appetite stimulant
How Supplied:	Oral: 4 mg (scored) tablets
Dose:	1–2 mg/cat PO sid–bid

CYTOSINE ARABINOSIDE, CYTARABINE
(Cytosar-U®)

Use:	Antineoplastic agent
How Supplied:	Injectable: 100 mg, 500 mg, 1g, and 2 g vials (reconstituted to 20 mg/ml)
Dose:	60–100 mg/m² IV (constant rate infusion) daily for 2–4 days; if no toxicity, increase to 150 mg/m² daily for 4 days
	OR
	10 mg/m² SQ sid–bid

DEXAMETHASONE (Azium®, Decadron®)

Use:	Corticosteroid therapy
How Supplied:	Injectable: 2 mg/ml in 100 ml vials
	Oral: 0.25 and 4 mg tablets
	0.1% Ophthalmic ointment with neomycin (3.5 mg/g) and polymyxin B (10,000 U/g) in 3.5 g tubes (Maxitrol®, Dexacidin®, AK-Trol®)
	0.1% Ophthalmic suspension in 15 ml bottles (Maxidex™)
	0.1% Ophthalmic suspension with neomycin (3.5 mg/ml) and polymyxin B (10,000 U/ml) in 5 ml tubes (Maxitrol®, Dexacidin®, AK-Trol®)
Dose:	0.28–2.2 mg/kg (0.125–1 mg/lb) PO or IM
	Screening dose: 0.1 mg/kg IV
	Suppression dose: 1.0 mg/kg IV
	Antiemetic dose: 1 mg/cat IV

DIAZEPAM (Valium®)

Use:	Tranquilizer, anticonvulsant, appetite stimulant
How Supplied:	Injectable: 5 mg/ml in 2 and 10 ml vials
Dose:	Anesthetic induction: 0.5–1 mg/kg IV (use with butorphanol for painful procedures)
	Appetite stimulant: 0.05–0.1 mg/kg IV
	Premedication: 0.2 mg/kg IV sid–bid
Note:	Schedule IV Controlled Substance

DIMENHYDRINATE (Dramamine®)

Use:	Antiemetic
How Supplied:	Injectable: 50 mg/ml in 1 ml vials
Dose:	8 mg/kg PO tid

DIPHENHYDRAMINE (Benadryl®)

Use:	Antiemetic, antihistamine
How Supplied:	Oral: 12.5 mg tablets and 25 mg capsules; 12.5 mg/ml oral elixir in 4 and 16 oz bottles
	Injectable: 10 mg/ml in 10 and 30 ml vials; 50 mg/ml in 1 and 10 ml vials
Dose:	2–4 mg/kg PO or IM tid

DOLASETRON MESYLATE (Anzemet®)

Use:	Antiemetic, antinausea
How Supplied:	12.5 mg ampules
Dose:	0.6–1 mg/kg IV slowly

DOXORUBICIN

(Adriamycin®, Doxorubicin®, Rubex®)

Use:	Antineoplastic agent
How Supplied:	Injectable: 2 mg/ml in 10, 20, 50, 150, and 200 mg vials
Dose:	1–1.1 mg/kg or 20–25 mg/m^2 IV slow infusion (over 30 min) q3wk
	Maximum cumulative dose: 180–240 mg/m^2 over lifetime
Note:	Dilute with NaCl solution prior to IV administration

DOXYCYCLINE (Vibramycin®)

Use:	Long-acting broad-spectrum tetracycline, metalloproteinase inhibitor
How Supplied:	Oral: 10 mg/ml suspension in 16 oz bottles; 100 mg tablets
Dose:	5 mg/kg (2.3 mg/lb) PO sid–bid

ENROFLOXACIN (Baytril®)

Use:	Broad-spectrum antibacterial (fluoroquinolone)
How Supplied:	Injectable: 22.7 mg/ml in 20 ml bottles
	Oral: 22.7 and 68 mg tablets
Dose:	5 mg/kg (1.13 mg/lb) PO or IM sid
	Dose may be increased to 20 mg/kg daily depending on infection and/or situation; daily dose may be divided and given bid
Note:	Per manufacturer, dosages greater than 5 mg/kg sid in cats may be associated with blindness, temporary blindness, partial blindness, and mydriasis.

ERYTHROPOIETIN, HUMAN RECOMBINANT

(Epogen®)

Use:	Stimulation of RBC production
How Supplied:	4000 U/ml in 1 ml vials
Dose:	Initial: 100 U/kg SQ 3 times/wk; may be decreased to twice weekly or increased in 50 U/kg increments depending on response
Note:	Antibody development to erythropoietin may cause anemia.

ERYTHROMYCIN

Use:	Macrolide antibiotic
How Supplied:	Oral: 250 mg tablets
Dose:	11–22 mg/kg (5–10 mg/lb) PO with small amount of food tid

ETOMIDATE

Use:	Anesthesia, hypnotic
How Supplied:	Injectable: 2 mg/ml in 20 ml vials
Dose:	1 mg/kg IV

FAMOTIDINE (Pepcid AC®)

Use:	H$_2$-receptor antagonist
How Supplied:	Injectable: 10 mg/ml in 20 ml vials
	Oral: 10 mg tablets
Dose:	0.5 mg/kg PO, SQ, or IV sid–bid

FATTY ACIDS (3V Caps®, Derm Caps Liquid®)

Use:	Fatty acid supplement
How Supplied:	Oral: Capsules in small, medium, and large animal sizes; Liquid (Derm Caps Liquid®) in 60 ml bottles
Dose:	Capsules (small animal size for patients up to 30 lb): 1–2/d PO
	Liquid: 0.5 ml/10 lb/d PO

FENTANYL (Sublimaze®)

Use:	Narcotic analgesic
How Supplied:	Injectable: 0.05 mg/ml in 5 ml ampules (20 and 50 ml vials available for research use only)
	Transdermal patch: 2.5 mg patches (also known as 25 μg/hr)
Dose:	0.0002–0.05 mg/kg IV q2–6h; administer as bolus prior to constant rate infusion
	0.001–0.004 mg/kg/hr IV (constant rate infusion)
	2.5 mg dermal patch (for a 4–5 kg cat); replace q3–5d
Note:	Schedule II Controlled Substance

5-FLUOROURACIL

(5-FU, Efudex®, Fluoroplex®, Fluorouracil)

Contraindicated in cats.

FUROSEMIDE (Lasix®)

Use: Diuretic
How Supplied: Injectable: 50 mg/ml in 100 ml vials
Oral: 12.5 and 50 mg tablets; 10 mg/ml solution in 60 ml bottles
Dose: 1–2 mg/kg (0.45–0.9 mg/lb) IM or IV sid–bid
2.2 mg/kg (1 mg/lb) PO sid–bid

GENTAMICIN (Gentocin®)

Use: Aminoglycoside antibiotic
How Supplied: Injectable: 100 mg/ml in 100 ml vials
0.3% Ophthalmic ointment in 3.5 g tubes
0.3% Ophthalmic solution in 5 ml bottles
0.3% Ophthalmic solution with betamethasone (0.1%) in 5 ml bottle (Gentocin® Durafilm®)
0.3% Otic solution with betamethasone (0.1%) in 7.5 ml bottles (Gentocin® Otic)
Dose: 2.2–4.4 mg/kg IV, IM, or SQ tid
Note: If given IV, administer slowly

HEPARIN SODIUM

Use: Anticoagulant (in vivo and in vitro)
How Supplied: Injectable: 1000 U/ml in 10 ml vials
Dose: Intraocular irrigation: 2 U/ml
To make heparinized saline: 1–2 U/ml
IV bolus: 200 U/kg

HETASTARCH

Use: Plasma volume expansion
How Supplied: 6% Injectable solution in normal saline in 500 ml vials
Dose: 10–15 ml/kg/d IV

HYDROCORTISONE

Use: Corticosteroid therapy
How Supplied: 1% Ophthalmic ointment with neomycin, polymyxin B, and bacitracin in 3.5 g tubes (Cortisporin®, TriOptic-S®)
1% Otic formulation with Burow's Solution in 1 oz bottles (Bur Otic® HC)
1% Topical conditioner in 8 oz bottles (ResiCORT®)
1% Astringent spray in 4 oz bottles (DermaCool® HC)

HYDROXYUREA (Hydrea®)

Use: Antineoplastic agent
How Supplied: Oral: 500 mg capsules
Dose: 80 mg/kg PO q3d

IDARUBICIN (Idamycin®)

Use: Antineoplastic agent
How Supplied: Oral: 2 mg tablets
Injectable: 5 and 10 mg vials (IV dose not established for cats)
Dose: 2 mg/cat/d PO for 3 consecutive days q3wk

IFOSFAMIDE (IFEX®)

Use: Antineoplastic agent
How Supplied: Injectable: 1 g vials
Dose: 900 mg/m^2 IV q3wk (investigational)
Note: Must give with IV saline diuresis and mesna (included in package)

INSULIN

Use: Diabetes mellitus, hyperkalemia
How Supplied: Injectable: 100 U/ml in 10 ml vials (plain crystalline regular, Lente®, NPH, and Ultralente®)
Dose: 0.5–1 U/kg (0.23–0.45 U/lb) of regular insulin SQ q12–24h, then adjust dosage to clinical response

IRON DEXTRAN

Use: Hematinic
How Supplied: Injectable: 100 mg iron/ml in 100 ml vials
Dose: 11–22 mg/kg (5–10 mg/lb) once only

KAOLIN/PECTIN (Kaopectate®)

Use: Antidiarrheal
How Supplied: Oral suspension: 6 oz bottles
Dose: 1–2 ml/kg PO q2–6h

KETAMINE (Ketaset®, Ketaved®, Vetalar®)

Use: Neuroleptanalgesia
How Supplied: Injectable: 100 mg/ml in 10 ml vials
Dose: Anesthesia/analgesia: 6–10 mg/kg (2.7–4.5 mg/lb) IV
Restraint: 11 mg/kg (5 mg/lb) IM
Anesthesia: 22–33 mg/kg (10–15 mg/lb) IM
Antianxiety: 0.5–1.0 mg/kg IM q30min

KETOPROFEN (Ketofen®)

Use:	Antiinflammatory
How Supplied:	Injectable: 100 mg/ml in 100 ml vials
Dose:	1–2 mg/kg IV, IM, or SQ; single postsurgical dose

LIDOCAINE (Xylocaine®)

Use:	Local and topical anesthetic, antiarrhythmic
How Supplied:	2% Injectable solution in 100 ml vials 2% Oral and topical preparations (viscous) in 100 ml bottles
Dose:	0.5 mg/kg 3 hr prior to bupivacaine for local anesthesia

LOMUSTINE (CCNU) (Ceenu®)

Use:	Antineoplastic agent
How Supplied:	Oral: 10, 40, and 100 mg capsules
Dose:	Initial: 50–60 mg/m² PO q6wk

MECHLORETHAMINE HCL (Mustargen®)

Use:	Antineoplastic agent
How Supplied:	10 mg powder for injection
Dose:	3 mg/m² IV or intracavitary prn

MECLIZINE (Bonine®)

Use:	Antiemetic (related to labyrinthitis)
How Supplied:	Oral: 12.5 and 25 mg tablets
Dose:	6.25–12.5 mg/cat PO sid

MEDETOMIDINE (Domitor®)

Use:	Small animal sedative, analgesic
How Supplied:	Injectable: 1 mg/ml in 10 ml vials
Dose:	5–20 µg/kg IM (combine with butorphanol for painful procedures) 0.001–0.01 mg/kg IM, SQ, or IV over 0.5–2 hr for anesthesia

MEGESTROL ACETATE (Ovaban®)

Use:	Appetite stimulant, feline dermatopathies
How Supplied:	Oral: 5 mg tablets
Dose:	0.25–0.5 mg/kg/d for 3-5 days, then q48–72h

MELPHALAN (Alkeran®)

Use:	Antineoplastic agent
How Supplied:	Oral: 2 mg tablets Injectable: 500 mg vials
Dose:	0.1 mg/kg sid for 10 days, then 0.05 mg/kg/d OR 2 mg/m² sid for 7–10, then no therapy for 2–3 wk. Usually results in 2 mg PO qod with or without prednisone at 20 mg/m² PO qod

MEPERIDINE (Demarol®)

Use:	Opioid agonist
How Supplied:	Injectable: 50 mg/ml in 30 ml vials
Dose:	2–5 mg/kg IM or SQ q2h

6-MERCAPTOPURINE (Purinethol®, 6MP®)

Use:	Antineoplastic agent
How Supplied:	50 mg tablets
Dose:	50 mg/m² PO sid

METHIMAZOLE (Tapazole®)

Use:	Antithyroid agent
How Supplied:	Oral: 5 mg tablets
Dose:	5 mg/cat tid for 2 wk, reduce to 5 mg/cat bid if euthyroid

METHOTREXATE (Rheumatrex®)

Use:	Antineoplastic agent
How Supplied:	Oral: 2.5 mg tablets Injectable: 5 mg, 20 mg, 50 mg, 100 mg, 200 mg, 250 mg, and 1 g vials
Dose:	2.5 mg/m² PO, IV, IM, or SQ sid

METHYLPREDNISOLONE (Depo-Medrol®)

Use:	Corticosteroid therapy
How Supplied:	Injectable: 20 mg/ml in 10 ml vials; 40 mg/ml in 5 ml vials
Dose:	5.5 mg/kg (2.5 mg/lb) to maximum of 20 mg IM or SQ

METOCLOPRAMIDE (Reglan®)

Use:	Antiemetic, GI disorders
How Supplied:	Injectable: 5 mg/ml in 20 ml vials Oral: 10 mg tablets; 1 mg/ml solution
Dose:	1–2 mg/kg/d IV (constant rate infusion over 24 hr) 0.2–0.4 mg/kg IM or SQ q8h 0.4–0.6 mg/kg PO q4h

MITOXANTRONE (Novantrone®)

Use:	Antineoplastic agent
How Supplied:	Injectable: 20, 25, and 30 mg multidose vials
Dose:	6.5 mg/m² IV q3wk
Note:	Give IV over at least 3 min

MORPHINE

Use: Analgesic
How Supplied: Injectable: 1 mg/ml (diluted strength
                    primarily for feline use); 1 mg/ml in
                    10 ml single-dose ampules (for
                    epidural use only); 15 mg/ml in 1
                    and 20 ml vials
Dose: 0.05–0.2 mg/kg IM or SQ q2–6h
                    0.05–0.2 mg/kg IV q1–4h
Note: Schedule II Controlled Substance

NALBUPHINE

Use: Narcotic agonist-antagonist
How Supplied: Injectable: 20 mg/ml in 10 ml
                    multiple-dose vials
Dose: Premedication: 0.2–0.4 mg/kg SQ or IM

NALOXONE

Use: Narcotic antagonist
How Supplied: Injectable: 0.4 mg/ml in 10 ml vials
Dose: 0.05–0.1 mg/kg IV
Note: The half-life of naloxone is shorter than
                    most other narcotics. If it is used for
                    reversal, animals must be watched
                    carefully for returning signs of
                    narcotic activity.

NYSTATIN

Use: Candidiasis
How Supplied: Oral: 100,000 U/ml suspension in 5
                    and 60 ml bottles
                    Cream: 100,000 U/g with neomycin,
                    thiostrepton, and triamcinolone in a
                    water-washable base in 7.5 g tubes
                    (Panolog® Cream)
                    Ointment: 100,000 U/g with
                    neomycin, thiostrepton, and
                    triamcinolone in an oil base in
                    7.5 ml tubes (Panolog® Ointment,
                    Derma-4®)
Dose: 100,000 U PO q6hr

OMEPRAZOLE (Prilosec®)

Use: Ulcer management
How Supplied: Oral: 20 mg sustained-release capsules
Dose: 0.7 mg/kg PO sid

ONDANSETRON (Zofran®)

Use: Prevent nausea and vomiting associated
                    with chemotherapy, surgery, etc.
How Supplied: Injectable: 4 mg/ml in 2 ml vials
                    Oral: 4 mg tablets
Dose: 0.1 mg/kg IV 15 min before and 4 hr
                    after chemotherapy
Note: Give slowly IV (over 2 to 5 min) or dilute

OXACILLIN SODIUM (Bactocill®, Prostaphlin®)

Use: Treat penicillinase-producing
                    Staphylococcus infections
How Supplied: Oral: 250 mg capsules
Dose: 12–24 mg/kg (5.5–11 mg/lb) PO tid

OXYMORPHONE (Numorphan®)

Use: Narcotic analgesic
How Supplied: Injectable: 1.5 mg/ml in 1 ml ampules
                    and 10 ml vials
Dose: 0.05–0.1 mg/kg IM or SQ q2–6h
                    0.02–0.05 mg/kg IV q2–4h
Note: Schedule II Controlled Substance

PACLITAXEL (Taxol®)

Use: Antineoplastic agent
How Supplied: 50 mg/5 ml in 5 ml vials
Dose: 5 mg/kg IV q3wk (investigational)
Note: Dilute with 0.9% NaCl to a
                    concentration of 0.6–0.7 mg/ml;
                    occasional collapse and anaphylaxis
                    can occur

PENICILLIN G POTASSIUM

Use: Gram-positive infections
How Supplied: Injectable: 1 million, 5 million, and 20
                    million U vials (contains 1.68 mEq
                    of potassium/million U)
Dose: 22,000 U/kg (10,000 U/lb) SQ, IM,
                    or IV q4–6h (minimum dose)
Note: Half-life is approximately 30 min

PENTOBARBITAL, SODIUM

Use: Sedative, anticonvulsant, IV anesthesia,
                    euthanasia
How Supplied: Injectable: 50 mg/ml in 50 ml vials;
                    400 mg/ml in 250 ml vials
                    (euthanasia solution)
Dose: Anesthesia: Approximately 25–30
                    mg/kg IV
                    Anticonvulsant: 3–15 mg/kg given
                    slowly IV until effect
                    Euthanasia: 88 mg/kg (40 mg/lb) IV
Note: Schedule II Controlled Substance

PHENOBARBITAL

Use:	Sedative, anticonvulsant
How Supplied:	Injectable: 130 mg/ml (sodium salt) in 1 ml vials
	Oral: 15, 30, 60, and 100 mg tablets
Dose:	2 mg/kg PO bid to start; base dose increases on serum levels
Note:	1. Schedule IV Controlled Substance
	2. One time loading dose: 6–20 mg/kg IV
	3. Diazepam (IV or rectally) may be given concurrently, since IV phenobarbital requires 20–30 min to exert an anticonvulsant effect

PIROXICAM (Feldene®)

Use:	Analgesic, antiinflammatory, antineoplastic agent
How Supplied:	10 and 20 mg capsules (2.5 mg and 5 mg capsules commonly compounded)
Dose:	Analgesia: 0.3 mg/kg PO sid for 4 days, then 0.3 mg/kg PO q48h
	Antineoplastic: 0.3 mg/kg PO q48h
Note:	Use cautiously—nephrotoxicity, GI ulceration common

POTASSIUM GLUCONATE (Tumil-K®)

Use:	Oral potassium supplement
How Supplied:	Oral: 2 mEq (468 mg) tablets
	Oral powder: 2 mEq (468 mg) potassium gluconate/0.25 teaspoon (0.65 g) in 4 oz bottles
Dose:	2.5–7.0 mEq/cat/d divided according to number of feedings

PREDNISOLONE

Use:	Corticosteroid therapy
How Supplied:	Injectable: 50 mg/ml acetate suspension in 30 ml vials
	Oral: 5 mg tablets
	1% Ophthalmic suspension: 10 ml bottles (Pred Forte™)
Dose:	0.5–2.2 mg/kg (0.23-1 mg/lb) IM or PO q24–48h

PREDNISOLONE SODIUM PHOSPHATE

Use:	Corticosteroid therapy
How Supplied:	Injectable: 20 mg/ml (14.8 mg prednisolone base/ml) in 50 ml vials
Dose:	0.5–2.2 mg/kg (0.23–1 mg/lb) IV q24–48h

PREDNISONE (Deltasone®, many generics available)

Use:	Corticosteroid therapy, antineoplastic agent
How Supplied:	Oral: 5, 10, 20, and 50 mg tablets and 1 mg/ml oral solution
	Injectable: 10 and 40 mg/ml
Dose:	0.5–2.2 mg/kg (0.23–1 mg/lb) PO sid
	Antineoplastic dose: 30–40 mg/m² IM or PO sid or eod for 21 days, then 1 mg/kg PO sid for 4 wk and 1 mg/kg eod thereafter

PROCARBAZINE

Use:	Antineoplastic agent
How Supplied:	Must be compounded
Dose:	10 mg/cat/d for 14 days as part of MOPP protocol

PROCHLORPERAZINE (Compazine®, Darbazine®)

Use:	Antiemetic
How Supplied:	Injectable: 5 mg/ml in 2 ml ampules
Dose:	Compazine®: 0.1–0.5 mg/kg IM or SQ q6–8h
	Darbazine®: 0.5–0.8 mg/kg IM or SQ q12h

PROPOFOL (Diprivan®, Rapinovet®)

Use:	Anesthesia
How Supplied:	Injectable: 10 mg/ml in 20 ml ampules
Dose:	2–6 mg/kg IV given slowly to effect
Note:	Repeated administration may cause anemia

RANITIDINE (Zantac®)

Use:	H_2-receptor antagonist
How Supplied:	Injectable: 25 mg/ml in 6 ml vials
	Oral: 15 mg/ml syrup; 150 and 300 mg tablets
Dose:	3.5 mg/kg PO bid
	2.5 mg/kg IV bid

SUCRALFATE (Carafate®)

Use:	Duodenal ulcer treatment
How Supplied:	Oral: 100 mg/ml solution; 1 g tablets
Dose:	0.25 g/cat PO tid 1 hr prior to feeding

THIOPENTAL SODIUM (Pentothal®)

Use:	Ultrashort-acting barbiturate
How Supplied:	Injectable: 5 g vials for preparation of 2.5% or 5% solution
Dose:	13.2–26.4 mg/kg IV to effect
Note:	Schedule III Controlled Substance

TILETAMINE AND ZOLAZEPAM (Telazol®)

Use:	Combination dissociative anesthetic/tranquilizer
How Supplied:	Injectable: 500 mg vial (100 mg/ml when reconstituted with 5 ml of diluent; follow directions on package insert)
Dose:	9.7–11.9 mg/kg IM for minor procedures of short duration
	10.6–12.5 mg/kg IM for mild to moderate levels of analgesia
Notes:	1. Schedule III Controlled Substance
	2. If supplemental doses are needed, total dose should not exceed 72 mg/kg
	3. Atropine (0.04 mg/kg) should be used concurrently to control hypersalivation

TRIAMCINOLONE (Kenalog®, Vetalog®)

Use:	Corticosteroid therapy
How Supplied:	Injectable: 2 mg/ml in 25 ml vials; 6 and 40 mg/ml in 5 ml vials
Dose:	0.1–0.2 mg/kg (0.045–0.09 mg/lb) IM or SQ sid

THIOTEPA

Use:	Antineoplastic agent
How Supplied:	Injectable: 15 mg vials
Dose:	Maximum systemic dosage: 9 mg/m^2 IM or SQ q3wk
	Bladder instillation: 30 mg/m^2 once q3–4wk, remove 1 hr later

TRIMETHOPRIM/SULFA

(Tribrissen®, Generics)

Use:	Antibacterial
How Supplied:	Combination product containing 1 part trimethoprim to 5 parts sulfamethoxazole
	Oral: 120 mg coated tablets (Tribrissen® 120); 480 and 960 mg tablets; 48 mg/ml oral suspension
Dose:	30 mg/kg PO bid up to 120 mg bid maximum
Note:	120 mg tablets and Uniprim® contain sulfadiazine, not sulfamethoxazole

General Oral Dosing Guidelines

Weight	Dose
Up to 10 lb	Oral suspension, 7 mg/lb bid
10 to 17 lb	120 mg tablet bid

TYLOSIN (Tylan®)

Use:	Macrolide antibiotic
How Supplied:	Oral powder: 25 g (base)/318.6 g bottle
	Oral: 30, 60, 130, 240, 345, and 430 mg compounded capsules
Dose:	6.6–11 mg/kg PO q12–24h

VINBLASTINE (Velban®)

Use:	Antineoplastic agent
How Supplied:	1 mg/ml in 10 mg vials
Dose:	2 mg/m^2 IV q2–3wk

VINCRISTINE (Oncovin®)

Use:	Antineoplastic agent
How Supplied:	Injectable: 1, 2, and 5 mg vials
Dose:	0.5–0.75 mg/m^2 IV once weekly

XYLAZINE (Rompun®, AnaSed®, Tranquived®)

Use:	α-2 agonist; sedative, analgesic; emetic in cats
How Supplied:	Injectable: 20 mg/ml in 20 ml vials; 100 mg/ml in 50 ml vials
Dose:	Sedation: 0.5–2 mg/kg IV, IM, or SQ
	Antianxiety: 0.05–0.2 mg/kg IV or IM q15–30min

YOHIMBINE (Antagonil®)

Use:	α-2 antagonist
How Supplied:	Injectable: 5 mg/ml in 20 ml vials
Dose:	0.1–0.5 mg/kg IV

This section contains information geared toward the owners of cats with cancer. The handouts are designed to be photocopied* and distributed to clients to help educate them about what to expect during the treatment of their pets. Because caregivers are important members of the veterinary health care team, it is critical that they understand what is being done for their cats and have the necessary knowledge to make informed decisions regarding the care and treatment of their beloved pets. They also need to know what to expect—and to be prepared to deal with reactions and complications of—diagnostic and/or therapeutic procedures. The more clients know about cancer and its treatment, the better able they are to focus on what is best for their cats.

The following handouts are provided:

- When Your Cat Has Cancer

- Healing Rays: Radiation Therapy for Your Cat with Cancer

- Nutritional Support of Your Cat with Cancer

- The Healing Power of Surgery for Your Cat with Cancer

- Combination Chemotherapy Protocol for Lymphoma: What You Need to Know

- When it is Time to Say Goodbye: Euthanasia and Your Cat

- Demystifying Cancer Care: A Glossary for Caregivers

---

*Permission is hereby granted to photocopy and distribute these forms to your clients for instructional purposes only.

When Your Cat Has Cancer

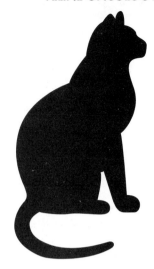

Cancer. The word is as dark and empty as the disease it defines. A diagnosis of cancer often brings with it feelings of overwhelming fear, loss of control, and hopelessness. This hopelessness is the most frightening thing of all. When we face the diagnosis of cancer in a beloved cat, we may feel weighted with a great responsibility. We must make important, life-changing decisions for a creature that relies totally on our judgment for its well-being. Your cat not only shares your home, your life, and your experiences, but also your heart. Seeking the most appropriate care will allow you to spend as much time as possible with your special friend.

Empower Yourself with Information

You can defeat the darkness of cancer with knowledge. Work with your veterinary health care team to learn as much about the disease and its treatment as possible. Be proactive. Ask questions and obtain resources to tear away the many misconceptions about cancer and cancer therapies. Tackling the emotional aspects of cancer can enhance your ability to think clearly, make decisions, and begin to find the hope and opportunities that lie before you as you deal with your cat's cancer.

Pick a Good Team

As your cat's primary caregiver, you are in the best position to know and meet your cat's needs and desires. Your greatest task is to find a veterinary health care team that is experienced in cancer care and committed to working with you as a member of that team. Once the right team is forged, everyone can provide true *compassionate care*. Compassionate care requires that your cat is as free as possible from the adverse effects that may be associated with cancer and cancer care. This includes freedom from pain, nausea, and loss of appetite. Ask your veterinary health care team about what supportive care measures can be undertaken to enhance the quality of your cat's life.

Empowerment Tips

■ **Write things down:** Record all discussions about your cat's disease or recommended treatments with the veterinary health care team. Repeat the information back to these people to ensure that you understand completely.

■ **Seek support:** Bring a friend or spouse with you when you talk to the veterinary health care team.

■ **Include the whole family:** All discussions should involve everyone who is intimately associated with your cat, including your children. Allow everyone to ask questions and to voice his or her opinions.

Some questions you may want to discuss with your veterinary health care team:

About your cat's cancer and treatment:

What is the scientific name of my cat's tumor?

Is the tumor benign or malignant (cancerous)?

How often does this type of tumor metastasize (spread to other parts of the body)?

If left untreated, what will the cancer do to my cat?

What diagnostic tests do we need to perform to determine the location and extent of the cancer (i.e., the stage of the disease)?

What are all the treatment options and what are the costs, side effects, time involved, and effectiveness of each treatment?

About your cat's pain management:

Is my cat in any discomfort?

How do you treat cancer pain?

Is pain management important at this practice?

What happens if my cat's pain is not relieved with the usual treatment?

Is severe pain considered an emergency at this practice?

Who do I call after hours?

Will I receive directions in writing?

Who can help when you are away?

What happens if my cat's pain does not go away?

Who will show me how to give pain medication to my cat?

About your cat's nutrition:

Is there anything special my cat should eat?

How much should my cat eat?

When should appetite stimulants be used?

What is "assisted tube feeding?"

How important is it to keep my cat from losing weight?

How can we prevent appetite loss in my cat?

About ensuring your cat does not have an upset stomach:

How can I tell if my cat has an upset stomach?

How can we prevent nausea and vomiting?

When should I call for help if my cat seems nauseated or is vomiting?

Who should I call?

What can be done if my cat seems nauseated or is vomiting?

What can we do to enhance appetite and ensure good nutrition?

Date and time of my next appointment: _____

Time required for the next appointment: _____

Purpose of my next appointment: _____

■ **Ask for printed materials or information:** Obtain resources to help you understand your cat's disease and the treatment options. The Internet can be a powerful resource for both the truth and misinformation. Work with your health care team to understand the validity of all information you obtain.

■ **Understand there are no correct decisions, only decisions that are right for you:** Do not worry what other people will think about your decisions. You know your cat better than anyone else in the world. *Once you are empowered with the information you need, listen to your heart and you will make the right decisions.*

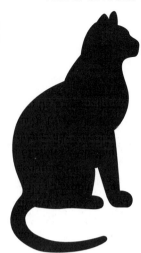

Healing Rays: Radiation Therapy for Your Cat with Cancer

How is Radiation Therapy Administered?

Whenever radiation therapy is planned for a cat with cancer, maintaining quality of life and freedom from discomfort are our highest goals. In order to minimize the adverse effects and to enhance the control of the cancer, small dosages of radiation are administered over several weeks. During each treatment, your cat will be placed under a light level of anesthesia and a machine will be used to safely and precisely direct the healing radiation therapy beams over a period of several minutes. The radiation therapist will determine the appropriate dosage and number of treatments to ensure the best outcome possible. When radiation is used with the intent of eliminating or controlling the cancer for a long period of time, 9 to 40 treatments are administered over 3 to 6 weeks. These treatments take only a few minutes to administer and they are not painful.

Are There Any Side Effects?

In the course of radiation treatment, some surrounding normal tissue will be affected. Radiation-induced effects to normal tissues usually do not begin until the end of the therapy period and they continue for weeks after the treatment has ended. These are called the acute side effects and they usually resolve within weeks after radiation has been completed. Other adverse effects associated with radiation therapy may occur months or years after radiation is complete. These are called delayed adverse effects. Interestingly, the adverse effects associated with radiation therapy are much less in cats than in most other species, including people. Indeed, the majority of these adverse effects are mild and self-limiting. We will work with you to ensure that your cat is as comfortable as possible during this 2 to 4 week period when adverse effects are noted. A few of the most common possible effects are listed below.

■ **Skin:** Radiation reactions that may appear toward the end of therapy include loss of hair and a sunburn-like effect to the skin, which may become itchy, dry, or moist. Most cats will keep the area clean. Oral or injectable medication to reduce itching or discomfort may be helpful. Applying oily creams or ointments usually reduces the rate of healing in cats. Most cats

Questions you may want to ask:

What is the probability for controlling my cat's tumor with radiation therapy?

For the average cat with this type of tumor, what, if anything, is known about how long the tumor will be controlled?

What additional therapies, such as chemotherapy, are recommended to enhance control of the cancer?

What are the possible acute adverse effects associated with my cat's radiation plan?

What are the possible delayed adverse effects associated with my cat's radiation plan?

I understand that the radiation treatments themselves do not hurt; however, what can be done to prevent or reduce the adverse effects associated with radiation therapy?

develop a change in the color of the skin and hair in the area being treated and, occasionally, hair will fall out and not regrow in that area. Other changes to the skin that are much less common include formation of a non-healing wound or thickened scar tissue in the treatment area.

- **Mouth:** If your cat is being treated for a tumor in or around the mouth, injury to this area can result in a sunburn-like effect to the tongue and the tissues lining the mouth. This can result in loss of appetite, altered tongue function, and tenderness to the lining of the mouth. In these cases, one of the best things that can be done to ensure your cat has a good quality of life is to consider assisted tube feeding. A small tube is placed into the swallowing pipe (esophagostomy tube), stomach (gastrostomy tube), or intestine (jejunostomy tube), bypassing the mouth area to allow the non-painful administration of food, water, and medicine. The key is to begin this assisted tube feeding before any weight loss is observed. During radiation therapy, you may want to gently rinse your cat's mouth out with a solution of salt and water (1 teaspoon salt in 1 quart of water). Some recommend adding Maalox® to this saltwater solution to coat the mouth. Some cats appreciate cool tea solutions to reduce the discomfort of the oral cavity and freshen the breath. Your veterinarian may recommend some additional therapies if your cat stops producing enough saliva (or "spit").

- **Large Intestine and Rectum:** Occasionally, the large intestine (colon) and rectum (area just inside the anal opening underneath the tail) are affected when tumors in that area of the body are being treated. Most cats have only mild, transient side effects that can include loose stool that may contain blood and perhaps some discomfort passing stool. A special diet, stool softeners, and, in some cases, steroid enemas may be beneficial in some cats. Whenever the anus and the area around it are injured by radiation therapy, the area should be gently cleansed using soap and water and dried thoroughly.

- **Eye:** The eye is often in the treatment field when tumors of the skin, sinuses, or nasal cavity are treated. While most cats do not show any adverse effects associated with damage to the eye, side effects can include cataract formation months to years after therapy is finished, damage to the retina (which is in the back of the eye), decreased tear production, and irritation to the tissues around the eye. Occasionally, an ulcer of the cornea (the outer layer of the eye) may be noted. In some cases, medicines may be needed to treat these conditions.

Nutritional Support of Your Cat with Cancer

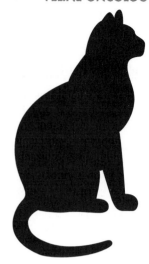

What Do I Feed My Cat with Cancer?

The answer is quite simple: anything your cat will eat! If your cat is eating, however, then you and your veterinarian should develop a dietary plan. While the ideal cancer diet for the cat is unknown, there are some simple guidelines that should be followed:

- Provide a diet with good aroma and taste.

- Minimize simple carbohydrates.

- Provide a diet that has high-quality protein sources.

- Whenever possible, consider enhancing the levels of n-3 fatty acids (your veterinarian can tell you what these are and what foods have them).

The single, biggest challenge for cats with cancer is the prevention and treatment of a finicky appetite. Therefore, be sure to:

- Provide a variety of fresh foods that are tasty and great smelling to cats. Warming the food to just below body temperature can enhance the appeal of many foods. Cats are intermittent eaters, so food should be available to them throughout the day.

- Work with your veterinary health care team to prevent and treat any discomfort. A painful cat often will not eat.

- Work with your veterinary health care team to prevent and treat nausea.

- Work with your veterinary health care team to prevent and treat dehydration. A dehydrated cat will often have a poor appetite. Your veterinarian may teach you how to administer fluids under the skin to prevent or treat dehydration.

- When necessary, consider the addition of appetite stimulants as prescribed by your veterinary health care team.

- Do not change the diet at the same time as chemotherapy or when other drugs are administered if these drugs have the chance of causing nausea. This results in "food aversion," a situation in which your cat may associate the uncomfortable feeling with the food rather than the true culprit, chemotherapy or other drugs or procedures.

What Do I Do If My Cat Won't Eat?

Assisted tube feeding can enhance both quality and length of life. This method also ensures that you can give medicines, fluids, and nutrition even when your cat will not eat. Assisted tube feeding is the placement of a small tube into the swallowing pipe (esophagostomy tube), stomach (gastrostomy tube), or intestine (jejunostomy tube) to allow the non-painful administration of food, water, and medicine. The key is to begin this type of feeding before any weight loss is observed. These techniques can prevent any decline in your cat's health and should be used early in the course of your cat's disease. Remember: You must be an advocate for your cat. Don't hesitate to contact your veterinary health care team to discuss your cat's nutritional care.

Additional Information

The Internet and other sources of information are brimming with promises of the health benefits of a wide variety of supplements. Most are unfounded and unproven, but your veterinary health care team welcomes any treatments that may help your cat. Discuss any and all treatments or supplements with your veterinarian before you administer them. They have some chance of being harmful as well as helpful. Our goal is to make your cat better regardless of the source of the treatment.

Instructions

Amount of food to feed my cat: _____

Recommended diets: _____

Appetite stimulants and dosage: _____

Anti-nausea medicine and dosage: _____

Supplements: _____

The Healing Power of Surgery for Your Cat with Cancer

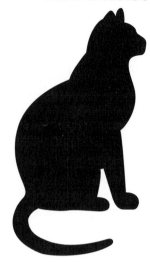

Surgery is the oldest form of cancer therapy in human and feline medicine and has been responsible for the cure of more patients than any other treatment. This great success is mainly due to the development of new surgical techniques. One of the greatest advantages of surgery, other than that it can be used to cure some cancers, is that it can make other treatments work better. Indeed, surgery plays an important role in the prevention, diagnosis, definitive treatment, and rehabilitation of the feline cancer patient.

While surgery is a critical step in the treatment of most feline malignancies, the surgical procedure can be frightening despite the fact that surgery will help your cat. We want to make sure that you understand the risks and benefits of the surgery. This can be done by first having a frank and open discussion with the entire veterinary health care team. This discussion may help dispel unfounded myths. For example, you may be afraid that the surgery will be disfiguring or that the procedure will result in a decreased quality of life. Your veterinary health care team can help you understand why this is not true.

There are many types of surgery that may be used to benefit the cat with cancer. For example:

■ **Prevention of Cancer:** Spaying and neutering in the cat is one example of a procedure that can help prevent some types of cancer and many noncancerous conditions, such as infection of the uterus (womb).

■ **Diagnosis of Cancer:** The veterinary surgeon plays an important role in determining the stage and extent of the cancer. A surgical biopsy is always required to make a definitive diagnosis. A biopsy may be obtained before the tumor is treated with the final procedure if it will change your willingness to treat or the way the veterinary health care team will treat the tumor. Surgery is then often employed to remove part or all of the cancer.

■ **Curative Surgery for Primary Cancer:** For the best chance of achieving a cure, a tumor must be removed with a properly executed surgical procedure the very first time the tumor is treated with definitive surgery. The curative surgery for primary cancer is the most common use of surgery for the cat with cancer.

■ **Surgery for Tumor Left after a Prior Surgery:** The best opportunity to cure a cat with a malignant disease is with the first surgery. However, tumors are sometimes incompletely removed, and subsequent surgery is required. "Debulking" surgery alone (i.e., surgery to reduce the size of a tumor rather than to completely remove it) is rarely an acceptable form of therapy unless it is used simply as a method to improve quality of life.

■ **Surgery for Metastatic Disease:** Surgical removal of metastases (cancer that has spread to other parts of the body) should be considered in select cases

POSTOPERATIVE INSTRUCTIONS

Next Appointment: _____
Suture Removal: _____

Medication Dispensed:
❑ Analgesic
❑ Antibiotic
❑ Other:_____
_____

Dosage: _____
_____

Give the Medication:
❑ Once a day
❑ Twice a day
❑ Three times a day
❑ Other: _____
_____

❑ By Mouth
❑ In the Food
❑ Other: _____
_____

Continue giving the medication
for:_____

Diet: _____
_____

Exercise:
❑ None
❑ Unlimited
❑ Other:_____
_____

Other Instructions:
_____
_____
_____

when it is obvious that the original cancer is not progressing rapidly and that the metastatic disease is restricted to a single site or a few sites that can be surgically excised. This is especially true when the surgery for the metastatic disease will improve quality of life or serve as a diagnostic tool for the management of your cat's disease.

■ **Surgery for Emergencies:** The most common applications for oncologic surgery in an emergency setting include the treatment of bleeding, perforation by a stomach ulcer, blockage of organs, or the drainage of an infected abscess.

■ **Surgery to Improve Quality of Life (Palliation):** When a tumor or its metastasis results in significant discomfort for your cat, surgery can be employed to improve or maintain the quality of life. In these patients, surgery should be used only if you are clearly aware that this procedure will not be curative.

Caring for Surgical Wounds

Surgery can result in some adverse effects, most of which are resolvable. You should inspect the incision every single day for excess swelling or discharge. Keep it clean, but be aware that the incision is tender to the touch. If you have questions, contact your veterinary health care team. Things to watch for include:

■ Mild "oozing" of blood or body fluids at the surgery site
　—Keep the area clean by gently washing with mild soap and water.

■ Visible, continued bleeding at the surgery site
　—Contact your veterinary health care team immediately.

■ Redness, swelling, and/or crusting of the stitches
　—Keep the area clean by gently washing with mild soap and water, and contact your veterinarian. Monitor your cat's body temperature and make sure it does not go above 102°F.

■ Infection of the surgery site can result in depression, loss of appetite, swelling, discharge, and fever (rectal temperature >102.2°F)
　—Contact your veterinary health care team immediately.

■ Stitches (sutures) that come untied or that your cat licks or scratches out
　—Contact your veterinary health care team and consider a "shirt" or an Elizabethan collar.

■ Discomfort
　—Contact your veterinary health care team to ensure your cat has appropriate pain control therapy.

■ Poor healing
　—Contact your veterinarian to consider possible therapies if the wound does not heal within the amount of time discussed.

© 2001 Veterinary Learning Systems

Combination Chemotherapy Protocol for Lymphoma: What You Need to Know

Chemotherapy is a word that creates an instant emotional response in everyone. Chances are that you, or someone you know, has experienced chemotherapy for the treatment of cancer. The reality of chemotherapy for animals is generally different from that for human cancer patients. Most people are pleasantly surprised at how well their cats seem to feel while undergoing chemotherapy.

"Protocol" is a chemotherapy treatment regimen. Most of the drugs in the regimen are administered by the veterinary health care team by injection (vincristine, doxorubicin, cyclophosphamide, L-asparaginase) or given orally (prednisone and sometimes cyclophosphamide). If therapy is to be administered by injection, the patient lies quietly on a padded table during administration and rarely needs any form of sedation.

Practically all anticancer drugs have side effects. However, their potential effect against the disease generally outweighs the possible risks. Although serious adverse effects can occur with any chemotherapy, there is less than a 5% chance that your cat will be hospitalized as a result of chemotherapy and less than a 1% chance of fatality. The possible benefits and side effects of the protocol are listed below. If you have questions about chemotherapy or any of its potential side effects, please ask your veterinarian.

Whisker or Hair Loss (Alopecia)

When a person loses hair as a result of chemotherapy, it can be devastating. Cats rarely lose their hair. Even if they do, they are rarely bothered by it. In cats, hair does not grow continually throughout their lives as it does in people. Therefore, hair loss in cats is rare. Cats may, however, temporarily lose all or most of their whiskers.

Low White Blood Cell Count (Neutropenia)

There are various types of cells in the blood. A decrease in the number of infection-fighting white blood cells is known as neutropenia. Many chemotherapeutic agents impair the bone marrow's ability to produce cells and, as a result, neutropenia may occur 7 to 10 days after chemotherapy. While neutropenia alone is not a danger to your cat, it can impair the animal's ability to fight off infection. For that reason, your cat is given a complete physical prior to each treatment, and a blood test, called a complete blood count (CBC), is performed. Should your cat have a significant reduction in the number of white blood cells, your veterinarian may wish to perform additional periodic blood tests and/or prescribe antibiotics to protect your cat from infection.

Stomach or Intestinal (Gastrointestinal) Discomfort

Many patients experience some form of stomach or intestinal discomfort 2 to 7 days after a chemotherapy treatment. Your veterinarian will prescribe medication to try to prevent or treat the discomfort. Steps you can take at home are listed on the next page.

Managing Gastrointestinal Problems at Home

■ Upset Stomach (Nausea)
  1. If your cat begins to show any signs of an upset stomach (drooling, "smacking" lips) or a loss of appetite, administer any medications your veterinarian may have prescribed for nausea.
  2. Offer ice cubes every few hours.
  3. After 12 hours, feed your cat small, frequent meals instead of infrequent large ones.
  4. Call your veterinarian if you have concerns or if the condition persists for more than 24 hours.

■ Vomiting
  1. Do not give your cat any food or water for 12 hours.
  2. After 12 hours, first offer your cat ice cubes, then water, and then small bland meals.
  3. Call your veterinarian if you have concerns or if the condition persists for more than 24 hours.

■ Loss of Appetite
  1. If your cat begins to show any signs of an upset stomach or loss of appetite, administer any medications your veterinarian may have prescribed for nausea.
  2. Offer your cat four small meals a day.
  3. Select foods your cat likes and add warm broth or animal fats to meals to improve flavor and appeal.

■ Diarrhea
  1. If your cat begins to show signs of diarrhea, administer any medications your veterinarian may have prescribed for diarrhea.
  2. Keep water available at all times.
  3. If your cat is not eating, offer chicken or beef broth.
  4. Call your veterinarian if you have concerns or if the condition persists for more than 24 hours.

Tissue Damage

If certain intravenous drugs are accidentally administered outside the vein, severe tissue reactions can result. Therefore chemotherapy drugs like Adriamycin® (doxorubicin) are handled with the utmost care and are administered only by highly trained professionals. If irritation develops at the injection site (for example, pain or redness), apply ice packs for 15 minutes every 3 hours. Call your veterinarian if you have concerns.

Allergic Reactions

Allergic reactions to chemotherapeutic agents are rare and develop only upon administration. Your veterinarian and the hospital staff are trained to treat such rare reactions.

Heart Damage

In some rare cases, Adriamycin® can irreversibly damage the heart muscle. The dose of Adriamycin® prescribed for your cat is below the dose that usually causes heart disease. This is an exceedingly rare adverse effect in cats and some specialists argue it is not a concern. Your veterinarian will discontinue the use of Adriamycin® if heart disease is detected at any time.

Each Visit

It is important to make an appointment for each chemotherapy administration. At each visit, a veterinarian or oncology nurse will admit your cat. Your veterinarian and hospital staff will work as a team to minimize the time you and your cat will spend at the hospital as well as maximize your cat's quality of care. While you may not see the same veterinarian or nurse at each visit, you will still receive the most comprehensive and compassionate care possible.

■ You will be asked how your cat has been doing since the last visit. This is a good time to express any concerns you may have about your cat's condition and let us know if you need refills of any medications.

■ Your cat will receive a complete physical examination by a veterinarian, and blood will be drawn for a complete blood count. Once the blood values have been reviewed and are determined to be within normal limits, your cat will receive the prescribed treatment. This entire process takes 2 to 3 hours. You may wait in the lobby during this time, or you may leave your cat in our care and return later in the day. Stop by the Business Office at the completion of each visit to keep your account current.

When It Is Time to Say Goodbye: Euthansia and Your Cat

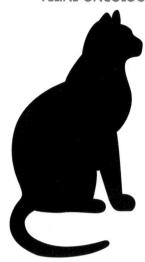

What is Euthanasia?

Euthanasia is the medical procedure of alleviating pain and suffering by administering intravenous drugs that stop the heart permanently to allow for a painless death. Every veterinary health care team performs euthanasia a bit differently, yet these different processes have many similarities. It is very important for you to realize that you are the ultimate decision maker. You have control of the decision-making process as well as the ability to guide and select options for this final step in the care of your beloved cat.

When Will I Know it is Time?

The actual "time" that euthanasia is performed is a very personal decision. There is no one correct decision. There is, however, a decision that will be right for you. There are many issues to take into account during this time. Some issues you may want to consider include, but are not limited to, your cat's quality of life, the cost of continued care, the time you must invest to care for your cat, and your desires for the kind of life you want your cat to live. Quality of life is a subjective assessment, but it can be judged in part by accounting for things such as appetite, activity and energy level, grooming habits, and attention to daily rituals, such as sleeping in favorite places. It is often very helpful for you to keep some sort of record of your cat's home "lifestyle." You may want to ask yourself questions such as:

- "Do the good days and times outnumber the bad?"
- "Is my cat able to do the things that in the past have made him or her happy?"
- "How does my cat's day differ now compared to days before he or she was sick?"

The decision to euthanize can profoundly affect your memories and actions for months to years. During this time of assessment, decision making, and action, it is important to realize that your cat's veterinary health care team can be a vital support system for you and any involved family and friends.

The first step of becoming comfortable with euthanasia is to realize that you can personalize this time to meet the needs of you, your family, and, most im-

Grief is a normal manifestation of loss regardless of whether the beloved friend is a person or a cat. There are many ways for you to work through the grief process. You should be aware that the loss of an animal, like the loss of a family member or friend, could cause physical and emotional changes that can last for weeks or months. You may wish to contact a pet loss support group, pet loss hotline, or local specialist who is knowledgeable about loss and receptive to helping people who have lost a beloved cat. Ask your veterinarian for a referral.

portantly, your precious cat. This is best done through advance planning whenever possible. Before the time of euthanasia, you may want to consider the following:

■ If comfortable for you and your cat, you may wish to spend some time doing some of those special activities or rituals that have held meaning to you during the lifetime of your cat. This may be something as simple as allowing your cat to bask in the sun in a favorite place or sit on your lap as you read the paper.

■ It is important that children not be "sheltered" from this important decision-making process and time. Many studies have shown that excluding children or making up stories (e.g., "Fluffy ran away") is destructive in the long run. It is also important for parents to appreciate the ability to comprehend the concepts of death and euthanasia at different ages.

■ You may wish to take pictures, clip hair, or make paw imprints (on paper or in clay) as a lasting memorial.

■ You may find it easier to discuss body care (cremation, burial, disposal, etc.) prior to euthanasia.

Many people decide they want to be present at the time of euthanasia, whereas others do not. Regardless of which path is chosen, the family needs to have an understanding of what will transpire. Every hospital performs euthanasia differently. The following is just one example of how the process may unfold:

■ A quiet time and place will be selected so that the veterinary health care team, you, and your family and friends can be involved. You should be comfortable stating how you would like this process to proceed.

■ A member of the veterinary health care team will describe the euthanasia process while other members of the team place a catheter in the vein. Euthanasia is the process of injecting an anesthetic agent into a catheter placed in the vein until unconsciousness occurs and the heart stops forever. The entire process is always accomplished in a quiet, tender, gentle manner with no pain, suffering, or struggle.

■ You may wish to spend some time alone with your special friend before and after euthanasia.

■ Euthanasia can be performed with many drugs. These medicines cause a smooth transition to a state of total relaxation, sleep, and then death within seconds to minutes. As your cat comes to this loss of consciousness, he or she may take a breath or make a slight movement in those last seconds. Some loss of bladder and bowel control is normal, and the eyes may remain open.

Although this can be an upsetting experience, you should take comfort in knowing you did what you could for your beloved pet, and that your cat is now at peace.

Demystifying Cancer Care: A Glossary for Caregivers

Cancer and cancer therapy are often viewed through a shroud of myths and misperceptions: Cancer is seen as a huge, dark, hopeless disease, and treatment is frequently thought to be worse than the disease. However, cancer is neither as big nor as dark as it seems. The first step toward dispelling the myths about cancer and its therapy is to demystify some of the words commonly used by the veterinary health care team.

A

Acute: Sudden in onset, such as symptoms that occur soon after detection of a cancer or soon after a treatment

Adenocarcinoma: A malignant or cancerous tumor arising from glandular tissue

Adenoma: A benign tumor made up of glandular tissue

Adjuvant chemotherapy: Chemotherapy given to kill any cancer cells that remain after all detectable tumor has been removed (e.g., by surgery or through radiotherapy)

Adrenal glands: Two small organs near the kidneys that release hormones

Alopecia: Loss of hair, which is an uncommon response to chemotherapy in cats

Analgesic: A pain-relieving drug

Anemia: A decreased number of red blood cells, which may cause tiredness and weakness

Anorexia: Loss of appetite

Antibody: A substance formed by the body to help defend it against infection

Antiemetic: A drug that prevents or controls nausea and vomiting

Antineoplastic agent: A drug that prevents, kills, or blocks the growth and spread of cancer cells

Arrhythmia: An irregular heartbeat

Aspiration: The process of removing fluid/tissue from a specific area using a needle and syringe

Autoimmunity: A condition in which the body's immune system mistakenly fights and rejects the body's own tissues

Axilla: The area where the foreleg joins the body wall; the "armpit"

B

Barium enema: The milky solution (barium sulfate) given by an enema to allow x-ray examination of the lower intestinal tract

Barium swallow: The milky solution (barium sulfate) given orally to allow x-ray examination of the upper intestinal tract

Basal cell carcinoma: The most common type of skin cancer

Benign tumor: A noncancerous swelling or growth that does not spread from one part of the body to another

Biopsy: Surgical removal of tissue for examination under a microscope to make a diagnosis

Blood cells: Minute structures made in the bone marrow, including red blood cells, white blood cells, and platelets

Blood count: The number of red blood cells, white blood cells, and platelets in a sample of blood

Bone marrow: The spongy material found inside the bones; most blood cells are generated in the bone marrow

Bone marrow aspiration: The procedure by which a needle is inserted into a bone to withdraw a sample of the marrow

Bone marrow suppression: A decrease in the production or number of blood cells

Bone scan: A picture of the bones made using a very small amount of a radioactive substance; it can reveal bone damage caused by cancer, other disease, or injury

Bronchogenic carcinoma: A cancer originating in the lungs or airways

Bronchoscopy: The insertion of a flexible, lighted tube through the mouth into the lungs to examine the lungs and airways

C

Cancer: A group of diseases in which malignant cells grow out of control and spread to other parts of the body

Cancer in situ: Cancer that has not invaded into surrounding tissues

Carcinogen: A substance that causes cancer; for example, cigarette smoke contains chemical carcinogens that cause lung cancer

Carcinoma: Cancer that starts in the skin or the lining of organs

Cardiomegaly: Enlargement of the heart

Cellulitis: Diffuse, subcutaneous inflammation of connective tissue

Central venous catheter: A special intravenous tubing that is surgically inserted into a large vein near the heart and exits from the chest or abdomen; the catheter allows medications, fluids, or blood products to be given and blood samples to be collected

Chemotherapy: The treatment of cancer with drugs designed to kill cancer cells

Chondrosarcoma: A malignant tumor of cartilage usually occurring near the ends of long bones

Chronic: Persisting over a long time

Colonoscopy: Endoscopy of the colon or large bowel

Colony stimulating factor (CSF): An injectable substance used to stimulate the bone marrow to produce more cells

Combination chemotherapy: The use of multiple anticancer drugs to treat cancer

Computed tomography (CT/CAT) scan: Use of computers and x-rays to create images of various parts of the body

Congestive heart failure: A buildup of fluid in the lungs and/or extremities (especially the legs); occurs because the heart cannot adequately pump blood

Cyst: An accumulation of fluid or semisolid material within a sac

Cystitis: Inflammation of the bladder

D

Drug resistance: Condition in which cancer cells have developed the ability to prevent being killed by cancer drugs

Dysphagia: Difficulty swallowing

Dyspnea: Difficult or painful breathing; shortness of breath

Dysuria: Difficult or painful urination

E

Edema: The accumulation of fluid in part of the body

Effusion: Collection of fluid in a body cavity, usually between adjoining tissues; for example, pleural effusion is the collection of fluid between two layers of the pleura (the lung's covering)

Electrocardiogram (EKG, ECG): A test that records the electrical activity of the heart

Endoscopy: A procedure for looking at the inside of body cavities, such as the esophagus (food pipe) or stomach

Erythema: Redness of the skin

Erythrocyte: Red blood cell; it carries oxygen to and removes carbon dioxide from body tissues

Esophagitis: Inflammation of the esophagus (food pipe)

Excision: Surgical removal of a tumor or growth

Extravasation: Inadvertent leakage of injectable medication into tissue surrounding the infusion site; extravasation of some cancer drugs, such as doxorubicin, vincristine, or vinblastine, may cause tissue damage

F

Feline immunodeficiency virus (FIV): Viral disease of cats transmitted primarily by bites between cats; infection with this virus can suppress the immune system

Feline leukemia virus (FeLV): Viral disease of cats transmitted by respiratory secretions; infection can suppress the immune system and, in rare circumstances, lead to the development of tumors in white blood cells (lymphocytes), lymph nodes, and other organs

Fine-needle aspiration: A procedure in which a needle is inserted into tissue to collect a sample; the sample is then examined under a microscope to obtain a specific diagnosis

Frozen section: Tissue sample prepared for microscopic analysis by cutting sections of fresh frozen tissue (rather than preserved tissue)

G

Grade: How aggressive or malignant a tumor appears when examined under the microscope

Granulocyte: A type of white blood cell that kills bacteria

H

Hematocrit (Hct): The percentage of red blood cells in the blood; a low hematocrit indicates anemia (similar to packed cell volume [PCV])

Hematologist: Veterinarian who specializes in hematology

Hematology: The study of blood and its diseases

Hematuria: Blood in the urine

Hormone: A substance that regulates growth, metabolism,

© 2001 Veterinary Learning Systems

and reproduction and is secreted by various organs in the body

Hospice: A concept of supportive care to meet the special needs of the pet and family during the terminal stages of illness; care may be delivered in the home or hospital by a specially trained team of professionals

I

Immunity, immune system: The body's ability to fight infections and disease

Immunosuppression: Weakening of the immune system, thereby decreasing the body's ability to fight infections and disease

Immunotherapy: Artificial stimulation of the body's immune system to treat or fight disease (also known as biologic response modifier)

Infiltration: Delivery of a drug into an area of the body or the cancer itself by injection; also refers to leakage of fluid or medicines into tissues, which can cause swelling

Infusion: Delivery of fluids or medications into the bloodstream over a specified time

Injection: Pushing a medication into the body with the use of a syringe and needle

Intramuscular (IM): An injection administered by a needle and syringe into a muscle

Intravenous (IV): An injection administered by a needle and syringe into a vein

L

Lesion: A lump or abscess caused by injury or disease, including cancer

Leukemia: Cancer of the blood; white blood cells may be produced in excessive amounts and are unable to work properly

Leukocyte: White blood cell

Leukopenia: A low number of white blood cells

Lumpectomy: Simple removal of a mass without resecting a substantial amount of tissue surrounding the lesion in question

Lymph nodes: Localized tissue that is part of the immune defense system; lymph nodes act as the body's first line of defense against infections and cancer

Lymphangiogram: A test to look at the lymph nodes

Lymphatic system: A network that includes lymph nodes, lymph, and lymph vessels; it serves as a filtering system for the blood

Lymphocytes: White blood cells; they kill viruses and defend against the invasion of foreign material

Lymphoma: Cancer of lymph nodes and white blood cells (lymphocytes); lymphoma is classified based on the type of cell involved in the tumor

M

Magnetic Resonance Imaging (MRI): A sophisticated test using magnetic energy to provide in-depth images of organs and structures in the body

Malignant tumor: A tumor composed of cancer cells that spread to other parts of the body; these tumors need to be treated

Mast cell tumor: A skin tumor that may involve the liver, spleen, lymph nodes, and/or bone marrow

Mastectomy: Surgical removal of the breast
  Lumpectomy: Removal of the lump and a small amount of surrounding breast tissue
  Simple mastectomy (modified mastectomy): Removal of the entire breast
  Radical mastectomy: Removal of the entire breast along with underlying muscle and possibly lymph nodes

Melanoma: Cancer of the pigment-forming cells of the skin or retina (part of the eye)

Metastasize: To spread from the original cancer site, such as bone cancer spreading to the lung

Mucosa (mucous membrane): The lining of the mouth and gastrointestinal tract

Myelogram: Use of a contrasting material to outline the spinal cord for radiographic examination

Myeloma: A malignant bone marrow tumor that is associated with the production of abnormal proteins (also known as *multiple myeloma* or *plasmal cell myeloma*)

Myelosuppression: Decrease in the production of red blood cells, platelets, and some white blood cells by the bone marrow

N

Neoplasm: A new growth of tissue or cells; a tumor that is generally malignant

Neutropenia: A decreased number of neutrophils, a type of white blood cell

O

Oncologist: A veterinarian who specializes in oncology

Oncology: The study and treatment of cancer

Osteosarcoma: A tumor of the bone

P

Palliative treatment: Treatment aimed at relieving pain

and other symptoms of disease but not intended to cure the disease

Pathologic fracture: A break in a bone usually caused by cancer or another disease condition

Pathology: The study of disease by the examination of tissues and body fluids under a microscope; a veterinarian who specializes in pathology is called a pathologist

Petechia: Tiny areas of bleeding under the skin, usually due to a low platelet count

Phlebitis: A painful inflammation of the vein

Photosensitivity: Extreme sensitivity to the sun, leaving the patient prone to sunburn; some cancer drugs and radiation have this side effect

Placebo: An inert substance often used in clinical trials for comparison

Platelet (Plt): Blood cells responsible for clotting

Platelet count: The number of platelets in a blood sample

Polyp: A growth of tissue protruding into a body cavity, such as a nasal or rectal polyp; it may be benign or malignant

Primary tumor: The original cancer site

Prognosis: The likely outcome of a disease or the life expectancy of a patient

Prosthesis: Artificial replacement of a missing body part, such as a limb

Protocol: The cancer treatment plan, which may involve radiation, chemotherapy, surgery, and/or supportive care

R

Radiation therapist: A veterinarian who specializes in the use of x-rays to treat disease

Radiation therapy: X-ray treatment that damages or kills cancer cells

Recurrence: The reappearance of cancer after a period of remission

Red blood cell (RBC; erythrocyte): Blood cells that carry oxygen to and remove carbon dioxide from body tissues

Red blood cell count: The number of red blood cells in a blood sample

Regression: Shrinkage of a cancerous growth

Relapse: Reappearance of cancer

Remission: Complete or partial disappearance of the signs and symptoms of disease

Risk factor: Anything that increases an animal's chance of developing cancer

S

Sarcoma: A malignant tumor of muscles or connective tissue, such as bone and cartilage

Side effects: Undesirable adverse effects of cancer treatment

Squamous cell carcinoma: Cancer arising from the skin or the surfaces of other structures, such as the mouth or lungs

Staging: Determination of extent of the cancer in the body

Steroid: A type of hormone

Stomatitis: Temporary inflammation and soreness of the mouth

Subcutaneous (SQ): An injection administered by a needle and syringe under the skin

Systemic disease: A disease that affects the whole body instead of a specific organ

T

Thoracentesis (pleural tap): A procedure to remove fluids from the area between the two layers (pleura) covering the lung

Thrombocytopenia: An abnormally low number of platelets; bleeding can occur when the platelet count is too low

Tracheostomy: A surgical opening through the trachea in the neck to provide an artificial airway

Tumor: An abnormal overgrowth of cells; tumors can be either benign or malignant

U

Ultrasound examination: The use of high-frequency sound waves for the purpose of imaging internal body structures and making a diagnosis

V

Venipuncture: Puncturing the vein to obtain blood samples, start an intravenous drip, or administer medication

Vesicant: An intravenous medication that, if leaked into tissues, could cause pain, swelling, and/or tissue damage

Virus: A tiny infectious agent that is smaller than bacteria

W

White blood cell (WBC): General term for a variety of cells responsible for fighting invading germs; specific white blood cells include granulocytes and lymphocytes

White blood cell count: The number of white blood cells in a blood sample

X

X-ray: Radiation used to diagnose and treat disease

INDEX

E

I

W

X

Y

Z

KEY TO ABBREVIATIONS

2,4D	2,4 dichlorophenoxyacetic acid		BUN	blood urea nitrogen
5-FU	5-fluorouracil		°C	celsius
5-HT-3	5-hydroxytryptamine		CBC	complete blood count
6-MP	6-mercaptopurine		CCNU	lomustine
AChRAb	acetylcholine-receptor antibody		CLL	chronic lymphocytic leukemia
ACT	activated clotting (coagulation) time		cm	centimeter(s)
ACTH	adrenocorticotropic hormone (corticotropin)		CML	chronic myeloid leukemia
			CNS	central nervous system
ADH	antidiuretic hormone		Co	cobalt
AG	alopecia, gastrointestinal toxicity		CO₂	carbon dioxide
AIGR	amended insulin:glucose ratio		COAP	cyclophosphamide (Cytoxan®), vincristine (Oncovin®), ara-c (cytosine arabinoside), prednisone
ALL	acute lymphoblastic leukemia			
ALP	alkaline phosphatase		COP	cyclophosphamide (Cytoxan®), vincristine (Oncovin®), prednisone
ALT	alanine aminotransferase			
AML	acute myeloid leukemia		COPA	cyclophosphamide (Cytoxan®), vincristine (Oncovin®), prednisone, doxorubicin (Adriamycin®)
AMM	anterior mediastinal mass			
ANLL	acute nonlymphoid leukemia			
APTT	activated partial thromboplastin time		CPR	cardiopulmonary resuscitation
ara-C	cytosine arabinoside		CR	complete response (remission)
AST	aspartate aminotransferase		Cs	cesium
AT	adrenal tumor		CSF	cerebrospinal fluid
AT-III	antithrombin III		CT	computed (computerized) tomography
ATLS	acute tumor lysis syndrome		CTZ	chemoreceptor trigger zone
ATP	adenosine triphosphate		DIC	disseminated intravascular coagulation
AV	atrioventricular		dl	deciliter(s)
BAG	bone marrow suppression, alopecia, gastrointestinal toxicity		DLH	domestic longhaired (cat breed)
			DM	diabetes mellitus
BCG	bacillus Calmette-Guerin		DNA	deoxyribonucleic acid
BCNU	carmustine		DPG	diphosphoglycerate
BER	basal energy requirement		DSH	domestic shorthaired (cat breed)
bid	twice a day		DTIC	dacarbazine
bpm	beats per minute		ECG	electrocardiogram
BRM	biologic response modifier		EDTA	ethylenediamine tetraacetic acid
BSA	body surface area		e.g.	for example

FDP	fibrin degradation product	L	liter(s)
FeLV	feline leukemia virus	lb	pound
FeSV	feline sarcoma virus	LDDS	low-dose dexamethasone-suppression
FIV	feline immunodeficiency virus	L-MTP-PE	liposome-encapsulated muramyltripeptide-phosphatidyethanolamine
FOCMA	feline oncornavirus-associated cell membrane antigen		
Fr	French	LRS	lactated Ringer's solution
g	gram(s)	M	distant metastasis (TNM classification)
ga	gauge	m^2	square meters
G-CSF	granulocyte colony-stimulating factor	m^3	cubic meters
GH	growth hormone	MBq	megabecquerel
GI	gastrointestinal	mCi	millicurie
GM-CSF	granulocyte-macrophage colony-stimulating factor	MCT	mast cell tumor
		MCV	mean corpuscular volume
Gy	gray (radiation dose)	MDB	minimum database; includes CBC, biochemical profile, urinalysis, FeLV/FIV serology, T_4 testing, and thoracic radiographs (three views)
H	hydrogen		
HDDS	high-dose dexamethasone-suppression		
HDL-CH	high-density lipoprotein cholesterol		
Hg	mercury	MDR	multiple drug resistance
HIV-1	human immunodeficiency virus-1	MDS	myelodysplasia
hr	hour	M:E	myeloid:erythroid ratio
I	iodine	mEq	milliequivalent
i.e.	that is	MeV	million electron volts
IER	illness energy requirement	MF	mycosis fungoides
IgA	immunoglobulin A	mg	milligram(s)
IgE	immunoglobulin E	μg	microgram(s)
IgG	immunoglobulin G	μl	microliter(s)
IgM	immunoglobulin M	μm	micrometer(s)
IL-1	interleukin-1	μU	micro unit(s)
IL-2	interleukin-2	min	minute(s)
IL-3	interleukin-3	ml	milliliter(s)
IM	intramuscular	MLO	multilobular osteochondrosarcoma
IP	intraperitoneal	mm	millimeter(s)
IU	international unit(s)	MOPP	mechlorethamine, vincristine (Oncovin®), procarbazine, prednisone
IV	intravenous		
K	potassium	MRC	Medical Research Council
Kcal	kilocalorie	MRI	magnetic resonance imaging
KCl	potassium chloride	n	number
kg	kilogram(s)	N	lymph node metastasis (TNM classification)

Na	sodium	qid	four times a day
NaCl	sodium chloride	qod	every other day
NaPO$_4$	sodium phosphate	RBC	red blood cell
Nd:YAG	neodymium:yttrium-aluminum-garnet	rcG-CSF	recombinant canine granulocyte colony-stimulating factor
ng	nanogram(s)	rhG-CSF	recombinant human granulocyte colony-stimulating factor
nM	nanomole(s)		
No.	number	RNA	ribonucleic acid
NSAID	nonsteroidal antiinflammatory drug	SCC	squamous cell carcinoma
OAF	osteoclast-activating factor	SD	stable disease
o,p'-DDD	mitotane	SIADH	syndrome of inappropriate secretion of antidiuretic hormone
OSHA	Occupational Safety and Health Administration		
		sid	once a day
OSPT	one-step prothrombin time	SQ	subcutaneous
OSPTT	one-step partial thromboplastin time	Sr	strontium
P	phosphorus	SUN	serum urea nitrogen
PAS	periodic acid–Schiff reaction	T	tumor size (TNM classification)
PCNA	proliferating cell nuclear antigen	T$_3$	triiodothyronine
PCV	packed cell volume	T$_4$	thyroxine
PD	progressive disease	TCC	transitional cell carcinoma
PDH	pituitary-dependent hyperadrenocorticism	tid	three times a day
PEG	polyethylene glycol	TNF	tumor necrosis factor
pH	negative logarithm of hydrogen ion activity	TNM	**T**umor size, lymph **N**ode metastasis, distant **M**etastasis (tumor staging)
PO	oral		
PR	partial response (remission)	TRH	thyrotropin-releasing hormone
PRN	according to circumstances; as needed	TSH	thyroid-stimulating hormone (thyrotropin)
PT	prothrombin time	TVT	transmissible venereal tumor
PTH-rP	parathyroid hormone-related peptide	U	unit(s)
PTU	propylthiouracil	WBC	white blood cell
PUVA	psoralen ultraviolet-A	WHO	World Health Organization
PVC	polyvinyl chloride	wt	weight
q	every		